First Aid®
Clinical Pattern Recognition
for the USMLE® Step 1

Asra R. Khan, MD
Associate Professor of Clinical Medicine
University of Illinois College of Medicine
Chicago, Illinois

Joseph R. Geraghty
MD/PhD Candidate
University of Illinois College of Medicine
Chicago, Illinois

 Mc Graw Hill

New York   Chicago   San Francisco   Athens   London   Madrid   Mexico City
Milan   New Delhi   Singapore   Sydney   Toronto

First Aid® Clinical Pattern Recognition for the USMLE® Step 1

1 2 3 4 5 6 7 8 9 LWI 26 25 24 23 22 21

ISBN 978-1-260-46378-1
MHID 1-260-46378-8

Notice

Medicine is an ever-changing science. As new research and clinical experience broaden our knowledge, changes in treatment and drug therapy are required. The author and the publisher of this work have checked with sources believed to be reliable in their efforts to provide information that is complete and generally in accord with the standards accepted at the time of publication. However, in view of the possibility of human error or changes in medical sciences, neither the author nor the publisher nor any other party who has been involved in the preparation or publication of this work warrants that the information contained herein is in every respect accurate or complete, and they disclaim all responsibility for any errors or omissions or for the results obtained from use of the information contained in this work. Readers are encouraged to confirm the information contained herein with other sources. For example and in particular, readers are advised to check the product information sheet included in the package of each drug they plan to administer to be certain that the information contained in this work is accurate and that changes have not been made in the recommended dose or in the contraindications for administration. This recommendation is of particular importance in connection with new or infrequently used drugs.

This book was set in Minion Pro by MPS Limited.
The editors were Bob Boehringer and Peter J. Boyle.
The production supervisor was Richard Ruzycka.
Project management was provided by Jyoti Shaw, MPS Limited.

This book is printed on acid-free paper.

Library of Congress Control Number: 2021945153

I am grateful to God for blessing me with so much…

I dedicate this book to:

—all the students who work so hard to seek knowledge and serve others

—our patients and teachers who inspire us to be the best we can be

—my inspirational and supportive colleagues at University of Illinois College of Medicine

—and my family and friends for their love and support

—Asra R. Khan

Contents

About the Editors

Asra R. Khan, MD
Editor-in-Chief

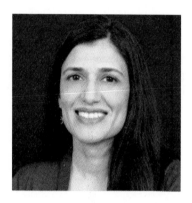

Asra is an Associate Professor of Clinical Medicine at the University of Illinois College of Medicine-Chicago. She earned her B.A. at the University of Chicago and was inducted into Phi Beta Kappa. She received her M.D. at The University of Chicago-Pritzker School of Medicine and completed her internal medicine residency at Northwestern University-McGaw Medical Center in Chicago. Asra has been involved in teaching residents and students since joining the University of Illinois College of Medicine-Chicago in 1998 where she currently serves as the co-Course Director of the Doctoring and Clinical Skills Course, Director of the Internal Medicine Clerkship, and Director of the Internal Medicine Sub-Internship. She was also an Associate Program Director of the internal medicine residency program. Inspired by her mission to increase student success in the USMLE Step Exams and to mentor better clinicians, she recruited and led a top-notch team of diverse and brilliant faculty, fellows, residents and students to develop this product. In addition to editing all the chapters, she created many of the algorithms, tables and cases throughout the book. It is her sincere hope that medical students will find this book useful for the USMLE Step 1, their pre-clinical years, and beyond.

Joseph R. Geraghty
Editor

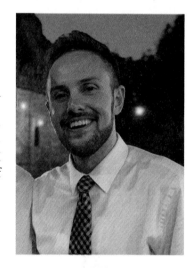

Joseph is an MD/PhD candidate in the Medical Scientist Training Program (MSTP) at the University of Illinois College of Medicine (UICOM)-Chicago who completed his PhD in Neuroscience and has since returned to medical school. He earned his bachelor's degree in biochemistry at the State University of New York (SUNY) College at Geneseo in 2014, graduating summa cum laude and being inducted into Phi Beta Kappa. He has published several peer-reviewed papers in neuroscience, clinical neurology, and medical education. He co-founded the UICOM Student Curricular Board which seeks to engage medical students as agents of change in medical education and has served as a peer tutor for USMLE Step 1 since 2016. In his spare time, he enjoys running and traveling.

Alfredo Mena Lora, MD
Associate Editor

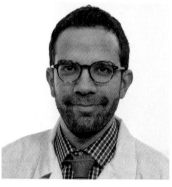

Alfredo is an Assistant Professor of Medicine at the University of Illinois College of Medicine-Chicago. He has a passion for medical education and currently serves as the Program Director for the Infectious Diseases Fellowship and Associate Program Director for the Internal Medicine Residency. Dr Mena Lora graduated from Universidad Iberoamericana in his native Dominican Republic. He moved to the United States for graduate medical education, completing residency, chief residency and fellowship training at the University of Illinois College of Medicine-Chicago.

Acknowledgments

We would like to acknowledge and give special thanks to Stuart J. Slavin, MD, who contributed to the initial idea and discussions around creating a pattern recognition book as a study aid for students studying for USMLE Step 1.

We would like to thank the faculty, fellows, residents, and students at the University of Illinois College of Medicine for their collaboration and contributions and the deans and department and division heads for their encouragement, guidance, and support. We would like to thank and acknowledge the numerous student and resident reviewers for providing their valuable feedback and input. We would like to thank our families for their love, support, patience, guidance, and encouragement over the last few years.

Finally, we are thankful and grateful to our publishing/editorial team led by Bob Boehringer and Peter Boyle for guiding and helping us throughout this process.

Chapter Leads

Javaneh Abbasian, MD
Department of Ophthalmology
Jesse Brown VA Medical Center
University of Illinois College of Medicine
Chicago, Illinois
Chapter 12

Saba Ahmad, MD
Department of Pediatrics
University of Illinois College of Medicine
Chicago, Illinois
Chapter 12

Waddah Alrefai, MD
Department of Medicine: Gastroenterology and Hepatology
University of Illinois College of Medicine
Chicago, Illinois
Chapter 9

Amer K. Ardati, MD, MSc
Department of Medicine: Cardiology
University of Illinois College of Medicine
Chicago, Illinois
Chapter 7

Rachel Bernard, MD, MPH
Department of Medicine: Academic Internal Medicine
Jesse Brown VA Medical Center
University of Illinois College of Medicine
Chicago, Illinois
Chapter 13

Sean Blitzstein, MD
Department of Psychiatry
Jesse Brown VA Medical Center
University of Illinois College of Medicine
Chicago, Illinois
Chapter 13

Ryan Bolton, MD
Department of Medicine: Academic Internal Medicine
University of Illinois College of Medicine
Chicago, Illinois
Chapter 9

Scott Borgetti, MD
Department of Medicine: Infectious Diseases
University of Illinois College of Medicine
Chicago, Illinois
Chapters 2 and 3

Claudia Boucher-Berry, MD
Department of Pediatric Endocrinology
University of Illinois College of Medicine
Chicago, Illinois
Chapter 8

Christie Brillante, MD
Department of Medicine: Pulmonary, Critical Care,
  Sleep and Allergy
University of Illinois College of Medicine
Chicago, Illinois
Chapter 16

Robert Carroll, MD
Department of Medicine: Gastroenterology and
  Hepatology
University of Illinois College of Medicine
Chicago, Illinois
Chapter 9

Michael Charles, MD
Department of Medicine: Academic Internal Medicine
University of Illinois College of Medicine
Chicago, Illinois
Chapter 11

Paul Chastain, PhD
Department of Health Sciences Education
University of Illinois College of Medicine
Rockford, Illinois
Chapter 1

Euna Chi, MD
Department of Medicine: Academic Internal Medicine
University of Illinois College of Medicine
Chicago, Illinois
Chapter 9

Rozina Chowdhery, MD
Northwest Cancer Center
Crown Point, Indiana
Chapter 10

Farheen Dojki, MD
Department of Endocrinology, Diabetes and
  Metabolism
Franciscan Health
Munster, Indiana
Chapter 8

Suzanne Falck, MD
Department of Medicine: Academic Internal Medicine
University of Illinois College of Medicine
Chicago, Illinois
Chapter 11

John Galvin, MD
Department of Medicine: Hematology and Oncology
University of Illinois College of Medicine
Chicago, Illinois
Chapter 10

Ananya Gangopadhyaya, MD
Department of Medicine: Academic Internal Medicine
University of Illinois College of Medicine
Chicago, Illinois
Chapter 12

Anna Marie Gramelspacher, MD
Department of Medicine: Academic Internal Medicine
University of Illinois College of Medicine
Chicago, Illinois
Chapter 6

Annette Hays, PharmD
University of Illinois College of Medicine
Rockford, Illinois
Chapter 5

Nuzhath Hussain, MD
Department of Obstetrics and Gynecology
Northwestern University Feinberg School of Medicine
Chicago, Illinois
Chapter 15

Elliot Kaufman, PhD
Department of Biochemistry and Molecular Genetics
University of Illinois College of Medicine
Chicago, Illinois
Chapter 1

George T. Kondos, MD
Department of Medicine: Cardiology
University of Illinois College of Medicine
Chicago, Illinois
Chapter 7

Amy Y. Lin, MD
Department of Pathology
University of Illinois College of Medicine
Chicago, Illinois
Chapter 4

Natalia Litbarg, MD
Department of Medicine: Nephrology
University of Illinois College of Medicine
Chicago, Illinois
Chapter 14

Claudia Lora, MD
Department of Medicine: Nephrology
University of Illinois College of Medicine
Chicago, Illinois
Chapter 14

Jonathan D. Meyer, MD
Department of Medicine: Cardiology
University of Illinois College of Medicine
Chicago, Illinois
Chapter 7

Noreen T. Nazir, MD
Department of Medicine: Cardiology
University of Illinois College of Medicine
Chicago, Illinois
Chapter 7

Samuel Ohlander, MD
Department of Urology
University of Illinois College of Medicine
Chicago, Illinois
Chapters 14 and 15

Mahesh C. Patel, MD
Department of Medicine: Infectious Diseases
University of Illinois College of Medicine
Chicago, Illinois
Chapters 2 and 3

Anne Polick, MD
Department of Medicine: Academic Internal Medicine
University of Illinois College of Medicine
Chicago, Illinois
Chapter 11

Azizur Rahman, MD
Glaucoma Associates of Illinois
Jesse Brown and Hines VA Medical Center
Department of Ophthalmology
University of Illinois College of Medicine
Chicago, Illinois
Chapter 12

Nimmi Rajagopal, MD
Department of Family and Community Medicine
Cook County Health and Hospitals System
Chicago, Illinois
Chapter 15

Ashima Sahni, MD
Department of Medicine: Pulmonary, Critical Care,
    Sleep and Allergy
University of Illinois College of Medicine
Chicago, Illinois
Chapter 16

Manpreet Samra, MD
Department of Medicine: Nephrology
Loyola University Medical Center
Maywood, Illinois
Chapter 14

Christopher Schriever, PharmD
Department of Pharmacy Practice
University of Illinois College of Medicine
Rockford, Illinois
Chapter 5

Neelofer Shafi, MD
Department of Neurology
University of Illinois College of Medicine
Chicago, Illinois
Chapter 12

Ardaman Shergill, MD, MSPH
Department of Medicine: Hematology/Oncology
The University of Chicago
Chicago, Illinois
Chapter 10

Radhika Sreedhar, MD, MS
Department of Medicine: Academic Internal Medicine
University of Illinois College of Medicine
Chicago, Illinois
Chapters 1 and 6

Anthony Vergis, MD
Department of Medicine: Pulmonary, Critical Care, and
    Sleep Medicine

University Hospitals Cleveland Medical Center,
    Case Western Reserve University
Cleveland, Ohio
Chapter 16

Catherine Wheatley, MD
Department of Obstetrics and Gynecology
University of Illinois College of Medicine
Chicago, Illinois
Chapter 15

R. Deepa Yohannan, MD
Department of Medicine: Academic
    Internal Medicine
Jesse Brown VA Medical Center
University of Illinois College of Medicine
Chicago, Illinois
Chapter 12

Contributors

Ivy Abraham, MD
Department of Hematology and Oncology
UChicago Medicine Ingalls Memorial
Harvey, Illinois
Chapter 10

Aneet Ahluwalia, MD
Department of Psychiatry and Internal Medicine
University of Illinois College of Medicine
Chicago, Illinois
Chapter 13

Tamika Alexander, MD, FACOG
Department of Obstetrics and Gynecology
University of Illinois College of Medicine
Chicago, Illinois
Chapter 15

Akika Ando, MD
Department of Medicine: Nephrology
University of Illinois College of Medicine
Chicago, Illinois
Chapter 14

Saad Arain, MD
Department of Medicine: Hematology and Oncology
University of Illinois College of Medicine
Chicago, Illinois
Chapter 10

Carrie Sharkey Asner, MD
Department of Family and Community Medicine
University of Illinois College of Medicine
Rockford, Illinois
Chapter 12

Katherine Aulis, MD
Department of Emergency Medicine
Cook County Health and Hospital System
Chicago, Illinois

Jalal Baig, MD
Department of Hematology and Oncology
Cancer Treatment Centers of America
Gurnee, Illinois
Chapter 10

Sylvia Biso, MD
Department of Medicine: Cardiology
University of Illinois College of Medicine
Chicago, Illinois
Chapter 7

Gianna Bosco, MD
Department of Internal Medicine and Pediatric
Rush University Medical Center
Chicago, Illinois
Chapter 14

Alexis Braverman, MD
Department of Obstetrics and Gynecology
University of Illinois College of Medicine
Chicago, Illinois
Chapter 15

Alina Brener, MD
Department of Medicine: Cardiology
University of Illinois College of Medicine
Chicago, Illinois
Chapter 7

Julia Brown, MD
Department of Medicine: Nephrology
University of Illinois College of Medicine
Chicago, Illinois
Chapter 14

Liliana Burdea, MD
Department of Pediatric Endocrinology
University of Illinois College of Medicine
Chicago, Illinois
Chapter 8

Mansoor Burhani, MD
Department of Internal Medicine
University of Colorado School of Medicine
Aurora, Colorado
Chapter 5

David Butler, PharmD
Department of Pharmacy Practice
Albany College of Pharmacy and Health Sciences
Albany, New York
Chapter 9

Erin Cavanaugh, MD
Department of Obstetrics and Gynecology
University of Illinois College of Medicine
Chicago, Illinois
Chapter 15

Wadih Chacra, MD
Department of Medicine: Gastroenterology and
   Hepatology
University of Illinois College of Medicine
Chicago, Illinois
Chapter 9

Sonia Christian, MD
Department of Hematology and Oncology
Illinois Cancer Specialists
Niles, Illinois
Chapter 10

Cheryl Conner, MD, MPH
Department of Medicine: Academic Internal Medicine
Jesse Brown VA Medical Center
University of Illinois College of Medicine
Chicago, Illinois
Chapter 11

Jissy Cyriac, MD
University of Illinois College of Medicine
Chicago, Illinois

Walaa Dabbas, MD
Department of Medicine: Nephrology
University of Illinois College of Medicine
Chicago, Illinois
Chapter 14

Susan J. Doh
University of Illinois College of Medicine
Chicago, Illinois

Andrew Donaldson, MD
Department of Surgery
Rush University Medical Center
Chicago, Illinois
Chapter 6

Venkata Dontaraju, MD
Department of Medicine
University of Illinois College of Medicine
Rockford, Illinois
Chapter 12

Yuval Eisenberg, MD
Department of Medicine: Endocrinology, Diabetes, and
   Metabolism
University of Illinois College of Medicine
Chicago, Illinois
Chapter 8

Jessica Gardiner, MD
Department of Psychiatry, Child and Adolescent
   Psychiatry
University of Illinois College of Medicine
Chicago, Illinois
Chapter 13

Kyle Geary, MD
Division of Gastroenterology
NorthShore University Health System
Evanston, Illinois
Chapter 9

Joseph R. Geraghty, MD/PhD candidate
Department of Neurology and Rehabilitation
University of Illinois College of Medicine
Chicago, Illinois

Krishna Ghimire, MD
Department of Medicine: Hematology and Oncology
University of Illinois College of Medicine
Chicago, Illinois
Chapter 10

Vivien Goh, MD
Department of Internal Medicine
McGaw Medical Center of Northwestern University
Chicago, Illinois
Chapter 11

Victoria Gotay, MD
Department of Psychiatry
University of Illinois College of Medicine
Chicago, Illinois
Chapter 13

Jennifer Grage, MD
Department of Pediatrics
Northwestern University McGaw Medical Center
Chicago, Illinois

John Groth, MD
Department of Pathology and Laboratory Medicine
Northshore University Health System
Evanston, Illinois
Chapter 4

Whitney Halgrimson, MD
Department of Urology
University of Illinois College of Medicine
Chicago, Illinois
Chapter 15

Ahmed Hassan, MD
Department of Neurology and Rehabilitation
University of Illinois College of Medicine
Chicago, Illinois
Chapter 12

Jacqueline Hirsch, MD
Department of Psychiatry and Behavioral Sciences
Northwestern University Feinberg School of Medicine
Chicago, Illinois
Chapter 13

Kelsey Holbert, MD
Department of Internal Medicine
University of Wisconsin Hospital
Madison, Wisconsin

Matthew Hooper, MD
Department of Orthopaedic Surgery
Marshall University School of Medicine
Huntington, West Virginia
Chapter 11

Ikuyo Imayama, MD, PhD
Department of Medicine: Pulmonary, Critical Care, Sleep
    and Allergy
University of Illinois College of Medicine
Chicago, Illinois
Chapter 16

Surbhi Jain, MD
Department of Obstetrics and Gynecology
University of Iowa Hospitals and Clinics
Iowa City, Iowa
Chapter 15

Ryan Kendziora, MD
Department of Laboratory Medicine and Pathology
Mayo Clinic Rochester
Rochester, Minnesota
Chapter 4

Deanne Kennedy Loube, MD
Department of Neurology and Neurological Sciences
Stanford University Hospital
Stanford, California
Chapter 12

Ambareen Khan, DO
Department of Medicine: Academic Internal Medicine
Jesse Brown VA Medical Center
University of Illinois College of Medicine
Chicago, Illinois
Chapter 11

Asra R. Khan
Department of Medicine: Academic Internal Medicine
University of Illinois College of Medicine
Chicago, Illinois

Fazal Khan, MD, JD
University of Georgia School of Law
Athens, Georgia
Chapter 6

Yasaman Kianirad, MD
Department of Neurology
University of Illinois College of Medicine
Chicago, Illinois
Chapter 12

Kenji Kobayashi, MD
Department of Otolaryngology-Head and Neck Surgery
Baylor College of Medicine
Houston, Texas
Chapter 12

Michael Kolozsvary-Kiss, MD
Department of Medicine: Academic
    Internal Medicine
Jesse Brown VA Medical Center
University of Illinois College of Medicine
Chicago, Illinois
Chapter 8

Vinod Kondragunta, MD
Department of Medicine: Hematology and
    Oncology
University of Illinois College of Medicine
Chicago, Illinois
Chapter 10

Marci Laragh, MD
Department of Medicine: Academic
    Internal Medicine
Jesse Brown VA Medical Center
University of Illinois College of Medicine
Chicago, Illinois
Chapter 12

Erik Liederbach, MD
Department of Internal Medicine
Oregon Health and Science University
Portland, Oregon
Chapter 10

Abby Litwiller, MD, FACOG
Department of Obstetrics and Gynecology
University of Illinois College of Medicine
Chicago, Illinois
Chapter 15

David M. Loeffler, DO
Department of Pathology
Oregon Health and Science University
Portland, Oregon
Chapter 4

Ikenna Madueke, MD, PhD
Department of Urology
University of Illinois College of Medicine
Chicago, Illinois
Chapter 15

Kiran Malhotra, MD
Department of Ophthalmology
University of California, Davis
Davis, CA

Isabella Marranzini-Rodriguez, MD
Department of Pediatrics
University of Illinois College of Medicine
Chicago, Illinois
Chapter 8

Mark McArthur, MD
Department of Radiological Sciences
University of California, Los Angeles
Los Angeles, California

Anne Meier, MD
Department of Medicine: Hematology and Oncology
University of Illinois College of Medicine
Chicago, Illinois
Chapter 10

Katie Mena, MD
Department of Medicine: Academic Internal Medicine
University of Illinois College of Medicine
Chicago, Illinois
Chapter 9

Alfredo J Mena Lora, MD
Department of Medicine: Infectious Diseases
University of Illinois College of Medicine
Chicago, Illinois

Dante Mesa, MD
Department of Internal Medicine
University of Colorado School of Medicine
Aurora, Colorado
Chapter 16

Yara Mikhaeil-Demo, MD
Department of Neurology
Northwestern University
Chicago, Illinois
Chapter 12

Diana Mnatsakanova, MD
Department of Neurology
University of Illinois College of Medicine
Chicago, Illinois
Chapter 12

Sarah Monick, MD
Department of Internal Medicine and Pediatrics
The University of Chicago Hospitals
Chicago, Illinois
Chapter 3

Vijeyaluzmy Motilal Nehru, MD
Department of Medicine: Hematology and Oncology
University of Illinois College of Medicine
Chicago, Illinois
Chapter 10

Tabassum Nafsi, MD FCCP
Department of Medicine: Pulmonary and Critical Care
University of Illinois College of Medicine
Rockford, Illinois
Chapter 16

Shelbi L. Olson, MD
Department of Surgery
University of Minnesota
Minneapolis, Minnesota

Diana Oramas Mogrovejo, MD
Department of Pathology
University of Texas MD Anderson Cancer Center
Houston, Texas
Chapter 4

Alexander Pan, MD
Department of Medicine: Gastroenterology and
    Hepatology
University of Illinois College of Medicine
Chicago, Illinois
Chapter 9

Steven Papastefan, MD
Department of Surgery
McGaw Medical Center of Northwestern University
Chicago, Illinois
Chapter 8

Devang S. Parikh, MD, MA
Department of Medicine: Cardiology
Houston Methodist
Houston, Texas
Chapter 7

Priyanka Patel, MD
Department of Dermatology
University of Illinois College of Medicine
Chicago, Illinois
Chapter 11

Lakshmi Kant Pathak, MD
Department of Medicine: Nephrology
University of Illinois College of Medicine
Chicago, Illinois
Chapter 14

Hannah Pennington
Department of Biochemistry and Molecular Genetics
University of Illinois College of Medicine
Chicago, Illinois
Chapter 1

Valentin Prieto-Centurion, MD
Department of Medicine: Pulmonary, Critical Care, Sleep
    and Allergy
University of Illinois College of Medicine
Chicago, Illinois
Chapter 16

Jonathan Radosta, MD
Department of Medicine: Academic Internal Medicine
University of Illinois College of Medicine
Chicago, Illinois
Chapter 9

Saud Rana, MD
Department of Medicine: Hematology and Oncology
University of Illinois College of Medicine
Chicago, Illinois
Chapter 10

Satyajit Reddy, MD, MEng
Department of Medicine: Cardiology
University of Illinois College of Medicine
Chicago, Illinois
Chapter 7

Jessica Richardson, MD
Department of Family Medicine
University of Illinois College of Medicine
Chicago, Illinois
Chapter 15

Mary Carolina Rodriguez Ziccardi, MD
Department of Medicine: Cardiology
University of Illinois College of Medicine
Chicago, Illinois
Chapter 7

Jason Ross, MD
Department of Internal Medicine
Barnes Jewish Hospital
St. Louis, Missouri
Chapter 5

Sarah Russel, MD
Department of Otolaryngology/Head and
    Neck Surgery
University of North Carolina–Chapel Hill
Chapel Hill, North Carolina
Chapter 2

Danil Rybalko, MD
Department of Orthopedic Surgery
MidAmerica Orthopaedics
Palos Hills, Illinois
Chapter 11

Kevin Rynn, PharmD
Department of Pharmacy Practice
University of Illinois College of Medicine
Rockford, Illinois
Chapter 5

Junaid Sandozi, MD
Department of Radiology
Georgetown University School of Medicine
Washington, DC

Candice Schwartz, MD
Department of Medicine: Hematology and Oncology
University of Illinois College of Medicine
Chicago, Illinois
Chapter 10

Ari Seifter, MD
Department of Medicine: Hematology and Oncology
University of Illinois College of Medicine
Chicago, Illinois
Chapter 10

Vinny Sharma, MD
Department of Neurology
University of Illinois College of Medicine
Chicago, Illinois
Chapter 12

Peggy W. Shiels, MD
Department of Medicine
University of Illinois College of Medicine
Rockford, Illinois
Chapter 8

Naina Singh, MD
Department of Medicine: Hematology and Oncology
University of Illinois College of Medicine
Chicago, Illinois
Chapter 10

Gordon Skeoch, MD
Department of Obstetrics and Gynecology
Advocate Illinois Masonic Medical Center
Chicago, Illinois
Chapter 15

Pavan Srivastava, MD
Departments of Medicine and Pediatrics
University of Illinois College of Medicine
Chicago, Illinois
Chapter 12

Nathan Stackhouse, MD, MPH
Department of Family Medicine
University of Illinois College of Medicine
Chicago, Illinois
Chapter 15

James Stinson, MD
Department of Urology
John H Stroger Hospital of Cook County
Chicago, Illinois
Chapter 15

Katrina Stumbras, MD, MPH
Department of Pediatrics
Children's National Medical Center
Washington, D.C.
Chapter 6

Hira Tanwir, MD
Department of Medicine: Academic Internal Medicine and
    Geriatrics
University of Illinois College of Medicine
Chicago, Illinois
Chapter 11

Stefan Tchernodrinski, MD
Department of Medicine: Academic Internal Medicine and
    Geriatrics
University of Illinois College of Medicine
Chicago, Illinois
Chapter 11

David Tofovic, MD
Department of Medicine: Cardiology
University of Illinois College of Medicine
Chicago, Illinois
Chapter 7

Daniel Toft, MD, PhD
Department of Medicine: Endocrinology, Diabetes, and
    Metabolism
University of Illinois College of Medicine
Chicago, Illinois
Chapter 8

Stephanie Toth-Manikowski, MD, MHS
Department of Medicine: Nephrology
University of Illinois College of Medicine
Chicago, Illinois
Chapter 14

Christen Vagts, MD
Department of Medicine: Pulmonary, Critical Care, Allergy
    and Sleep Medicine
University of Illinois College of Medicine
Chicago, Illinois
Chapter 16

Maidah Yaqoob, MD
Department of Medicine: Pulmonary, Critical Care, Allergy
    and Sleep Medicine
University of Illinois College of Medicine
Chicago, Illinois
Chapter 16

Akira Yoshii, MD, PhD
Department of Anatomy and Cell Biology, Department of
    Pediatrics
University of Illinois College of Medicine
Chicago, Illinois
Chapter 12

Gardner Yost, MD
Division of Cardiothoracic Surgery
University of Michigan
Ann Arbor, Michigan
Chapter 7

Annette Zacharia, MD
Department of Medicine: Academic Internal Medicine
University of Illinois College of Medicine
Chicago, Illinois
Chapter 11

Joseph Zapater, MD, PhD
Department of Medicine: Endocrinology, Diabetes and
    Metabolism
University of Illinois College of Medicine
Chicago, Illinois
Chapter 8

Brian Zobeck, PharmD, BCPS
Department of Pharmacy Practice
University of Illinois College of Medicine
Rockford, Illinois
Chapter 5

Introduction

Joseph R. Geraghty and Asra R. Khan

Congratulations! By using this book, you are one step closer to developing your skills as a future physician and in preparation for the USMLE Step 1 exam and the practice of medicine.

Why Use This Book?

- USMLE Step 1 has increasingly used clinical case-based approaches to licensing exam questions, translating into a need for medical students to rapidly recognize clinical patterns, to develop a differential diagnosis, and to use clinical reasoning and basic science skills to answer questions. Cases or vignettes provided on Step 1 are usually given in their most classic presentation. *First Aid for USMLE Step 1* is the most commonly used resource by medical students as they prepare for USMLE Step 1. Given the goals and sheer volume of material necessary to include in the book, the text often only provides a list of signs, symptoms, tests, and findings for a given condition, without providing the context that ties all of these features together. What is often missing is a discussion of the subtle similarities and differences between conditions that initially may not seem related. Further, given the need for USMLE Step 1 to test many basic science concepts, many of the conditions tested are quite rare, greatly limiting the chances that medical students will have encountered cases like these in the clinic or hospital setting during their early years of medical training.

- The *First Aid Clinical Pattern Recognition (CPR)* book presents classic "textbook" vignettes of high-yield syndromes and cases commonly tested on USMLE Step 1 and encountered in clinical practice. This resource provides context that ties different symptoms, signs, and conditions together, encouraging medical students to consider a differential diagnosis for a given chief concern, the relationships between different conditions, and more. Ultimately, this book will help medical students learn to recognize patterns and start building illness scripts for various high-yield conditions. While several books on the market provide selected cases designed to address single high-yield points about a given condition, this book goes beyond that. By partnering with the *First Aid for USMLE Step 1* book, we combine classic clinical scenarios with basic science concepts that are tested on USMLE Step 1. The chapters are organized similarly to *First Aid for USMLE Step 1,* but the vignettes are presented in a way that students would encounter in the real world and exam setting.

- This book is designed to be used in tandem with *First Aid for USMLE Step 1* throughout preclinical curricula and leading up to the USMLE Step 1 exam. In this book, we introduce general approaches to initial presenting signs and symptoms, offer guidance for evaluating these in the context of answering a USMLE Step 1 question, provide high-yield cases that highlight major buzzwords and findings, and supply detailed discussions that compare and contrast cases, as well as schematics, tables, and algorithms that will help individual learners recognize clinical patterns commonly tested on USMLE Step 1.

- The second overarching goal of this book goes beyond just USMLE Step 1 by helping medical students build a strong clinical foundation so they can excel in medical school. By acknowledging the importance of obtaining a focused history and physical examination, developing a differential diagnosis, and understanding the purpose of common tests and general treatment concepts for various conditions, students will recognize common patterns, build illness scripts, and improve their clinical reasoning skills.

How Should I Use This Book?

- Start using this book as early as possible during your preclinical education, during which you learn basic medical sciences.

- When you learn about a particular condition in a class or encounter an interesting case in the clinic, it is helpful to go back to this book to reference what a classic textbook case would look like. Did your patient have all of these findings? They may not have. Did they have a unique or unusual presentation? Annotate this into the book!

- This book will serve as your go-to resource for identifying what features of a given condition are the most commonly tested on USMLE Step 1.

- As such, this book is a great accompaniment to your clinical experiences throughout the first two years of medical training and beyond.

- Students are encouraged to use pens and highlighters of different colors to develop their own system for annotating this book. Perhaps you can annotate based on your preclinical coursework, on your clinical experiences thus far, and on material covered in other high-yield resources.

- You may also consider removing the binding of the book and inserting with individual chapters in the larger *First Aid for USMLE Step 1* book.

- Keep in mind that this is not a question book. Instead, the vignettes highlight what a classic presentation of a particular case would look like: who gets the disease; the common symptoms and physical exam findings; other conditions that may present similarly; tests that will help confirm the diagnosis (and what the typical findings will be) or help refute the other conditions; and what the standard treatment is. The discussion portion reinforces the common presentations and expands on these and on pertinent basic science principles.

- The cases build on each other. Simple, more straightforward cases are followed by less common and more complex vignettes. It is important to note that many cases will present with more than one symptom. For instance, a patient with gastroesophageal reflux disease (GERD) may present with classic heartburn symptoms, atypical chest pain, or a chronic cough. This information will be conveyed in the discussion session.

Anatomy of the Cases

CASE 1	Actual Case or Key Features Being Highlighted
The vignette includes classic demographics (who gets the disease), common symptoms and signs, other relevant history, and physical exam findings.	
Evaluation/Tests	This section includes important tests to confirm the diagnosis and highlights the classic findings. If the diagnosis is typically made based on history and physical exam findings, then "clinical diagnosis" is written, followed by other tests that may be done to confirm or refute alternative diagnoses.
Treatment	Standard treatment for the presented case is explained.
Discussion	This section reinforces salient features of the case, elaborates on other reasonable differential diagnoses, includes more detailed treatment options, and—most importantly—links the basic sciences relevant to USMLE Step 1.
Additional Considerations	When applicable, this section highlights other similar conditions or complications that are important to consider for Step 1 and beyond. Common symptoms, signs, evaluation, and treatment are presented in an abbreviated format.

Example Case

CASE #	Stable Angina
A 65-year-old man with a history of hypertension, type 2 diabetes, hyperlipidemia, and tobacco use presents with intermittent chest pain for the past 2 months. He describes it as a squeezing pressure sensation in his left parasternal to mid-clavicular area with radiation down his left arm that is associated with mild shortness of breath. The symptoms occur each time he climbs more than two flights of stairs and it improves after he rests for a few minutes. His vital signs, as well as his cardiovascular, pulmonary, and abdominal exams, are normal. There is no reproducible chest wall tenderness or lower extremity edema.	
Evaluation/Tests	Clinical diagnosis. If ordered, exercise ECG would show ≥ 1 mm ST depression in more than 1 contiguous lead. A stress echo would show induced regional wall motion abnormalities consistent with ischemia.
Treatment	Treat with aspirin, statin, and antianginal medications (beta blockers, calcium channel blockers, and/or nitroglycerin). Optimize risk factors (i.e., diabetes, hypertension) and encourage lifestyle modifications (i.e., diet, exercise, smoking cessation). Patients that have persistent symptoms despite optimal medical therapy can safely be offered revascularization.
Discussion	Stable angina typically occurs when there is an obstructive atherosclerotic lesion in the coronary arteries that is over 70% occlusive. Cardiac risk factors include age (male patients >45, female patients >55), male sex, HTN, DM, dyslipidemia, family history of premature CAD (males <55, females <65), smoking, and abdominal obesity. At times, the chest pain is described as a discomfort or pressure sensation rather than pain. Additional symptoms can include dyspnea, nausea, diaphoresis, lightheadedness, dizziness, and easy fatigability. Typical angina is provoked by exertion and relieved with rest or nitroglycerin. Physical exam findings are often normal. If a patient has atypical or vague symptoms, an exercise test stress test can confirm the diagnosis.

CASE # | Stable Angina *(continued)*

Discussion	The relatively short duration of pain and association with exertion makes **acute coronary syndrome** (ACS) (unstable angina, NSTEMI, and STEMI) less likely. New onset angina, chest pain at rest, or change in previous predictable angina in a patient with known CAD or cardiac risk factors are characteristic features of ACS. Physical exam findings are often normal.
	Unstable angina (UA) occurs secondary to coronary atherosclerosis plaque rupture and subsequent thrombus formation without complete occlusion of the coronary artery. The pain associated with UA tends to be more severe and typically lasts for 15 min or more. Patients with UA should be hospitalized on a telemetry unit to be stabilized, monitored for arrhythmias, and initiated on a protocol to rule out an MI, which includes checking serial ECGs and cardiac biomarkers. ECG may show ST depression and T wave inversions, and cardiac biomarkers would be normal. Once the patient is stabilized and asymptomatic, they may either undergo stress testing or proceed to coronary angiogram if they are at high risk of ischemia.
Additional Considerations	**Vasospastic (aka Variant or Prinzmetal) angina** is a condition in which chest pain results from transient vasospasm in the coronary arteries, limiting blood flow and causing transient ischemia. The chest pain typically occurs at rest and may be triggered by drugs or substances such as triptans (e.g., sumatriptan), cocaine, cannabis, ephedrine-based products, or alcohol. It is a diagnosis of exclusion, and it is important to rule out a fixed obstructive coronary artery lesion.

What Is the Anatomy of a Typical USMLE Step 1 Question?

- Many students feel overwhelmed by the idea of taking USMLE Step 1 and addressing clinical vignettes successfully. However, there is a specific anatomy to Step 1 questions, and once you become familiar with the format and begin to recognize clinical patterns, you will feel more comfortable answering these questions.

- Many USMLE Step 1 questions are presented in the form of a short clinical vignette that can range from a few sentences to a full paragraph.

A 48-year-old man with past medical history of hypertension and type 2 diabetes mellitus is hospitalized following a significant burn injury from a fire at home. Upon arrival to the emergency room, the patient is stabilized and transferred to the burn unit, where he then recovers over the course of the next week. Ten days after admission, the patient's vital signs are recorded as follows: temperature 38.1°C, respirations 28/min, pulse 110/min, and blood pressure 148/90 mmHg. Though his burn appears to be recovering well, he is tachypneic, and lung exam is notable for crackles bilaterally and bronchial breath sounds. He is tachycardic, but the rest of his cardiac exam is normal. Sputum culture shows a motile, gram negative rod that is oxidase-positive and produces a blue-green pigment. Which of the following best describes the toxin released by this particular pathogen?

A) Stimulates nonspecific activation of T lymphocytes
B) Inactivates elongation factor 2 via ribosylation
C) Activates adenylate cyclase via ADP ribosylation of Gs protein to increase host cell cAMP
D) Inhibits adenylate cyclase via ADP ribosylation of Gi protein to decrease host cell cAMP
E) Induces actin depolymerization leading to mucosal cell death

- **IDENTIFYING STATEMENT:** These vignettes often begin with an identifying or power statement that introduces the patient, including their age, gender, significant past medical history, and chief concern that brought them into the physician's office or hospital. If you are paying careful attention to this statement alone, you may already have an idea of what the question will ask and what limited number of conditions you should have on your differential, or you may have already arrived at an accurate diagnosis. Keep in mind that certain themes and concepts tend to be tested more heavily.

- Everything matters until you are sure it doesn't. Consider why a test writer may have chosen to include certain pieces of information (i.e., geographical location, gender, age). Oftentimes, there is a reason.

- **ADDITIONAL HISTORY/COURSE OF ILLNESS:** After presenting the initial identifying statement, USMLE Step 1 vignettes will often provide additional context clues. Does this patient have underlying cardiovascular risk factors (e.g., smoking, hypertension, diabetes, hyperlipidemia) that might predispose them to myocardial infarction or stroke? Is the patient from a developing country where they may not have received proper immunizations? Did the patient recently travel or eat something associated with particular infections? These types of statements will often allow you to start narrowing down your differential diagnosis and figuring out exactly what the vignette is testing.

- **PHYSICAL EXAM FINDINGS:** Physical exam findings are often brief in USMLE Step 1 vignettes. Typically, you are presented with one sentence providing key physical exam findings, including key findings that are normal on exam. Some physical exam maneuvers are quite specific to a particular condition, so pay attention to how things are worded. Oftentimes, test writers will not use the exact buzzword that may be most familiar to you. For example, in a pediatric patient with Tay-Sachs disease, an exam item will likely never mention "cherry red spot in the macula" on fundoscopy; however, you should be prepared to be presented with a description of this classic finding rather than the term itself. A vignette may be more likely to note, "On fundoscopy, you note a central area of reddening in the retina."

- **LABORATORY FINDINGS:** Laboratory findings are commonly presented on USMLE Step 1 questions, and you will be expected to interpret these. You are provided with a list of common laboratory values to use for reference, and it is worthwhile to spend some time familiarizing yourself with what is provided in this list and what is not. If you are given a lab value in a vignette that is not provided on this list, the vignette may indicate whether the result is normal or abnormal. However, it is important to note that not all questions will rely on your interpreting each lab value provided. Sometimes a long list of lab values is provided, which may take a long time to go through but may ultimately be less helpful than the remainder of the vignette. If presented with a long list of lab values, it may be helpful to go on to read the rest of the question and then go back to the list with an idea of which lab values are most relevant to the case. Cases dealing with hematology, oncology, or renal and endocrine systems commonly list multiple lab results, so it will be important to train yourself to work quickly through these items.

- **IMAGING:** Images are commonly provided on USMLE Step 1, including both radiological images and pathological specimens (gross anatomical specimens and histology sections). While knowing the normal appearance of a particular specimen or tissue type is helpful, it is often not needed to adequately answer the exam item. Consider that the test writer chose to provide this image for a reason and that that a principal finding is likely to be obtained from the image that would not be clear from the text alone. *First Aid for USMLE Step 1* provides a large number of radiological and pathological images, and it would be a good use of time to familiarize yourself with these key images. You may be able to determine the answer to a question just by looking at the image and not the text, while other times you may be able to rely on the text alone without the image. This works to your advantage, as there are often several context clues in a Step 1 vignette that will allow you to successfully answer an item without using all of them.

- **THE QUESTION:** Now you arrive at the actual question. Many students are often dismayed when they have read the entire vignette and are 100% certain of the diagnosis, only to have the question give the diagnosis away and then be asked a more basic science question related to the mechanism of action of a drug or molecular cause of a particular finding. For example, a microbiology case may present a sick patient who recently ate potato salad at a company picnic and is now suffering from vomiting and diarrhea. From this statement alone, you may have already narrowed down particular pathogens that may be the culprit, and you would likely arrive at a quick diagnosis with additional context clues in the vignette. When you reach the actual question, it may ask you about the mechanism of the pathogen's toxin or virulence factor instead of asking you what bug is the causative pathogen. These are the types of questions that USMLE Step 1 prefers to ask because it will require higher-order critical reasoning skills and incorporate basic science questions into clinical vignettes.

- Should you read the whole vignette first or the actual question at the end of the vignette? Up to you! Different students have different strategies for this. Some students prefer to skip the entire vignette and first read the question and scan the answer choices. These students will then return to the beginning of the vignette and, having an idea of the question, search for pertinent context clues that may support their hypothesis of what the answer may be. This works well for many students, and it is reported to help decrease the amount of time you spend on a given test item because you are not spending time interpreting irrelevant lab values or physical exam findings before knowing the question. Other students prefer to read the vignette from beginning to end, using basic science and clinical reasoning skills to build a case in their head of what the question and answers might be before directly reading them. This is more similar to how you would approach patients in the clinic, and it provides a more logical flow to addressing test items.

- **THE ANSWER CHOICES:** The number of answer choices provided in a Step 1 exam item vary, but most questions have a minimum of 5 answer choices. The best approach to this section of the exam item is to arrive at what you think the answer is after reading the question (and/or the case, as just described). Then look through the answer choices and see whether that answer is present. If it is, select it! If it is not, you may need to do some rethinking, reviewing the vignette for key words or significant findings that you may have missed. There will be a single best answer, given the nature of multiple-choice exam items, even though, in medicine, you may actually do several things in the real world. So you have to pick a single answer if a question asks you about the next step.

We hope that this book is helpful to medical students as they master the material needed to find success on the USMLE Step 1 examination and beyond. As medicine is an ever evolving discipline where new mechanisms are discovered and new treatments are developed every year, we welcome suggestions to improve the clarity, accuracy, and completeness of this work. Good luck!

1

Biochemistry

Radhika Sreedhar, MD, MS
Paul Chastain, PhD
Elliot Kaufman, PhD

Knowledge of biochemistry is essential to detecting and understanding the consequences of disordered metabolism. In general, symptoms occur due to the accumulation of substrates upstream from a defective enzyme or due to a lack of production of important substrates downstream from the deficient enzyme. It is important to understand the key regulatory steps in metabolic pathways and areas in the pathways that can be impacted by pharmaceutical agents. Biochemical pathways are interconnected; interruption in one pathway can cause other pathways to be affected, resulting in manifestations or exacerbation of a disease.

By knowing what happens when a pathway is interrupted and the intermediate metabolites that are affected, one can predict some of the typical patient presentations. For instance, lactate builds up in a defect in pyruvate dehydrogenase complex, causing metabolic acidosis. This, in turn, leads to an increased respiratory rate to compensate for the acidosis.

Most patients have some characteristic features in their mode of inheritance, clinical presentation, and tests that should help narrow the differential and determine if there is a biochemical reason for their symptoms. Often, patients present in early or late childhood, so a pediatric or newborn presentation should raise suspicion for biochemical or genetic disorders. As the defects presented here occur at the genetic or molecular level, these disorders frequently present with numerous symptoms, making definitive grouping into a single category more challenging. These disorders are grouped on the basis of main presenting symptoms or signs. Where possible, the text highlights other ways in which the condition may manifest.

FAILURE TO THRIVE

Inborn errors of metabolism occur in important biochemical pathways involved in the synthesis, regulation, and breakdown of important nutrients. Defects in these pathways can result in "failure to thrive," which can be described as inadequate weight gain, weight loss/deceleration, or falling consistently below the 5th percentile for growth in a child, despite meeting adequate nutritional requirements. Many of these disorders present with symptoms that include poor feeding, vomiting, irritability, or lethargy.

Typical pathways that, when disturbed, can lead to failure to thrive include:

- **Glucose metabolism**—Glucose provides an essential source of energy for various aerobic and anaerobic processes in all cells. Complex carbohydrates are broken down into monosaccharide forms such as glucose, which then enter glycolysis for the production of pyruvate (and 2 ATP). Pyruvate can then enter the Krebs cycle (also called the tricarboxylic acid or TCA cycle) and electron transport chain, ultimately producing a large amount of ATP to supply the energy needed to carry out cellular functions. It is important to keep in mind that the metabolism of glucose is highly regulated. Defects in key enzymes in these pathways can, therefore, have severe consequences, often resulting from a switch from aerobic to anaerobic respiration and leading to a buildup of lactic acid throughout the body.

- **Fructose metabolism**—Fructose is another monosaccharide, often obtained from the diet in the form of sucrose (glucose + fructose). Compared to the tight regulation of glucose metabolism, the metabolism of fructose and other monosaccharides (e.g., galactose) is not as well regulated. Metabolism of fructose, occurring primarily in the liver, requires phosphorylation to fructose-1-phosphate before it can be acted on by the key rate-limiting enzyme, aldolase B, to ultimately form glyceraldehyde-3-phosphate for energy production (shuttled to glycolysis or gluconeogenesis). Disruption of this pathway can, therefore, result in phosphate trapping and thus hypoglycemia. Generally, disorders of fructose metabolism are milder than those involving galactose metabolism (discussed under visual problems).

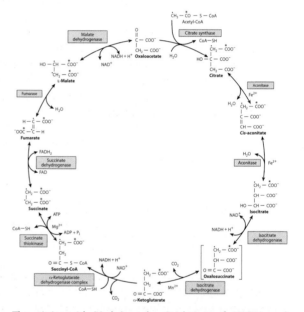

The citric acid (Krebs) cycle. Oxidation of NADH and FADH$_2$ in the respiratory chain leads to the formation of ATP via oxidative phosphorylation. In order to follow the passage of acetyl-CoA through the cycle, the two carbon atoms of the acetyl moiety are shown labeled on the carboxyl carbon (*) and on the methyl carbon (·). Reproduced with permission from Rodwell VW, Bender DA, Botham KM, et al: Harper's Illustrated Biochemistry, 31st ed. New York, NY: McGraw Hill; 2018.

- **Glycogen storage**—Glycogen storage is important because it acts as a buffer to provide glucose until gluconeogenesis is fully functional. When infants have disorders of glycogen regulation, it can present as hypoglycemia and alteration in mental status secondary to hypoglycemia. Some glycogen storage diseases only affect the liver, causing hepatomegaly with hypoglycemia. If muscle is affected, it manifests as weakness and difficulty with exercise as a result of the inability to increase glucose entry into glycolysis during exercise (also covered in myopathy section). A characteristic feature of glycogen storage disorders is a "second wind phenomenon," whereby after a period of rest, if the patient resumes exercise, increased blood flow to muscle can provide other substrates, such as glucose and free fatty acids instead of glycogen, that can lead to improvement in symptoms.

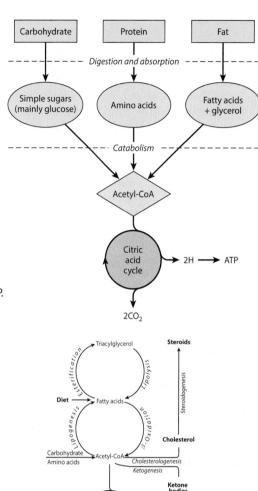

Catabolism of carbohydrate, protein, and fat. Lead to the production of acetyl-CoA, which is oxidized in the citric acid cycle, ultimately yielding ATP. Reproduced with permission from Rodwell VW, Bender DA, Botham KM, et al: Harper's Illustrated Biochemistry, 31st ed. New York, NY: McGraw Hill; 2018.

- **Fatty acid metabolism**—Fatty acids are an additional source of energy, especially in circumstances where glucose is low, such as prolonged fasting or in the onset of illness. Acetyl-CoA from the beta oxidation of fatty acids can be shuttled to the Krebs cycle and also results in formation of ketone bodies, which can be used as energy sources as well. Defects in beta oxidation inhibit the use of fatty acid for energy production. Defects cause hypoketotic hypoglycemia and elevated levels of dicarboxylic acids.

The ketone bodies are acetoacetate, 3-hydroxybutyrate, and acetone. Reproduced with permission from Rodwell VW, Bender DA, Botham KM, et al: Harper's Illustrated Biochemistry, 31st ed. New York, NY: McGraw Hill; 2018.

- **Amino acid metabolism**—When amino acids cannot be degraded, intermediates in their metabolism can build up and cause organic acidurias and metabolic acidosis. The metabolites normally produced may become limited, and important products like L-DOPA, dopamine, epinephrine, norepinephrine, and melanin are not produced. Excess amino acids can also interfere with normal amino acid transport across the blood–brain barrier and limit protein and neurotransmitter synthesis in the brain. Some of the metabolites that build up have a distinctive smell/urine color (see the following table), which is considered a hallmark of each disorder. Organic acidemias have metabolic acidosis and urine ketones, which helps differentiate them from urea cycle defects.

Smell/Color	Disease	Amino Acid
Mousy smell	Phenylketonuria	Phe
Maple syrup smell	Maple syrup urine disease	BCAA
Cabbage smell	Tyrosinemia type 1	Phe, Tyr
Rancid butter smell	Tyrosinemia type 1	Phe, Tyr
Black urine color	Alkaptonuria	Phe, Tyr

- **Urea cycle and transport of ammonia**—Excess organic acids may also interfere with the urea cycle and cause increased levels of ammonia. Urea cycle disorders cause primary hyperammonemia, and organic acidemias cause secondary hyperammonemia. Ammonia diffuses freely across the blood–brain barrier and leads to impaired cerebral function. Both of these disorders can present as altered mental status due to elevated ammonia.

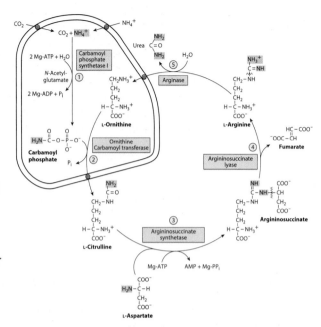

The nitrogen-containing groups that contribute to the formation of urea are shaded. Reactions ① and ② occur in the matrix of liver mitochondria and reactions ③, ④, and ⑤ in liver cytosol. CO_2 (as bicarbonate), ammonium ion, ornithine, and citrulline enter the mitochondrial matrix via specific carriers (see red dots) present in the inner membrane of liver mitochondria.
Reproduced with permission from Rodwell VW, Bender DA, Botham KM, et al: Harper's Illustrated Biochemistry, 31st ed. New York, NY: McGraw Hill; 2018.

CASE 1 | Pyruvate Dehydrogenase Complex (PDC) Deficiency

A mother brings her 1-year-old boy for a well-baby checkup. She is worried because her son seems "extra tired." He doesn't seem to be getting ready to walk, sitting on his own, or babbling as much as her older children did at this age. He also has not been eating as much, and when she tries to feed him, he becomes quite fussy. She reports no history of trauma or injury. On physical exam, he is afebrile but has rapid breathing.

Evaluation/Tests	Labs show normal CBC and glucose and low serum pH. Lactate, pyruvate, and alanine levels are high. Enzyme testing reveals a deficiency in the pyruvate dehydrogenase complex (PDC).
Treatment	Cofactor supplementation with thiamine and lipoic acid stimulates the PDC and may prevent acute worsening of the syndrome. Increase intake of ketogenic nutrients (high fat, low carbohydrate, moderate protein) to promote use of fat and amino acid instead of glucose.
Discussion	Pyruvate dehydrogenase complex (PDC) is an enzyme complex that converts pyruvate to acetyl-coenzyme A (CoA), which is one of the first steps of the Krebs, or tricarboxylic acid (TCA) cycle. In PDC deficiency, this enzyme has an X-linked defect that affects the transition from glycolysis to the TCA cycle, resulting in a buildup of pyruvate. The pyruvate then gets converted into lactate and alanine. Increased lactate results in metabolic acidosis, which can lead to a compensatory respiratory alkalosis in attempts to rid the body of excess acid in the form of carbon dioxide. The buildup of these substrates and the lack of energy (from blocking the TCA and thus electron transport cycle) results in fatigue, poor feeding, and tachypnea, especially during times of illness, stress or high carbohydrate intake. Characteristic findings include neurological deficits, lactic acidosis, and increased serum alanine starting in infancy. Given the young age of the patient, suspicion should be raised for other biochemical defects like **von Gierke disease** and **medium-chain acyl-CoA dehydrogenase (MCAD) deficiency**. Many of these conditions can be ruled in or out by genetic or enzyme testing.

CASE 2 | Hereditary Fructose Intolerance

A 4-year-old boy is brought for evaluation of acute vomiting and lethargy shortly after attending a birthday party. He had several bouts of vomiting in the past, usually after consuming fruit juice. On exam, hepatomegaly and jaundice are noted.

Evaluation/Tests	Labs show low glucose, lactic acidemia, ketosis, hypophosphatemia.
Treatment	Decrease intake of fructose and sucrose (glucose + fructose).
Discussion	Hereditary fructose intolerance is an autosomal recessive disorder involving a deficiency in aldolase B, the rate-limiting enzyme in fructose metabolism. Fructose is commonly found in fruits, juice, and processed sugary foods. When consumed, it is first converted by fructokinase to fructose-1-phosphate. This phosphorylation step traps fructose-1-phosphate inside of cells. Aldolase B then acts on fructose-1-phosphate, converting it into dihydroxyacetone phosphate (DHAP) and glyceraldehyde, which can be used downstream in glycolysis or

CASE 2 | Hereditary Fructose Intolerance (continued)

Discussion	glycerol synthesis. Defects in aldolase B result in accumulation of fructose-1-phosphate inside of cells, leading to a decrease in available phosphate for other processes such as glycogenolysis and gluconeogenesis. This results in hypoglycemia. Symptoms develop shortly after consuming fructose-containing foods. Left untreated, it can lead to further metabolic disturbances including lactic acidemia, hypophosphatemia, and hyperuricemia. It can also progress to liver and renal damage unless fructose intake is reduced.
	Essential fructosuria is a similar disorder that is a benign, asymptomatic condition due to a defect in fructokinase. Fructose may appear in blood or urine, but it can still be used for metabolism because hexokinase (which normally phosphorylates glucose to glucose-6-phosphate) can also act on fructose. Compared to disorders of galactose metabolism (galactokinase deficiency or classic galactosemia), disorders of fructose metabolism tend to be milder.
	Disorders of galactose metabolism may present following ingestion of breast milk or other dairy products while those of fructose metabolism present after ingestion of fruit, high-fructose corn syrup, or other fructose-containing products.

CASE 3 | Von Gierke Disease (Glycogen Storage Disorder Type 1)

A 4-month-old infant is brought to the emergency room with irritability, rapid breathing, and cold-like symptoms. Parents report that episodes of fussiness occur when the baby doesn't feed for >4 hours. Exam is significant for clear rhinorrhea, pharyngeal erythema, tachypnea, with clear breath sounds. The abdomen is protuberant, and the liver edge is palpable 10 cm below the costal margin.

Evaluation/Tests	Labs show severe fasting hypoglycemia, elevated lactate, elevated pyruvate, hyperuricemia, hyperlipidemia, hypertriglyceridemia, and elevated AST and ALT.
Treatment	Frequent oral glucose or cornstarch to sustain blood sugar levels. Avoidance of fructose and galactose (to decrease glycogenesis).
Discussion	Von Gierke disease (glycogen storage disease type I) occurs when a patient has an autosomal recessive defect in the glucose-6-phosphatase enzyme. This defect prevents glucose-6-phosphate from being converted to glucose during gluconeogenesis. This failure in glycogenolysis and gluconeogenesis ultimately results in hypoglycemia. The excess glucose-6-phosphate can enter the pentose phosphate pathway (also called the hexose monophosphate or HMP shunt), causing an increase in ribose formation and purine turnover, which leads to hyperuricemia. The excess glucose-6-phosphate can also be metabolized by glycolysis, leading to increased pyruvate and thus increased lactate and alanine levels. The hypoglycemia causes physiologic epinephrine release, resulting in activation of lipoprotein lipase (LPL), which causes fatty acid release and hypertriglyceridemia. Other features include hepatomegaly and enlarged kidneys (glucose-6-phosphatase is also used in the kidneys for glycogenolysis, although to a lesser extent than the liver).
	Cori disease (type III glycogen storage disease) presents similarly to Von Gierke disease but is usually much milder. Cori disease is caused by a defect in the α-1,6-glucosidase debranching enzyme. Gluconeogenesis remains intact, so lactate levels remain normal. Patients with Cori disease also have muscle weakness and hypotonia.

CASE 4 | Medium-Chain Acyl-CoA Dehydrogenase (MCAD) Deficiency

A 4-month-old infant is brought in for evaluation because she was not acting like herself, and her body went limp suddenly. She had a fever, poor appetite, and was vomiting and lethargic most of the day. She was diagnosed with a viral infection a few days earlier. Physical exam is significant for hypotonia and hepatomegaly.

Evaluation/Tests	Labs show hypoketotic hypoglycemia, increased medium-chain fatty acids (C6, C8, and C10), and hyperammonemia.
Treatment	Avoid fasting and place patient on a special diet.
Discussion	MCAD deficiency is the most common genetic defect in fatty acid beta oxidation and involves an autosomal recessive mutation in the medium chain acyl-CoA dehydrogenase enzyme. Following entry of fatty acyl-CoA into the mitochondrial matrix via the carnitine shuttle, fatty acids normally undergo beta oxidation via acyl-CoA dehydrogenase enzymes, eventually being converted into acetyl-CoA.

CASE 4 | Medium-Chain Acyl-CoA Dehydrogenase (MCAD) Deficiency *(continued)*

Discussion	Acetyl-CoA is then used for ketogenesis or the TCA cycle. In MCAD, the defective medium chain acyl-CoA dehydrogenase enzyme impairs the ability to break down medium chain fatty acids (ones with 6–10 carbons) to acetyl-CoA. Infants typically develop symptoms between 3 and 24 months, as they are weaned from nighttime feedings and experience longer fasts, or in the setting of viral illness and decreased food intake. Lack of acetyl-CoA causes impairment in ketogenesis and gluconeogenesis, resulting in a characteristic hypoketotic hypoglycemia during these times. This can lead to neurologic dysfunction including weakness, lethargy, seizures, and fat accumulation in the liver that causes hepatomegaly, hyperammonemia, and liver injury.
Additional Considerations	**Maple syrup urine disease (MSUD)** is an autosomal recessive disorder involving a mutation in the branched-chain α-ketoacid dehydrogenase enzyme, which is responsible for the degradation of isoleucine, leucine, and valine. Patients may present with signs of central nervous system toxicity (seizures, hypotonia, spasms, lethargy, and intellectual disability), poor feeding, and a distinct sweet odor to the urine that smells like maple syrup or burnt sugar. Treatment includes strict dietary restriction of all three branched-chain amino acids. To differentiate between fatty acid disorders, pay attention to the particular lab findings and the length of the fatty acid chains. **Primary carnitine deficiency (PCD)** is a condition that prevents the body from using fatty acids for energy, which is needed during fasting. PCD results from an autosomal recessive mutation in the *SLC22A5* gene. Carnitine is involved in the shuttling of long-chain fatty acids into the mitochondria for subsequent beta oxidation and production of energy. PCD often appears during infancy or early childhood and can result in neurologic symptoms like weakness and confusion due to encephalopathy, dyspnea, fatigue due to cardiomyopathy, decreased ketogenesis, and low blood glucose levels (hypoketotic hypoglycemia). Although the severity varies, everyone with PCD is at risk for heart failure, liver disease, and sudden death. Symptoms are often triggered by periods of fasting, including sleeping or illness. PCD is quite similar in manifestations to medium-chain acyl-CoA dehydrogenase (MCAD) deficiency; however, labs will show reduction in total and free carnitine levels without an increase in medium-chain fatty acids. Patients with PCD are also at higher risk for rhabdomyolysis, skeletal hypotonia, and cardiomyopathy. PCD can often be mistaken for Reye syndrome, which is caused by the use of aspirin during viral infections like chicken pox or flu. An adequate history can be used to rule out Reye syndrome. Although symptoms may be similar to glycogen storage disorders, disorders of fatty metabolism typically manifest after prolonged exercise and do not improve with rest periods (no second-wind phenomenon).

CASE 5 | Ornithine Transcarbamylase Deficiency (OTC) (Urea Cycle Disorders)

A 7-day-old boy is brought in for evaluation of poor feeding, lethargy, vomiting, and irritability. Physical examination is significant for hypotonia and hepatomegaly.

Evaluation/Tests	Labs show high ammonia, low citrulline in the blood, and high orotic acid in urine.
Treatment	Limit dietary protein intake, advise high-calorie diet and essential amino acid supplements.
Discussion	Ornithine transcarbamylase (OTC) deficiency is the most common urea cycle disorder caused by an X-linked recessive complete or partial deficiency of ornithine transcarbamylase, which is needed for the breakdown and removal of nitrogen in the urea cycle. The first step of the urea cycle involves conversion of CO_2 and ammonia into carbamoyl phosphate. OTC then combines carbamoyl phosphate with ornithine to form citrulline, allowing for entry into the remainder of the urea cycle. Defects in OTC thus prevent progression through the cycle, resulting in accumulation of ammonia and decreased citrulline in the blood. Excess carbamoyl phosphate is then converted to orotic acid (part of the pyrimidine synthesis pathway). Deficiency results in hyperammonemia, which affects the CNS and stimulates increased respiration. Symptoms can vary based on the degree of enzyme deficiency and in the severe form can occur within 24 hours after birth, after a protein feed. Symptoms include poor suckling, vomiting, lethargy, irritability, and seizures. Hypotonia, hepatomegaly, and respiratory difficulties can lead to intellectual disability, developmental delay, coma, and death if untreated. **Orotic aciduria** is an autosomal recessive disorder that may present similarly to OCT deficiency but instead involves an enzyme deficiency in the *de novo* pyrimidine synthesis pathway, whereby orotic acid cannot be converted to uridine monophosphate (UMP) due to a mutation in UMP synthase. Orotic aciduria will result in orotic acid crystals in urine, megaloblastic anemia, and failure to thrive, but it lacks the hyperammonemia seen in OTC deficiency.

DEVELOPMENTAL DELAY OR REGRESSION

Many inborn errors of metabolism can present with either developmental delay or regression. While these terms are often used interchangeably, they are discrete entities. Developmental delay refers to failure of a child to meet specific milestones related to speech, motor, or cognitive development. Developmental regression is used to describe a condition in which a child who has already met normal developmental milestones then loses that function or reverts back to an earlier stage.

Developmental delay is seen in various inborn errors of metabolism such as lysosomal storage diseases, a group of inherited disorders caused by deficiencies in key lysosomal enzymes. These deficiencies result in accumulation of abnormal metabolic products that can become toxic to cells. Depending on the condition, accumulation of these abnormal products in cells (e.g., neurons) can take some time before they begin to interfere with normal physiologic processes, at which point regression may occur. Another group of disorders where developmental delay or regression may be observed is in the metabolism of amino acids. Disruption in the synthesis of essential amino acids can result in toxic accumulation of metabolites and disrupt normal cellular processes.

CASE 6 | Tay-Sachs Disease

A 10-month-old infant is brought in for evaluation of new-onset seizures and change in her ability to perform activities. This was first noticed after 6 months when she gradually lost her ability to sit and could no longer grasp objects. She became less interactive and lost interest in eating. On exam, she is underweight and her funduscopic exam reveals a central area of reddening in the retina bilaterally ("cherry-red spot"). She has exaggerated reactions to loud noises, muscle weakness, and movement problems.

Evaluation/Tests	Genetic testing reveals a deficiency in hexosaminidase A and accumulation of GM2 ganglioside.
Treatment	No cure; goal of treatment is support and comfort.
Discussion	Tay-Sachs disease is an autosomal recessive lysosomal storage disorder caused by a defect in the enzyme hexosaminidase A. This results in accumulation of GM2 ganglioside, particularly in neurons. A classic feature observed in the retina is a "cherry-red spot" in the macula. This is due to the accumulation of GM2 ganglioside within the ganglion cell layer of the retina, which is thicker within the macula. This makes the spot appear red in color, while the rest of the retina is pale. Other characteristic features include developmental regression, muscle weakness, hypotonia, seizures, blindness, macrocephaly, and abnormal startle reflexes. Lysosomal accumulation occurs predominantly in cells and organs that have the highest rates of biosynthesis or uptake of the undegradable sphingolipids and their precursors. Biopsy of affected tissue would show lysosomes with an "onion skin" morphology. The reticuloendothelial system (encompassing macrophages in lymphoid organs, liver, spleen, and more) is unaffected, so there is no hepatosplenomegaly. **Niemann-Pick disease** is an autosomal recessive lysosomal storage disorder caused by a defect in the enzyme sphingomyelinase. This results in accumulation of sphingomyelin, which can lead to cellular malfunction, particularly in the brain, spleen, liver, and lungs. Characteristic features include progressive neurodegeneration, hepatosplenomegaly, cherry-red spot on the macula, and loss of previously acquired milestones; blood smear will show lipid-laden macrophages or "foam cells." Cherry-red spots on the macula can also be seen in **central retinal artery occlusions**; however, this is typically seen in adults with underlying cardiovascular risk factors and typically presents unilaterally.

CASE 7 | Hurler Syndrome (Mucopolysaccharidosis Type I)

A 3-year-old boy is brought in for evaluation of developmental delay in milestones and hearing loss. The child is cognitively delayed for his age, as he is only able to say a few words. He has coarse facial features with a large head, flattened nasal bridge and large lips, corneal clouding, short stature for his age, hepatosplenomegaly, umbilical hernia, limited joint mobility, and cognitive impairment.

Evaluation/Tests	Enzyme assay shows a deficiency of α-L-iduronidase. There is an accumulation of glycosaminoglycans/mucopolysaccharides in urine.
Treatment	Enzyme replacement therapy and human stem cell transplantation.
Discussion	Hurler syndrome is a lysosomal storage disease under the subcategory of mucopolysaccharidoses caused by an autosomal recessive mutation in the gene encoding α-L-iduronidase. Mutation results in the accumulation of mucopolysaccharides, including heparan sulfate and dermatan sulfate. Clinical features of Hurler syndrome present in infancy or early childhood with coarsening of facial features, corneal clouding, dysostosis multiplex (skeletal anomalies), hearing loss, and neurological deterioration. Developmental delay is a key feature. The accumulation of glycosaminoglycans increases with age. At a certain point, this accumulation interferes with the normal biologic function of the tissue. This is responsible for developmental regression.

CASE 7 | Hurler Syndrome (Mucopolysaccharidosis Type I) *(continued)*

Discussion	A similar defect is seen in **Hunter syndrome**, another mucopolysaccharidosis that is X-linked recessive and that is often milder than Hurler syndrome, where patients lack corneal clouding but display aggressive behavior. Hunter syndrome is caused by a defect in iduronate-2-sulfatase.

CASE 8 | Phenylketonuria (PKU)

A 2-year-old boy is brought in for evaluation of progressive developmental delays and growth retardation over the last year. He was born at-term after an uneventful pregnancy. His parents state that he took a much longer time to hold his head up, sit, walk, and talk compared to his older siblings. His parents noted a distinct musty body odor. On physical exam, his height and weight are below the 5th percentile for age, and he has light-colored hair and eyes and eczema.

Evaluation/Tests	Cognitive testing consistent with significant delays. Phenylalanine levels are elevated, and urine is positive for phenylketones. Tyrosine and tetrahydrobiopterin levels are low. Genetic testing shows a mutation in phenylalanine hydroxylase.
Treatment	Restrict phenylalanine and increase tyrosine in the diet. Tetrahydrobiopterin cofactor supplementation.
Discussion	Phenylketonuria (PKU) is an autosomal recessive disorder involving a mutation in the enzyme phenylalanine hydroxylase (PAH), which converts phenylalanine to tyrosine. PKU can also be caused in rare instances by disorders of tetrahydrobiopterin (BH4) synthesis, which is a PAH cofactor. Deficiency of phenylalanine hydroxylase leads to toxic accumulation of phenylalanine and its metabolite phenylpyruvic acid. Newborns have no symptoms due to clearance of phenylalanine by the placenta. If left untreated, it will manifest in delayed development, microcephaly, seizures, and behavioral problems. Affected individuals are hypopigmented due to deficiency of tyrosine, which is the starting point in melanin synthesis. Patients may also have a musty body odor, which comes from phenylalanine metabolites. Newborn screening is widely practiced, allowing initiation of a phenylalanine-restricted diet before the onset of neurological damage.

INTELLECTUAL DISABILITY

Several genetic disorders can result in intellectual disability. Compared to developmental delay, intellectual disability is used to describe patients with broad impairments in cognition that limit their ability to learn at the expected level for their age and function in everyday life. It is typically associated with an intelligence quotient (IQ) less than 70 (median IQ is 100) and is diagnosed prior to the age of 18.

Here, we will cover two groups of genetic abnormalities: trinucleotide repeat expansion diseases and disorders of genomic imprinting. **Trinucleotide repeat expansion diseases** are the result of mutations in which repeats of three nucleotides result in an increase in copy number. Many of these trinucleotide repeats occur naturally; however, once their copy number exceeds a given threshold, they can cause chromosome instability and altered gene expression, which leads to manifestation of different disease types. Not all trinucleotide-repeat diseases present with intellectual disability because it is highly dependent on the particular gene involved.

Genomic imprinting is a normal phenomenon in some genes whereby epigenetic modifications (typically methylation) result in the transcriptional silencing of one gene copy from either maternal or paternal origin, leading to expression in a parent-specific fashion. The two classic disorders of genomic imprinting are Prader-Willi syndrome and Angelman syndrome. The disease phenotype of the patient depends on whether the maternal- or paternal-derived genes are silenced. When the remaining nonsilenced gene undergoes a microdeletion, the disease will occur. These diseases may also be caused by **uniparental disomy**, whereby both chromosome copies are inherited from a single parent. This can result in the silencing of both copies, resulting in disease.

CASE 9 | Prader-Willi Syndrome

A 14-year-old boy is brought to the clinic for evaluation of hypotonia and intellectual disability. His mother notes that he had feeding difficulties as an infant, but since then has developed an insatiable appetite and behavioral problems. The boy has dysmorphic facial features including almond-shaped eyes, narrow forehead, short stature, and small hands and feet, but he is also obese with a BMI of 31. Neurologic exam reveals diminished muscle tone and poor reflexes. Remainder of the exam is normal except for hypogonadism.

CASE 9 | Prader-Willi Syndrome (continued)

Evaluation/Tests	Genetic testing showed deletion of the paternal chromosome 15q11-13 and DNA methylation studies were positive on maternal chromosome 15q.
Treatment	Symptomatic treatment and strict supervision of food intake. Genetic counseling and growth hormone supplementation.
Discussion	Prader-Willi syndrome is a disorder of genomic imprinting. Genomic imprinting is a normal phenomenon whereby certain gene segments inherited from either the mother or father normally undergo methylation to silence that gene copy. Normally, certain segments of chromosome 15q11-13 show methylation and silencing of maternal gene copies. In addition to this normal imprinting, in Prader-Willi syndrome there is either a deletion or mutation in the corresponding paternal allele that is normally expressed. Some cases are also caused by maternal uniparental disomy (25% of cases), whereby the child receives two maternal chromosomes, which are then both silenced through genomic imprinting mechanisms. Either of these genetic alterations results in the absence of the normal paternal gene contribution to this chromosome. Clinical features of Prader-Willi syndrome at birth include hypotonia, lethargy, and feeding difficulties. Some of these features gradually resolve, but patients develop hyperphagia by early childhood, which results in (often significant) obesity. There is also intellectual disability and hypogonadism. Genetic testing is key to confirming the diagnosis and ruling out other causes.
Additional Considerations	**Fragile X syndrome (FXS)** is an X-linked dominant disorder caused by an expansion of a CGG triplet repeat in the promoter region of the *FMR1* gene. Repeat number ranges from 6 to 40 in the general population. Individuals with this syndrome have more than 200 repeats, accompanied by methylation of the promoter, which leads to silencing of the gene. FXS is the most common cause of inherited intellectual disability. Additional manifestations include developmental delay, behavioral problems (attention deficits, hyperactivity, autism spectrum disorder, etc.), dysmorphic facial features (long, narrow face, prominent forehead and chin, large head circumference, large everted ears, etc.), and macroorchidism. Patients are also at risk of developing mitral valve prolapse. **Angelman syndrome** is a disorder of genomic imprinting resulting from the absence or mutation of maternal alleles on chromosome 15. The most common gene affected is *UBE3A*. Normally, children inherit one allele from each parent, the paternally derived copy is methylated and silenced, and the maternally derived copy is expressed. In Angelman syndrome, there is a mutation or deletion in the maternal copy. Clinical features include severe intellectual disability, movement disorders, seizures, developmental delays, learning disabilities, ataxia, tremulousness, and decreased to absent speech. A distinct pattern of unprovoked episodes of laughter and smiling is observed in the disease. Similar to Angelman syndrome, **Rett syndrome** is seen almost exclusively in girls and is due to an X-linked *de novo* mutation in *MECP2*. Affected males die *in utero* or shortly after birth. Symptoms appear in early childhood and include developmental regression, ataxia, seizures, and stereotypical hand-wringing, but lack episodes of inappropriate laughter seen in Angelman syndrome.

DYSMORPHIC FEATURES

Several syndromes present with dysmorphic features, the recognition of which will help identify the underlying abnormality. Dysmorphic features are differences in normal structural development and may involve facial structures, upper or lower extremities, or other areas of the body. The presence of multiple dysmorphic features increases the likelihood of a single unifying cause such as genetic syndrome or congenital birth defect. However, sometimes it is difficult to actually resolve dysmorphic features because they may be subtle, so comparison to parents or siblings may be helpful. Further, genetic testing should be performed to confirm any suspicions.

The most pathognomonic syndromes associated with dysmorphic features are the chromosomal abnormalities resulting in inheritance of three copies of a chromosome (trisomy) rather than two. Karyotype analysis will be diagnostic, although ultrasonography and other serum tests are available. Most trisomies are not viable and will result in spontaneous miscarriage, typically within the first trimester. The only viable trisomies are trisomies 21, 18, and 13. In addition to trisomies, other chromosomal abnormalities may involve translocations, deletions, or microdeletions.

CASE 10 | Down Syndrome (Trisomy 21)

A newborn baby boy born to a 42-year-old mother is noted to have hypotonia and dysmorphic features. The child's length is low for gestational age, and he has a flat occiput with bilateral epicanthal folds. His neck is short with loose skin at the nape. Hands are short and broad with a curved fifth digit and a single palmar crease.

CASE 10 | Down Syndrome (Trisomy 21) *(continued)*

Evaluation/Tests	Chromosomal karyotype—47,XY+21
Treatment	Supportive—early childhood intervention, screening for common problems (heart and cognitive issues), work-related training.
Discussion	Down syndrome (Trisomy 21) is an autosomal trisomy involving the presence of three copies of chromosome 21. It is the most common viable chromosomal disorder and the most common cause of noninherited genetic intellectual disability (vs. inherited, which is Fragile X syndrome). Most often Down syndrome is due to maternal meiotic nondisjunction. Risk of meiotic nondisjunction increases with advanced maternal age as in this case. Rarely, cases can be due to an unbalanced Robertsonian translocation between chromosome 21 and another chromosome, usually 14. First-trimester ultrasound shows increased nuchal lucency and hypoplastic nasal bone with increased free beta-HCG. Second-trimester ultrasound shows decreased alpha-fetoprotein, increased beta-HCG, decreased estriol, and increased inhibin A. Children have weak muscle tone (hypotonia) at birth and may have congenital anomalies, especially cardiac and gastrointestinal. In childhood, duodenal atresia and congenital heart defects (e.g., atrial septal defect) predominate, along with atlantoaxial instability as the child grows. Hirschsprung disease and Brushfield spots in the iris are often present. Characteristic facial features include flat facies, prominent epicanthal eye folds and furrowed tongue. Other characteristics include short fingers and toes, curved fifth finger (clinodactyly), and a wide space between the first and second toes. Intellectual disability is common with delayed cognitive development, although this can vary. There is an increased risk of respiratory infection during childhood and a higher risk of leukemia (AML and ALL) than the general population. Adults are at risk of early-onset Alzheimer disease because the amyloid precursor protein is found on chromosome 21.
Additional Considerations	**Edwards syndrome (Trisomy 18)** is an autosomal trisomy involving the presence of three copies of chromosome 18 due to meiotic nondisjunction. This is one of the three viable trisomies; however, death usually occurs by age 1. Infants with trisomy 18 are born with multiple congenital anomalies. Most notable are low birth weight, prominent occiput, low set ears, a small jaw (micrognathia), and tightly clenched fingers. Internal organ malformations, especially congenital heart disease, are common. Serum marker screening shows decreased alpha-fetoprotein, decreased beta-HCG, decreased estriol, and decreased or normal inhibin A. Clenched fists and rocker bottom feet are often seen on ultrasonography and after birth. **Patau syndrome (Trisomy 13)** is the rarest viable autosomal trisomy involving the presence of three copies of chromosome 13 due to meiotic nondisjunction. This is one of the three viable trisomies; however, death usually occurs by age 1. Infants with Trisomy 13 are born with low birth weight and have multiple congenital anomalies, affecting the heart (congenital heart disease), brain (holoprosencephaly), and kidneys (polycystic kidney disease). Most notable are facial anomalies, including hypotelorism (eyes are closer together than normal), cleft lip and palate, microphthalmia (small eyes), and microcephaly. There may be areas of deficient or absent skin in the scalp (cutis aplasia), polydactyly and "rocker bottom feet." The first-trimester screen shows decreased free beta-HCG and decreased PAPP-A.

PEDIATRIC OPHTHALMOLOGIC ABNORMALITIES

Ophthalmologic abnormalities in a newborn should raise suspicion for genetic or biochemical abnormalities. Inborn errors of galactose metabolism commonly present with ophthalmologic abnormalities including cataracts or leukocoria (loss of red reflex) in newborns. Similar to the metabolism of fructose, galactose metabolism is not well regulated; however, symptoms tend to be more severe in disorders of galactose metabolism compared to analogous ones of fructose metabolism. This is related to the formation of galactitol, an osmotically active form of galactose which can be trapped in cells such as the lens of the eye, retina, kidneys, and Schwann cells. Genetic mutations that may give rise to visual deficits include mutation of the tumor suppressor gene *Rb*, giving rise to retinoblastoma. Identification of specific features may help narrow the differential diagnosis and focus in on the genetic or biochemical pathways involved.

CASE 11 | Classic Galactosemia

A 1-week-old girl who is breast-fed is brought in for evaluation due to poor feeding, vomiting, and lethargy. The baby also is failing to thrive. Physical exam is notable for hepatomegaly, jaundice, and presence of opacification of the lens in each eye.

CASE 11 | Classic Galactosemia *(continued)*

Evaluation/Tests	Galactose is present in the blood and urine. Blood chemistry reveals elevated liver enzymes and hypoglycemia. Feeding with a glucose solution is well tolerated, but formula causes vomiting.
Treatment	Remove lactose and galactose from the diet.
Discussion	Classic galactosemia is an autosomal recessive disorder due to the absence of the rate-limiting enzyme of galactose metabolism, galactose-1-phosphate uridyltransferase. This enzyme converts galactose-1-phosphate to glucose-1-phosphate, which can then undergo glycolysis or glycogenesis. Deficiency in this enzyme results in accumulation of two toxic substances (vs. only one seen in galactokinase deficiency): galactose (and osmotically active galactitol, which can accumulate in the lens) and galactose-1-phosphate, which can also be toxic. Symptoms of classic galactosemia begin much earlier and are more severe compared to those seen in galactokinase deficiency. Symptoms develop when an infant begins feeding (lactose is present in breast milk and formula) and include failure to thrive, jaundice, hepatomegaly, infantile cataracts, and intellectual disability. This can predispose neonates to *E. coli* sepsis. Patients with galactosemia become hypoglycemic within several hours of ingestion of galactose. Galactose is one of the degradation products of lactose (along with glucose) found in dairy products, breast milk, and many baby formulas. **Galactokinase deficiency** is an autosomal recessive disorder involving the first step in galactose metabolism, by which galactose is normally converted to galactose-1-phosphate by the enzyme galactokinase. Galactose accumulates in many tissues and can be converted by aldose reductase to the osmotically active substance galactitol. This can drive fluid accumulation in certain tissues such as the lens. Galactokinase deficiency is relatively mild, but characteristic features include galactosemia, galactosuria, infantile cataracts, failure to track objects, and failure to develop a social smile, which is normally present by 6–8 weeks of age. It can be distinguished from classic galactosemia by the fact that there is no accumulation of galactose-1-phosphate.

CASE 12 | Retinoblastoma

A 2-year-old boy is referred to the ophthalmologist because the right pupil appears white on examination. He has right-sided strabismus, leukocoria (pupil appeared white), nystagmus, a bulging of the eyeball, and decreased visual acuity.

Evaluation/Tests	Ophthalmoscopic examination under anesthesia reveals a chalky, off-white retinal mass with a soft, friable consistency. Lens appears normal. Ultrasound reveals a normal-sized globe with calcification of the mass. MRI shows no involvement of the optic nerve. Biopsy is contraindicated due to risk of tumor seeding. Molecular genetic testing reveals a mutation in the *Rb* gene.
Treatment	Local and systemic chemotherapy, cryotherapy, laser photoablation, radiotherapy, and, rarely, enucleation and genetic counseling.
Discussion	Retinoblastoma is a cancer of the retina caused by a mutation in the *Rb* tumor suppressor gene, which results in loss of heterozygosity. Loss of heterozygosity is an important concept for tumor suppressor genes and supported by the "two-hit hypothesis" whereby both alleles must be mutated or deleted before a cancer is able to develop. Normally, a patient inherits two functional copies or alleles of a tumor suppressor gene. If a patient inherits a single dysfunctional allele, the remaining allele is often sufficient to protect against neoplastic transformation. However, mutations are quite common in somatic cells, and these patients have an increased risk of acquiring a "second-hit" mutation in their remaining allele, predisposing them to the development of retinoblastoma in later childhood or adolescence. Those who inherit two defective alleles (hereditary retinoblastoma) will develop retinoblastoma much earlier in life. Both familial and *de novo* cases can occur. Leukocoria of the left eye caused by retrolental membrane (persistent hyperplastic primary vitreous or persistent fetal vasculature). Reproduced with permission from Hay WW Jr, Levin MJ, Abzug MJ, et al: Current Diagnosis & Treatment: Pediatrics, 25th ed. New York, NY: McGraw Hill; 2020.

CASE 12 | Retinoblastoma (continued)

| Discussion | Retinoblastoma is often detected due to the reflection of light off the tumor, which causes the pupil to appear white (leukocoria). This is sometimes noticed in photographs. Affected children are at increased risk for developing second cancers (commonly osteosarcoma, specifically in hereditary retinoblastoma) in addition to consequences of systemic chemotherapy like hearing loss with carbo-platin therapy. The *Rb* gene on chromosome 13 encodes a nuclear protein that regulates the G1 to S checkpoint of the cell cycle. Normally it is in an active, hypophosphorylated state that prevents progression to the S phase by binding to the E2F transcription factor; however, mutations result in abnormal hyperphosphorylation, resulting in release of E2F and unregulated progression through the cell cycle. |

MUSCLE WEAKNESS

Muscle weakness, or myopathy, is a presenting feature of several disorders of metabolism or neurologic disorders. Approaches to a patient with myopathy can be based on the age of the patient, family history, pattern of involvement, associated signs and symptoms, and diagnostic test results.

Muscular dystrophies are genetic disorders with various forms of inheritance that result in progressive weakness and muscle atrophy due to defects in proteins important in the structure and function of muscle cells. To distinguish between different forms of muscular dystrophy, pay attention to the pattern of inheritance (X-linked, autosomal dominant, etc.) and pattern of myopathy (starts with proximal vs. distal muscles).

Mutations in mitochondrial DNA (mtDNA) are inherited from the mother and can result in a heterogenous group of disorders called mitochondrial myopathies. Although all children inherit the mutation from the affected mother, only the daughters can pass it on to their children. The difference in expression of mitochondrially inherited disease among different members of the same family (heteroplasmy) is due to involvement of different organs and the uneven distribution of normal and mutant mtDNA in different tissues. The systems that tend to be affected the most are the central nervous system, cardiac, respiratory, eye, and endocrine in addition to muscles because they contain the most metabolically active cells.

Another common cause of myopathy or hypotonia (decreased muscle tone) are inborn errors of metabolism affecting glycogen and lipid storage and transport pathways. Glycogen is an important storage source of carbohydrates; breakdown of glycogen via glycogenolysis is used to maintain blood sugar, especially during times of increased need such as exercise or stress. Failure to adequately break down glycogen and convert to glucose results in characteristic features including exertional myalgias, rhabdomyolysis, cardiorespiratory involvement, and exercise intolerance. Some patients may experience a "second wind" phenomenon whereby after a period of rest, if the patient resumes exercise, increased blood flow to muscle can provide other substrates such as glucose and free fatty acids instead of glycogen, leading to improvement in symptoms. Lipids are an additional important source of energy that can be used by the body under periods of prolonged exercise, fasting, or stress when normal glycogen stores have been depleted via conversion to ketone bodies. Patients with defective lipid metabolism are unable to produce ketone bodies so they present with hypoketotic hypoglycemia.

CASE 13	Duchenne Muscular Dystrophy (DMD)
A 5-year-old boy is brought in for evaluation of progressive difficulty in getting up from a sitting position. His father says every time he tries to sit up, he needs to "walk up his legs with his hands." He has also been unable to keep up with his playmates for the last couple of years. On exam, there is weakness and wasting of muscles of upper legs, arms and shoulder, hypertrophy of calf muscles, waddling gait, and significant difficulty climbing stairs.	
Evaluation/Tests	Serum CK is elevated. Muscle biopsy showed muscle fiber degeneration and necrosis and complete absence of dystrophin. Genetic tests were positive for a frameshift mutation in the *DMD* gene.
Treatment	There is no cure. Symptomatic treatment includes physical therapy and steroids to improve muscle strength.
Discussion	Duchenne muscular dystrophy (DMD) is an X-linked recessive disorder caused by a frameshift mutation in the *DMD* gene, which encodes the muscle membrane protein dystrophin. Frameshift mutations involve a deletion or insertion of a number of nucleotides not divisible by 3, therefore disrupting the reading of all downstream codons. In DMD, this leads to a complete lack of dystrophin production. Dystrophin normally

CASE 13 | Duchenne Muscular Dystrophy (DMD) *(continued)*

Discussion	helps anchor muscle fibers in cardiac and skeletal muscle. Lack of dystrophin causes myonecrosis, resulting in weakness and atrophy of the muscles commonly starting around 3–5 years of age, starting in the proximal muscles such as the pelvic girdle and then progressing superiorly. There is often associated cardiomyopathy, and there may be cognitive dysfunction. Features include waddling gait, difficulty climbing stairs, using upper extremities to stand up from a sitting position (Gower sign), and repeated falling. Calf pseudohypertrophy occurs due to replacement of muscle by fibrofatty tissue. Serum CK levels are at least 10–20 times (often 50–200 times) the upper limit of normal. Due to early onset, affected children are usually wheelchair-bound by adolescence. Death is common in the twenties, often due to dilated cardiomyopathy. **Becker muscular dystrophy (BMD)** is also an X-linked recessive muscular dystrophy; however, it results from nonframeshift deletions in the dystrophin gene, resulting in partial loss of function. BMD is therefore less severe, may present later in life (adolescence or early adulthood), progresses more slowly, and patients may survive into their forties or beyond.

CASE 14 | Myotonic Dystrophy Type 1

A 32-year-old man presents with progressive distal muscle weakness. Symptoms started when he was 20 years old. He has difficulty releasing objects after he grasps them and notes declining strength in upper and lower extremities. Family also reports memory loss and hypersomnia. His father had similar symptoms that began much later in his life. Physical exam is notable for ptosis, cloudy opacity in his lenses, and frontal balding. He has wasting in his proximal and distal muscles, prolonged muscle tension (myotonia), and testicular atrophy. No upper motor neuron defects are noted.

Evaluation/Tests	Creatinine kinase is elevated. Muscle biopsy shows a high number of nuclei and marked variation in fiber diameter with splitting fibers and adipose deposition. Genetic testing shows expansion of unstable CTG trinucleotide repeat in the *DMPK* gene on the long arm of chromosome 19.
Treatment	Supportive care with braces, scooters, or wheelchairs.
Discussion	An autosomal dominant inherited expansion of a CTG trinucleotide in the noncoding region of the DMPK gene, results in Myotonic dystrophy type 1. When this gene with expanded CTG repeats is transcribed, the abnormal RNA produced causes cellular dysfunction leading to the symptoms of myotonic dystrophy. Normal alleles include 5–35 repeats; full penetrance alleles are >50 repeats. During meiosis in germ cells, these unstable repeats can be expanded, thus increasing the number of repeats in offspring through a process known as genetic anticipation that may increase the severity of disease and lower the age of onset from generation to generation. Patients with myotonic dystrophy type 1 typically present at 20–40 years old, and men and women are equally affected (as opposed to DMD and BMD where primarily men are affected because of their X-linked inheritance patterns). Besides myotonia, affected individuals exhibit muscle weakness, wasting effect, frontal balding, cataracts, and testicular atrophy. A key feature is difficulty releasing objects after grasping them due to myotonia (delayed relaxation after muscle contraction). More distal muscles (lower legs, hands, face, etc.) are often affected first. They often develop dysphagia, generalized weakness, and respiratory failure. Cardiac conduction defects, resulting in arrhythmia, are common.

CASE 15 | Mitochondrial Encephalomyopathy Lactic Acidosis and Stroke-Like Episodes (MELAS) Syndrome

A 6-year-old girl is brought to clinic for evaluation of left-sided muscle weakness in her face, arm, and leg. Per her mother, the patient had complained of a bad headache and had convulsions the night prior to presentation. Her brother had a similar disorder and passed away a few years ago. On exam, she appears confused, is tachypneic, and aphasic, and her strength is diminished on the left side.

Evaluation/Tests	CBC and CMP are normal, and lactate level is high. ABG shows pH 7.3, PO2 72 mmHg, and PCO2 50 mmHg. MRI shows multiple small infarcts in the parietal and occipital lobes on the right side. EEG shows prominent and diffuse periodic epileptiform discharges. Genetic testing reveals a mutation in the mitochondrial DNA gene *MT-TL1*. Muscle biopsy reveals the presence of ragged red fibers.
Treatment	No specific treatment. Anticonvulsants are used to help prevent and control seizures.

CASE 15 | Mitochondrial Encephalomyopathy Lactic Acidosis and Stroke-Like Episodes (MELAS) Syndrome *(continued)*

Discussion	A mutation of mitochondrial genes (*MT-TL1* is most common) results in a maternally transmitted myopathy of variable expression (heteroplasmy) affecting energy metabolism in multiple tissues and is known as **MELAS** (Mitochondrial encephalomyopathy, lactic acidosis, and stroke-like episodes). It often presents as stroke like episodes in childhood with focal neurologic deficits and imaging findings suggestive of infarctions. Other presenting symptoms include seizures, ataxia, myopathy and lactic acidosis with gradual loss of cognitive function. **Myoclonic epilepsy with ragged red fibers (MERRF)** is another mitochondrial myopathy caused by a mutation in the *MT-TK* gene encoding mitochondrial lysine-tRNA. It differs from MELAS in that the strokes are more generalized and myoclonic jerks are seen. Additionally, optic atrophy, hearing loss, and cardiomyopathy are commonly present. Muscle biopsy for both MELAS and MERRF show ragged red fibers on Gomori trichrome stain. mtDNA mutations associated with MERRF are diagnostic and can usually be detected in white blood cells.

CASE 16 | McArdle Disease (Glycogen Storage Disease Type V)

A 20-year-old man presents with myalgias, cramps, and easy fatigability since childhood. Symptoms are worse with moderate exercise and improve after a brief period of rest. He also notes red urine after moderate activity.

Evaluation/Tests	Blood glucose is normal. Forearm exercise test (patient performs maximal effort handgrips for one minute, then blood samples are drawn) shows inability to produce lactate (deficient glycogenolysis). Muscle biopsy–PAS staining shows increased glycogen-containing vacuoles. Genetic testing shows defect in *PYGM* gene encoding muscle glycogen phosphorylase (myophosphorylase).
Treatment	No cure, but diet and exercise strategies such as consuming sucrose before low-moderate activity can help control symptoms.
Discussion	This individual has McArdle disease (glycogen storage disease type V), an autosomal recessive deficiency of skeletal muscle glycogen phosphorylase (myophosphorylase). Glycogen phosphorylase removes glucose-1-phosphate off of branched glycogen until four glucose units remain. Defects in glycogen phosphorylase, therefore, prevent the quick liberation of glucose-1-phosphate molecules during periods of exercise or stress. Because it only involves skeletal muscle, blood glucose levels are typically unaffected (unlike in von Gierke disease). The key features are exercise intolerance, myoglobinuria with exercise, and a characteristic "second wind" phenomenon in young adults due to increased blood flow and conversion of glycogen metabolism to other sources of energy. Ischemic forearm exercise test shows no increase in pyruvate and lactate levels in venous blood from contracting ischemic forearm muscles. The lack of increase in pyruvate and lactate levels is because the muscles cannot utilize their glycogen stores. **Carnitine palmitoyltransferase (CPT) II deficiency** can present similarly and results in low carnitine levels and inability of muscles to use certain long-chain fatty acids (LCFAs) as an energy source. This results in a breakdown of muscle fibers. Labs would show decreased CPT II activity, increase in long-chain C16 and C18 plasma acylcarnitine levels, hypoketotic hypoglycemia, elevated creatine phosphokinase (CPK), and myoglobinuria.

CASE 17 | Pompe Disease (Glycogen Storage Disease Type II)

A newborn is noted to have hypotonia and a heart murmur after an uncomplicated birth. On physical exam, notable findings included macroglossia, hepatomegaly, and severe hypotonia.

Evaluation/Tests	Echocardiogram shows severe biventricular cardiac hypertrophy. Labs notable for normal glucose and increased serum lactate, AST, and ALT. Lysosomal enzyme acid-α-1,4-glucosidase activity is low.
Treatment	Treat with enzyme replacement therapy.
Discussion	Pompe disease (GSD type II) is an autosomal recessive condition involving deficiency in the lysosomal acid α-1,4-glucosidase (acid maltase) enzyme. Early-onset Pompe disease presents in the first year, typically as a floppy-baby with severe hypotonia. Unique to this form of GSD, patients present with cardiac abnormalities including cardiomegaly and hypertrophic cardiomyopathy. Other symptoms

Discussion	include exercise intolerance, hypotonia, failure to thrive, hepatomegaly, and other systemic findings such as respiratory failure, which can lead to early death. Glycogen deposits can be observed in muscle, liver, and cardiac tissue. Later-onset Pompe disease can present with difficulty rising from a chair or climbing stairs or with morning headaches and fatigue. Pompe disease patients often have elevated lactic acid and CK levels.
	Glucose levels are often normal in Pompe disease, helping differentiate it from hypoglycemia in **Von Gierke disease**, in which glucose cannot be released due to deficiency of glucose-6-phosphatase.

BONE AND JOINT ABNORMALITIES

Several types of biochemical disorders present with abnormalities in bone, cartilage, and joints. One such group involves mutations in extracellular matrix proteins such as collagen or fibrillin. Given the important role of extracellular matrix proteins in forming the basement membrane underlying blood vessels, these disorders may also present with bruising and vascular damage.

Another group of disorders involves defects in metabolic pathways that lead to the accumulation of crystals that can deposit in joints and induce an inflammatory response. They typically have abnormalities in urine, behavioral disturbances, and systemic manifestations, which suggest a systemic process and helps distinguish them from other types of arthritis.

CASE 18 | Osteogenesis Imperfecta

A 13-year-old boy is referred by the school nurse to clinic for suspicion of child abuse. He has a history of recurrent fractures in the forearms and legs after minor falls, which started when he was 1 year old. These fractures healed without significant delays. Physical exam reveals blue sclera, decreased hearing, an overbite, and bowing of tibia and fibula.

Evaluation/Tests	X-rays show multiple fractures. Audiogram confirms bilateral hearing loss. Genetic testing reveals mutations in type I collagen (*COL1A1* gene).
Treatment	Supportive care, exercise, physical therapy, and surgery for fractures.
Discussion	Osteogenesis imperfecta (OI) is a genetic bone disorder often caused by mutations in genes encoding components of type I collagen (*COL1A1* and *COL1A2*). The mutation impairs triple helix formation and is commonly inherited in an autosomal dominant fashion. The basic phenotype of OI is the occurrence of brittle bones with high tendency to fracture even with minimal trauma, which occurs because type 1 collagen is the main type of collagen in osteoid. Fractures occur in locations that are not typical and can occur as early as *in utero* or at childbirth. In some instances, it is associated with short stature. Other features include blue sclera due to translucent connective tissue overlying choroidal veins, hearing loss from abnormal ossicle formation, and dentinogenesis imperfecta (weakening of the teeth). There is a wide range of variable expression, including neonatal onset with lethality early in life, to relatively mild symptoms.

CASE 19 | Ehlers-Danlos Syndrome (EDS)

A 30-year-old woman presents for evaluation of increased bruising, achy muscles and increased fatigue. As a teenager, she had recurrent dislocations of her shoulder when playing softball. On physical exam, she has a high-arched palate, hypotonia, and flat feet. She is able to place her hands flat on the floor without bending her knees. She can bend her thumb to touch her forearm. Dermatologic exam shows cigarette paper–like scars over her knees and hyperelastic skin that can be pulled about an inch without any pain.

Evaluation/Tests	Skin biopsy shows a relative increase in the elastic fibers with scant collagenous fibers showing cauliflower-like degeneration. Genetic tests and electron microscopy show collagen structure abnormalities.
Treatment	Monitor for complications and provide physical therapy.

CASE 19 | **Ehlers-Danlos Syndrome (EDS)** (continued)

Discussion	Ehlers-Danlos syndrome (EDS) has multiple forms and can be genetically heterogeneous with most forms being autosomal dominant. The classic form of EDS has mutations in the genes encoding peptides involved in forming type V collagen (*COL5A1* and *COL5A2*). There is joint hypermobility and instability, as well as soft, velvety, hyperelastic skin. There is delayed, abnormal wound healing and generalized tissue fragility. The vascular form of EDS results from a mutation in type III procollagen and has more systemic tissue fragility affecting large vessels such as aorta, muscles, and other organs. Vessel fragility in the vascular form of the disease makes them prone to rupture, and affected patients can have berry aneurysms and aortic aneurysms.

CASE 20 | Marfan Syndrome

A 13-year-old boy presents for evaluation of poor vision. On exam, he is in the >99th percentile for his height, is very thin, and has myopia. Additionally, he has disproportionately long, slender arms, legs, fingers, and toes (arachnodactyly); pectus carinatum with protruding chest; joint hypermobility (able to bend his fingers back to touch the dorsum of his hands); flat feet; and scoliosis. On cardiac auscultation, he is noted to have a high-pitched "blowing" early diastolic murmur heard best over the left sternal border.

Evaluation/Tests	Echocardiogram shows aortic root dilatation and aortic regurgitation. Detailed eye exam reveals lens dislocation. Genetic testing is positive for a mutation in the *FBN1* gene.
Treatment	Avoidance of competitive, contact sports and prophylactic surgery when aorta reaches 5 cm in diameter and valve surgery when indicated.
Discussion	Marfan syndrome is an autosomal dominant connective tissue disorder caused by a mutation in the *FBN1* gene encoding the glycoprotein fibrillin-1. Fibrillin forms a sheath around elastin, and together they form microfibrils that provide strength and flexibility to the extracellular matrix and connective tissues. Clinical features affect the bones, joints, eyes, blood vessels, and heart. The most common findings are increased height and arm span due to overgrowth of the long bones of the extremities, scoliosis, pectus deformity of the chest wall (pectus carinatum or pectus excavatum), dislocation of the lenses of the eyes, and myopia. Complications include widening and tearing of the aorta and valve deformities resulting in aortic regurgitation or mitral valve prolapse. Mitral valve prolapse can be asymptomatic or can be associated with arrhythmias and mitral regurgitation. Aneurysm of the aorta has to be monitored closely because it can cause aortic rupture if untreated. Hypoplastic iris and retinal detachment can occur, and these patients are prone to cataracts and glaucoma. Pneumothorax is another complication that can occur in these individuals. The range of manifestations is varied, and the syndrome progresses with age in most cases.

CASE 21 | Alkaptonuria

A 40-year-old man presents with pain in the low back, hips, and knees, which is significantly affecting his ability to walk. He has a history of ruptured Achilles tendon and kidney stones. He has previously passed tiny black stones in his urine and notes that his urine turns black on exposure to air. On physical exam, there is a bluish-black discoloration over the pinna and parts of his sclera, and he has restricted spine, hip, and knee mobility.

Evaluation/Tests	Urine testing reveals the presence of homogentisic acid.
Treatment	Symptomatic therapy.
Discussion	Alkaptonuria is an autosomal recessive disorder caused by a mutation in the gene encoding homogentisate oxidase. This enzyme is involved in the normal pathway of degradation of tyrosine by converting homogentisic acid (an intermediate in the breakdown of tyrosine) into maleylacetoacetic acid, which is then normally converted to fumarate to be recycled into the TCA cycle. Mutation in homogentisate oxidase results in accumulation of homogentisic acid, which can undergo oxidation and accumulate in the connective tissues of the skin, eyes, and ears. Ochronosis can occur with oxidation resulting in bluish-black discoloration of these areas and pigmented ear wax. This disease tends to be benign but can cause arthralgias due to deposition of pigment in cartilage. It can also cause cardiac valve abnormalities and formation of kidney stones. A key lab finding is the excretion of homogentisic acid in the urine, which results in black-colored urine on exposure to air.

CASE 22 | Gaucher Disease

A 22-year-old man of Ashkenazi Jewish descent presents with fatigue, easy bruising with minor trauma, and pain over the left hip. Physical exam is significant for skin pallor, hepatosplenomegaly, and bruises over his forearms and thighs. External rotation of the left hip is limited, and there is tenderness over the hip joint.

Evaluation/Tests	CBC shows pancytopenia. An ultrasound shows hepatosplenomegaly. X-rays show avascular necrosis of the femur, and DEXA scan is consistent with osteopenia/osteoporosis. Enzyme testing shows reduced activity of β-glucosidase (glucocerebrosidase).
Treatment	Enzyme replacement therapy with recombinant glucocerebrosidase.
Discussion	Gaucher disease is the most common lysosomal storage disease and is caused by an autosomal recessive mutation in the gene encoding the lysosomal enzyme glucocerebrosidase (β-glucosidase). This results in accumulation of glucocerebrosidase within lysosomes and can affect multiple organ systems. There are three major clinical subtypes. The most common form is characterized by bone disease (lytic lesions, osteopenia, avascular necrosis of the femur, osteoporosis), hepatosplenomegaly, pancytopenia, and lung disease. Destruction of bone occurs from the release of hydrolytic lysosomal enzymes and inflammatory mediators. Bleeding and bruising are secondary to the thrombocytopenia. Other less common forms involve a progressive neurological impairment. Biopsy typically shows Gaucher cells, which are lipid-laden macrophages resembling crumpled or crinkled tissue paper. Lipid-laden macrophages can be observed in both Gaucher and **Niemann-Pick disease**. Gaucher disease is distinguished from **Tay-Sachs** and Niemann-Pick by lack of ocular findings. It may present anytime from childhood to adulthood while these other disorders most often present in infancy or childhood.

CASE 23 | Lesch-Nyhan Syndrome

A 3-year-old boy is brought to the office for evaluation of pain and swelling over his joints, which has been worsening over the last year. His family reports that he has had self-destructive behavior and often bites his lips and fingers over the past year. He has a pronounced limp when he walks. Range of motion of his knees and small joints of hands is reduced. He has multiple lumps on hands and feet and has swollen and deformed nose, lips, wrists, and fingers.

Evaluation/Tests	Labs show elevated serum uric acid. Joint fluid aspiration shows negatively birefringent crystals. Enzyme testing reveals absence of hypoxanthine guanine phosphoribosyltransferase (HGPRT).
Treatment	Allopurinol or febuxostat (2nd line), symptomatic, and behavioral therapies.
Discussion	Lesch-Nyhan syndrome is caused by an X-linked recessive mutation in the gene encoding the HGPRT enzyme. Due to its pattern of inheritance, it is almost exclusively seen in men. Defects in this enzyme cause a deficiency in the purine salvage pathway, where purine metabolites such as guanine and hypoxanthine are normally recycled back to precursors for reuse in the synthesis of nucleic acids. Due to lack of purine salvage capabilities, these precursors are instead broken down into xanthine and then uric acid by the enzyme xanthine oxidase, resulting in the accumulation of these products and hyperuricemia. Hypotonia and developmental delay are the presenting symptoms seen in infancy. This is followed by progressive motor symptoms due to pyramidal and extrapyramidal system involvement. Uric acid is deposited in joints and urinary tract with infant diapers revealing sand like orange sodium urate crystals. Aggression, compulsive behavior, neurologic and renal dysfunction are other manifestations. Reduction of uric acid production via the inhibition of xanthine oxidase using allopurinol or febuxostat is the cornerstone of treatment of Lesch-Nyhan syndrome.

ALTERED MENTAL STATUS

Certain vitamin deficiencies can cause altered mental status, or a reversible form of dementia. This is important to identify in elderly patients who might otherwise be suspected of having more irreversible forms of dementia such as neurodegenerative diseases like Alzheimer disease. Altered mental status in the setting of additional skin and/or hematologic findings may indicate a vitamin deficiency or systemic process involving deposition diseases. The key to differentiating these disorders is to identify the characteristic skin and hematologic manifestations or knowing the pathways where vitamins are needed as cofactors.

CASE 24 | Niacin (B3) Deficiency (Pellagra)

A 60-year-old man with a past medical history of chronic alcoholism presents with abdominal pain and diarrhea. He is homeless and has not eaten in a few days. On exam, he is irritable, anxious, alert, and oriented to name only. He has a reddish-brown rash over his face, chest, and arms. The skin is rough and brittle over the areas of the lesions. The abdominal exam is unremarkable.

Evaluation/Tests	Labs show low levels of erythrocyte nicotinamide adenine dinucleotide (NAD^+), niacin plasma metabolites, and urine niacin metabolites.
Treatment	Treat with oral nicotinamide and correct other nutritional deficiencies.
Discussion	This patient is presenting with pellagra, caused by vitamin B3 (niacin) deficiency. Niacin, or nicotinic acid, is derived from tryptophan and is a component of NAD^+ and $NADP^+$. It serves as a cofactor for coenzymes in oxidation-reduction reactions and plays a crucial role in ATP synthesis, glycolysis, and metabolism of fatty and amino acids. Niacin deficiency causes pellagra, which is commonly seen in people who are chronically malnourished such as those who are homeless, abuse alcohol or drugs, or suffer from anorexia. Pellagra can also be seen in patients with Hartnup disease, malignant carcinoid, and those taking isonizaid (because this medication causes decreased B6 levels, which is a cofactor required for synthesis of B3). Pellagra is characterized by diarrhea, dementia, dermatitis, and rarely death (the four D's). The dermatitis is often reddish-brown, hyperkeratotic, and photosensitive. It often presents as a broad collar of circumferential rash along the C3/4 dermatome, called Casal necklace. The sunburn becomes darker with time instead of fading and results in hyperpigmentation of sun-exposed areas. If untreated, this can result in death.
Additional Considerations	**Thiamine (B1) deficiency** can lead to Wernicke-Korsakoff syndrome. Thiamine is a water-soluble vitamin that is a component of thiamine pyrophosphate (TPP), a cofactor for several key dehydrogenase enzyme reactions. This cofactor is used by pyruvate dehydrogenase (converts pyruvate from glycolysis to acetyl-CoA for entry into TCA cycle), alpha-ketoglutarate dehydrogenase (in TCA cycle), and transketolase (involved in HMP shunt). Thiamine deficiency can thus result in impaired ability to break down glucose to ATP. **Wernicke-Korsakoff syndrome** is an encephalopathy characterized by a triad of confusion, ataxia, and ophthalmoplegia (nystagmus and conjugate gaze palsies). It is a clinical diagnosis, and supplementation of thiamine can result in resolution of symptoms. If a patient is given glucose without thiamine, symptoms can acutely worsen, and patients can have acute onset neuropsychiatric symptoms. This is because of thiamine's key role as a cofactor that allows for progression through the TCA cycle. Without thiamine, increased glucose will be shuttled to the formation of more lactic acid, precipitating an acute worsening of the patient's symptoms. Risk factors contributing to deficiency include alcohol abuse, hyperemesis, and chronic diuretic use. Severe and chronic thiamine deficiency is known as beriberi, and it can have two forms. **Wet beriberi** affects the heart and can lead to dilated cardiomyopathy, high-output cardiac failure, and severe edema. **Dry beriberi** primarily affects the nervous system and can cause polyneuropathy, symmetric muscle wasting, and other neurologic symptoms. Over time, this can lead to Korsakoff's psychosis, which is characterized by amnesia, confabulation (fabricated or misinterpreted memories but without an intent to deceive), and personality changes. **Hartnup disease** is an autosomal recessive deficiency in neutral amino acid transporters in the gut and kidney, which results in low levels of tryptophan and pellagra-like symptoms. Niacin can also be used therapeutically to treat dyslipidemia by increasing HDL and lowering VLDL. Niacin causes a prostaglandin-dependent facial flushing on ingestion, which can be avoided by pretreatment with aspirin. In addition to facial flushing, excess niacin (podagra) can cause hyperglycemia and hyperuricemia.

NEUROPATHY

Neurons are highly active, nonreproducing cells that require a large amount of energy to satisfy their metabolic demands. As such, certain vitamin deficiencies, cellular organelle defects, and inborn errors of metabolism can present with signs and symptoms related to nervous system damage. One of the more common presenting symptoms is peripheral neuropathy due to damage of peripheral nerves. Peripheral neuropathy can present with weakness, hypotonia, tingling or burning sensations, numbness, or paresthesia. Additional dermatologic and/or hematologic findings make biochemical defects more likely compared to other causes of peripheral neuropathy.

CASE 25 | Vitamin B12 (Cobalamin) Deficiency

A 56-year-old woman presents with numbness and tingling in her hands and feet, persistent fatigue, and decreased memory. The woman has been consuming a strict vegan diet without dairy products or eggs for the past 20 years. Physical exam is notable for conjunctival pallor, loss of pinprick sensation and touch distal to the wrist and ankles, decreased vibration sense, and mild cognitive impairment.

Evaluation/Tests	CBC is normal except for Hgb of 11.0 and MCV 120, and peripheral blood smear shows hypersegmented neutrophils. Serum folate is normal, vitamin B12 levels are low, and homocysteine and methylmalonic acid levels are elevated. Serum testing for intrinsic factor antibodies is negative.
Treatment	Vitamin B12 supplementation.
Discussion	This patient is presenting with a vitamin B12 (cobalamin) deficiency. Vitamin B12 is found mainly in animal products. It is a cofactor for two essential enzymatic reactions: the remethylation of homocysteine to methionine and the conversion of methylmalonyl-CoA to succinyl-CoA. B12 deficiency can be caused by poor dietary intake (which occurs with vegan diets), malabsorption (which can occur in alcoholism), loss of intrinsic factor (as seen in pernicious anemia), gastric bypass surgery, and destruction or loss of the terminal ileum (such as in Crohn's disease), all of which result in depletion of the storage pool of vitamin B12 in the liver. It takes many years for this deficiency to develop as the liver has abundant B12 stores. In addition to its important role in DNA synthesis, vitamin B12 is a cofactor in odd-chain fatty acid metabolism through the conversion of methylmalonyl CoA to succinyl CoA. Without B12, increased methylmalonyl CoA and its precursors can disrupt lipids in plasma membranes. This can occur in cells of the nervous system, resulting in demyelination commonly affecting the dorsal columns and lateral corticospinal tract, known as subacute combined degeneration. Hematologic changes are characterized by megaloblastic anemia (large immature and dysfunctional red blood cells) and hypersegmented neutrophils. Prolonged B12 deficiency can result in irreversible nerve damage. Testing for intrinsic factor and parietal cell antibodies helps determine if pernicious anemia is the cause of the B12 deficiency. Pernicious anemia is often associated with other autoimmune diseases and atrophic gastritis.
Additional Considerations	**Folate deficiency** often coexists with other nutrient deficiencies, including B12 deficiency. It can be caused by poor nutrition or medications such as tetrahydrofolate analogs (e.g., methotrexate) and dihydrofolate reductase inhibitors (e.g., trimethoprim). Folate is normally metabolized to tetrahydrofolate (THF), a coenzyme in single carbon transfer and methylation reactions in the metabolism of nucleic or amino acids. Serum folate can decline within three weeks of decreased folate intake due to a small reserve pool in the liver. Folate deficiency results in macrocytic, megaloblastic anemia due to the diminished synthesis of purines and TMP, which inhibits the cell from making adequate amounts of DNA. Folate deficiency and vitamin B12 deficiency both cause megaloblastic anemias. However, there are several key differences between them: (1) Vitamin B12 deficiency can lead to neurologic symptoms, but folate deficiency has no neurologic symptoms; (2) vitamin B12 deficiency leads to elevated homocysteine and methylmalonic acid, whereas folate deficiency has elevated homocysteine and normal methylmalonic acid levels; and (3) vitamin B12 deficiency takes years to develop, but folate deficiencies can develop in weeks. If B12 deficiency is misdiagnosed as folate deficiency and a patient is started on folic acid, the hematologic symptoms may resolve but the neurologic symptoms will not resolve and may worsen.

CASE 26 | Vitamin B6 (Pyridoxine) Deficiency

A 43-year-old woman presents with burning pain in her legs over the past three months. She has been on treatment for latent tuberculosis with isoniazid for the last four months. On physical exam, she is irritable and has fissuring at the angles of her mouth and beefy red bald/smooth tongue. There is diminished peripheral pinprick sensation and loss of monofilament sensation in both feet.

Evaluation/Tests	Serum and urine B6 levels were low, CBC shows microcytic anemia, and a peripheral blood smear shows microcytic hypochromic red blood cells with sideroblasts.
Treatment	Pyridoxine supplementation.
Discussion	This patient is presenting with a pyridoxine (vitamin B6) deficiency. Pyridoxine is converted to pyridoxal phosphate, which is a cofactor used in transamination (synthesis of ALT and AST), decarboxylation, and glycogenolysis. It is involved in the synthesis of neurotransmitters, heme, niacin, and histamine. Common manifestations of pyridoxine deficiency include irritability, peripheral neuropathy, seizures, and sideroblastic anemia due to impaired heme synthesis and iron excess. Isoniazid, used in the treatment of tuberculosis, can induce vitamin B6 deficiency by forming an inactive derivative of pyridoxal phosphate. Deficiency is commonly seen in this setting, as well as in infants fed formulas low in B6 and in patients with alcoholism.

CASE 27 | Fabry Disease

A 20-year-old man presents with burning pain in his hands and feet, abdominal pain with alteration in bowel movements, and clusters of small red spots on his skin. He reports feeling excessively hot with dry skin and says he never sweats. His family history is significant for a maternal uncle who died at age 55 from progressive kidney damage and heart failure. On exam, he is short, has hearing loss, and has a heaving apical impulse and systolic ejection murmur over the left sternal border. Clusters of erythematous red-purple papules with a slightly keratotic surface are seen in the groin, and absence of sweat in the axilla is noted. Ophthalmic exam is notable for corneal opacities (pale gray, brownish, or yellowish streaks in the cornea of the eye).

Evaluation/Tests	Labs show low levels of α-galactosidase A enzyme, and elevated levels of ceramide trihexoside (globotriaosylceramide). Echocardiogram shows left ventricular hypertrophy.
Treatment	Enzyme replacement therapy.
Discussion	Fabry disease is a lysosomal storage disorder caused by an X-linked recessive mutation of gene encoding α-galactosidase A. Deficiency or inactivity of this enzyme leads to an accumulation of glycolipids, such as ceramide trihexoside, in lysosomes throughout the body, especially in blood vessels, the eyes, heart, kidney, and peripheral nerves. Symptoms usually appear early in life but may present in adulthood. Symptoms are exacerbated by exercise, stress, or fatigue. Patients may present with burning pain in extremities (acroparesthesias), decreased sweating (hypohidrosis), and small, dark red, nonblanching skin lesions (angiokeratomas). Major organ complications occur in the second to third decade, including kidney failure, heart irregularities, and/or progressive neurological abnormalities.

CASE 28 | Zellweger Syndrome

A newborn baby girl is evaluated for several abnormalities including hypotonia, dysmorphic features, difficulty breathing, and seizures. The pregnancy and birth were uncomplicated. On physical exam, the baby is noted to have a flattened face, high forehead, large fontanelles, hypotelorism, corneal clouding, and nystagmus. There is a broad nasal bridge with a small nose and upturned nostrils. The palate has a high arch, and she has extra folds of skin in the neck.

Evaluation/Tests	Blood testing reveals elevation of very-long-chain fatty acids (VLCFAs). Genetic testing reveals a mutation in the peroxisome biogenesis factor 1 (*PEX1*) gene.
Treatment	Poor prognosis; supportive management along with genetic counseling.
Discussion	Zellweger syndrome is caused by an autosomal recessive mutation in the *PEX1* gene involved in the biogenesis of peroxisomes. Peroxisomes play important roles in beta-oxidation of very-long-chain fatty acids (VCLFAs), catabolism of branched-chain fatty acids, and synthesis of cholesterol, bile acids, and plasmalogens—the latter of which are important membrane phospholipids, especially in white matter of the nervous system. Nervous system symptoms are common and include hypotonia, hearing loss, vision problems, and seizures. Other features include hepatosplenomegaly, respiratory failure, and progressive liver and kidney dysfunction. Testing for peroxisomal disorders can be done by chorionic villus sampling or amniocentesis in the first or second trimester.
Additional Considerations	**Refsum disease** is another disorder of peroxisomal biogenesis; however, it involves an autosomal recessive defect in the alpha-oxidation of phytanic acid, a branched-chain fatty acid typically obtained from dairy, beef, and certain types of fish. Refsum disease presents with retinitis, peripheral neuropathy, gait ataxia, scaly skin, cataracts/night blindness, and skeletal abnormalities. **Adrenoleukodystrophy** is an X-linked recessive disorder of beta-oxidation whereby very-long-chain fatty acids (VLCFAs) accumulate in the adrenal glands, white matter of the brain, and testes, which can result in adrenal crisis, coma, and death. The most common presentation is that of a degenerative neurologic disorder that begins in childhood or adolescence; progresses to severe dementia with loss of vision, hearing, speech, and gait; and results in death within a few years. ALD is characterized by high ratios of C26 to C22 VLCFA in plasma and tissues. Genetic testing (*ABCD1* gene mutation) confirms the diagnosis.

HEMATOLOGIC ABNORMALITIES

Various vitamin deficiencies and metabolic defects can give rise to hematologic abnormalities. Broadly, these abnormalities can be divided into bleeding/coagulopathies or anemias. Bleeding can occur due to conditions that lower the platelet count

(Gaucher disease), the inability of blood to clot (vitamin K deficiency), or unstable collagen (vitamin C). Biochemical disorders resulting in anemia may include:

1. Deficiency of enzymes like G6PD and delta-aminolevulinic acid synthetase;
2. Deficiency of coenzymes like vitamin B12, folate;
3. Defective proteins like in hereditary spherocytosis.

Some of these defects can result in changes in red blood cell shape and subsequent hemolysis. While a few select biochemistry-relevant cases are presented in this chapter, the remainder of anemias and coagulopathies will be discussed in the "Hematology and Oncology" chapter.

CASE 29	Vitamin C Deficiency (Scurvy)
	A 53-year-old man presents for evaluation of a new rash over his legs that has progressively worsened over the last year. He also notes fatigue, pain in his knees, and bleeding every time he brushes his teeth. His wife died a year and a half ago, and since then his diet consists primarily of microwaved rice and beans. On exam, he has friable and swollen gingiva with loss of teeth, corkscrew hair, ecchymosis, and nonblanching erythematous perifollicular petechiae over his lower extremities.
Evaluation/Tests	CBC with peripheral smear is normal; prothrombin time (PT) and partial thromboplastin time (PTT) are normal; labs are notable for low serum vitamin C levels.
Treatment	Oral vitamin C supplementation.
Discussion	Scurvy is caused by a deficiency of vitamin C (ascorbic acid). Vitamin C has many functions: It is an antioxidant and cofactor needed for hydroxylation of proline to lysine in collagen synthesis; it helps absorb iron by reducing it to the Fe^{2+} state; and it is a cofactor for dopamine beta-hydroxylase, which converts dopamine to norepinephrine. Vitamin C deficiency typically develops within 8–12 weeks of inadequate intake of fresh fruits and vegetables. Vitamin C deficiency affects blood vessels, skin, and basement membranes separating the epidermis and dermis. Patients can have poor wound healing, gum swelling, loss of teeth, corkscrew hair, petechiae and ecchymosis, and hemarthrosis. Petechial hemorrhages are common in lower extremities due to capillary fragility and gravity-dependent hydrostatic pressure. Brittle bones occur due to disruption of endochondral bone formation. Ocular manifestations can include hemorrhages, papilledema, and optic atrophy.

CASE 30	Vitamin K Deficiency
	A 3-week-old baby boy is brought to clinic for evaluation of increased sleepiness, difficulty breast-feeding, irritability, and emesis. The patient had a normal delivery; however, his parents refused vitamin K injection due to their religious beliefs. He did not have any complications with circumcision on the tenth day of his life. There is no family history of unusual illnesses or sick contacts. Physical exam reveals an irritable baby with increased heart and respiratory rate, ecchymosis over the thighs, sluggish pupils, and full fontanelles.
Evaluation/Tests	Labs show a normal CBC; coagulation studies reveal prolonged PT and aPTT, normal bleeding time, normal von Willebrand factor (vWF), and fibrinogen degradation products; CT head revealed a small intracranial bleed.
Treatment	Vitamin K injection.
Discussion	This patient is presenting with vitamin K deficiency. Vitamin K is a fat-soluble vitamin needed for the synthesis and maturation of blood clotting factors II, VII, IX, and X, and proteins C and S. It is activated by epoxide reductase to the reduced form and acts as a cofactor for gamma-carboxylation of glutamic acid residues on proteins involved in the coagulation cascade. It is present in green leafy vegetables and can also be produced by intestinal flora. Vitamin K deficiency occurs relatively quickly in the newborn because of the short half-life, limited stores of vitamin K (not in breast milk), and immature GI tracts. Neonates are given an intramuscular vitamin K injection at birth to prevent bleeding and potentially fatal intracranial hemorrhage. Vitamin K deficiency can also occur because of prolonged use of broad-spectrum antibiotics, destroying gut microorganisms. Warfarin inhibits vitamin K–dependent synthesis of clotting proteins. Correction of coagulopathy and supplementation of vitamin K are the treatment. Patients with DIC or sepsis typically will have other signs or symptoms consistent with infection, such as fever or elevated WBC count. The first step in treating prolonged PT and aPTT is to give vitamin K to make sure prolonged times are not due to nutritional deficiencies. If PT and aPTT are not corrected with vitamin K, then it is important to search for other causes of abnormal coagulation studies.

CASE 31	Pyruvate Kinase Deficiency
\	A 16-year-old boy presents with fatigue and yellow color of the skin and sclera. His mother states he had insufficient weight gain as a child. Physical exam is notable for yellowing of the white of the eyes (scleral icterus), jaundice, and splenomegaly.
Evaluation/Tests	CBC shows low hemoglobin, normal MCV, and reticulocytosis. Peripheral blood smear reveals spiculated red blood cells (echinocytes or "burr cells"). Labs are notable for increased levels of unconjugated bilirubin and a negative Coombs test.
Treatment	People with severe anemia may need blood transfusions.
Discussion	Pyruvate kinase deficiency is an autosomal recessive disorder resulting from a defect in pyruvate kinase. Pyruvate kinase is one of several key enzymes in glycolysis as it catalyzes the last step by converting phosphoenolpyruvate (PEP) to pyruvate. RBCs rely almost exclusively on glycolysis for ATP production due to lack of mitochondria, so they are the most significantly affected by this deficiency. Decreased ATP from this deficiency, therefore, has a significant effect on RBCs. Normally, Na^+/K^+ ATP pumps help RBCs maintain their unique shape by regulating water content inside the cell. With decreased ATP, this pump cannot function, and thus the RBC becomes rigid and abnormally shaped, resulting in spicule formation and extravascular hemolysis. While RBCs are most heavily affected, pyruvate kinase is also used by all cells throughout the body. Without efficient glycolysis, cells will rely on fatty acid oxidation, producing ketones and upregulating gluconeogenesis. Acute infections or stressors may therefore increase these processes, resulting in hemolysis.

DERMATITIS OR RASH

Dermatologic abnormalities are common in vitamin deficiencies and specific genetic abnormalities affecting DNA repair pathways. Vitamin deficiencies may present with rash or dermatitis, but typically are associated with additional systemic features. Dermatitis may be limited to a specific location (e.g., the angle of the mouth) or may be more widespread. Mutations in DNA repair pathways limit the ability of cells to repair spontaneously or induce mutations. Given the exposure of skin to the environment, it is particularly susceptible to accumulation of mutations such as from UV radiation in sunlight.

CASE 32	Vitamin A (Retinol) Deficiency
\	A 32-year-old man presents with a progressive rash over his face, arms, and legs and difficulty seeing at night. He underwent a Roux-en-Y gastric bypass surgery, a type of weight-loss surgery that involves creating a small pouch from the stomach and connecting the newly created pouch directly to the small intestine, several months ago. He has dry eyes, a triangular spot on the bulbar conjunctiva, and dry skin with hyperkeratotic papules over face, shoulders, buttocks, and extremities.
Evaluation/Tests	Vitamin A levels are decreased.
Treatment	Treat with vitamin A as retinol or retinyl esters supplementation.
Discussion	Vitamin A is an essential part of vision pigments and is needed for the growth, maintenance, and differentiation of epithelial cells. Retinoic acid binds to receptor proteins and regulates retinoid-specific RNA synthesis. This controls the expression of the gene for keratin and rhodopsin, the visual pigments in rods and cones. Deficiency can occur in the setting of fat malabsorption (e.g., following gastric bypass as seen in this case), alcoholism, or protein-energy malnutrition. Night blindness is one of the earliest symptoms of vitamin A deficiency, which can progress and be irreversible. Xerophthalmia, inability to produce tears, and white foamy spots on conjunctiva due to sloughing (bitot spots) are characteristic features; if untreated, they can lead to corneal ulceration and blindness. The skin manifestation, called phrynoderma, is characterized by dry, hyperkeratotic papules symmetrically distributed over the face, extensor surface of shoulders, and extremities. Additionally, retinol and retinal are needed for spermatogenesis in men, so deficiency in vitamin A can result in fertility problems. Acute toxicity due to excess vitamin A causes nausea vomiting and blurred vision. Chronic toxicity can result in alopecia, dry skin, liver toxicity, and pseudotumor cerebri. Oral isotretinoin, commonly used to treat acne, requires two forms of contraception because it is teratogenic and can cause cleft palate and cardiac abnormalities. *All-trans* retinoic acid (ATRA) is used to treat acute promyelocytic leukemia (APL) because it forces APL cells to differentiate and lose proliferation capacity.

CASE 33 | Xeroderma Pigmentosum (XP)

A 14-year-old girl is referred to a dermatologist for evaluation of recurrent blistering sunburns since childhood. The sunburns occur even when she has only been outside for a few minutes. She also has increased light sensitivity and itching of her eyes. Physical exam reveals dry, parchment-like skin, skin atrophy, and telangiectasias with several freckles in the sun-exposed areas. There is inflammation of the conjunctiva with some clouding of the cornea.

Evaluation/Tests	Molecular testing for mutations in the xeroderma pigmentosum genes involved in nucleotide excision repair was positive.
Treatment	Treat complications.
Discussion	Xeroderma pigmentosum (XP) is a genetically heterogeneous disorder caused by mutations in various genes involved in DNA nucleotide excision repair. This type of DNA repair is important in repairing DNA pyrimidine dimer mutations, which form upon exposure to ultraviolet (UV) light. XP is characterized by increased sensitivity to the damaging effects of UV light and typically affects the skin, eyes, and nervous system. Blistering burns on sun-exposed skin after minimal exposure is characteristic. Characteristic long-term features include dry parchment-like skin, a mixture of increased and decreased skin pigmentation (poikiloderma), skin thinning, and telangiectasias. Actinic keratosis and skin cancer are common complications. Eye involvement consists of increased light sensitivity, dry eye, inflammation of the cornea, resulting in opacification and vascularization that leads to blindness. Some patients may display neurologic symptoms. Cancers occur at a higher rate, including those of the skin, oral cavity, glioblastoma, and astrocytomas. Prevention and rigorous UV protection is critical. **Porphyria cutanea tarda** and albinism may also present with photosensitivity. Porphyria cutanea tarda typically manifests in adulthood, is associated with hepatitis C, is exacerbated by alcohol consumption or other oxidative stressors, and commonly involves hyperpigmentation of the skin. **Albinism** can be distinguished from XP by the lack of any pigmentation (hypopigmentation) due to decreased production of melanin.

RESPIRATORY DISTRESS

Several genetic defects can impair normal function of the respiratory tract in the clearance of mucous and potential pathogens. Important in this role is the mucociliary elevator maintained by the ciliated pseudostratified columnar epithelia and mucous-secreting Goblet cells lining the respiratory tract. Formation and excretion of mucous are a tightly regulated process involving the exchange of ions and fluids across the respiratory epithelia. Inherited mutations that disrupt the normal function of any of these important cells can lead to recurrent respiratory or sinus infections and respiratory distress.

CASE 34 | Kartagener Syndrome/Primary Ciliary Dyskinesia

A 22-year-old man presents for evaluation of infertility. On review of systems, he mentions that he has had recurrent sinus infections and productive cough with thick sputum all his life. He also notes thick nasal discharge and a decreased sense of smell. On physical exam, his nasal mucosa is not visible due to thick nasal secretions, and bilateral sinus tenderness is present. The apical impulse is on the right fifth intercostal space, and hepatic dullness is percussed on the left side.

Evaluation/Tests	Chest X-ray shows dextrocardia and a gastric fundus on the right with elevated left hemidiaphragm. CT sinuses shows mucosal thickening. Biopsy of sinus cavities or airway shows ciliary abnormalities. Semen analysis shows immotile spermatozoa.
Treatment	Airway clearance therapy to help loosen thick mucus. Antibiotics to treat respiratory, sinus, or ear infections.
Discussion	Kartagener syndrome is a form of primary ciliary dyskinesia that is caused by autosomal recessive mutations that affect the proteins involved in the dynein arm of cilia. Defects in ciliary movement lead to frequent middle ear, sinus, and lung infections, conductive hearing loss and infertility. In women, there is an increased risk of ectopic pregnancy. Headache, anosmia, and corneal abnormalities can also occur. It is also characterized by situs inversus (mirror image reversal of internal organs including dextrocardia).

CASE 35 | Cystic Fibrosis

An 8-month-old male infant who recently migrated from a remote fishing town in Iceland presents with a cough productive of dark brown, thick sputum. His past medical history is significant for pneumonia 1 month ago and an admission to a hospital days after birth because he was unable to have a bowel movement. On exam, the patient is fussy, underweight, and grunting and tachypneic. His temperature is 38.5°C, respirations are 40/min, pulse is 120/min, and pulse oximetry on room air shows an oxygen saturation of 89%. He has decreased breath sounds, crackles, and dullness to percussion in the left lower lung field.

CASE 35 | Cystic Fibrosis (continued)

DDx	Cystic fibrosis, pneumonia, primary immunodeficiency, respiratory syncytial virus, asthma, bronchiolitis.
Evaluation/Tests	Chest X-ray shows consolidation in the left lower lung field. Sweat chloride testing reveals an elevated chloride concentration of 115 mmol/L. Fecal elastase is low. Nasal transepithelial potential difference is elevated. Genetic testing confirms a Phe508 deletion in the *CFTR* gene on chromosome 7.
Treatment	Treat pneumonia with antibiotics and start chest physiotherapy.
Discussion	This patient has cystic fibrosis (CF), an autosomal recessive disorder involving a defect in the cystic fibrosis transmembrane conductance regulator (*CFTR*) gene on chromosome 7. One of the more common mutations is a deletion of the amino acid, phenylalanine, at codon 508. *CFTR* encodes an ATP-gated chloride channel involved in the secretion of chloride in the lungs and GI tract and the reabsorption of chloride in sweat glands. The abnormal chloride regulation also leads to abnormal water regulation, which can lead to thick secretions. In the lungs, patients can have abnormally thick mucus. Clearance is disrupted and increases risk of recurrent infection. In the GI tract, thickened secretions can lead to pancreatic insufficiency (steatorrhea, fat-soluble vitamin deficiencies). Additional complications include biliary cirrhosis, liver disease, infertility, nasal polyps, digital clubbing, and meconium ileus in newborns. Screening involves searching for mutations in the *CFTR* gene. The diagnostic test of choice is the chloride sweat test, which will reveal an elevated chloride concentration in the sweat. Confirmation is typically done with genetic testing. Recent advances in CF therapy include lumacaftor, which helps correct misfolding of the CFTR protein, and ivacaftor, which helps promote opening of chloride channels. However, these are only effective in CF patients with homozygous Phe508 mutation. Otherwise, treatment is mostly supportive and aimed at limiting or preventing complications. A history of unexplained, recurrent infections in a child should also raise suspicion for **primary immunodeficiencies** (e.g., severe combined immunodeficiency syndrome). Unlike CF, the pathology in primary immunodeficiencies can often be explained by specific infections (e.g., sinus or GI infections) and will show decreased white blood cell count on CBC.

DYSLIPIDEMIAS

Dyslipidemias are a class of diseases related to the transport and uptake of lipids throughout the body. Acquired lipid disorders are very common in adulthood and result mainly from lifestyle habits such as poor diet, lack of exercise, and excessive alcohol intake. Here, we will focus on inherited dyslipidemias, which involve genetic defects in key enzymes or proteins involved in the transport and uptake of dietary and endogenous lipids. Typical features of inherited dyslipidemias include:

1. Severe hypercholesterolemia and/or hypertriglyceridemia, often appearing at a younger age than typically expected;
2. Family history of dyslipidemias;
3. Dermatologic manifestations related to lipid deposits in the skin or tendons (as well as the eye);
4. Increased risk of premature coronary heart disease, peripheral arterial disease, and stroke due to accelerated atherosclerosis;
5. GI manifestations including pancreatitis (related to severe hypertriglyceridemia) and hepatic steatosis.

The dyslipidemia disorders may look very similar to one another. Pay close attention to the pathogenesis and specific clinical presentations to help differentiate among them.

CASE 36 | Familial Hyperchylomicronemia (Hyperlipidemia Type I)

A 30-year-old woman was admitted to the ICU a week ago for severe pancreatitis. Her labs showed significant hypertriglyceridemia. Plasmapheresis was performed to rapidly reduce triglyceride (TG) and chylomicron levels in her blood, and her symptoms resolved. On further investigation, numerous family members also suffer from recurrent pancreatitis, but not myocardial infarctions. On physical exam, the patient has eruptive xanthomas on her back (lipid deposits in the skin and subcutaneous tissue) and milky appearance of retinal veins and arteries (lipemia retinalis).	
Evaluation/Tests	Triglycerides and chylomicrons are elevated. When blood is drawn, it has a creamy layer in the vial.
Treatment	Lifestyle modification, cholesterol-lowering drugs including fibrates and/or statin.

CASE 36 | Familial Hyperchylomicronemia (Hyperlipidemia Type I) *(continued)*

Discussion	Familial hyperchylomicronemia is a type of familial dyslipidemia caused by an autosomal recessive defect in lipoprotein lipase (LPL) or apolipoprotein C-II (Apo CII), which results in reduced clearance of chylomicrons from the plasma. LPL is found on the surface of vascular endothelial cells and degrades TGs in circulating chylomicrons to release free fatty acids. The free fatty acids are then taken up by adipocytes for storage. Apo CII is a cofactor for LPL that helps catalyze this cleavage. A defect in either of these causes triglycerides and chylomicrons to accumulate in the plasma. Patients have eruptive xanthomas (lipid deposits in the skin and subcutaneous tissue), severely elevated triglycerides, hepatosplenomegaly, lipemia retinalis, and they may develop abdominal pain due to acute pancreatitis. Total cholesterol levels may also be elevated. **Familial hypertriglyceridemia** (hyperlipidemia type IV) is caused by an autosomal dominant defect in apolipoprotein A V (Apo AV), which results in hepatic overproduction of very-low-density lipoproteins (VLDLs). VLDLs are secreted by the liver and deliver hepatic TGs to peripheral tissues. Compared to other lipoproteins such as LDL and HDL, VLDLs contain the highest amount of TGs. In familial hypertriglyceridemia, elevation in VLDLs causes a severe hypertriglyceridemia and chylomicron levels are normal. This condition can also cause acute pancreatitis and is often related to insulin resistance so is seen more often in diabetics and obese patients.

CASE 37 | Familial Hypercholesterolemia (Hyperlipidemia Type IIa)

An 18-year-old man presents for a yearly physical exam, but he is very concerned about his strong family history of early heart attacks and high levels of "bad" cholesterol. Physical exam is significant for yellowish deposits on his Achilles tendon and a light-colored ring around the edge of the cornea.

Evaluation/Tests	A lipid panel shows high levels of total cholesterol and LDL but normal triglyceride levels.
Treatment	Statins.
Discussion	Familial hypercholesterolemia is caused by an autosomal dominant defect in LDL receptors or in Apo B-100. Apo B-100 is an apolipoprotein found in lipoproteins originating from the liver and helps bind to LDL receptors found on peripheral cells. The LDL receptor on peripheral cells allows for peripheral cholesterol uptake. Most patients with hyperlipidemia are asymptomatic and are often diagnosed after a routine lipid profile; however, there is commonly accelerated atherosclerosis with premature coronary artery and peripheral vascular disease. Patients also typically have tendon xanthomas (especially in the Achilles tendon), corneal arcus, and xanthelasmas on the eyelids. There are two types of familial hypercholesterolemia: IIa involves elevated LDL and cholesterol, while IIb also has elevated VLDLs. **Familial dysbetalipoproteinemia** (hyperlipidemia type III) involves an autosomal recessive defect in apolipoprotein E (ApoE). ApoE helps mediate the uptake of remnants of chylomicrons, VLDL, IDL, and HDL back into the liver. A defect in ApoE results in accumulation of these remnants, especially chylomicrons and VLDLs, in the serum. Clinical features include premature atherosclerosis leading to coronary artery and peripheral vascular disease; palmar xanthomas, which are yellowish plaques or nodules that deposit on the palm and elsewhere; and tuberoeruptive xanthomas. Symptoms are generally more severe when there is a secondary genetic or environmental factor that causes an increase in lipids such as obesity, hypothyroidism, and diabetes. Lipid panel shows elevated chylomicron and VLDL remnants. Treat with fibrates and/or statins.

2

Immunology

Mahesh C. Patel, MD

PRIMARY IMMUNODEFICIENCIES

Primary immunodeficiency diseases are a group of disorders that most commonly result from inherited defects that impair the immune system. Although over 300 of these disorders have been described, most are rarely encountered by the practicing clinician. They appear fairly commonly on board exams, however, because they are relatively distinctive diseases in which the pathophysiology is relatively well understood. The vast majority of these immunodeficiencies present in the first year of life or early childhood, but a few milder ones are diagnosed in later childhood or adulthood. The typical presentation is that of recurrent and/or chronic infections, sometimes with opportunistic organisms. These disorders can be most easily classified by the main component of the immune system that is absent, deficient, or defective, which can broadly be categorized into primary problems of the innate or adaptive immune system. Problems with the innate immune system include neutrophil/phagocyte and complement protein deficiencies. Problems with the adaptive immune system include B-cell, T-cell, or mixed-cell deficiencies.

Primary Immunodeficiency Disorders Grouped by Component Deficiency/Absence

Phagocyte/Neutrophil	Complement	B-Cell	T-Cell	B- and T-Cell
- Leukocyte adhesion deficiency (type 1) - Chronic granulomatous disease (CGD) - Chédiak-Higashi syndrome	- C1 esterase inhibitor deficiency - Terminal complement deficiency (C5–C9 deficiency)	- IgA deficiency - X-linked (Bruton) agammaglobulinemia - Common variable immunodeficiency (CVID)	- Thymic aplasia (DiGeorge syndrome) - Autosomal dominant hyper-IgE syndrome (Job syndrome) - IL-12 receptor deficiency - Chronic mucocutaneous candidiasis	- Severe combined immunodeficiency (SCID) - Wiskott-Aldrich syndrome - Ataxia-telangiectasia - Hyper-IgM syndrome

In addition to problems with chronic and opportunistic infections, patients with immunodeficiency may present with failure to thrive, chronic diarrhea, mucosal abnormalities, lymphadenopathy, and skin abnormalities.

Understanding the functions of phagocytes and complement, B-cells, and T-cells is important prior to learning about these immunodeficiencies.

Several immune cells have the ability to phagocytose pathogens and cellular debris. These include neutrophils, macrophages, and dendritic cells. Neutrophils, in particular, often serve as the "first responders" to infection, tissue damage, or inflammation. Deficiencies in phagocytic cells such as neutrophils constitute approximately 10% of primary immunodeficiencies. Phagocytic cell deficiencies typically arise early in a child's life and are characterized by a wide range of infections (from mild skin infections to sepsis) due to fungi, parasites, and bacteria. In particular, children with these deficiencies are prone to infections with *Staphylococcus* spp., *Serratia*, *Nocardia*, *Pseudomonas aeruginosa*, *Burkholderia cepacia*, *Candida* spp., *Aspergillus*, and *Mucor*. They are not at increased risk from viral infections as viruses exist largely within intact host cells and therefore are not as easily recognized by phagocyte pattern recognition receptors.

In addition to cellular components of the innate immune system, several secreted proteins are instrumental in coordinating the immune response. Examples of secreted proteins include chemokines, cytokines, and complement proteins. Deficiencies in complement proteins are observed to constitute approximately 5% of primary immunodeficiencies. Complement deficiencies are typically diagnosed after a patient has recurrent, severe infections with encapsulated bacteria such as *N. meningitidis*, *H. influenzae*, and *S. pneumoniae*. Complement proteins play an important role in the binding to and subsequent opsonization of pathogens, particularly encapsulated bacteria.

The two major cell types of the adaptive immune system include B- and T-lymphocytes. B-cell defects make up approximately 65% of all primary immunodeficiencies and therefore represent the most common form of primary immunodeficiency. B-cell defects often do not present in the first 6 months of life as maternal antibodies are still present. The most common of the B-cell defects is immunoglobulin A (IgA) deficiency. Pure B-cell defects lead to recurrent and severe sinopulmonary infections and otitis media with encapsulated organisms such as *S. pneumoniae* and *H. influenzae*. Patients are often infected with **extracellular** bacteria. B-cell deficient patients are also more prone to infection with enteroviruses and giardiasis and may present with chronic diarrhea and malabsorption.

T-cell defects make up approximately 5% of the primary immunodeficiencies. Most patients are affected in the first 6 months of life. Various viruses, protozoa, fungi, mycobacteria, and **intracellular** bacteria infect patients with T-cell defects. In particular, T-cell deficient patients are more prone to fungal and viral infections as T-lymphocytes play a large role in the detection of infected host cells. Similar to patients with AIDS, these patients are predisposed to opportunistic infections such as *Pneumocystis jiroveci*, *Cryptococcus*, cytomegalovirus (CMV), JC virus, *Mycobacterium* spp., and *Candida* spp. They are also prone to chronic infection with respiratory and GI viruses.

Combined B- and T-cell defects have features of both of the preceding defects and make up approximately 15% of all primary immunodeficiencies.

Key Findings and Primary Immunodeficiency Differential Diagnosis

Primary Immunodeficiencies with Key Associated Findings	Diagnoses
Boy (X-linked)	Bruton agammaglobulinemia, SCID (commonly), hyper-IgM, Wiskott-Aldrich, CGD
Absent B-cells in peripheral blood; _BTK_ (a tyrosine kinase gene) defect	Bruton agammaglobulinemia
Severe pyogenic infections early in life; additionally, patient develops opportunistic infections with organisms such as _Pneumocystis_ and CMV. Normal or increased IgM with low IgG, IgA, and IgE; no germinal centers; defective _CD40L_ on Th-cells	Hyper-IgM syndrome
Infections with catalase positive organisms (e.g., _Staph aureus_, _Nocardia_, _Aspergillus_, etc.) Abnormal dihydrorhodamine test; negative nitroblue tetrazolium dye reduction test	CGD
Triad of thrombocytopenia, eczema, and recurrent pyogenic infections	Wiskott-Aldrich syndrome
"Global" immunodeficiency (recurrent viral, bacterial, fungal, and protozoal infections) Defective IL-2 receptor	SCID
Sinopulmonary infections, lymphoma in a patient >2 years old Decreased plasma cells and subsequent decreased immunoglobulins; **normal B-cell number**	CVID
Asymptomatic _or_ autoimmune, atopy, anaphylaxis to IgA-containing products Giardia infection	IgA deficiency
Tetany due to hypocalcemia, recurrent viral or fungal infections Absent thymus and parathyroids; congenital heart and great vessel defects Decreased PTH, calcium, T-cells; no thymic shadow on CXR	Thymic aplasia (DiGeorge)
Disseminated mycobacterial infections Poor interferon-γ function	IL-12 receptor deficiency
FATED: coarse **F**acies, cold **A**bscesses, retained primary **T**eeth, increased Ig**E**, and **D**ermatologic problems (e.g., eczema)	Hyper-IgE syndrome (Job syndrome)
Noninvasive _Candida_ infections of the skin and mucous membranes	Chronic mucocutaneous Candidiasis
Difficulty with balance and walking, delayed onset of walking, cutaneous telangiectasias, recurrent infections particularly sinopulmonary infections, malignancy at a young age Cerebellar ataxia, ocular and cutaneous telangiectasias, growth retardation, immune deficiency, radiation sensitivity, increased rates of malignancy	Ataxia-telangiectasia
Recurrent skin infections _without_ pus; impaired wound healing; **delayed umbilical cord separation**	Leukocyte adhesion deficiency (type 1)
Albinism, peripheral neuropathy, recurrent pyogenic infections with _Staph_ and _Strep_ Giant granules in granulocytes and platelets	Chédiak-Higashi syndrome
Hereditary angioedema	C1 esterase inhibitor deficiency
Increased IgE levels; increased eosinophils	Hyper-IgE syndrome (Job syndrome)
C5–C9 deficiency	Recurrent _Neisseria_ infections

CASE 1 | X-linked (Bruton) Agammaglobulinemia

A 2-year-old boy is brought to clinic for evaluation of fever and right ear pain over the past 2 days. Review of his medical records reveals frequent visits for otitis media and several episodes of pneumococcal pneumonia over the last 18 months. In addition, his maternal uncle had many infections as a child, one of which ultimately led to his death. The patient's temperature is 39.2°C, pulse is 138/min, respirations are 26/min, and blood pressure is 100/52 mmHg. Bulging of the right tympanic membrane with obscured landmarks is present. Examination of the oropharynx reveals very small tonsils. No skin lesions are noted.

Evaluation/Tests	Clinical diagnosis. Labs reveal low immunoglobulin levels. A mutation is seen in the Bruton tyrosine kinase (*BTK*) gene. Absence of B-cells in peripheral blood.
Treatment	Treat with immune globulin replacement therapy at regular intervals.
Discussion	This patient with recurrent sinopulmonary infections most likely has a B-cell defect. His exam shows lymphoid hypoplasia (e.g., small tonsils, absent lymph nodes), a common finding in X-linked agammaglobulinemia. These patients lack germinal centers in their lymph nodes and do not have B-cells in their peripheral blood. Defects in the *BTK* gene lead to failure of B-cell development. Inheritance is X-linked recessive. Immunoglobulins of all classes are decreased. Patients are prone to recurrent bacterial, enteroviral, and giardia infections, which start after 6 months of age when maternal immunoglobulins have decreased. These patients should not receive live vaccines. **Common variable immunodeficiency (CVID)** involves a defect in B-cell maturation and differentiation. Patients with CVID subsequently have decreased plasma cells and decreased immunoglobulins of all classes. CVID presents *after* patients are 2 years old, which is later than X-linked agammaglobulinemia. CVID may not be diagnosed until after puberty, and patients are at increased risk for autoimmune disease, lymphoma, sinopulmonary infections, and bronchiectasis. In this case, the patient has already demonstrated recurrent infections before age 2 with a pattern of inheritance that suggests an X-linked condition, which makes X-linked agammaglobulinemia more likely.

CASE 2 | Thymic Aplasia (DiGeorge Syndrome)

A newborn girl is observed by a nurse to have a seizure. The girl's mother reports poor feeding and a "bluish" appearance to the skin, especially when the child becomes agitated. The patient's temperature is 37.3°C, pulse is 160/min, respirations are 42/min, and blood pressure is 90/52 mmHg. She appears sleepy and has mild cyanosis of the lips, and a harsh systolic murmur is heard at the left upper sternal border.

Evaluation/Tests	T-cells, parathyroid hormone, and serum calcium levels are decreased. Phosphorus is high. Thymic shadow is absent on chest X-ray. Genetic testing reveals a 22q11 deletion.
Treatment	Treat infections and calcium and vitamin D deficiency. Surgical correction of cardiac defects and possible thymic or hematopoietic cell transplantation.
Discussion	DiGeorge syndrome is the most likely diagnosis in this newborn with seizure due to hypocalcemia (secondary to absent parathyroids), episodes of cyanosis, a harsh murmur (likely due to tetralogy of Fallot), and no thymic shadow on CXR. DiGeorge syndrome results from failure of development of the third and fourth pharyngeal pouches, which leads to absent thymus and parathyroid glands. Patients with DiGeorge syndrome can present with seizures or tetany due to hypocalcemia, conotruncal abnormalities of the heart, and recurrent viral and fungal infections due to T-cell deficiency. DiGeorge syndrome is caused by a chromosomal deletion at 22q11.2. Other features include abnormal facies (small chin, overfolded ear helices) and cleft palate. **Severe combined immunodeficiency (SCID)** often presents in early infancy as this is a combined immunodeficiency with involvement of all lymphocytes (T- and B-cells). SCID can be X-linked due to a defective IL-2R gamma chain or autosomal recessive due to an adenosine deaminase deficiency. Patients may present with failure to thrive, chronic diarrhea, thrush, and recurrent infections from viruses, bacteria, fungi, and protozoa. Findings include the absence of a thymic shadow on chest X-ray, lack of germinal centers on lymph node biopsy, and absent T-cells and decreased T-cell receptor excision circles (TRECs). While SCID also presents with an absent thymic shadow and recurrent infections, the conotruncal anomalies and deficient calcium and PTH present in this vignette suggest DiGeorge syndrome. DiGeorge patients will predominantly become infected with viruses and fungi, so a pattern of infections that includes bacteria and protozoa would be more indicative of SCID rather than DiGeorge.

CASE 3 | Chronic Granulomatous Disease

A 5-year-old boy is brought to his primary care doctor for evaluation of multiple abscesses on his buttocks. On review of the medical records, it's noted that the child has had previous infections with *Aspergillus* and *Nocardia* and was treated for a *S. aureus* lung abscess last year. Patient's temperature is 38.6°C, pulse is 138/min, respirations are 26/min, and blood pressure is 92/54 mmHg. He has a 5-cm-round, painful, fluctuant bump on his right buttocks that is draining purulent material. The abscess drainage is positive for gram positive cocci in clusters.

Evaluation/Tests	The dihydrorhodamine test demonstrates decreased green fluorescence. Nitroblue tetrazolium dye reduction test does not turn blue.
Treatment	Treat acute infections.
Discussion	This patient is presenting with chronic granulomatous disease (CGD). Important clues include recurrent infections with *S. aureus* and less typical organisms such as *Aspergillus* and *Nocardia* (catalase positive organisms). Patients with CGD are prone to infection with catalase positive organisms due to a defect in NADPH oxidase, which produces the reactive oxygen species superoxide (precursor to H_2O_2) in the respiratory burst in neutrophils. Catalase negative organisms will produce their own H_2O_2 that CGD patients' cells can utilize to generate the hypochlorite needed to kill pathogens. Catalase positive organisms, however, use catalase to neutralize their own H_2O_2, so the neutrophils cannot use this to overcome their inability to produce H_2O_2 and thus cannot produce hypochlorite. Patients with CGD have normal responses to viral infections. CGD is most commonly X-linked recessive, so vignettes may include a history of men in the family with similar patterns of infection.
	Patients with **leukocyte adhesion deficiency (type 1)** (LAD-1) have an absence of neutrophils (pus) at sites of infection. This disease results from an autosomal recessive defect in LFA-1 integrin protein on phagocytes, so adhesion to the vascular wall cannot occur properly, causing transmigration and chemotaxis to be impaired. Consequently, neutrophils cannot adhere fully to the vessel wall, detect the chemical attractants necessary to find the site of infection, or cross the interstitium to reach the site of infection. Patients with LAD-1 have an elevated neutrophil count but will lack neutrophils at sites of infection. They will therefore be less likely to have pus formation at infection sites. These patients often present with delayed separation of the umbilical cord, absent pus, impaired wound healing, and recurrent skin and mucosal bacterial infections.
	Individuals with the autosomal recessive disease **Chédiak-Higashi syndrome** have microtubule dysfunction due to a defect in the lysosomal trafficking regulator gene (*LYST*). This causes impairment in phagosome-lysosome fusion, giant granules in granulocytes and platelets, and an increased risk of bacterial infections with *Staphylococci* and *Streptococci* and defects in primary hemostasis. Patients with Chédiak-Higashi also have pancytopenia, albinism, and peripheral neuropathy. In addition, they are at risk of developing hemophagocytic lymphohistiocytosis (HLH). Infections with *Aspergillus* and *Nocardia*, as in this vignette, would be uncommon.

CASE 4 | Terminal Complement Deficiency (C5–C9)

A 22-year-old woman is brought to the emergency department for evaluation of altered mental status and fever. Her friend said the patient had been complaining of a headache and neck pain for the last 12 hours and developed a strange rash. Her past medical history is notable for recurrent sexually transmitted infections with *N. gonorrhoeae*. The patient's temperature is 39.1°C, pulse is 123/min, respirations are 24/min, and blood pressure is 84/42 mmHg. She is obtunded and not responding to commands.

Evaluation/Tests	Cerebrospinal fluid cultures reveal a gram negative diplococcus suggestive of *Neisseria meningitidis*. CH50 and C5–C9 levels are decreased.
Treatment	Treat with antibiotics, and patient should be vaccinated against meningococcus.
Discussion	Terminal complement deficiency is the most likely immunodeficiency disorder in this patient presenting with recurrent *Neisseria* infections. Patients with terminal complement deficiency have recurrent *Neisseria* infections, especially with *N. meningitidis*. In particular, patients have a defect in the formation of the membrane attack complex (MAC), which is a combination of C5b, C6, C7, C8, and C9 complement components. MAC defends against gram negative bacteria through lysis and cytotoxicity.
	Early complement deficiencies (C1–C4) typically result in severe, recurrent pyogenic sinus and respiratory infections such as *Streptococcus pneumoniae* and less frequently with *Haemophilus influenzae*.

CASE 5	Hyper-IgM Syndrome
	A 2-year-old boy is brought to clinic for evaluation of fever and a cough for 4 days. The patient has a history of recurrent episodes of acute otitis media and has been hospitalized for pneumonia in the past. The patient's temperature is 39.0°C, pulse is 140/min, respirations are 36/min, and blood pressure is 85/44 mmHg. Chest X-ray reveals diffuse, ground-glass opacities bilaterally. A lung biopsy stained with methenamine silver stain demonstrates disc-shaped yeast.
Evaluation/Tests	IgM levels are normal. IgG, IgA, and IgE are all severely decreased.
Rx	Treat acute *Pneumocystis jirovecii* infection and continue antibiotic prophylaxis to prevent future infections. Definitive treatment is with a stem cell transplant.
Discussion	Hyper-IgM syndrome is an X-linked recessive disease most commonly due to defective CD40L on T-helper (Th) cells. In B-cell activation and class switching, the B-cell presents the antigen on MHC II to the T-cell receptor (TCR) on the Th-cell. CD40 on the B-cell then binds CD40 ligand (CD40L) on the Th-cell. Both signals are necessary for the Th-cell to secrete cytokines that induce B-cells to undergo Ig class-switching. In hyper-IgM syndrome, the second signal does not occur, so B-cells cannot undergo class switching and thus can only continue to produce IgM. This leads to low levels of IgA, IgG, and IgE, which leads to poor opsonization. This makes patients prone to recurrent pyogenic infections particularly with encapsulated organisms as well as opportunistic infections such as *Pneumocystis*, *Cryptosporidium*, and CMV. These patients also fail to make germinal centers, which is typically where class-switching and plasma cell differentiation occurs. IgM levels are normal to elevated in these patients. **SCID** also presents with recurrent infections early in life. However, the presence of normal to elevated IgM levels would be unusual in SCID. **Selective IgA deficiency** is the most common primary immunodeficiency and places patients at increased risk for mucosal infections. Most IgA-deficient patients are asymptomatic, but they are at increased risk of autoimmune disease, allergies, and anaphylaxis to IgA-containing products, such as blood products. They are also at increased risk for giardiasis. IgA levels are decreased, but other immunoglobulin levels are normal. **Wiskott-Aldrich syndrome** is due to an X-linked recessive mutation in the *WASP* gene, which prevents proper reorganization of the actin cytoskeleton. This causes defective antigen presentation and leads to defective humoral and cellular immunity. This defect also puts patients at increased risk for autoimmune diseases and cancer. Patients may present with the triad of thrombocytopenia, eczema, and recurrent infections. **Ataxia-telangiectasia** is an autosomal recessive disorder. Patients may have decreased IgA, IgG, and IgE levels, but this illness typically presents with the triad of ataxia, telangiectasia, and IgA deficiency. It is due to a defect in the ATM gene that encodes a DNA repair enzyme. Individuals are not able to repair breaks in DNA prior to cell division, which leads to the accumulation of various somatic mutations, which in turn leads to an increased risk of certain cancers, specifically lymphomas and acute leukemias.

HYPERSENSITIVITY REACTIONS

Hypersensitivity reactions occur when genetically predisposed individuals develop an overactive immune response to an innocuous/harmless antigen. The inflammation from these responses can cause serious tissue damage and disease. Hypersensitivity reactions are commonly grouped into four types: type I (acute, IgE antibody–mediated), type II (cytotoxic, IgG antibody–mediated), type III (immune complex–mediated), and type IV (delayed, T-cell-mediated). Understanding the underlying immunology associated with these reactions is very important for testing.

Examples of Hypersensitivity Reactions

Type I	Type II	Type III	Type IV
Systemic anaphylaxis	Autoimmune hemolytic anemia	Systemic lupus erythematous	Type I diabetes mellitus
Angioedema	Acute thrombocytopenic purpura	Cryoglobulinemia	Steven-Johnson syndrome/toxic epidermal necrolysis/erythema multiforme
Urticaria	Goodpasture's disease	Poststreptococcal glomerulonephritis	
Asthma	Graves' disease	Serum sickness	Drug rash, eosinophilia, systemic symptoms (DRESS)
Allergic rhinitis	Myasthenia gravis	Polyarteritis nodosa	Contact dermatitis
	Pemphigus vulgaris	Arthus reaction	Graft vs. host disease
	Hemolytic disease of the newborn		PPD test
	Rheumatic fever		
	Hyperacute transplant rejection		

- Type I hypersensitivity reactions are the classic IgE-mediated, allergic reactions that occurs secondary to preformed antibodies and occurs very quickly (within minutes) after exposure to an antigen. Fever is typically **absent**, and the severity of reaction ranges from urticaria (hives) to systemic anaphylaxis (hypotension and angioedema).

- Type II hypersensitivity reactions are caused by IgG antibodies against cellular antigens. Clinical examples include autoimmune hemolytic anemia, and autoimmune diseases such as Graves' disease (autoimmune cause of hyperthyroidism).

- Type III reactions involve the deposition of immune complexes (antigen–antibody complexes) and can cause diseases such as poststreptococcal glomerulonephritis.

- Type IV reactions are T-cell-mediated and present in a more delayed fashion (as it takes time to activate sensitized T-cells). Contact dermatitis and drug reactions such as Steven-Johnson syndrome are examples.

Key Findings and Hypersensitivity Reaction Differential Diagnosis

Hypersensitivity Reactions and Key Associated Findings	Diagnosis
Immediate development of symptoms: urticaria (raised, erythematous, papules and plaques that are pruritic), wheezing, flushing, hypotension, angioedema (swelling of lips/mouth/tongue/throat), anaphylaxis History of allergies, asthma (atopy)	Type I
Febrile reaction after blood transfusion (without anaphylaxis)	Type II
Neutropenia (agranulocytosis) in patient being treated for hyperthyroidism	Type II (propylthiouracil adverse effect)
Young, male smoker with hematuria and acute kidney injury (AKI)	Type II (Goodpasture syndrome)
Progressively worsening ptosis through the course of a day	Type II (myasthenia gravis)
Bulging eyes (exophthalmos) with weight loss, tremor, dry skin, diarrhea, fatigue	Type II (Graves' disease)
Flaccid blistering rash	Type II (Pemphigus vulgaris – flaccid bullae as opposed to the tense bullae of bullous pemphigoid)
Sore throat and fever followed by hematuria and AKI days to weeks later	Type III (poststreptococcal glomerulonephritis)
Fever, rash, lymphadenopathy, arthralgia, proteinuria about 5 days after starting a new drug	Type III (serum sickness reaction)
Poor dentition and fever followed by AKI injury and hematuria	Type III (glomerulonephritis secondary to subacute bacterial endocarditis)
Malar rash (erythema on face sparing nasolabial folds)	Type III (systemic lupus erythematosus)
Exposure to forested area/outdoors followed by rash several days later	Type IV (contact dermatitis)
Fever, rash, eosinophilia with hepatic and/or renal injury after starting a new drug several days to weeks ago	Type IV (DRESS)
Severe, blistering/desquamating rash involving the mucous membranes (mouth/lips, etc.) after starting a drug	Type IV (Steven-Johnson syndrome)
"Target" rash after starting new drug	Type IV (erythema multiforme)

CASE 6 | Type I Hypersensitivity—Anaphylaxis

An 18-year-old woman with asthma and seasonal allergies is given amoxicillin for an ear infection. Within 30 minutes of taking the medication, she develops lightheadedness, hives, facial swelling, and nausea and presents for evaluation. She has never had this reaction before. She took amoxicillin once before as a child. On exam, the patient's temperature is 37.0°C, pulse is 118/min, respirations are 22/min, and blood pressure is 80/45 mmHg. She is flushed, in acute distress, and has notable swelling of the lips and face (angioedema). She has audible wheezing and a diffuse raised, erythematous rash that is pruritic (urticaria).

Evaluation/Tests	Clinical diagnosis. However, there can be elevated serum tryptase, an inflammatory mediator released from mast cells.

CASE 6 | Type I Hypersensitivity—Anaphylaxis *(continued)*

Treatment	Administer intramuscular epinephrine immediately. H1 and H2 blockers can be given as adjunctive therapy. Albuterol and prednisone can help treat bronchospasm and delayed anaphylaxis.
Discussion	The patient has classic symptoms of anaphylaxis with hypotension, angioedema, bronchospasm, and urticaria. Anaphylaxis is the most severe form of **type I hypersensitivity reaction**. Any patient who has an episode of anaphylaxis should be provided with an epinephrine injector for home use so they can initiate therapy if an attack develops. Type I hypersensitivity reactions occur due to free antigens that cross-link IgE on mast cells and basophils. This causes an immediate release of histamine, which causes vasodilation at postcapillary venules. The delayed phase results from mast cells and basophils releasing cytokines that cause cellular inflammation. This hypersensitivity reaction develops rapidly after initial exposure to the antigen because the body preforms antibodies against it, so anaphylaxis occurs on the second exposure but not the first (as in this patient). **Delayed drug reactions (type IV)** can present with rash, but the other symptoms are typically lacking. Also, the patient clearly had a very immediate onset of symptoms, which makes anaphylaxis and type I hypersensitivity more likely. **Serum sickness (type III)** would also present with urticaria, but it would be accompanied by fever, arthralgias, and lymphadenopathy, which are not present in this patient. It would also occur 5–10 days after antigen exposure rather than within 30 minutes.

CASE 7 | Type II Hypersensitivity—Hemolytic Disease of the Newborn

A 26-year-old pregnant woman with limited prenatal care comes to the doctor because she is in labor. She has been pregnant once before and carried the baby to term without complications. The baby is born via spontaneous vaginal delivery. His APGAR scores are 8 and 9, but he appears jaundiced. The mother's blood type is O–, and the baby's type and screen are pending.

Evaluations/Tests	The infant's blood type is found to be B+. Hyperbilirubinemia is confirmed.
Treatment	The infant should be treated with phototherapy.
Discussion	**Hemolytic disease of the newborn is a type II hypersensitivity reaction** that results from maternal IgG that crosses the placenta. This can occur in one of two situations: (1) An Rh– mother who has previously been exposed to Rh+ blood, such as during a previous pregnancy, develops anti-D IgG antibodies, which can cross the placenta in subsequent pregnancies. (2) A mother with type O blood with anti-A or anti-B IgG antibodies that cross the placenta and can affect the first and later pregnancies. In both cases, the neonate can present with jaundice in the first 24 hours and anemia in the most severe cases. This occurs because IgG antibodies can cross the placenta and bind to antigens on the erythrocyte surface, causing opsonization of the red blood cells. This leads to activation of complement as well as natural killer cell–mediated cytotoxicity, lysing erythrocytes and releasing their contents into the bloodstream. Other examples of type II hypersensitivity include autoimmune hemolytic anemia and acute hemolytic transfusion reactions, both of which have a similar mechanism of action. In myasthenia gravis and Graves' disease, IgG antibodies bind to cell surface receptors and block their function. Type II hypersensitivity also includes diseases in which antibodies bind to cell surfaces and cause complement activation and inflammation, such as in Goodpasture syndrome and rheumatic fever. While **Gilbert syndrome** and **Crigler-Najjar syndrome** can both cause jaundice, they would be less likely to present this early. Additionally, the incompatible blood types between the mother and the infant make hemolytic disease of the newborn more likely.

CASE 8 | Type III Hypersensitivity—Serum Sickness

A 65-year-old man with coronary artery disease presents to the emergency department with acute onset of severe, substernal chest pain. An ECG demonstrates ST-segment elevations in leads V1–V4, and his troponins are elevated. The patient undergoes percutaneous coronary intervention and is started on abciximab. Ten days later, the patient presents with joint pains, fever, and a pruritic rash. On exam, the patient's temperature is 38.6°C, pulse is 110/min, respirations are 18/min, and blood pressure is 132/82 mmHg. The patient is noted to have urticaria on his arms, torso, and back.

Evaluation/Tests	Clinical diagnosis. Urinalysis shows proteinuria, and serum C3 level is decreased.
Treatment	Stop abciximab and use a different antiplatelet agent.

CASE 8 | Type III Hypersensitivity—Serum Sickness (continued)

Discussion	This patient is experiencing **serum sickness**, a **type III hypersensitivity reaction**. Serum sickness results from antibodies that form against foreign proteins. As in other type III hypersensitivity reactions, these antibodies form immune complexes, which are deposited into membranes. Immune complexes fix complement thus activating this cascade and releasing C5a, which attracts neutrophils. This reaction generates inflammation and damages surrounding tissues. Serum sickness is typically caused by drugs, such as chimeric monoclonal antibodies, acting as haptens that activate this response.
	The **Arthus reaction** is another form of type III hypersensitivity that can occur in response to drug administration. In individuals who have IgG against a particular antigen, intradermal administration of a drug with that antigen will cause immune complex formation in the skin and underlying small blood vessels, which leads to complement activation and neutrophil recruitment. This causes small vessel fibrinoid necrosis with neutrophil infiltration. The affected area will have edema, erythema, and even necrosis. This rare reaction is often associated with vaccine boosters.
	While urticaria would be typical of an **atopic reaction** to a medication, proteinuria and arthralgias would be unlikely.

CASE 9 | Type IV Hypersensitivity—Tuberculin (PPD) Skin Test

A 24-year-old nursing student receives his annual PPD skin test to screen for tuberculosis infection. Approximately 72 hours later, he develops an area of induration at the injection site measuring 16 mm.

Evaluation/Tests	For the general population, the cutoff for a positive PPD skin test (performed 48–72 hours after injection) is an area of induration at least 15 mm in transverse diameter. For health care workers, the cutoff is a minimum of 10 mm. For AIDS and transplant patients, who are expected to have a decreased immune response to tuberculin, the cutoff is a minimum of 5 mm.
Treatment	A positive test would be followed with a chest X-ray to rule out active tuberculosis. Treat latent tuberculosis (if CXR is negative) with isoniazid or rifampin.
Discussion	The **tuberculin skin test is an example of type IV hypersensitivity** induced by intradermal injection of the purified protein derivative (PPD) tuberculin from *Mycobacterium tuberculosis*. Type IV hypersensitivity reactions are T-cell-mediated reactions and thus do not involve antibodies, which differentiates type IV from the other forms of hypersensitivity reactions. Type IV hypersensitivity reactions occur through (1) direct cytotoxicity via CD8+ T-cells against targeted cells and (2) delayed-type hypersensitivity via sensitized CD4+ T-cells that release cytokines in response to an antigen. In patients with prior tuberculosis exposure, upon reexposure to similar antigens with the PPD skin test, antigen-presenting cells within the skin will reintroduce the antigen to memory T-cells, resulting in a rapid and strong secondary immune response. These memory T-cells, most of which are CD4+, can release chemokines and cytokines, which then coordinate a robust immune response. One such cytokine is interferon-γ (IFN-γ), which stimulates macrophages within the skin to phagocytose the injected protein. Macrophages can further secrete tumor necrosis factor-α (TNF-α), a potent activator of endothelium that drives further immune cell influx into tissue. Swelling and phagocytic cell infiltration near the site of injection results in induration. The PPD test will be positive in situations of current or past exposure and negative in patients without exposure. False positives may be seen in patients with a previous BCG vaccination or nontuberculosis mycobacterial infection. False negatives can be seen in patients with HIV infection (especially if their CD4+ cell counts are low) or in sarcoidosis. Another test for *M. tuberculosis* infection includes the IFN-γ release assay (IGRA), a blood-based test that exposes blood samples to TB antigens or controls and measures release of IFN-γ. IGRA does not require a follow-up visit and is not affected by BCG vaccination status.

BLOOD TRANSFUSION REACTIONS

Blood transfusion reactions are potentially serious complications that can occur within minutes to hours of initiating a transfusion. When facing a question that sounds like a potential blood transfusion reaction, the time course is important to consider when trying to determine the etiology of the reaction. Additionally, which symptoms predominate can help suggest a specific diagnosis. While several reactions can include fever, the accompanying symptoms will help determine which type of transfusion reaction is occurring and thus help narrow down the etiology.

CASE 10	Anaphylactic Blood Transfusion Reaction
	A 36-year-old previously healthy woman loses a significant amount of blood during a vaginal delivery. Bleeding is controlled and transfusion of packed red blood cells is initiated. Fifteen minutes after the transfusion is started, the patient reports itching and develops a rash on her arm through which she is receiving the transfusion. Within minutes, the rash spreads over her entire body, and she reports difficulty breathing. The patient's temperature is 37.9°C, pulse is 116/min, respirations are 24/min, and blood pressure is 82/44 mmHg. Wheezes are heard in bilateral lung fields.
Evaluation/Tests	Clinical diagnosis. Urinalysis and CBC are within normal limits.
Treatment	Treat with epinephrine and antihistamines. Albuterol and prednisone can help decrease the delayed phase of anaphylaxis. Vasopressors may be needed for hypotension.
Discussion	Anaphylactic blood transfusion reactions are type I hypersensitivity reactions against proteins in the plasma of administered blood products. This can occur in patients with IgA deficiency who produce anti-IgA antibodies upon receipt of IgA in a transfusion. As patients with selective IgA deficiency are typically asymptomatic, they may not know that they have this condition. Patients present as quickly as 15 minutes from the initiation of their transfusion and experience pruritus, urticaria, wheezing, hypotension, and shock. Epinephrine acts quickly while albuterol and prednisone help prevent the delayed phase of anaphylaxis that results from mast cell and basophil degranulation and release of other cytokines that further potentiate the inflammatory response.
	While the other transfusion reactions should be considered, the rapid onset of symptoms in this case makes anaphylaxis the most likely diagnosis. It can be further distinguished from other reactions with the presence of urticaria and pruritus, which suggest a type I hypersensitivity reaction.
	Febrile nonhemolytic transfusion reactions (FNHTRs) present with fever and chills approximately 1–6 hours after receiving a transfusion. These patients do not have hemolysis or hemodynamic instability. FNHTRs are a type II hypersensitivity reaction with host antibodies to donor human leukocyte antigens (HLA) and WBCs. Host antibodies bind to donor HLA, causing a cytotoxic response to donor white blood cells. Donor cells can then release cytokines, which causes an inflammatory response, including fever, chills, flushing, and/or headache. These cytokines are created and accumulate during the storage of blood products. FNHTR is the most common of the transfusion reactions and is not life-threatening. Management is symptomatic.
	Acute hemolytic transfusion reactions (AHTR) are type II hypersensitivity reactions in response to foreign antigens on erythrocytes. This typically occurs in response to ABO blood type incompatibility. For instance, if a patient with blood type A receives type B blood, the anti-B IgM antibodies in the patient's blood will react to the B antigens on the surface of donor RBCs. This leads to complement activation and formation of MAC on the RBC surface. Complement-mediated lysis causes cellular destruction and intravascular hemolysis, which causes an increase in unconjugated (indirect) bilirubin, decreased hemoglobin, and decreased haptoglobin since haptoglobin binds free hemoglobin from lysed cells. The additional cytokines from complement activation cause fever, tachypnea, tachycardia, and hypotension, which should be treated urgently with aggressive IV fluid resuscitation. These reactions are rare because patients are typically typed and screened so that they can receive properly matched blood products. AHTR could present with hypotension and tachypnea, but the patient in this vignette does not have signs of hemolysis, such as flank pain and jaundice.
	Transfusion-related acute lung injury (TRALI) is an adverse blood transfusion reaction due to donor antileukocyte antibodies attacking recipient pulmonary endothelial cells and neutrophils. Donor antibodies bind to antigens on intravascular neutrophils, which causes the release of cytokines and thus further neutrophil activation. Since the neutrophils are intravascular, their activation also causes endothelial damage, which leads to vascular leakage and pulmonary edema. The release of cytokines also causes vasodilation of pulmonary vasculature and further inflammatory pulmonary edema. This occurs within 6 hours of the transfusion. Patients with TRALI present with respiratory distress and pulmonary infiltrates due to noncardiogenic pulmonary edema. Chest X-ray would demonstrate inflammatory, noncardiogenic pulmonary edema. TRALI patients typically do not have urticaria and pruritus. Anaphylaxis would also occur more quickly than TRALI and would present with wheezing rather than the crackles of pulmonary edema.

TRANSPLANT REJECTION

Transplant grafts can be divided into autografts (the graft is from the patient), syngeneic grafts (from a clone or identical twin), allografts (from another human that is not an identical twin), and xenografts (from another species). Graft rejection is a common and potentially dangerous complication of transplants. Pretransplant workup and post-transplant immunosuppression are aimed at preventing transplant rejection, but even optimal preparation and postoperative immunosuppression cannot always prevent this complication. When determining which type of transplant rejection is occurring, the time course and key features of the rejection are important factors to consider. Some opportunistic infections in transplant recipients include CMV, BK virus, *Candida* spp., and *Aspergillus*.

CASE 11 | Acute Transplant Rejection

A 54-year-old woman who received a kidney transplant 2 months ago presents for follow-up of her transplanted kidney. She is doing fairly well but has experienced malaise over the past week. The patient has been compliant with her immunosuppressant therapy. Her vital signs are within normal limits, and her physical exam is unremarkable. Her labs show a creatinine of 2.1, which is increased from a level of 1.2 at her last visit.

Evaluation/Tests	Kidney biopsy demonstrates vasculitis of renal vessels and a dense, lymphocytic, interstitial infiltrate.
Treatment	The patient's immunosuppressants should be increased in an effort to reverse the acute rejection.
Discussion	Acute transplant rejection most commonly occurs within 6 months of organ transplantation. It is the most common failure of transplantation and is prevented through immunosuppression. Acute transplant rejection can occur in one of two ways: (1) Cellular—In a type IV hypersensitivity reaction, CD8+ T-cells are activated against donor MHC's, which causes a vasculitis in the graft vessels with interstitial mononuclear cell infiltration. (2) Humoral—The recipient develops antibodies against the donor tissue, which leads to a type II hypersensitivity and subsequent necrotizing vasculitis. Complement activation also leads to release of chemokines for neutrophils, so a neutrophilic infiltrate may be seen on biopsy (in contrast to mononuclear cells seen in the cellular type). Symptoms depend on the organ that was transplanted, but patients may be asymptomatic. **Hyperacute transplant rejection** is a type II hypersensitivity reaction in which recipient preformed antibodies react to antigens on vascular endothelial cells in the grafted organ. The formation of antibody–antigen complexes leads to the activation of complement and adhesion of immune cells to the vascular wall. Endothelial damage activates the coagulation cascade and causes widespread thrombosis of the grafted organ vessels. As blood supply to the donor organ becomes compromised, the organ undergoes ischemia and subsequent necrosis, rapidly rendering the graft nonviable. Hyperacute transplant rejection occurs within minutes and will likely be seen before the patient leaves the operating room. Pretransplant screens aim to match organ recipients and organ donors such that the recipient would not have antibodies to antigens in the donated organ. Treatment of hyperacute rejection involves removal of the graft. **Chronic transplant rejection** occurs over months to years and is irreversible. The time course and histological findings can help differentiate between chronic and acute transplant rejection. While both may happen after a few months, acute transplant rejection will have a lymphocytic or neutrophilic vasculitis on biopsy. In contrast, chronic transplant rejection will have biopsy findings consistent with arteriosclerosis, parenchymal atrophy, and interstitial fibrosis rather than vasculitis. Inflammatory cells are an uncommon finding in chronic transplant rejection biopsies. Chronic transplant rejection manifests in various ways depending on the affected organ—vanishing bile duct syndrome in the liver, chronic graft nephropathy in the kidney, bronchiolitis obliterans in the lungs, and atherosclerosis in the heart. **GVHD** is less common in kidney transplants and would have more disseminated findings.

CASE 12 | Graft-Versus-Host Disease (GVHD)

A 68-year-old man who received a bone marrow transplant for multiple myeloma 1 month ago presents with a rash, nausea, and diarrhea for the past week. He has been compliant with his immunosuppressive therapy. The rash started on his neck and arms but has spread to his entire body. His diarrhea is watery and has been increasing in volume. On exam, the patient has a maculopapular rash covering his whole body. His sclerae are icteric. His abdomen is soft but diffusely tender to palpation, and hepatosplenomegaly is noted.

Evaluation/Tests	Clinical diagnosis. Histologic confirmation by biopsy of affected site (e.g., skin, GI tract, etc.). Direct bilirubin and alkaline phosphatase levels are elevated.
Treatment	Systemic glucocorticoids. Topical corticosteroids can be used with mild GVHD involving only the skin, with additional immunosuppression in steroid-refractory cases.

CASE 12 | Graft-Versus-Host Disease (GVHD) *(continued)*

Discussion	Graft-versus-host disease (GVHD) is typically a complication of allogeneic bone marrow transplants. In GVHD, a type IV hypersensitivity reaction occurs in which donor T-cells proliferate in the immunosuppressed recipient and attack host cells. Because the donor cells are multiplying in the host, they are not localized to the graft and thus cause systemic disease. The most commonly involved organs are the skin (maculopapular rash), GI (nausea, diarrhea), and liver (destruction of bile ducts, increased bilirubin and alkaline phosphatase). These disseminated findings help differentiate GVHD from other types of transplant rejection. GVHD can occur at any point, but the classic acute form typically occurs within the first 100 days after transplantation. Chronic GVHD typically presents much later. **Infectious** causes of **diarrhea** may also cause rash (e.g., *Salmonella typhi*), but the findings of hepatosplenomegaly and hepatic dysfunction are less likely.

3

Microbiology

Mahesh C. Patel, MD
Scott Borgetti, MD

Infectious diseases are caused by a variety of organisms that can be viral, bacterial, fungal, or parasitic. Through the innate and adaptive immune system, immunocompetent hosts can deter many pathogens. However, when an organism is able to evade some of our defenses and cause disease, these same host defenses tend to drive the symptoms we see in a patient. Inflammation is the hallmark of infectious diseases, with *calor* (heat), *rubor* (redness), *dolor* (pain), and swelling as a consequence. Organ-specific inflammation can be a clue to infectious diseases, such as pyuria in genitourinary infections or pleocytosis (increased cell count) in central nervous system infections. It is important to define the infectious syndrome by identifying the anatomical compartment or the organ involved. An anatomical compartment or organ can have a variety of infectious syndromes associated with it (e.g., the lung (organ) can be the location of a pneumonia (infectious syndrome). The general approach to patients with suspected infectious diseases is to obtain a full history, exploring activities that may have exposed the patient to a pathogen and comorbidities that may affect the ability of the patient to defend against organisms. An immunocompetent host may have a community-acquired (CAP) or hospital-acquired pneumonia (HAP), while a patient with advanced AIDS may have CAP, HAP, or an opportunistic infection such as *Pneumocystis jirovecii* pneumonia. A thorough physical exam can help localize the anatomical compartment, and useful initial labs and tests include WBC and/or inflammatory markers such as ESR (erythrocyte sedimentation rate) or CRP (C-reactive protein), imaging, and cultures. A careful history, exam, confirmatory tests, and cultures will help narrow the differential diagnosis and guide treatment and management.

FEVER AND HEADACHE

Fever and headache in combination are concerning for infections involving the central nervous system (CNS) and should prompt immediate evaluation, diagnosis, and treatment. A variety of pathogens can cause infection of the brain, the meninges, or the spinal cord. The presentations of patients infected with different pathogens may be quite similar. Brain abscesses are space-occupying infections that can also present with fever and headache and likewise can be due to a host of pathogens. A thorough evaluation of risk factors for given pathogens, as well as CNS imaging and cerebrospinal fluid (CSF) sampling, is paramount to making an accurate diagnosis.

There is some overlap between the CSF studies among these syndromes, but the basic patterns are very important to be familiar with to help narrow the differential diagnosis.

Pathogen	Cell Count (cells/μl)	Protein (mg/dL)	Glucose (mg/dL)
Bacterial	1000–5000 (>80% PMNs/neutrophils)	100–500	<40 (can even be <10)
Fungal/TB	100–1000 (mostly lymphocytes)	50+	<40 (in TB especially)
Viral	5–500 (mostly lymphocytes)	50+	Normal

Differential Diagnosis (DDx) for CNS Infections

Meningitis	Tick-borne Illness	Encephalitis	Brain Abscess

Bacterial
  S. pneumoniae
  N. meningitidis
  Listeria
  Tuberculosis
Fungal
  Cryptococcus
  Coccidiosis
Viral
  HSV-2
  VZV
  Enteroviruses (e.g., Coxsackie)
	- CNS Lyme Disease
	- Rocky Mountain spotted fever (RMSF)
		- HSV-1
		- West Nile virus
		- VZV
		- Other (e.g., St. Louis encephalitis, Eastern equine)
		- JC virus (PML in immunocompromised patients)
			- S. aureus
			- Viridans group Streptococci
			- Anaerobes
			- Toxoplasmosis
			Noninfectious
			- CNS Lymphoma

Meningitis and encephalitis represent a spectrum of disease of the CNS involving the brain and/or spinal cord. There is significant crossover in the presentation of these syndromes; fever, headache, and neck pain may be present in both. Classically, encephalitis patients also have altered mental status, which suggests involvement of the brain parenchyma.

Key Findings and CNS Infections Differential Diagnosis

Fever and Headache with Key Associated Findings	Diagnosis
Tick exposure, New England, Northeastern United States/Wisconsin states travel	Lyme disease
Tick exposure, petechial rash Appalachian states/Southeastern United States	RMSF
College student living in a dormitory, petechial rash	*N. meningitidis*
Associated vesicular rash	HSV, VZV
- Mosquito exposure in summer months - Flaccid paralysis	West Nile virus
- Older patient, >50 years old - Contaminated milk products	*Listeria* meningitis
- Recent dental infection, oral abscess - History of bacterial endocarditis, new heart murmur - History IV drug use - Focal neurologic deficit	Pyogenic brain abscess
- Altered mental status - Focal neurologic deficit	Encephalitis
- Homeless, incarcerated, travel to developing world - Cranial nerve deficits (if involving basilar brain structures)	TB meningitis
HIV/AIDS (CD4 <50) Focal, ring-enhancing lesions on imaging	CNS toxoplasmosis or CNS lymphoma
HIV/AIDS (CD4 <50) Meningitis or encephalitis	Cryptococcal meningitis or progressive multifocal leukoencephalopathy (from JC virus)
- Travel to the Southwestern United States - Eosinophilic meningitis (on CSF or serum)	Coccidioidomycosis
- Travel to Latin America	Paracoccidioidomycosis
- Travel to Mississippi and Ohio River Valley	Histoplasmosis
- Travel to Eastern and Central United States	Blastomycosis

CASE 1 | *Streptococcus Pneumoniae* Meningitis

A 45-year-old man presents with fever, rigors, headache, and neck pain of a few hours duration. He has no significant medical history and denies recent travel or sick contacts. He is ill appearing but remains alert, responding appropriately to questions, and has no focal neurologic deficits. On exam his temperature is 39.5°C, pulse 110/min, respirations 24/min, blood pressure 95/60 mmHG. He has a stiff neck and flexes his hips and knees when his neck is passively flexed (positive Brudzinski's sign) and when hip and knee are flexed to 90° and then extension of the knee is attempted, there is restriction and pain in the neck (positive Kernig's sign).

Evaluation/Tests	CSF analysis reveals increased opening pressure, cell count of 2500 cells/µl, with 85% polymorphonuclear cells, protein 156 mg/dL, glucose 35 mg/dL. Gram stain of CSF shows gram positive diplococci. CSF and blood cultures ordered and pending. CT head without contrast is negative for space-occupying lesions.
Treatment	Rapid initiation of empiric antibiotics (usually vancomycin and ceftriaxone). Steroids (dexamethasone) may be added in select cases to reduce inflammation-associated neurologic deficits.
Discussion	**Bacterial meningitis** presents with classic features including rapid onset of fever, headache, and neck pain or stiffness. Generally, meningitis caused by bacterial or fungal pathogens is more severe than aseptic meningitis caused by viral pathogens. Bacterial meningitis can be diagnosed by CSF analysis, which would demonstrate increased opening pressure, neutrophils, and protein with low glucose (<40 mg/dL). When discussing meningitis, it is often said "time is brain" and the workup and initiation of empiric antibiotics should not be delayed. The most common pathogen causing bacterial meningitis across adults of all ages is **Streptococcus pneumoniae**, followed by *N. meningitidis*. In older or immunocompromised patients, *Listeria monocytogenes* is commonly seen. *S. pneumoniae* is a gram positive, α-hemolytic, lancet-shaped, encapsulated diplococci. In addition to being the most common cause of bacterial meningitis, it is also the most common cause of otitis media (in children), pneumonia, and sinusitis. *S. pneumoniae* meningitis may follow a pulmonary infection or mild upper respiratory tract infection, and those with underlying medical conditions (e.g., sickle cell disease) are at higher risk.

CASE 1 | *Streptococcus Pneumoniae* Meningitis *(continued)*

| Discussion | Given the lack of focal neurologic deficits or altered mental status in this patient, **bacterial encephalitis** is less likely.
Viral (aseptic) meningitis would show lymphocyte predominance and may have normal or elevated opening pressure and protein, with normal glucose on CSF analysis. Viral meningitis is often accompanied by inflammation of the brain parenchyma and therefore may involve mental status or subtle personality changes.
A **brain abscess** typically has focal neurologic deficits and can be ruled out with a normal CT scan. |

CASE 2 | *Neisseria Meningitidis* Meningitis

An 18-year-old man with a history of asthma develops 12 hours of fever, severe headache, neck pain, myalgias, and rash. He lives in a college dormitory and is sexually active with women, but he always uses condoms. On exam, his temperature is 39.4°C, pulse is 125/min, respirations are 22/min, and blood pressure is 98/68 mmHg. He is awake and alert but extremely uncomfortable. He has a stiff neck and a petechial, nonblanching rash on his legs that has not migrated. He has no focal findings on neurologic exam.

| Evaluation/Tests | CSF analysis reveals a white blood cell count of 2500 cells/µl (85% PMNs), protein 156 mg/dL, glucose 28 mg/dL, and Gram stain reveals gram negative diplococci. Culture is pending. |
| Discussion | ***Neisseria meningitidis***, an encapsulated, gram negative diplococcus, is the etiology of the patient's bacterial meningitis. The classic presentation of *N. meningitidis* meningitis, also called **meningococcal meningitis**, is a teenager living in a college dormitory who presents with severe, abrupt onset meningitis and a petechial rash. This pathogen is spread by respiratory droplets and can cause outbreaks in compressed living spaces such as dormitories, military barracks, prisons, etc. *N. meningitidis* has several virulence factors, including an antiphagocytic polysaccharide capsule and the presence of lipooligosaccharide, which can induce significant cytokine production and sepsis. *Neisseria* does require special culturing methods using Thayer-Martin agar, which includes vancomycin, trimethoprim, colistin, and nystatin to inhibit growth of other organisms. One complication of infection is bilateral adrenal cortical hemorrhage, known as **Waterhouse-Friderichsen syndrome**. The meningococcal vaccine is recommended for all adolescents between 11 and 18 years old.
Rocky Mountain spotted fever (RMSF), caused by the zoonotic bacteria *Rickettsia rickettsii* and transmitted by the *Dermacentor* dog tick, can also cause fever, headache, altered mental status, and a rash. However, this patient lacks risk factors for tick exposure and the pattern of rash in RMSF typically starts at the distal extremities and then spreads proximally. |

CASE 3 | Herpes Simplex Virus (HSV) Encephalitis

A 35-year-old woman presents to the emergency department with 3 days of fever, headache, confusion, and now an episode of "shaking" seen by her husband. She has no other medical problems and reports no recent travel or sick contacts. On exam, the patient is febrile to 38.5°C. Vitals are otherwise normal. She is minimally responsive and cannot participate in the neurologic exam, but she spontaneously moves all of her extremities, and no rashes are noted. She has a witnessed generalized seizure during the evaluation.

Evaluation/Tests	CSF analysis reveals a normal opening pressure, numerous red blood cells, white blood cell count of 325 cells/µl, with 80% lymphocytes, protein 70 mg/dL, and glucose 62 mg/dL. Gram stain is negative. PCR for HSV-1 in the CSF would return positive. MRI brain reveals numerous hyperintense lesions on the temporal lobes bilaterally with evidence of edema and hemorrhage. Scalp EEG shows numerous periodic epileptiform discharges originating from the temporal lobe bilaterally.
Treatment	Stabilize airway, breathing, and circulation (ABCs); rapid initiation of empiric therapy with vancomycin, ceftriaxone, and acyclovir until CSF results return. After diagnosis, treat with targeted antimicrobials.
Discussion	**Herpes simplex virus encephalitis** is an infection of the brain parenchyma that often results in headache, altered mental status, focal neurologic deficits, seizures, and/or subtle personality changes. Viral infections of the CNS often result in combined infection of the meninges and brain parenchyma, resulting in meningoencephalitis. The most common cause of spontaneous encephalitis is **herpes simplex virus-1 (HSV-1)**. HSV-1 is an enveloped, linear, double-stranded DNA virus. CSF findings are similar to other viral meningitis presentations (moderately elevated cell count (100–500, lymphocyte predominance), moderately elevated protein, and normal glucose). However, one unique feature of HSV-1 encephalitis is that it is often hemorrhagic, and therefore the presence of numerous RBCs in the

CASE 3 | Herpes Simplex Virus (HSV) Encephalitis (continued)

Discussion	CSF is a common manifestation. HSV encephalitis is one of the few viral causes with specific treatment (IV acyclovir). HSV-1 infection results from an initial oropharyngeal infection that travels via the olfactory nerves and tract to the brain or from reactivation of latent virus within the trigeminal ganglion of cranial nerve V. This results in hemorrhagic necrosis of the temporal lobes, which can be unilateral or bilateral and may result in symptoms such as temporal lobe seizures, Wernicke's (receptive) aphasia, olfactory hallucinations, and more. Other causes of viral encephalitis may present similarly, so diagnosis is based on CNS imaging and CSF studies. **HSV-2** is typically spread by sexual contact and establishes latency in the sacral ganglia. It actually is a more common cause of viral meningitis than HSV-1 but typically does not cause accompanying encephalitis. **Enterovirus** is the leading cause of viral meningitis and is a member of the picornavirus family of positive-sense, single-stranded, icosahedral RNA viruses.

CASE 4 | Malaria

A 35-year-old woman with no past medical history presents with intermittent fevers, shaking chills, sweats, myalgias, and headaches. She returned from Africa 1 week ago and did not take any immunizations or prophylaxis medications during her trip. Her symptoms last 4–5 hours and recur every 2–3 days. On exam, she has a fever of 41.5°C, is tachycardic, and has splenomegaly.

Evaluation/Tests	Parasitological testing of peripheral blood smear with Giemsa stain would detect: *Plasmodium*: trophozoite ring form in RBC. CBC notable for mild normocytic anemia and thrombocytopenia. Thin blood films of Plasmodium falciparum. Young trophozoite. Reproduced with permission from Bench Aids for the Diagnosis of Malaria Infections, 2nd ed. World Health Organization; 2000.
Treatment	Treat uncomplicated *infection* with chloroquine (if sensitive) or mefloquine or atovaquone/proguanil (if resistant) or oral artemisinin combination therapy (ACT) and severe cases with intravenous artesunate.
Discussion	**Malaria** is transmitted by infected *Anopheles* mosquitos and is caused by *Plasmodium species* (*P. falciparum* is the most common and potentially deadliest). Complications include cerebral malaria, hemolytic anemia, hypoglycemia, lactic acidosis and cardiopulmonary, renal, and liver damage. Therefore, timely diagnosis and treatment are important. Other species include *P. vivax, P. ovale, P. malariae,* and *P. knowlesi.* When traveling to endemic areas, it is important to prescribe prophylaxis treatment.
Additional Considerations	**West Nile virus (WNV) encephalitis** is a form of viral meningoencephalitis that can present with fever, altered mental status, and flaccid paralysis. WNV is an arbovirus spread by the female *Culex* mosquito and is seen in the summer months. WNV initially appeared in the United States in New York City but now occurs throughout the country. There is no specific therapy for WNV, but supportive care can help improve outcomes. Those at highest risk of severe disease include the elderly, very young, or immunocompromised patients. Infections in immunocompetent, healthy adults are mostly asymptomatic. **Dengue fever** is caused by another flavivirus (dengue virus), is transmitted by the *Aedes* mosquito, and presents with flu-like symptoms, headache, fever, myalgias, arthralgias, and retro-orbital pain. It is prevalent in tropical and subtropical regions. ***Naegleria fowleri*** is a free-living protozoan/amoeba found in freshwater that can cause rapid-onset and fatal primary amebic meningoencephalitis when inhaled during activities such as swimming. Wet mount of CSF would show motile trophozoites.

CASE 5 | CNS Toxoplasmosis

A 29-year-old man with HIV nonadherent to antiretroviral medications presents with 2 weeks of fever, headache, lethargy, and now left arm weakness. He has had no recent travel or sick contacts and lives alone at home with his pet cat. On exam, he has a temperature of 38.4°C, pulse 93/min, respirations 14/min, and blood pressure 105/74 mmHg. He is awake but confused and falls asleep easily. He is able to participate in the neurologic exam, which is unremarkable aside from 4/5 left upper extremity strength and hyperreflexia of left biceps reflex. No rashes are noted.

CASE 5 | CNS Toxoplasmosis *(continued)*

Evaluation/Tests	CD4 count is low at 45. CSF analysis reveals a white blood cell count of 3 cells/µl, protein 28 mg/dL, and glucose 54 mg/dL. Gram stain of CSF is negative. Brain MRI with and without contrast shows multiple ring-enhancing lesions. Serology is positive for antitoxoplasma IgG antibodies; other microbiological tests like serum cryptococcal antigen would be negative. Toxoplasma gondii Infection. Contrast head CT showing typical multiple ring-enhancing lesions seen in T gondii CNS infection. Reproduced with permission from Knoop KJ, Stack LB, Storrow AB, et al: The Atlas of Emergency Medicine, 5th ed. New York, NY: McGraw Hill; 2021. Photo contributor: Edward C. Oldfield III, MD.
Treatment	First-line treatment is sulfadiazine and pyrimethamine, supplemented with leucovorin (folinic acid) to reduce adverse side effects. If a patient fails to respond, consider brain biopsy to evaluate for CNS lymphoma.
Discussion	**CNS toxoplasmosis** is an encephalitis common in HIV/AIDS patients that classically presents with multiple ring-enhancing brain lesions on MRI and relatively unremarkable CSF findings. Severely immunocompromised patients are at risk of a variety of opportunistic infections such as *Cryptococcus*, toxoplasmosis, and PML (JC virus). Toxoplasmosis is caused by ***Toxoplasmosis gondii,*** an obligate intracellular protozoan that causes mononucleosis-like symptoms in immunocompetent patients but can lead to formation of brain abscesses and encephalitis in AIDS patients. *T. gondii* is transmitted most commonly from cysts in undercooked meat, but the classic picture is transmission via food or water contaminated with oocysts in cat feces as the cat is the host of the protozoan. Brain biopsy can provide a definitive diagnosis, but it is a risky procedure, so treatment is initiated empirically, and the diagnosis is confirmed if there is a positive response. *T. gondii* can also infect developing fetuses, resulting in **congenital toxoplasmosis** presenting with a classic triad of chorioretinitis, hydrocephalus, and intracranial calcifications. **Primary CNS lymphoma** can also present as ring-enhancing lesions in the brain. Patients who fail to respond to sulfadiazine and pyrimethamine therapy for toxoplasmosis should be considered to have CNS lymphoma, a diffuse, large-cell non-Hodgkin's lymphoma of B-cell origin. Primary CNS lymphoma is more likely to show up as a solitary lesion but can be multiple and would show uptake on PET scan. **Progressive multifocal leukoencephalopathy (PML)** from reactivation of the JC virus will show nonenhancing areas of demyelination on MRI rather than a clearly demarcated lesion. Infection with the opportunistic fungus ***Cryptococcus neoformans*** can result in meningoencephalitis with characteristic "soap bubble" lesions in the brain on MRI. These lesions are usually small, and CSF culture would reveal a heavily encapsulated, round yeast with peripheral clearing on India ink or mucicarmine stain.

FEVER AND COUGH

Fever and cough make up a clinical syndrome that generally is associated with infections of the upper respiratory tract (bronchitis) and/or lower respiratory tract (pneumonia). As the clinical consequences of lower respiratory tract infections are much more important, we will focus on pneumonia here. The differential diagnosis for acute infections of the respiratory tract is extremely broad and ranges from extremely common, mild infections that almost all humans have experienced (viral infections) to rare, life-threatening etiologies (e.g., *Pneumocystis, Aspergillus*). As with most infectious diseases, developing the differential diagnosis for pulmonary infections requires a thorough understanding of the patient's epidemiology and risk factors (health care exposure, prior antibiotic exposure, structural lung disease, etc.), as well as local geographic epidemiology (endemic mycoses, areas where TB is endemic, etc.).

In general, the diagnosis of pneumonia is based on symptoms (fever, cough, sputum production, dyspnea, chest pain) and signs (fever, tachypnea, hypoxemia, rales, egophony) in combination with a new pulmonary infiltrate on chest imaging (typically CXR or sometimes CT chest).

Differential Diagnosis for Pneumonia

Immunocompetent, Community-acquired	Immunocompetent, Health Care–associated	Immunocompromised (in addition to other etiologies already listed)

More Common
Bacterial (typical)
✗Streptococcus pneumoniae
  Staphylococcus aureus
  Klebsiella spp.
  Haemophilus influenzae
  Anaerobes (aspiration)
Bacterial (atypical)
  Legionella pneumophila
  Mycoplasma pneumoniae
  Chlamydophila pneumoniae
Viral
  Rhinovirus
  Influenza
  RSV
  SARS-CoV-2
Less Common
Fungal
  Coccidioides
  Histoplasma
  Blastomyces
Mycobacterium tuberculosis (TB)
	Most Common
	Bacterial
	- Staphylococcus aureus (MRSA)✱
	- Pseudomonas aeruginosa✦
	- Klebsiella spp.
	- Escherichia coli
	- Acinetobacter spp.
	- Enterobacter spp.
		Bacteria
		- Nocardia
		Fungal
		- Aspergillus
		- Pneumocystis jirovecii
		- Cryptococcus

Categorizing patients by their general immune status and by the setting in which they developed pneumonia can greatly aid in narrowing the differential diagnosis. The first distinction to be made is between immunocompetent and immuno-compromised (e.g., HIV/AIDS, transplant patients) hosts, as the latter group can be infected with opportunistic pathogens in addition to more common causes. A second important differentiation is between community-acquired infection and health care–associated/hospital-acquired infection because the microbiologic epidemiology is quite different. Community-acquired pneumonia is most likely due to *Streptococcus pneumoniae*, atypical pathogens such as *Mycoplasma*, and common viruses (RSV, *Influenza*). Health care–associated or hospital-acquired infections are more likely to be due to resistant bacterial pathogens such as methicillin-resistant *Staphylococcus aureus* (MRSA), *Pseudomonas*, and other drug-resistant gram negatives.

Key Findings and Lung Infection and Pathogen Differential Diagnosis

Fever and Cough with Key Associated Findings	Diagnoses and Pathogens
Alcohol-dependent patient	Anaerobes (aspiration pneumonia) or *Klebsiella pneumoniae*
Recent *Influenza* infection	*Staphylococcus aureus*
Pneumonia develops while patient is hospitalized or on the ventilator.	Typical bacterial pneumonia (e.g., *Staphylococcus aureus*), resistant bacterial pathogens (e.g., MRSA, *Pseudomonas*, or other drug-resistant gram negatives)
Cystic fibrosis, bronchiectasis	*Pseudomonas aeruginosa*
- Exposure to water source (air conditioner, etc.) - Hyponatremia, diarrhea, and pneumonia	*Legionella pneumophila*
Rash and pneumonia	*Mycoplasma pneumoniae* or blastomycosis
Erythema multiforme, bullous myringitis (inflammation of tympanic membrane)	*Mycoplasma pneumoniae*
Pulse–temperature dissociation (high fever without much change in pulse)	Atypical pathogens (*Mycoplasma, Legionella, Chlamydia*)
Subacute (prolonged) symptoms	Atypical pathogens, fungal, or TB
HIV/AIDS (CD4 <200)	Typical bacterial pneumonia, *Pneumocystis jirovecii* pneumonia (PJP), or TB

(continued)

Key Findings and Lung Infection and Pathogen Differential Diagnosis (*continued*)

Fever and Cough with Key Associated Findings	Diagnoses and Pathogens
- Stem cell or organ transplant recipients - Leukemia/lymphoma	Typical bacterial pneumonia, fungal infections (e.g., *Aspergillus fumigatus*), or rare bacterial pathogens (e.g., *Nocardia*)
Travel to Southwestern United States, California	Coccidioidomycosis
Mississippi or Ohio River Valley travel	Histoplasmosis or blastomycosis
- Squamous cell carcinoma type skin lesion - Travel to Central and Eastern United States	Blastomycosis
Travel to Latin America	Paracoccidioidomycosis
Bird exposure	Psittacosis, histoplasmosis, or *Cryptococcus neoformans*
New regurgitant heart murmur	Pulmonary septic emboli from endocarditis (*S. aureus* most common)

CASE 6 | Community-Acquired Pneumonia (*Streptococcus Pneumoniae*)

A 71-year-old man with a history of hypertension presents with 1 day of fever, dyspnea, pleuritic chest pain, and productive cough. He says he felt "well one minute and sick the next." No sick contacts or travel reported. On exam, the patient has a temperature of 39.7°C, pulse 110/min, respirations 24/min, blood pressure 90/60 mmHg, and oxygen saturation 90% on room air. He appears ill, and crackles are auscultated posteriorly over the lower right lung field. Dullness to percussion and egophony are noted over the left lower lobe. No rashes are seen.

Evaluation/Tests	Chest X-ray shows right lower lobe consolidation. Sputum Gram stain reveals gram positive, lancet-shaped diplococci that are sensitive to optochin. Blood cultures pending. 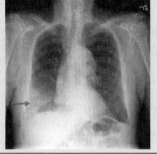 Lobar pneumonia caused by Streptococcus pneumoniae. Arrow points to area of consolidation in right lung. Reproduced with permission from McKean SC, Ross JJ, Dressler DD, et al. Principles and Practice of Hospital Medicine, 2nd ed. New York, NY: McGraw Hill; 2017.
Treatment	Hospitalize the patient and treat him with ceftriaxone and azithromycin or doxycycline and oxygen (outpatient treatment in less severe presentations: amoxicillin or doxycycline).
Discussion	**Community-acquired pneumonia (CAP) secondary to *Streptococcus pneumoniae*** presents with relatively rapid onset with severe symptoms (hypotension, toxic appearing). In adults, *S. pneumoniae* is the most common pathogen in lobar pneumonias; other common bacterial pathogens include *Legionella* and *Klebsiella*. *S. pneumoniae* is a gram positive lancet-shaped, encapsulated diplococcus. It is the most common cause of CAP, meningitis, otitis media in children, and sinusitis. Pneumococcal pneumonia is associated with a productive "rusty" sputum, and patients with sickle cell disease or asplenia are at increased risk of sepsis. Consolidation seen on CXR may involve an entire lobe or the whole lung. The natural history of lobar pneumonia involves congestion, red hepatization, gray hepatization, and resolution of the infection, which occurs on average about 8 or more days. *S. aureus*, *H. influenzae*, *Klebsiella*, and *Moraxella catarrhalis* can also cause bronchopneumonia. CXR may show patchy distribution involving >1 lobe. *Mycoplasma*, *Chlamydophila pneumoniae*, *Chlamydophila psittaci*, *Legionella*, and viruses such as influenza, adenovirus, RSV, or CMV may cause interstitial or atypical pneumonias (also called "walking pneumonia") and CXR may show diffuse patchy infiltrates in interstitial areas. ***Legionella pneumophila*** typically infects following exposure to a water source and can present with pulse–temperature dissociation. *Legionella* urine antigen testing can assist in diagnosis. ***Mycoplasma pneumoniae*** typically causes more diffuse, interstitial infiltrates and a more subacute course. Sputum Gram stain and culture may be helpful in guiding therapy, especially in patients with severe illness that necessitate hospitalization (e.g., patients presenting with concerning vital signs such as tachypnea, tachycardia, and hypoxia).

CASE 6 | Community-Acquired Pneumonia (*Streptococcus Pneumoniae*) *(continued)*

Additional Considerations	Community acquired pneumonia (CAP) secondary to **SARS-CoV-2 (COVID-19)** presents with a prodromal syndrome that often includes fever, anosmia (loss of smell), GI symptoms (abdominal pain, diarrhea, anorexia), fatigue and myalgias. Majority of patients (~80%) will recover and never develop pneumonia or severe disease. For those who do develop progressive disease, symptoms of lower respiratory tract infection (dyspnea and cough) occur about a week into the illness. The diagnosis is made if a patient with clinically compatible syndrome tests positive for SARS-CoV-2 by PCR (or by an antigen test) performed on a nasal or nasopharyngeal specimen. Patients typically have diffuse, bilateral opacities on CXR and significant hypoxemia. CT chest would reveal bilateral ground-glass opacities. Laboratory work-up will often reveal lymphopenia and elevated inflammatory markers (ferritin, d-dimer, C-reactive protein, LDH). Treatment for hospitalized patients requiring oxygen consists of antiviral therapy to stop viral replication (remdesivir) and anti-inflammatory therapy to control the dysregulated inflammatory response the virus induces (dexamethasone).

CASE 7 | Hospital-Acquired Pneumonia (*Pseudomonas Aeruginosa*)

A 75-year-old man with a history of congestive heart failure presents with increased dyspnea, dry cough, and lower extremity swelling and is admitted for decompensated heart failure. He is started on IV diuretics and initially improves. On hospital day 3, his dyspnea worsens, and his cough becomes productive of sputum. On exam he has a temperature of 39.5°C, pulse 110/min, respirations 24/min, and blood pressure 95/60 mmHg. His oxygen saturation is 93% on 3 L of oxygen via nasal cannula. Crackles are noted in the left posterior lung base. No lower extremity edema or jugular venous distension is noted.

Evaluation/Tests	Left lower lobe consolidation noted on chest X-ray. Sputum culture is positive for a motile, oxidase positive, gram negative rod.
Treatment	Given the initial chest X-ray findings, empiric antibiotics for MRSA (vancomycin) and *Pseudomonas* (antipseudomonal β-lactams such as piperacillin-tazobactam or cefepime). Once *Pseudomonas* is confirmed from culture, antibiotic coverage should be narrowed.
Discussion	The patient has a **hospital-acquired pneumonia** (pneumonia that developed >48 hours after admission) with gram negative rods seen on sputum culture, which is highly suggestive of pneumonia caused by the bacterium ***Pseudomonas aeruginosa***. The two most common pathogens to cause hospital-acquired pneumonia are MRSA and *Pseudomonas*. *P. aeruginosa* is an aerobic, motile, gram negative rod that is oxidase positive and nonlactose fermenting with a thick mucoid polysaccharide capsule. In culture, it gives off a characteristic grape-like odor and produces blue-green pigments pyoverdine and pyocyanin, which can be used to generate reactive oxygen species. Two important virulence factors are exotoxin A (which inactivates the EF-2 translation elongation factor via ADP ribosylation) and phospholipase C (degrades cell membranes). Since it is a gram negative bacterium, it also produces the endotoxin lipopolysaccharide that can lead to fever and shock. Classic *Pseudomonas* presentations are often nosocomial or hospital acquired, but additional presentations include ecthyma gangrenosum, otitis externa, urinary tract infections, and skin infections (hot tub folliculitis or wound infections in burn victims). Patients with a typical community-acquired bacterial pneumonia usually have acute findings and a sudden deterioration, while **aspiration pneumonia** is usually anaerobic and will likely be more chronic. For aspiration pneumonia, patients will likely have risk factors such as alcoholism, seizures, or disorders that can alter their gag reflex or mentation.

CASE 8 | Pulmonary Tuberculosis

A 64-year-old man with hypertension and type 2 diabetes presents with six weeks of fever, night sweats, weight loss, and productive cough. He was born in Mexico and moved to Chicago 10 years ago. He has no history of IV drug or tobacco use. He denies recent sick contacts or animal exposure. On exam, the patient has a temperature of 38.6°C, pulse 95/min, respirations 22/min, and blood pressure 107/81 mmHg, with oxygen saturation 93% on room air. Pulmonary auscultation reveals coarse crackles in the right upper lobe posteriorly and increased tactile fremitus.

Evaluation/Tests	Chest X-ray shows a cavitary lesion in the left upper lobe and hilar lymphadenopathy. Sputum culture with acid-fast (Ziehl-Neelsen) stain is positive for acid-fast bacilli.

CASE 8 | Pulmonary Tuberculosis *(continued)*

Treatment	First-line treatment for TB involves four drugs: rifampin, isoniazid, pyrazinamide, and ethambutol (RIPE). Treatment is for at least 6 months.
Discussion	The patient has classic **pulmonary tuberculosis (TB)** symptoms and is from an endemic area. He has a subacute presentation (6 weeks of symptoms) of fever, cough, night sweats, and weight loss (constitutional symptoms). Other risk factors in patients who have not immigrated from endemic areas include homelessness, incarceration, health care work, and HIV/AIDS. Pulmonary tuberculosis can present in several ways. Initial infection (primary tuberculosis) presents with classic TB symptoms in addition to development of ipsilateral hilar adenopathy and a middle or lower lobe lesion known as a Ghon complex. Most cases, if untreated, will develop latent TB, during which the patient is asymptomatic and no longer contagious. Latent TB is diagnosed if an asymptomatic individual has a positive result on the tuberculin skin test or the interferon-γ release assay. Chest X-ray is subsequently ordered to rule out active infection, at which point patients with latent TB can be treated with isoniazid (9 months), rifampin (4 months), or combined isoniazid and rifapentine (3 months). Reactivation of TB can occur (secondary tuberculosis), and this results in formation of a fibrocaseous cavitary lesion often within the upper lobes, as is seen in this patient. Secondary TB can lead to localized destruction with caseation and scar formation. Rarely, primary or secondary tuberculosis can cause progressive lung disease or bacteremia, which can lead to miliary TB with extrapulmonary manifestations. This progressive form of TB is more common in immunocompromised patients with HIV/AIDS or malnutrition. Other complications of TB include **tuberculous spondylitis (Pott disease)**. Endemic fungal infections such as histoplasmosis and blastomycosis can present in a similar fashion to TB. **Histoplasmosis** is more commonly seen in individuals living in the Ohio and Mississippi River Valley regions. Histoplasmosis is usually transmitted in bird and bat droppings, so it is important to ask about the patient's hobbies such as spelunking. On microscopy, histoplasmosis can be found within macrophages. **Blastomycosis** is more commonly seen in Eastern and Central United States and can form granulomatous nodules and cause verrucous skin lesions when spread. On microscopy, broad-based buds can be seen. **Anaerobic lung infections** typically are subacute as well, but patients would have risk factors such as poor dentition, seizure history, or gag reflex abnormalities.

CASE 9 | *Pneumocystis Jiroveci* Pneumonia (PJP)

A 28-year-old woman with HIV who is not adherent to therapy presents with 3 weeks of fever, dyspnea, and dry cough. She denies night sweats, weight loss, history of IV drug use, homelessness, incarceration, or recent travel. On exam, the patient has a temperature of 38.7°C, pulse 100/min, respirations 22/min, blood pressure 110/70 mmHg, and oxygen saturation 88% on room air. Faint crackles are appreciated bilaterally on pulmonary auscultation.

Evaluation/Tests	CD4+ T-cell count is 136 cells/mm^3, serum lactate dehydrogenase is elevated. Chest X-ray reveals bilateral diffuse pulmonary infiltrates and ground-glass opacities distributed in a "bat-wing" pattern. Bronchoscopy with bronchoalveolar lavage (BAL) reveals a disc-shaped yeast on Gomori methenamine silver stain. PJP direct-fluorescent antibody (DFA) is positive on the BAL fluid.
Treatment	Since PJP is confirmed, trimethoprim-sulfamethoxazole (TMP-SMX) is the first line. Alternative agents include pentamidine and atovaquone. Steroids should be added for severe PJP with hypoxemia.
Discussion	***Pneumocystis jirovecii* pneumonia (PJP)** presents as a subacute pneumonia with bilateral pulmonary infiltrates on chest X-ray in the setting of AIDS. *Pneumocystis jirovecci*, formerly known as *Pneumocystis carinii* (hence the commonly used acronym PCP), was originally classified as a protozoan but is in fact a yeast-like fungus. PJP is an opportunistic infection seen in immunocompromised patients, typically in HIV/AIDS patients with a CD4+ cell count <200 cells/mm^3. Once a patient's CD4+ count drops below 200, PJP prophylaxis should be initiated with TMP-SMX. Dapsone may also be used for prophylaxis in certain patients. **Tuberculosis** and other **fungal infections** such as aspergillosis typically have a more prolonged clinical course and present with cavitary lung disease rather than interstitial infiltrates. **Aspergillosis** is typically seen in patients with CD4 <100 cells/mm^3. **CMV pneumonitis** would present with ground glass opacities and pleural effusion on chest X-ray and is typically seen in patients with CD4 <100 cells/mm^3.

CASE 10	Invasive Pulmonary Aspergillosis

A 44-year-old woman on chemotherapy for acute myeloid leukemia who underwent an allogeneic stem cell transplant 2 weeks ago develops fever and cough. Her cough was productive with evidence of hemoptysis. She was placed on vancomycin and cefepime, but her fevers persist for 72 hours. On exam, the patient has a temperature of 38.8°C, pulse 105/min, respirations 18/min, blood pressure 107/81 mmHg, and oxygen saturation 94% on room air. Some scattered crackles are noted on posterior lung fields. No rashes are noted.

Evaluation/Tests	CBC shows an absolute neutrophil count (ANC) of 0 cells/mm^3. Chest X-ray does not show obvious infiltrates. CT chest without contrast shows a cavitary lesion in the right middle lobe with nodular infiltrates and surrounding ground glass opacities (halo sign). Serum galactomannan and 1,3-β-D-glucan are positive. Bronchoalveolar lavage reveals monomorphic, septate hyphae that branch at 45° angles.
Treatment	Voriconazole is the drug of choice for invasive aspergillosis. In neutropenic fever, antibacterial coverage is also continued until the fevers and neutropenia resolve.
Discussion	**Invasive pulmonary aspergillosis (IPA)** is caused by *Aspergillus fumigatus*, which is a ubiquitous, airborne saprophytic fungus; IPA typically occurs in immunocompromised patients, especially in those with neutropenia or individuals with chronic granulomatous disease with neutrophil dysfunction. Biopsy demonstrating tissue invasion with aspergillus is the gold standard for diagnosis but is often difficult to obtain. Thus diagnosis relies on imaging and culture/antigen testing. Serum galactomannan and 1,3-β-D-glucan, when positive, are nonspecific signs of fungal infection. *Aspergillus* has a characteristic morphology with acute-angle septate hyphae and conidiospores that may have a "broom-like" appearance when grown in culture. *Aspergillus* also has a tendency to invade vasculature, which can lead to widespread disease and to manifestations such as hemoptysis from pulmonary blood vessel invasion. Other clinical manifestations of aspergillosis include **aspergillomas**, which typically form in preexisting lung cavities such as from a prior tuberculosis infection. The differential diagnosis for pneumonia in immunocompromised patients is broad. Persistence of fever despite broad-spectrum antibiotics suggests fungal or viral etiology. In addition to *Aspergillus*, neutropenic patients are at risk for PJP, mucormycosis, etc. **PJP** would have bilateral infiltrates that are more likely ground glass opacities. **Mucormycosis** typically presents in a rhinocerebral pattern with frontal lobe abscess, cavernous sinus thrombosis, and necrotic black eschar on the face. **Nocardiosis** also can cause pneumonia and brain abscesses (lung-brain syndrome).
Additional Considerations	**Allergic bronchopulmonary aspergillosis (ABPA)**, a hypersensitivity response to *Aspergillus*, presents with wheezing, fever, eosinophilia, and bronchiectasis, classically in patients with asthma or cystic fibrosis. Susceptible individuals develop an abnormal T-lymphocyte cellular immune response to *A. fumigatus*, which results in activation of the complement cascade that leads to inflammation. Damage can progress to bronchiectasis, pulmonary cavities, focal emphysema, and fibrosis. Patients will usually have peripheral eosinophilia, elevated *Aspergillus*-specific IgG antibodies, high total serum IgE, and positive immediate and delayed skin reactions to *Aspergillus* antigens. On CXR, fleeting parenchymal opacities that respond to corticosteroids are typical. End-stage ABPA will manifest with cavitation and fibrosis.

FEVER AND NIGHT SWEATS

Night sweats are a very common outpatient complaint. For the purposes of this discussion, this will be defined as drenching sweats (requiring changing of clothes). In clinical practice, many patients will have "night sweats" if asked, but on further questioning few actually have drenching sweats. More often, patients have some mild–moderate sweating at night due to their room being too hot, for example. Flushing—warmth and redness of the face and/or body—can be associated with sweating and is difficult to cleanly distinguish from night sweats clinically. We will thus include notable causes of flushing in this discussion as well. If the patient also has fever, then the differential shrinks considerably, and many of the potential diagnoses can be quite consequential and need to be effectively worked up. Obtaining additional history related to symptoms that suggest a specific disease—unintentional weight loss, cough, enlarged lymph nodes, localized pain—is very important to guide the laboratory and imaging evaluation.

The following are some of the key diagnoses.

Differential Diagnosis for Night Sweats

Infections	Malignancy	Other

Mycobacteria
  Tuberculosis
  Nontuberculous mycobacteria
Bacterial
  Brucellosis
  Subacute bacterial endocarditis
  Osteomyelitis
Fungal
  Blastomycosis
  Histoplasmosis
  Coccidioidomycosis
Viral
  HIV
	Lymphoma
	  Hodgkin's lymphoma
	  Non-Hodgkin's lymphoma
	Solid Tumors
	  Prostate cancer
	  Renal cell cancer
	  Germ cell tumors
		Endocrine
		  Carcinoid tumors (flushing)
		  Hyperthyroidism
		  Pheochromocytoma
		Menopause
		Medications
		  Antidepressants
		  Cholinergics

Malignancy and infections are the most serious broad categories of diagnoses that can present as night sweats. Among malignancies, lymphoma is the most likely to cause night sweats and is the most important etiology to remember even though some solid tumors cause night sweats as well, though rarely (e.g., renal cell carcinoma). In fact, night sweats are one of the constitutional or "B" symptoms seen in Hodgkin's lymphoma. Tuberculosis is the infection most associated with night sweats; therefore, a thorough history related to TB symptoms (cough, weight loss, fever) and TB risk factors (travel, homelessness, incarceration, etc.) should be obtained. Endemic fungi such as histoplasmosis, blastomycosis, coccidioidomycosis, or paracoccidioidomycosis can mimic TB clinically but are limited to certain geographic regions. The acute retroviral syndrome caused by new HIV infection includes symptoms of fever, diarrhea, rash, headache, and night sweats as well; it should be on the differential, especially in young, sexually active patients. Causes of symptoms difficult to distinguish from night sweats (such as flushing) should be considered as well.

Key Associated Findings and Night Sweats Differential Diagnosis

Fever and Night Sweats with Key Associated Findings	Diagnoses
Travel to developing world, homelessness, incarceration, health care worker - Lung exam with rales (crackles), especially upper lobe	Tuberculosis
Sexually active, IVDU	Acute HIV infection
Lymphadenopathy	Lymphoma, TB, or acute HIV
Valvular heart disease, history of rheumatic fever, poor dentition - Heart murmur, Osler nodes, Janeway lesions, splinter hemorrhages, Roth spots, conjunctival petechiae	Subacute bacterial endocarditis
Chronic lung disease, bronchiectasis	Nontuberculosis mycobacteria such as *M. avium-intracellulare* (MAI)
HIV/AIDS and other immunocompromised hosts	TB, disseminated MAI, disseminated histoplasmosis, or non-Hodgkin's lymphoma
Hypercalcemia (increased vitamin D 1,25)	Lymphoma
Animal exposure (sheep, cattle, goats), unpasteurized milk and cheese consumption	Brucellosis (*Brucella* (rare cause of endocarditis))
- Eastern and Central United States, Great Lakes region - Rales (crackles), especially upper lobe	Blastomycosis
Mississippi and Ohio River Valleys (overlap with blastomycosis)	Histoplasmosis
Southwestern United States, California	Coccidioidomycosis
Central and South America	Paracoccidioidomycosis
Wheezing	Carcinoid syndrome
Severe hypertension	Pheochromocytoma
Splenomegaly	Lymphoma (most likely), disseminated TB, or fungal disease
Exophthalmos, hair thinning, tremor	Hyperthyroidism (Grave's disease)

CASE 11 | Subacute Bacterial Endocarditis (*Streptococcal*)

A 45-year-old woman with mitral valve prolapse presents with fevers, sweats, decreased appetite, weight loss, malaise, and arthralgias for 2 weeks. She recently had dental work for an infected dental implant. On exam, she appears ill, and her vital signs are temperature 38.4°C, pulse 110/min, blood pressure 90/60 mmHg, RR 22, and SpO2 98% on room air. Fundoscopic exam shows round white spots surrounded by hemorrhage (Roth spots). A systolic murmur is heard at the cardiac apex. There are several tender, raised lesions on her finger and toe pads (Osler nodes); small, nontender, erythematous lesions on palms and soles (Janeway lesions); and the nail beds have splinter hemorrhages.

Evaluation/Tests	Echocardiography shows an echogenic, mobile mass on the mitral valve (vegetation). WBCs, ESR, and CRP are elevated. Two out of two blood cultures reveal gram positive, α-hemolytic, optochin-resistant cocci.
Treatment	Prolonged IV antibiotics with an agent such as ceftriaxone. If the valve is seriously damaged (resulting in heart failure or embolism), valve replacement should be considered.
Discussion	The patient has a classic presentation of **subacute bacterial endocarditis**. She has night sweats and fever in the setting of a new heart murmur along with positive blood cultures and mobile vegetations on echocardiogram. She has underlying valvular heart disease, a recent dental procedure, and gradual onset of symptoms. Viridans group *Streptococci* are part of the normal flora of the oropharynx, but they can enter the bloodstream and infect patients with underlying damaged heart valves during dental procedures. Species within this group include *Streptococcus mutans, S. mitis,* and *S. sanguinis*. Diagnosis of bacterial endocarditis is done via the modified Duke major and minor criteria. Major criteria include (1) multiple positive blood cultures with a typical endocarditis-causing organism and (2) echocardiogram showing vegetations, abscess, and new regurgitation of a native or prosthetic valve or new dehiscence of a prosthetic valve. Minor criteria include (1) history of IV drug use or predisposing valvular disease; (2) fever >38°C; (3) vascular phenomena including Osler nodes, painful red lesions found on hands and feet due to immune complex deposition; (4) embolic phenomena including Roth spots on retina, painless Janeway lesions on palms or soles, due to septic emboli; (5) blood culture suggestive of endocarditis but not meeting the preceding criteria. Endocarditis is diagnosed with 2 major criteria, 1 major and 3 minor, or 5 minor criteria. **Acute bacterial endocarditis** has a much more rapid onset, involves large vegetations on previously normal hearts, and is most commonly caused by *S. aureus*. Patients with a history of IVDU may present with tricuspid valve endocarditis because this is the first valve encountered in the heart by bacteria traveling in the bloodstream. Other causes of tricuspid valve endocarditis in the setting of IVDU include *Pseudomonas* and *Candida*. Blood cultures that are positive for *Streptococcus bovis* (*gallolyticus*) will require evaluation for underlying colon cancer. Lastly, patients with prosthetic valves are vulnerable to endocarditis from coagulase-negative species such as *Staphylococcus epidermidis*. **Nonbacterial endocarditis**, also called marantic or thrombotic endocarditis, can be seen secondary to underlying malignancy, hypercoagulable states, or lupus. High-grade **bacteremia** or **fungemia** may also have similar features without valve involvement.

Potential Clues to Etiology of Endocarditis

History of	Potential organism(s)
Dental procedures	Viridans group *Streptococcus*
Colon cancer	*S. bovis*
GI/GU procedure	*Enterococcus*
Prosthetic valves	*S. epidermidis*
IV drug use	*S. aureus, Pseudomonas, Candida albicans*
Negative cultures	*Coxiella burnetti, Bartonella,* HACEK (*Haemophilus, Aggregatibacter, Cardiobacterium, Eikenella, Kingella*)
SLE, metastatic cancer, hypercoagulable states	Consider noninfectious endocarditis

FEVER AND ARTHRITIS

Fever and arthritis can be due to a variety of infectious and noninfectious conditions, and they can affect one joint (monoarticular) or multiple joints (polyarticular). Determining the duration of symptoms (acute vs. chronic) can help to risk-stratify the patient and narrow the differential diagnosis. The most urgent and important monoarticular diagnosis to make is septic arthritis (acute bacterial arthritis). Bacterial septic arthritis is both joint threatening and potentially life-threatening and can be mimicked by noninfectious causes such as gout making accurate workup and diagnosis paramount. Interestingly, a sizable percentage of patients with true septic arthritis may lack fever (about 50%), but if present, fever should raise suspicion. Arthrocentesis and synovial fluid analysis are the primary means of discerning the etiology of a joint with arthritis; in general, the following patterns of cell count and differential are useful for making a diagnosis.

Differential Diagnosis for Arthritis Based on Arthrocentesis and Synovial Fluid Analysis

Measure	Normal	Inflammatory (gout, etc.)	Septic (bacterial)
Color	Clear/transparent	Yellow/opaque	Yellow/opaque
WBC	<200	>2000	>50,000
PMNs (%)	<25	>50%	>75%
Culture	Negative	Negative	Positive
Crystals	Negative	Positive (uric acid, CPPD)	Negative

Fever and Arthritis Differential Diagnosis

Acute Monoarticular Arthritis	Chronic Monoarticular	Polyarticular arthritis
Bacterial	Bacterial	Bacterial
Staphylococcus aureus	Lyme	Lyme disease
Gonococcal	Fungal	– Disseminated gonococcal disease
Streptococcus spp.	Blastomycosis	Viral
Crystal-induced arthropathy	Histoplasmosis	Parvovirus
Gout	Coccidioides	Chikungunya
Pseudogout	Candida	Autoimmune disease
Autoimmune disease	Tuberculosis	Rheumatoid arthritis
Psoriatic arthritis		Reactive arthritis
Inflammatory bowel disease		

Common findings present in patients with an inflammatory or infective arthritis are pain, swelling, warmth, redness, and reduced range of motion of the affected joint(s). The first key to delineate the patient's diagnosis is defining the number of joints involved.

Monoarticular arthritis is much more likely to be secondary to a typical bacterial pathogen (most commonly *S. aureus*) than polyarthritis. In young, sexually active patients with monoarticular arthritis, gonococcal arthritis should be suspected. Due to improved diagnosis and treatment of gonorrhea urethritis, the incidence of gonococcal arthritis is decreasing. The main noninfectious causes of monoarticular arthritis are gout and pseudogout, and, in fact, they are much more common than septic arthritis. However, the presence of gout or another inflammatory condition in a joint does not rule out septic arthritis, and it puts the patient at higher risk of infection.

Chronic monoarticular arthritis is more likely to be due to less virulent pathogens such as fungi or TB. Polyarthritis is much more likely to result from viral pathogens or noninfectious causes, including rheumatoid arthritis or reactive arthritis (arthritis, conjunctivitis, urethritis).

Key Findings and Fever and Arthritis Differential Diagnosis

Fever and Arthritis with Key Associated Findings	Diagnoses
Multiple, symmetric small joint arthritis	Rheumatoid arthritis
- Metabolic syndrome, obesity, alcohol use - Arthritis of the 1st metatarsophalangeal joint (MTP)	Gout
Young, sexually active, monoarticular arthritis	Gonorrhea
Triad of tenosynovitis, rash (pustular/necrotic), polyarthralgia	Disseminated gonococcal infection

(continued)

Key Findings and Fever and Arthritis Differential Diagnosis (*continued*)

Fever and Arthritis with Key Associated Findings	Diagnoses
Recent diarrheal illness or STI	Reactive arthritis (e.g., *Campylobacter* or *Chlamydia*)
- Exposure to sick child - Lacy, reticular rash	Parvovirus
Homeless, incarcerated, travel to developing world	Tuberculosis
- IVDU - New regurgitant heart murmur	Septic arthritis secondary to endocarditis (*Staphylococcus aureus* most common), *Candida albicans*, *Pseudomonas*
Prosthetic joint	*S. aureus*, other gram positives (e.g., *Propionibacterium acnes*, coagulase-negative staphylococci such as *S. epidermidis*), as well as gram negatives if the infection occurs postoperatively
- History of erythema migrans ("bulls-eye" rash) - Northeast United States or Wisconsin/tick exposure	Lyme disease (*Borrelia burgdorferi*)
Travel to the Southwestern United States	Coccidioidomycosis
Mississippi or Ohio River Valley travel	Histoplasmosis or blastomycosis
Central or Eastern United States	Blastomycosis
Travel to Caribbean country, mosquito bite	Tropical diseases such as Chikungunya or Dengue virus

---

CASE 12 | Septic Arthritis (*Staphylococcus Aureus*)

A 65-year-old man with type 2 diabetes presents with right knee pain, swelling, redness, and difficulty walking for 2 days. He has no history of arthritis, gout, IVDU, or recent sexual activity. On exam, he has a temperature of 38.5°C, pulse 110/min, respirations 18/min, and blood pressure 128/78 mmHg. His right knee is edematous, warm, erythematous, and he has restricted active and passive range of motion.

Evaluation/tests	Arthrocentesis reveals yellow-opaque, cloudy synovial fluid with low viscosity, 150,000/mm³ WBCs (85% PMNs). Gram stain of the fluid reveals gram positive, catalase positive, coagulase positive cocci in clusters. Negative for crystals. Synovial fluid and blood cultures pending.
Treatment	Drain knee fluid, and start empiric antibiotics. Include MRSA coverage (vancomycin).
Discussion	**Septic arthritis** presents with acute monoarticular arthritis and synovial fluid analysis showing high WBC count, positive Gram stain, and no crystals. Findings on Gram stain in this case (gram positive cocci in clusters) are highly suggestive of **Staphylococcus aureus** as the causative pathogen. *S. aureus* is a gram positive, β-hemolytic organism with several virulence factors and clinical manifestations. It normally colonizes the nares, ears, axilla, and groin. Protein A is used by the bacteria to bind Fc-IgG and therefore inhibit complement activation and phagocytosis. Beyond septic arthritis, *S. aureus* can cause numerous other diseases including skin infections, organ abscesses, pneumonia, endocarditis, osteomyelitis, toxic shock syndrome, food poisoning, and scalded skin syndrome. Methicillin resistant *S. aureus* (MRSA) is an important cause of both nosocomial and community-acquired infections. Other pathogens that commonly cause septic arthritis include *Streptococcus* spp. and *Neisseria gonorrhoeae*. **Gout** or **pseudogout** could present this way, but gout would present with needle-like crystals in the knee aspirate, and pseudogout would present with rhomboid-shaped crystals in the synovial fluid.

CASE 13 | Disseminated Gonococcal Infection

A 28-year-old woman presents to clinic with right wrist, left wrist, and left ankle swelling for 3 days. She also has pain when she moves her fingers, and she has noticed some "spots" on her hands and feet. She is sexually active with multiple male partners and intermittently uses condoms. She has no history of IVDU. She denies dysuria, vaginal discharge, recent illnesses, sick contacts, or recent travel. She resides in Texas. On exam, she has a temperature of 38.2°C, pulse 100/min, respirations 16/min, and blood pressure 110/70 mmHg. Mild swelling, warmth, redness, and reduced active range of motion are noted in both wrists and her left ankle. She has pustules on her hands and feet. She has pain with flexion of her fingers and tenderness over flexor tendons bilaterally.

CASE 13 | Disseminated Gonococcal Infection (*continued*)

Evaluation/Tests	Arthrocentesis reveals a clear yellow synovial fluid with low viscosity, 10,000/mm³ WBCs (65% PMNs), and Gram stain reveals gram negative intracellular diplococci. Synovial fluid and blood cultures are pending, but urine nucleic acid amplification tests for *Neisseria gonorrhoreae* are positive.
Treatment	Ceftriaxone and appropriate drainage of the septic joint.
Discussion	**Disseminated gonococcal infection (DGI)** presents with the triad of tenosynovitis (pain/inflammation insertion sites), dermatitis, and polyarthralgias in a sexually active patient. The causative pathogen is *Neisseria gonorrhoeae,* a gram negative diplococcus that is often found intracellularly inside neutrophils. *N. gonorrhoeae* lacks a polysaccharide, metabolizes glucose but not maltose (vs. *N. meningitidis,* which metabolizes both), and is transmitted sexually or perinatally. Positive blood culture or synovial fluid culture confirms the diagnosis, and urine NAAT supports it. In addition to disseminated gonococcal infection and septic arthritis, infection with *N. gonorrhoeae* can cause urethritis, neonatal conjunctivitis, pelvic inflammatory disease, and Fitz-Hugh-Curtis syndrome.
	Reactive arthritis presents with a triad of urethritis, arthritis, and conjunctivitis ("can't see, can't pee, can't bend my knee"). This clinical syndrome has a strong association with HLA-B27. Given this patient's lack of urethritis and conjunctivitis, this diagnosis is unlikely. Furthermore, reactive arthritis is more often seen after *Shigella, Yersinia, Chlamydia, Campylobacter,* and *Salmonella* infections.
	Lyme disease, caused by the spirochete *Borrelia burgdorferi* and transmitted by the *Ixodes* deer tick, can cause migratory myalgias and transient arthralgias in its early disseminated stage and chronic arthritis in its late disseminated stage. The lack of other symptoms in this patient (erythema migrans, flu-like symptoms, facial nerve palsy, cardiac abnormalities, etc.) and geographical location make this less likely. Lyme disease is highly endemic to the Northeastern United States.
	Parvovirus can also present with rash and polyarthritis, but the rash has a lacy-reticular pattern.

FEVER AND SORE THROAT

Sore throat is common in outpatient medicine and may or may not be accompanied by fever. This discussion will focus on the causes of fever and acute-onset sore throat. Almost all of these result from a viral (most commonly) or bacterial pathogens. Note that many viruses cause a sore throat, but we will focus on the most common viruses that present with this complaint.

Differential Diagnosis for Fever and Sore Throat

Viral	Bacterial

Pharyngitis
    Adenovirus
    EBV (causing mononucleosis)
    Coxsackievirus (causing herpangina and hand-foot-mouth disease)
    Influenza
	Pharyngitis
	    Streptococcus pyogenes
	    Corynebacterium diphtheriae
	    Chlamydia trachomatis
	    Neisseria gonorrhoeae
	Epiglottitis
	    Haemophilus influenzae B
	Retropharyngeal abscess (mixed aerobes and anaerobes)
	    Group A *Streptococcus pyogenes*
	    Staphylococcus aureus
	    Fusobacterium
	    Haemophilus
	Peritonsillar abscess (mixed aerobes and anaerobes)
	    Group A *Streptococcus pyogenes*
	    Staphylococcus aureus
	    Streptococcus pneumoniae
	    Haemophilus

Although pharyngitis can be caused by many viruses and bacteria, these viruses also tend to cause systemic symptoms or are associated with other illnesses (e.g., adenovirus: pharyngitis with conjunctivitis or pneumonia; EBV: sore throat, malaise, myalgias). It is important to remember that adenovirus-induced pharyngitis is similar to streptococcal pharyngitis on clinical presentation and examination. Coxsackievirus is responsible for two distinct clinical entities that can cause sore throat and fever: (1) herpangina, a febrile illness that causes papulovesicular lesions in the back of the throats of infants and young children and (2) hand-foot-mouth disease, characterized by low-grade fever, anterior tongue and buccal mucosa, and hand and foot lesions in children. Streptococcal pharyngitis in the setting of fever and sore throat can lead to devastating immunologic sequelae such as rheumatic fever or glomerulonephritis if left untreated. Finally, epiglottitis is uncommon but can be life-threatening and should always be considered in the differential for fever and sore throat.

Key Associated Findings and Sore Throat Differential Diagnosis

Fever and Sore Throat with Key Associated Findings	Diagnoses and Pathogens
- Conjunctivitis - School-age child	Adenovirus
- Tonsillar exudates in a school-age child - Scarlatiniform rash	Streptococcal pharyngitis (Strep throat)
- Pharyngitis, extreme fatigue - Posterior cervical lymphadenopathy, hepatosplenomegaly, atypical lymphocytosis - Teens to young adults	Infectious mononucleosis (EBV) ("kissing disease")
- Grayish-white membranes (pseudomembranes) in oropharynx; often with lymphadenopathy, myocarditis, arrhythmias - Airway obstruction - Unvaccinated patient from developing country or former Soviet Union	*Corynebacterium diphtheriae* aka diphtheria (obstruction of airway secondary to pseudomembranes)
- Drooling, difficulty breathing leading to respiratory distress - "Tripod" or "sniffing" posture, "cherry red" epiglottis - Unvaccinated patient	Epiglottitis (classically due to *Haemophilus influenza* type b)
Men who have sex with men, history of anogenital gonorrhea	Gonococcal pharyngitis
- Neck swelling, trismus - "Hot potato" voice	Peritonsillar abscess or retropharyngeal abscess

CASE 14 | Streptococcal Pharyngitis (Scarlet Fever)

An 8-year-old girl is brought to clinic for evaluation of fever and sore throat for 2 days. She has no cough. She also has a fine, lacy rash that began in the groin and spread to her trunk and extremities. She has had no recent travel and is up-to-date on her vaccinations. On exam, her temperature is 39.2°C, pulse is 112/min, respirations are 14/min, and blood pressure is 110/68 mmHg. She has white exudates on her tonsils bilaterally, and her posterior oropharynx is erythematous. Her anterior cervical lymph nodes are tender. She has a red, "sandpaper"-like rash on her trunk and extremities.

Evaluation/Tests	Rapid streptococcal antigen test is positive.
Treatment	Penicillin V or amoxicillin.
Discussion	This patient is presenting with **streptococcal pharyngitis**, a common infection seen in children 6–12 years old that also can occur across all ages. A clinical diagnosis can be established using the CENTOR criteria, which are fever, absence of cough, and presence of tender anterior cervical lymphadenopathy. Pain is rapid onset, and fever is typically greater than 38.3°C. This is caused by Group A *Streptococcal pyogenes*, a gram positive cocci in chains that is bacitracin sensitive, β-hemolytic, and pyrrodinoyl arylamidase (PYR) positive. In addition, this patient is experiencing **scarlet fever**, a syndrome seen in streptococcal pharyngitis in children that also presents with a blanching, sandpaper-like body rash, circumoral pallor, and a strawberry tongue. Scarlet fever is induced by the pyrogenic exotoxin secreted by *S. pyogenes*. The rash most commonly is found on the neck, armpits, and groin. As it is difficult to differentiate streptococcal pharyngitis from adenoviral pharyngitis, a throat culture or rapid streptococcal antigen test is usually employed. Note that antibiotic treatment is instituted to prevent noninfectious sequelae of streptococcal pharyngitis, such as rheumatic fever and glomerulonephritis, more than to speed up resolution of the febrile pharyngitis. These are immunologic reactions related to host antibody production to the streptococcal M protein, which shows molecular mimicry with proteins on heart valves in the context of rheumatic fever.

CASE 14 | Streptococcal Pharyngitis (Scarlet Fever) *(continued)*

Discussion	**Adenovirus** can cause fever and sore throat, but patients typically have a viral prodrome and other sick contacts. Conjunctivitis is also commonly seen in adenovirus infections.
	Diphtheria would be uncommon in someone who is up-to-date on their immunizations, and grayish-white exudates would be visible in the posterior oropharynx.
	A **peritonsillar abscess** is a deeper infection of the head and neck and would present with a "hot potato" voice, along with swelling noted in lateral wall of the oropharynx on the affected side. Usually, the pain is more severe on one side of the neck than the other in peritonsillar abscess–often with referred pain to the ipsilateral ear.

CASE 15 | Epiglottitis (*H. Influenzae* Type B)

A 3-year-old previously unvaccinated boy is brought for evaluation of sore throat, fever, and drooling for 1 day. His parents report that he has had increased difficulty breathing and sounds hoarse but has not had a cough. On exam, the patient is acutely ill and anxious. His vitals are as follows: temperature 38.9°C, pulse 128/min, respirations 30/min, and blood pressure 100/64 mmHg. When examined, he refuses to lay back, appears anxious, and has intercostal retractions and stridor.

Evaluation/Tests	Nasolaryngoscopy reveals a cherry-red, edematous epiglottis. Lateral neck radiograph shows a "thumb sign" due to an enlarged epiglottis with narrowing of the airway.
Treatment	Stabilize his airway, start antibiotics such as ceftriaxone, and consider steroids.
Discussion	This patient is presenting with **epiglottitis**, most commonly caused by the small gram negative rod *Haemophilus influenzae* **type b**. Any child with the three Ds—dysphagia, drooling, and distress (respiratory)—should be suspected of having epiglottitis and impending airway obstruction, which needs to be treated urgently. Although it is quite rare in the modern era following the widespread use of *H. influenzae* type b (Hib) vaccination, it can still be seen in unvaccinated children. Patients typically appear "toxic" and have severe respiratory distress (often with stridor) requiring them to sit in a "tripod" position (trunk leaning forward, elbows on knees, neck extended, and chin forward to maximize air intake). Confirmation of diagnosis may be required using a fiberoptic laryngoscope, but it must be carefully undertaken after the airway is stabilized. Laryngoscopy will reveal the classic "cherry-red" epiglottis. Lateral neck radiographs will show the "thumbprint" sign, which reflects an enlarged epiglottis. *H. influenzae* is transmitted by respiratory droplets and is cultured on chocolate agar containing the growth factors V (nicotinamide adenine dinucleotide, NAD) and X (hemin). *H. influenzae* can also cause meningitis, otitis media, and pneumonia. Most *Haemophilus* infections in vaccinated patients come from nontypeable strains.
	Retropharyngeal abscess typically will present with a history of pharyngitis with exudates and lack of improvement with antibiotics. Trismus (locking of the jaw) may also be present.
	Croup is caused by the parainfluenza virus and presents with a "seal-like" barking cough, normal-appearing epiglottitis, and narrowing of the upper trachea and subglottis that give rise to a steeple sign on X-ray.
	Respiratory syncytial virus (RSV) bronchiolitis is seen most often in children <2 years old and presents with cough, low-grade fever, and poor feeding.

CASE 16 | Infectious Mononucleosis (Epstein-Barr Virus)

A 19-year-old woman presents with sore throat, fever, and fatigue for the last 10 days. She has been unable to attend her classes and has been resting in bed in her college dormitory. She denies recent travel. She has a new boyfriend but denies having oral or vaginal intercourse. On exam, the patient has a temperature of 38.7°C, pulse 95/min, respirations 16/min, and blood pressure 119/74 mmHg. She has bilateral pharyngeal exudates as well as palpable tender lymph nodes in the posterior neck region. On abdominal exam, her spleen tip is felt.

Evaluation/Tests	CBC shows WBC 15,500/mm³ (predominantly lymphocytes), Hgb 13g/dL, hematocrit 39%, platelets 230,000/mm³, and peripheral blood smear is notable for the presence of atypical lymphocytes. HIV and rapid streptococcal antigen tests are negative. Heterophile antibody test is positive.
Treatment	Symptomatic and supportive care. Avoid contact sports to avoid splenic rupture.
Discussion	**Infectious mononucleosis** typically presents with fever, pharyngitis, posterior cervical lymphadenopathy, and fatigue. Often referred to as the "kissing disease," it can be spread by other means which involve exposure to saliva or respiratory secretions. Peripheral blood smear reveals atypical lymphocytes that are reactive cytotoxic T lymphocytes (not B-cells). Patients will have a positive Monospot test that looks for heterophile antibodies detected by agglutination of sheep or horse red blood cells. Mononucleosis is most commonly caused by the **Epstein-Barr virus (EBV)**, a member of

CASE 16 | Infectious Mononucleosis (Epstein-Barr Virus) *(continued)*

Discussion	the herpes viruses that are enveloped, double-stranded, linear DNA viruses. EBV infects B lymphocytes through the CD21 receptor. Virally infected cells can be recognized through antigen presentation on MHC Class I, which can lead to activation of CD8+ cytotoxic T lymphocytes (forming "atypical" lymphocytes). EBV is also associated with other conditions including Burkitt lymphoma, nasopharyngeal carcinoma, and lymphoproliferative disease in transplant patients. **Viral pharyngitis** or **streptococcal pharyngitis** is unlikely given the chronicity of symptoms and presence of splenomegaly on physical exam. **Acute retroviral (HIV) syndrome** can present as a mono-like illness, but the patient's negative test rules this out. Symptoms of mononucleosis in the setting of a negative Monospot test may indicate **cytomegalovirus (CMV)** infection.

FEVER AND HIV/AIDS

The differential diagnosis for fever in a patient with HIV/AIDS is broad. Infection is the most common cause of fever in most immunocompetent patients, and this is no different in persons living with HIV. Practically any bacteria, virus, fungus, or parasite can cause fever in any patient. The focus here will be on infectious and noninfectious causes of fever in immunocompromised patients. Not only are patients who are infected with HIV more likely to present with common pathogens, but they will have additional causes of infectious fever that are not seen in the immunocompetent host.

Differential Diagnosis for Fever and HIV/AIDS

Bacterial	Viral	Fungal	Parasitic
• Pulmonary or disseminated tuberculosis • Disseminated MAC (*Mycobacterium avium* complex) • Bacillary angiomatosis (*Bartonella henselae*) • Secondary syphilis	• Progressive multifocal leukoencephalopathy (PML) • Cytomegalovirus (CMV) retinitis, colitis, esophagitis, (rarely) encephalitis • Genital HSV, recurrent • Dermatomal zoster (VZV) • Acute retroviral (HIV) syndrome (aka primary HIV infection)	• *Pneumocystis jirovecii* pneumonia (PJP) • Disseminated histoplasmosis • Disseminated blastomycosis • Disseminated coccidioidomycosis • Aspergillosis, invasive • Cryptococcal meningitis • Candida esophagitis	• CNS toxoplasmosis • Cryptosporidiosis (*Cryptosporidium parvum*)

Given the variety of infections causing fever in patients with HIV/AIDS, it can be helpful to categorize them by type of pathogen (as just shown). Alternatively, one can categorize them by body system (e.g., skin, CNS, pulmonary, disseminated, etc.). Keep in mind that certain infections only present in patients with AIDS and should serve as a clue when narrowing the differential. Remember that a few noninfectious entities can result in fever such as malignancy or adverse drug reactions.

 Key Findings and Fever and HIV/AIDS Differential Diagnosis

Fever and HIV/AIDS and Key Associated Findings	Diagnosis
Fever, diffuse lymphadenopathy, sore throat, +/− rash (mono-like syndrome)	Acute retroviral (HIV) infection
Demyelination, multiple white matter changes, JC virus	Progressive multifocal leukoencephalopathy (PML)
Headache, meningoencephalitis, increased ICP, + India Ink smear	Cryptococcal meningitis
Focal neurological deficit, multiple well-circumscribed lesions (basal ganglia)	Central nervous system (CNS) toxoplasmosis
Cotton wool spots on fundoscopy, intraretinal hemorrhage, "ketchup and mustard" retina	Cytomegalovirus (CMV) retinitis
Odynophagia, oral thrush	Candida esophagitis

(continued)

Key Findings and Fever and HIV/AIDS Differential Diagnosis (*continued*)

Fever and HIV/AIDS and Key Associated Findings	Diagnosis
Cavitary lung lesion, positive PPD or IGRA, often foreign-borne person	Pulmonary tuberculosis
Cough, fever, oxygen desaturation with activity, diffuse bilateral infiltrates on CXR or "groundglass" opacities on chest CT	*Pneumocystis jirovecii* pneumonia (PJP)
Hemoptysis, pleuritic chest pain, pulmonary nodules, acute angle branching septate hyphae	Invasive aspergillosis
- Systemic illness, elevated LFTs, hepatosplenomegaly, residence/travel to Mississippi or Ohio River Valley	Disseminated histoplasmosis
- Systemic illness, skin lesions, CNS disease, residence/travel to Mississippi or Ohio River Valley - Squamous cell carcinoma-type skin lesion	Disseminated blastomycosis
Systemic illness, skin lesions, CNS disease, residence/travel to Southwestern United States	Disseminated coccidioidomycosis
Linear ulcers on GI endoscopy, bloody stools	CMV colitis
Diarrhea, severe anemia (<10 g/dL), and fever without localizing symptoms	Disseminated *Mycobacterium avium* complex (MAC)
Diarrhea, "acid-fast" oocysts	Cryptosporidiosis
Skin lesions and cat scratch	Bacillary angiomatosis
Rash on palms and soles, sexually active	Secondary syphilis
Painful genital ulcers, inguinal lymphadenopathy	Herpes simplex virus (HSV), recurrent
Vesicular, painful rash in different stages in a dermatomal distribution	Dermatomal *Varicella zoster*

CASE 17 | Disseminated *Mycobacterium Avium/Intracellulare* Complex (MAC)

A 28-year-old man with a history of HIV/AIDS presents with fever, night sweats, weight loss, and diarrhea over the last month. He reports excessive fatigue. There are no skin lesions. On exam, he has a temperature of 39.5°C, pulse 121/min, respirations 18/min, and blood pressure 102/72 mmHg. He has mild diffuse abdominal pain. Diffuse lymphadenopathy and hepatosplenomegaly are noted.

Evaluation/Tests	CBC shows WBC 2200/mm³, CD4+ cell count 32/mm³, Hgb 11 g/dL, hematocrit 33%, platelets 150,000/mm³. HIV viral load is 10,000 copies/mL. Liver function tests show AST 25 U/L, ALT 32 U/L, alkaline phosphatase 437 U/L, total bilirubin 0.7 mg/dL, and direct bilirubin 0.2 mg/dL. Serum lactate dehydrogenase (LDH) is elevated. Gram stain from blood culture is positive for acid-fast bacilli.
Treatment	Treat with a combination of clarithromycin, rifampin, and ethambutol.
Discussion	**Disseminated *Mycobacterium avium/intracellulare* complex (MAC)** is an infection caused by one of two nontuberculous mycobacteria (*M. avium* or *M. intracellulare*). Although the preceding symptoms are nonspecific, the constellation of findings of fever, night sweats, weight loss, and diarrhea in the setting of AIDS is most consistent with disseminated MAC. Patients also have diffuse lymphadenopathy, hepatosplenomegaly, and anemia with elevated serum alkaline phosphatase and LDH. Mycobacteria can affect both immunocompetent and immunocompromised patients; however, disseminated disease is most commonly seen in HIV+ patients with a CD4 count <50. Ultimately, the diagnosis is made after AFB blood cultures are positive, but patients are often treated presumptively prior to culture results. In addition to disseminated disease, MAC can also cause a **focal lymphadenitis.** Disseminated fungal infections such as **histoplasmosis** and **blastomycosis** may have other symptoms such as lung and skin involvement. Patients with histoplasmosis typically have transaminitis and gastrointestinal involvement. Blastomycosis typically presents as verrucous skin lesions and granulomatous skin nodules. Diagnosis is often made by detecting fungal antigens in the urine or via culture of affected organs. Although patients with **lymphoma** have fever, night sweats, and weight loss, lymph node biopsy with typical features consistent with lymphoma would help with differentiation in this setting.

CASE 18 | Secondary Syphilis (*Treponema Pallidum*)

A 34-year-old man with HIV presents with fever and a diffuse rash for the last week. He has been busy with work and has not participated in any recreational outdoor activities or travel recently. He reports having five male sexual partners over the last 6 months and uses condoms inconsistently. On exam, the patient has a temperature of 38.9°C, pulse 106/min, respirations 14/min, and blood pressure 121/81 mmHg. He has diffuse lymphadenopathy. He has a maculopapular rash on his trunk as well as on the palms and soles of his feet. He has smooth, painless, wart-like lesions on the genitals (condylomata lata).

Evaluation/Tests	CBC reveals a CD4 count of 597 cells/mm³. Chlamydia and gonorrhea urine nucleic antigen amplification tests (NAATs) are both negative. VDRL antigen test is positive, followed by a positive FTA-ABS test.
Treatment	Treat with long-acting penicillin (benzathine penicillin G). Pregnant patients with secondary syphilis who have an IgE-mediated hypersensitivity reaction to penicillin should still be given penicillin *after* desensitization.
Discussion	**Secondary syphilis** is a sexually transmitted infection caused by the spirochete *Treponema pallidum*. The patient has systemic/constitutional symptoms including maculopapular rash, fever, and diffuse lymphadenopathy. The rash of secondary syphilis can be varied in appearance but often involves the palms and soles. Patients may or may not recall the preceding painless chancre of primary syphilis. Secondary syphilis can manifest several weeks after primary syphilis. Additional manifestations of secondary syphilis include wart-like condylomata lata on the genitals and patchy hair loss. *T. pallidum* is diagnosed with serologic tests including the sensitive but nonspecific VDRL or RPR tests, followed by a confirmatory specific test, such as FTA-ABS. Although not performed often, the gold standard for diagnosis of primary syphilis is visualization of spirochetes using fluorescent or dark-field microscopy. **Viral exanthem** is less likely because this patient does not report sick contacts or a viral prodrome. Although viral exanthems can also cause similar rashes, diffuse lymphadenopathy is not as common with most viruses. **Rocky Mountain spotted fever (RMSF)** is often accompanied by a rash, but the distribution and evolution would be different. Lack of exposures to ticks or outdoor activities makes tick-borne infections less likely.
Additional Considerations	**Primary syphilis** begins as a single, round, painless chancre (aka ulcer) that can last for 3–6 weeks. The chancre will involute whether or not it has been treated. If primary syphilis is untreated, it can develop into secondary syphilis within 6–8 weeks after initial infection and will present with systemic symptoms. Without treatment, the infection can enter a latent stage where the individual may not have any signs and symptoms of syphilis. This stage may last for years. They may also progress to **tertiary syphilis**. Tertiary syphilis can occur 10–30 years after the initial infection and can affect multiple organ systems, with the most significant systems being the cardiovascular and nervous systems. Individuals may present with aortic regurgitation, ascending thoracic aortic dilation/aneurysm, or **neurosyphilis** consisting of general paresis, dementia, tabes dorsalis, Argyll Robertson pupils, and/or uveitis. Patients with tertiary syphilis may also present with gummas, irregular granulomatous lesions found on skin, bone, or internal organs that ulcerate. Pregnant women can transmit syphilis to their fetus up to 4 years after initial infection, leading to **congenital syphilis**. Congenital syphilis may cause stillbirth or premature delivery. Clinical manifestations after birth include failure to thrive, hepatomegaly, lymphadenopathy, maculopapular rash, nasal discharge, sensorineural deafness, and characteristic facial abnormalities such as notched teeth, saddle nose deformity, etc. Treatment of syphilis at any stage (but most commonly in primary and secondary and in pregnant persons) can cause an acute syndrome characterized by fever, headache, myalgias, and hypotension known as the **Jarisch-Herxheimer reaction**. This is due to the release of lipopolysaccharide (LPS) from dying spirochetes.

CASE 19 | *Candida Albicans* Esophagitis

A 42-year-old man with a history of HIV/AIDS presents with a 1-week history of pain with swallowing and feeling like food is getting stuck in his throat. On exam, the patient has a temperature of 38.3°C, pulse 102/min, respirations 16/min, and blood pressure 118/82 mmHg. He is cachectic in appearance. His oropharynx shows diffuse white plaques on his tongue, palate, and bilateral buccal mucosa that can be scraped off with a tongue depressor. His most recent CD4 cell count was 46 cells/mm³.

Evaluation/Tests	Clinical diagnosis.
Treatment	Antifungal therapy with fluconazole for 14–21 days.

CASE 19 | *Candida Albicans* Esophagitis *(continued)*

Discussion	This patient is presenting with **Candida esophagitis**, which is caused by the opportunistic fungus *Candida albicans*. Patients with profoundly low CD4 counts (<100 and often <50) with odynophagia and white scrapable plaques/pseudomembranes almost always have *Candida* esophagitis. *Candida* is a dimorphic fungus that forms pseudohyphae and budding yeasts and is present normally in low numbers on the skin, in the oral cavity, and in gastrointestinal and genitourinary tracts. It typically causes only minor infections in immunocompetent patients. Risk factors for more severe disease include HIV, diabetes, or other immunosuppressed populations. In immunocompetent patients, *Candida* can cause diaper rash, vulvovaginitis, and endocarditis (in IV drug users). In immunocompromised patients, *Candida* can cause oral thrush, esophagitis, or disseminated disease that may affect any organ system and can lead to sepsis. It is also a common cause of fungemia in the blood of patients with intravascular catheters.
	Given the patient's history of HIV/AIDS, noninfectious causes of esophagitis are less likely. In immunosuppressed patients, the differential should include viral pathogens such as HSV and CMV. **HSV esophagitis** would cause punched-out round ulcerations, and **CMV esophagitis** would present with deep linear ulcerations, especially in the lower esophagus. Definitive diagnosis would be made by upper endoscopic biopsy of the esophagus. Both HSV and CMV esophagitis can be seen in solid organ and bone marrow transplant recipients, as well as in HIV+ patients with CD4 <50.

CASE 20 | Cryptococcal Meningoencephalitis (*Cryptococcus Neoformans*)

A 39-year-old woman with AIDS presents with a 2-week history of worsening headache and fever. Her family reports that she has been getting progressively confused and is having difficulty with her activities of daily living. The patient has not traveled anywhere recently and has no pets. On exam, the patient has a temperature of 39.4°C, pulse 122/min, respirations 18/min, and blood pressure 102/68 mmHg. The patient is cachectic and not oriented to person, place, or time. No rashes are noted. Examination of her lungs, abdomen, and heart is unremarkable except for tachycardia. There are no focal neurologic deficits.

Evaluation/Tests	CD4 cell count is 16 cells/mm^3. Head CT is unremarkable. Lumbar puncture reveals a CSF cell count of 30/mm^3, protein 75 mg/dL, and glucose 40 mg/dL. CSF opening pressure is 38 cm H$_2$O. Gram stain of CSF is negative. India ink stain shows the presence of spherical yeast buds with clear surrounding halos (peripheral clearing). Mucicarmine stain reveals a thick red-stained capsule. 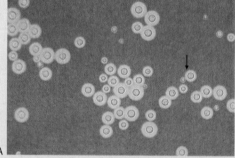 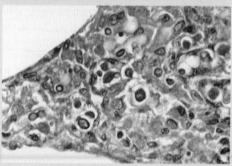
	A. Cryptococcus neoformans—India ink preparation. Arrow points to a budding yeast of Cryptococcus neoformans. Note the thick, translucent polysaccharide capsule outlined by the dark India ink particles. Used with permission from Dr. L. Haley, Public Health Image Library, Centers for Disease Control and Prevention. **B.** Cryptococcus neoformans—Mucicarmine stain. Note many red, oval yeasts of C. neoformans in lung tissue of patient with AIDS. Used with permission from Dr. Edwin P. Ewing, Jr, Public Health Image Library, Centers for Disease Control and Prevention.
Treatment	Start dual antifungal therapy with amphotericin B and flucytosine; lumbar puncture (LP) to remove CSF to decrease intracranial pressure, if present. Once clinical status improves, treat with fluconazole for long-term maintenance. Antiretroviral (ARV) therapy for HIV should not be started until at least 2 weeks of antifungal therapy have been given due to risk of immune reconstitution inflammatory syndrome (IRIS), which can result in increased intracranial pressure in the "closed space" of the CNS following more rapid initiation of ARVs.

CASE 20 | Cryptococcal Meningoencephalitis (*Cryptococcus Neoformans*) (*continued*)

Discussion	A fever, headache, and altered mental status in an AIDS patient is very suggestive of **cryptococcal meningoencephalitis** caused by the opportunistic fungal pathogen *Cryptococcus neoformans*. *Cryptococcus* is found in soil and pigeon droppings and can be acquired via inhalation. After inhalation, it can enter the bloodstream and spread to the meninges and brain. The current method of diagnosis involves a latex agglutination test for cryptococcal antigen. In addition to meningoencephalitis, immunocompromised patients may also present with **pulmonary cryptococcosis**. Typically, **bacterial** (and most viral) causes of **meningitis** would progress more rapidly than the 2-week progressive worsening seen in this patient, and CSF analysis would differ. Noninfectious causes of meningitis and/or encephalitis can be the result of **paraneoplastic syndromes** secondary to malignancy, lupus, or other autoimmune diseases.

DYSURIA

Dysuria (broadly defined as burning, tingling, pain, and/or discomfort associated with voiding) is a very common complaint, particularly in the outpatient setting. Refer to Chapter 14, "Renal," and Chapter 15, "Reproductive (OB/GYN and Urology)," for additional cases.

Urethritis is inflammation of the urethra. Urethritis classically presents with urethral discharge, but some patients may be asymptomatic. In clinical practice, the term often implies infection-induced urethral inflammation though noninfectious etiologies exist. Urethral infections are typically sexually transmitted. Stemming from historical diagnosis by gram staining of urethral discharge for gram negative diplococci, urethritis is categorized as gonococcal and nongonococcal. Gonococcal infections are the result of *N. gonorrhea*. The most common organism of nongonococcal urethritis (NGU) is *Chlamydia trachomatis.* Symptoms will present approximately 1 day to 2 weeks after exposure. Gonococcal urethritis will typically present more quickly and abruptly than nongonococcal urethritis. Men will present with symptoms more frequently than women, and symptoms are usually local rather than systemic. Nucleic acid amplification test (NAAT) is the recommended test to evaluate for male urogenital infections. This is done through a urine specimen, which can be tested for both gonorrhea and chlamydia because there is a high asymptomatic coinfection rate. If urine is not available, a urethral swab may be obtained. Other common STIs include syphilis, HIV, and HSV.

Differential Diagnosis for Dysuria

Infectious	Noninfectious, Inflammatory	Noninflammatory
Both men and women • Cystitis • Pyelonephritis • Urethritis (secondary to STI or non-STI causing organisms) Men • Prostatitis (acute and chronic) • Epididymo-orchitis Women • Vulvovaginitis • Cervicitis	Dermatologic • Contact/irritant • dermatitis • Behçet syndrome Foreign body (e.g., stone) Urethritis (aseptic) secondary to reactive arthritis	Both men and women • Urethral stricture • Interstitial cystitis • Bladder or renal cancer • Pelvic irradiation • Horseback or bicycle riding • GU instrumentation • Foreign body Men • Benign prostatic hyperplasia (BPH) • Prostate or penile cancer Women • Atrophic vaginitis • Endometriosis • Vaginal or vulvar cancer

Patients should be assessed for and treated with appropriate antibiotics if the etiology is infectious. If infectious causes are not found, then noninfectious inflammatory and noninflammatory causes should be sought. It is important to remember that there are male and female differences in infectious and noninfectious causes for dysuria. Treatment of noninfectious causes involves treatment of the underlying disorder that is causing the dysuria, along with pain control. Reactive arthritis can result from enteric organisms or genitourinary infections; in the case of aseptic urethritis, there is typically an antecedent enteric infection.

Key Findings and Dysuria Differential Diagnosis

Dysuria and Key Associated Findings	Diagnosis
- Urinary urgency, increased frequency, possible suprapubic pain - Suprapubic tenderness on exam	Cystitis
- Urinary urgency, increased frequency, fever and flank pain - Costovertebral angle (CVAT) present	Pyelonephritis
- Fever, myalgias, "tip of penis" pain - Enlarged, tender prostate	Acute prostatitis
- Dribbling, decreased stream, hesitancy, urinary incontinence - Enlarged, nontender prostate	Benign prostatic hyperplasia (BPH)
- Testicular pain, possible scrotal swelling - Scrotal tenderness	Epididymo-orchitis
- Vulvovaginal dryness, dyspareunia (pain with sexual intercourse) - Vaginal atrophy	Atrophic vaginitis, UTI
- Vaginal discharge	Vulvovaginitis
- Purulent discharge from cervix	Cervicitis
- Urethral discharge	Urethritis (typically associated with STI)
- Urethritis (aseptic), arthritis and enthesitis, following an enteric infection	Urethritis secondary to reactive arthritis
Prior treatment with cyclophosphamide	Interstitial cystitis
Oral and genital ulcers, uveitis	Behçet syndrome
Perineal rash or irritation	Contact/irritant dermatitis

CASE 21 | Acute Pyelonephritis

A 43-year-old woman presents with a 1-day history of fever, flank pain, nausea, and several episodes of vomiting. Three days prior to these symptoms, she began to have dysuria, increased urinary frequency, and urgency. On exam, the patient is acutely ill and has chills. Her vitals are as follows: temperature 38.9°C, pulse 106/min, respirations 16/min, and blood pressure 110/70 mmHg. Her abdominal exam is notable for suprapubic tenderness, and she has left costovertebral angle tenderness. Her pelvic exam is normal.

Evaluation/Tests	Urinalysis shows a specific gravity of 1.015, cloudy color, leukocyte esterase and nitrites positive, numerous WBCs and WBC casts present, some RBCs present, and is negative for protein, glucose, and ketones. Urethral swab for gonorrhea and chlamydia NAAT tests is negative. Urine culture reveals gram negative, indole positive rod-shaped bacteria.
Treatment	Hospitalize patient and treat with ceftriaxone. Milder cases can be treated with a fluoroquinolone as an outpatient.
Discussion	Acute **pyelonephritis** is a bacterial infection of the renal parenchyma that often leads to renal scarring and (as with all UTIs) is much more common in women than in men because the shorter urethra in women facilitates colonization by fecal flora such as *E. coli*. Bacteria usually ascend from the lower urinary tract but may also reach the kidney via the bloodstream. Common pathogens include *Escherichia coli* followed by *Staphylococcus saprophyticus*, *Klebsiella pneumoniae*, *Enterococcus* spp., and other gram negative rods. Evaluation includes a urinalysis, urine culture, and sensitivity. CBC will often show an elevated WBC count. Blood cultures should be obtained in hospitalized patients. Imaging with ultrasound or CT to rule out perinephric abscess should be considered if there is no clinical improvement after 48 hours of appropriate treatment. Complications include bacteremia, sepsis, renal abscess, renal papillary necrosis, or chronic pyelonephritis causing scarring and chronic kidney disease. **Cystitis** frequently causes dysuria, frequency, and urgency consistent with an uncomplicated urinary tract infection (UTI), but the presence of flank pain, back pain, costovertebral tenderness, fever, chills, and nausea makes pyelonephritis (an upper tract UTI) more likely in this patient. Patients with **pelvic inflammatory disease (PID)** typically have vaginal discharge and cervical motion tenderness on exam.
Additional Considerations	Consider **kidney stones** as a potential diagnosis if antecedent colicky pain radiating to the groin, hematuria, or history of stones is present. For men, consider **prostatitis** in the case of recurrent UTI or pelvic/perineal pain in the setting of pyelonephritis.

CASE 22 | Gonococcal Urethritis (*Neisseria Gonorrhoeae*)

A 26-year-old man reports severe burning with urination and "white" discharge from his penis. He reports having had five different partners over the last 6 months and uses condoms infrequently. He reports no testicular pain. On exam, he is afebrile, and his vital signs are normal. There are no areas of fluctuance upon palpating the urethra, but mild tenderness is noted on the most distal aspect, and a mucopurulent discharge is milked from the urethra.

Evaluation/Tests	Urine gonorrhea NAAT test is positive, chlamydia NAAT test negative. HIV test is negative.
Treatment	Ceftriaxone and azithromycin.
Discussion	This patient is presenting with **gonococcal urethritis** caused by the gram negative diplococci *Neisseria gonorrhoeae*. Gonorrhea is a common sexually transmitted infection and may coinfect with *Chlamydia trachomatis*. Purulent urethritis is most likely due to gonococcal urethritis. In order to better manage gonorrhea in an era of increasing cephalosporin resistance, the CDC recommends treatment of gonorrhea with both ceftriaxone and azithromycin. Unlike its close relative *Neisseria meningitidis*, *N. gonorrhoeae* lacks a polysaccharide capsule, does not ferment maltose, and has no vaccine due to antigenic variation of its pilus proteins. **Nongonococcal urethritis (NGU)** presents as a nonpurulent urethritis and is typically due to *Chlamydia trachomatis*. Gonococcal urethritis is typically more purulent and painful than Chlamydia urethritis in men. Additional causes of NGU include *Mycoplasma genitalium* and *Ureaplasma urealyticum*. In patients who engage in insertive anal intercourse, consider enteric gram negative rods (e.g., *E. coli*) as a cause of NGU as well. **HSV** should be considered as a rare cause of NGU, but a history of vesicles, recurrent HSV, and/or ulceration will be clues to the diagnosis. **Acute bacterial prostatitis** is usually seen in older men from *E. coli* infections. Younger individuals with acute bacterial prostatitis are typically infected with *N. gonorrhoeae* or *C. trachomatis*. Patients with acute bacterial prostatitis will present with pelvic pain, fever, and a tender prostate along with dysuria and increased frequency.
Additional Considerations	*N. gonorrhoeae* can also cause septic arthritis, neonatal conjunctivitis, and pelvic inflammatory disease (PID) in women. Perihepatic inflammation due to ascending infection can be seen in PID and is known as the **Fitz-Hugh-Curtis syndrome**. "Violin string" adhesions of the peritoneum to the liver are classically seen in this syndrome.

GENITAL LESIONS AND STI

The vast majority of genital lesions, particularly ulcerative lesions, can be attributed to sexually transmitted infection (STI). Despite this, lesions that do not respond appropriately to treatment should always prompt further evaluation, often including biopsy.

Pathogen	Classic Presentation
Herpes simplex (HSV)	Multiple small painful vesicular lesions that erupt and leave behind a shallow ulcerative base; may have constitutional symptoms like malaise, fever, lymphadenopathy with primary outbreak
Primary syphilis	Typically singular painless ulcer (chancre) with a clear/clean base and raised border; may have associated mild tender lymphadenopathy
Chancroid	Typically singular painful ulcer with a friable/exudative base; often with suppurative and tender lymphadenopathy
Lymphogranuloma venereum (LGV)	Small, shallow, and painless ulcers or papules which may be genital or rectal; tender lymphadenopathy; rectal symptoms (pain, discharge)
Granuloma inguinale (donovanosis)	Persistent painless hypertrophic red papules or ulcers; no lymphadenopathy noted but can have granulomas

CASE 23 | Genital Herpes

A 28-year-old woman presents with a new onset cluster of painful pimple-like bumps on her labia. Before the bumps appeared, she had 1 day of tingling and a burning sensation in the area. On exam, there is a cluster of vesicles on the labia majora that are tender to light palpation and associated inguinal lymphadenopathy.

CASE 23 | Genital Herpes (continued)

Evaluation/Tests	Real-time PCR assay of the vesicle/open ulcer positive for HSV-2. RPR and other STI screening negative.
Treatment	Acyclovir (or its pro-drugs, valacyclovir or famciclovir).
Discussion	Both HSV-1 and HSV-2 can cause genital herpes, though historically HSV-2 has been more common in the genital area. HSV-1 also causes gingivostomatitis, keratoconjunctivitis, herpes labialis, and temporal lobe encephalitis. Both types can reactivate and cause recurrent disease as they establish latency in sensory ganglia. HSV-1 typically causes cold sores or keratitis (reactivation from trigeminal ganglia), while HSV-2 typically causes genital herpes (reactivation from lumbosacral dorsal root ganglia). Consider daily antiviral medication for suppression, which will reduce symptom severity, duration, recurrence, and transmission. **Syphilis** is an STI caused by *Treponema pallidum*. The lesion of primary syphilis is initially a painless chancre that develops on average 21 days after the infection. Secondary syphilis develops weeks to months later and is noted by a fever, lymphadenopathy, rash (includes palms and soles), and condyloma lata. After this, syphilis enters a latent stage where there are no symptoms. Tertiary syphilis is noted for gummatous disease with possible CNS and cardiovascular involvement. All stages of syphilis are treated with different regimens of penicillin G. **Genital warts** are caused by HPV types 6 and 11, and the lesions range from small flat papules to large cauliflower-like lesions on anogenital mucosa and surrounding skin. They tend not to be painful and do not form clusters of vesicles or ulcerate.

VAGINAL DISCHARGE AND PELVIC INFECTIONS

The normal vaginal ecosystem in the reproductive age patient can vary greatly depending on the timing of the menstrual cycle, pregnancy, use of hormonal contraception or medication, hydration status, and infections. Alterations in the ecosystem can result in variations in the amount, color, and consistency of the usual normal physiologic vaginal discharge.

Vaginitis is the general term for inflammation or changes in the vaginal environment causing discharge, irritation, pain, and odor. Common diagnosis/causes include candida vulvovaginitis, bacterial vaginosis, trichomonas, and vaginal atrophy. While there can be a myriad of ways in which patients with different vaginitis/infectious etiologies present, there are some classic associations.

Pathogen/Condition	Key Words/Phrases
Bacterial vaginosis (BV)	Vaginal pH >4.5, gray discharge, amine ("fishy") odor, clue cells
Candida vulvovaginitis	Itch/burn, "curdy" or "cottage cheese" white discharge, hyphae
Trichomonas vaginalis	Vaginal pH >4.5, frothy green discharge, cervical petechiae ("strawberry cervix"), motile flagellated organism on wet prep
N. gonorrhoeae/ C. trachomatis	Mucopurulent cervical discharge, "chandelier sign" (aka cervical motion tenderness, only in ascending infection); or asymptomatic
Atrophic vaginitis	Vaginal pH >4.5, menopausal patient, pale pink vaginal wall and loss of rugae

Patients with more serious infections such as pelvic inflammatory disease (PID), tubo-ovarian abscess, and toxic shock syndrome typically present with severe systemic sequelae such as severe pain, nausea and vomiting, fever, and in some cases, sepsis that may require prolonged hospitalization or surgery. Potential complications of these infections include chronic pelvic pain, infertility, and death.

CASE 24 | Bacterial Vaginosis (*Gardnerella Vaginalis*)

A 31-year-old sexually active woman presents with increased foul smelling vaginal discharge for three days. The discharge is white and thin. The patient is in a monogamous relationship with her husband. On exam, there is no vulvar inflammation or cervical motion tenderness. Thin discharge with fishy odor is noted.

CASE 24 | Bacterial Vaginosis (*Gardnerella Vaginalis*) (continued)

Evaluation/Tests	Wet mount of the vaginal discharge: clue cells present, pH >4.5.
Treatment	Metronidazole or clindamycin.
Discussion	**Bacterial vaginosis** (BV) is caused by *Gardnerella vaginalis* as well as an overgrowth of anaerobic bacteria in the vagina. Patients present with painless, gray vaginal discharge with a fishy odor. This odor can be enhanced with the addition of 10% potassium hydroxide (KOH) to the vaginal discharge (the so-called "amine whiff test"). Risk factors for acquisition include vaginal douching, smoking, new or multiple sexual partners, and unprotected intercourse. Clue cells and vaginal epithelial cells stippled with *Gardnerella* bacteria are seen on microscopy. Treat with topical or oral metronidazole or oral clindamycin. **Candida vulvovaginitis** discharge is odorless, thick white cottage cheese discharge, with normal pH (4–4.5) and pseudohyphae and is treated with azoles such as topical clotrimazole or oral fluconazole. **Trichomonas** may present with an inflamed or "strawberry cervix," frothy, foul-smelling thick yellow discharge with motile flagellated organisms (trichomonas), with pH >4.5. Patients and sexual partners should be treated with oral metronidazole.

CASE 25 | *Chlamydia Trachomatis*

A 21-year-old woman presents to the clinic for a routine pelvic exam. She has had two male partners in the last 12 months and uses condoms intermittently. On review of systems, she says she has had mild dysuria for the last 3 days. On exam, there is no abdominal or cervical motion tenderness, but a creamy purulent vaginal discharge is seen.

Evaluation/Tests	NAAT is positive for chlamydia. Testing for gonorrhea, HSV, trichomonas is negative, and urine dipstick is unremarkable for UTI.
Treatment	Azithromycin *or* doxycycline.
Discussion	Patients infected with *Chlamydia trachomatis* can be asymptomatic or present with cervicitis, PID, urethritis, conjunctivitis, or reactive arthritis. Untreated cases can lead to PID and infertility; therefore, women should be tested for asymptomatic infection. Coinfection with gonorrhea is common. Sexual partners should be treated as well. Patients should be tested for HIV. Chlamydia are obligate intracellular organisms because they cannot make their own ATP. They exist in two forms: the infectious form (known as the "elementary body") and the replicative form (known as the "reticulate body"). Chlamydia trachomatis has numerous serotypes. Types A–C are associated with conjunctivitis, while types L1–L3 can cause lymphogranuloma venereum (LGV), a genital infection that is characterized by painful inguinal lymphadenopathy that ulcerates to form "buboes." Other *Chlamydia* spp. can cause pneumonia. **Cervicitis** results from infectious and noninfectious etiologies. In this case, positive NAAT for *Chlamydia* confirms the diagnosis.

CASE 26 | Pelvic Inflammatory Disease (PID)

A 22-year-old woman presents with lower abdominal/pelvic pain for 3 days. She also notes an abnormal vaginal discharge and pain with sexual intercourse. The patient has had multiple male sexual partners and uses condoms intermittently. She denies dysuria, diarrhea, or fevers. She has intermittent nausea but no vomiting. On exam, she has a low-grade fever, tenderness to palpation in the lower abdominal/pelvic area, cervical motion and bilateral adnexal tenderness, and mucopurulent cervical discharge. Her last menstrual period was 2 weeks ago.

Evaluation/Tests	Clinical diagnosis. NAAT for chlamydia/gonorrhea are often positive. Quantitative hCG is negative.
Treatment	Ceftriaxone with either azithromycin or doxycycline.
Discussion	**Pelvic inflammatory disease (PID)** is a clinical diagnosis and may include endometritis, salpingitis, and/or tubo-ovarian abscess. It is typically caused by bacterial infection with *Chlamydia trachomatis* and/or *Neisseria gonorrhoeae*. Women with PID can develop infertility from tubal scarring, and they are at increased risk for ectopic pregnancy and chronic pelvic pain. Indications for inpatient treatment include being unable to follow or tolerate outpatient oral medications, lack of clinical response, pregnancy, nausea and vomiting, high fever, or tubo-ovarian abscess. Treatment with antibiotics should not be postponed while waiting for culture confirmation. Perihepatitis (**Fitz-Hugh-Curtis syndrome**) is a complication ("violin string" adhesions of peritoneum to liver). Ultrasound imaging or abdominal/pelvic CT are helpful to rule out appendicitis and ovarian torsion if the diagnosis is not clear.

CASE 26 | Pelvic Inflammatory Disease (PID) *(continued)*

Discussion	Pelvic pain is common with **ovarian torsion** and presents very acutely. These patients typically have nausea and vomiting with an adnexal mass. They usually do not have vaginal or endocervical discharge. **Ectopic pregnancy** causes abdominal pain and/or vaginal bleeding with a positive quantitative hCG. **UTI** typically presents with dysuria, urinary frequency, and suprapubic pain.

CASE 27 | Toxic Shock Syndrome

A 20-year-old woman with a history of light menses presents to the emergency department after rapid onset of fever with chills, muscle aches, abdominal pain, nausea, and vomiting over the past 6 hours. Her last menstrual period began 2 days ago. She notes she had been camping at an outdoor festival the past 3 days and placed a tampon at the start of her menses but had been unable to replace it since she forgot to bring extra with her. The patient appears ill with a temperature of 40.0°C and is tachycardic with a blood pressure of 76/42 mmHg. She has a diffuse macular erythematous rash and on pelvic exam is noted to have vaginal hyperemia with significant odor from the retained tampon.

Evaluation/Tests	CBC with elevated WBC and low platelets and BMP notable for elevated BUN and creatinine. LFTs with elevated transaminases and bilirubin and elevated creatine kinase levels. Urinalysis normal. Serologies negative for Rocky Mountain spotted fever, leptospirosis, and measles.
Treatment	Removal of foreign body; supportive care/treatment of shock; empiric multidrug antibiotic therapy that includes anti-MRSA antibacterials; possible debridement (when focal infection is present).
Discussion	**Toxic shock syndrome (TSS)** is classified as menstrual or nonmenstrual. TSS is not common but is life-threatening when it occurs. TSS is secondary to exotoxin production (toxic shock syndrome toxin (TSST-1)) by *Staphylococcus aureus*. TSST-1 is a "superantigen" that is capable of cross-linking the Beta region of a T-cell receptor (TCR) to an MHC Class II molecule on antigen-presenting cells (APCs) outside of the antigen binding site. This cross-linking leads to massive release of various cytokines such as IL-1, IL-2, IFN-gamma, and TNF-alpha, which leads to shock. Menstrual-related cases are most classically attributed to prolonged retention of a vaginal foreign body, such as a tampon. Patients typically present with fever, rash, and shock. Patients will often have multiorgan system involvement as well. Approximately half of TSS cases are due to nonmenstrual causes such as postoperative wound infections and burns. Toxic shock-like syndrome presents with fever, shock, and rash much like TSS but is due to the erythrogenic exotoxin A produced by *Streptococcus pyogenes*. This syndrome is typically associated with soft tissue infections and is not common with retained tampons. **Rocky Mountain spotted fever (RMSF)** presents with fever, shock, and rash, but the rash typically begins at the wrists and ankles and spreads to the trunk and evolves from macular to petechial. Furthermore, patients with RMSF often have fever, headache, myalgias, and arthralgias early on in the presentation. Because this is a tick-borne illness, patients have some outdoor exposure to ticks.

TRANSPLACENTAL INFECTIONS

ToRCHeS	Other Infections
Toxoplasma gondii	*Streptococcus agalactiae*
Rubella	*Escherichia coli*
Cytomegalovirus (CMV)	*Listeria monocytogenes*
Herpes simplex virus (HSV)	Tuberculosis
Syphilis	Parvovirus
	Varicella zoster virus
	Malaria
	Fungal

CASE 28	Congenital Rubella Syndrome

A 27-year-old primigravida woman at 11 weeks gestation presents with fever, malaise, and rash. The rash is macular, started on her face, and has spread to her trunk. She recalls having chicken pox and measles as a child. She is a teacher and has no obstetric complaints but is concerned about how her illness might affect her pregnancy. On exam, she has a macular rash from the face to the trunk that blanches with pressure, generalized lymphadenopathy, and arthralgias.

Evaluation/Tests	Rubella-specific IgM antibodies; check fetal ultrasound.
Treatment	None. Symptomatic management.
Discussion	Since the onset of consistent vaccination against **rubella**, infection in pregnancy is rare. Titers are routinely checked in early pregnancy to establish a patient's immunity status. Most infants are asymptomatic but develop symptoms over time. Twenty to fifty percent of maternal infections are asymptomatic; the remaining patients present with fever, malaise, rash, and arthralgias. Worsening manifestations of congenital rubella syndrome are noted with earlier gestational age at the time of infection, with 80% vertical transmission noted in the first trimester. Fetal infection is associated with miscarriage, intrauterine growth restriction, eye defects, sensorineural hearing loss, purpuric "blueberry muffin" rash, patent ductus arteriosus, and cerebral palsy. The classic triad is cataracts, deafness, and congenital heart disease.
Additional Considerations	**Congenital toxoplasmosis** is transmitted via undercooked meat and occasionally cat feces. Most mothers are asymptomatic, as are most infants. Symptomatic neonatal infections present with the classic triad of chorioretinitis, hydrocephalus, and intracranial calcifications. **Congenital syphilis** is transmitted sexually. Prenatal testing routinely includes syphilis in the first trimester or at time of presentation. Fetal infection is associated with stillbirth, hydrops fetalis, prematurity, congenital deafness, and facial abnormalities (notched teeth, saddle nose), though most neonates are asymptomatic at birth. **Congenital cytomegalovirus** is the most common congenital viral infection. It is frequently transmitted via contact with children, such as in day care facilities. Maternal infection is typically asymptomatic. Neonatal infection classically presents with sensorineural hearing loss, seizures, "blueberry muffin" rash, and periventricular calcifications. **HSV** is acquired perinatally or, rarely, in utero. Most cases are perinatally acquired during vaginal delivery. Mothers with active genital infection should deliver via cesarean section. Mothers with a history of infection are prescribed antiviral therapy for suppression at 36 weeks. Neonatal infection is characterized by either localized mucocutaneous disease (vesicles that may lead to scarring and eye damage), CNS disease, or disseminated disease. **Invasive listeriosis** is rare, though pregnant patients are 13 times more likely to be affected than the general population. Primarily a foodborne illness, pregnant women are advised not to consume foods with a high risk for listeria contamination, including processed meats, unpasteurized milk and soft cheese, and unwashed raw produce. While asymptomatic exposed pregnant women can be managed expectantly, women with high suspicion for invasive listeriosis should be treated with 14 days of high-dose IV ampicillin. Fetal/neonatal sequelae can be severe, including fetal loss, preterm labor, neonatal sepsis and meningitis, and neonatal demise.

DIARRHEA (INFECTIOUS)

Diarrhea is a very common clinical problem and is categorized by duration of symptoms. Acute diarrhea is, by definition, present for <2 weeks and is overwhelmingly secondary to infectious causes. The majority of cases of acute, infectious diarrhea are viral in etiology. Patients with acute, bloody diarrhea are more likely to have a bacterial pathogen such as *Shigella*, *Salmonella*, or *Campylobacter*. Diarrhea that lasts >2 weeks is categorized as persistent or chronic and is more likely to be secondary to a noninfectious cause. We will focus primarily on the few infectious causes when discussing chronic diarrhea in this section. Of note, several of the causes listed here can also cause emesis (emesis with diarrhea = gastroenteritis), which will be noted in individual cases, but diarrhea will be the main symptom in this section.

Differential Diagnosis for Diarrhea

Acute Watery Diarrhea	Acute Bloody Diarrhea	Persistent Diarrhea

Bacterial
  Enterotoxigenic (ETEC) *E. coli* (traveler's diarrhea)
  Clostridium difficile
  Listeria monocytogenes
Viral
  Norovirus
  Rotavirus
  Other enteric viruses (astrovirus, etc.)
  Cytomegalovirus (CMV) (in immunocompromised hosts)
	Bacterial
	  Salmonella
	    Typhoid
	    Nontyphoidal
	  Shigella
	  Campylobacter
	  Yersinia spp.
	  Enterohemorrhagic (EHEC) *E. coli*
	  Vibrio spp. ?.
	Protozoan
	  Entamoeba histolytica
		Parasites
		  Giardia lamblia
		  Cryptosporidium parvum
		  Strongyloides stercoralis
		Noninfectious
		  Inflammatory bowel disease
		  Celiac disease
		  Irritable bowel syndrome

Most acute diarrheal infectious causes are very difficult to distinguish from one another. However, getting a good history with regard to food exposures, travel, animal exposures, sick contacts, antibiotic use, etc. can help pin down a diagnosis. Additionally, the presence of fever and/or bloody diarrhea may also provide clues to the underlying etiology as well and may reflect infection with an organism that is more invasive (able to cross intestinal epithelia). Immunocompromising conditions such as HIV/AIDS and organ transplantation broaden the differential to include opportunistic causes of diarrhea such as *Cryptosporidium* and cytomegalovirus (CMV). Ultimately, most causes of acute diarrhea are managed with supportive care, so identifying causes that require antimicrobial therapy, such as *Clostridium difficile*, is important.

Key Findings and Diarrhea Differential Diagnosis

Diarrhea with Key Associated Findings	Diagnoses and Pathogens
- Recent antibiotic exposure, recent hospitalization - "Pseudomembranous colitis" appearance on colonoscopy	*C. difficile*
- Severe abdominal distention, systemic toxicity	*C. difficile* with toxic megacolon
Hemolytic uremic syndrome (HUS)	EHEC
Travel abroad	ETEC *E. coli*, *E. histolytica*, Typhoid fever, or *Strongyloides stercoralis*
Cruise ship outbreak	Norovirus
- Freshwater exposure, time in the woods/hiking - Common variable immune deficiency (CVID, IgA deficiency)	*Giardia lamblia*
Day care center exposure	*Giardia lamblia* or rotavirus
- Unpasteurized milk - Pregnancy	*Listeria monocytogenes*
- Undercooked poultry - Fever	*Campylobacter*, *Shigella* or *Salmonella*
Reptile/turtle exposure	*Salmonella*
"Rose spot" rash on abdomen	*Salmonella enterica* serotype *typhi*—Typhoid fever
- Diarrhea followed by polyarticular arthritis, conjunctivitis	Reactive arthritis, which is associated with *Campylobacter*, *Shigella*, *Salmonella*, *Yersinia*
- Hemochromatosis - Severe RLQ pain: "pseudoappendicitis" due to severe ileocolitis	*Yersinia* spp.
Diarrhea followed by flaccid, ascending weakness on exam	*Campylobacter* (the most associated diarrheal cause with Guillain-Barre syndrome)
- Men who have sex with men - Diarrhea and liver abscess	*Entamoeba histolytica*
Eosinophilia on labs	*Strongyloides stercoralis*
Cirrhosis	*Vibrio* spp.
Orthostatic hypotension, frank hypotension	Any diarrhea if severe enough can cause hypovolemia, which can manifest as hypotension.

Clues for Special Populations

Clue	Diagnosis
HIV/AIDS and other immunocompromised hosts	Patients with AIDS are at risk of all the common causes of acute diarrhea but are at increased risk of cryptosporidiosis, which can be slowly fatal if the patient does not receive antiretroviral medications. CMV colitis can affect immunocompromised hosts as well, and presentations vary from subacute watery diarrhea to hematochezia from colonic mucosal hemorrhage.
Hospitalized patient, chronically ill patients	In patients who are hospitalized or have a lot of health care exposure and who develop new diarrhea, *C. difficile* should be at the top of the differential.
Travel to developing nations	Patients who travel abroad, especially to unindustrialized countries, are at risk of several infections that are not common in the United States like ETEC (traveler's diarrhea), typhoid fever, *E. histolytica*, and strongyloidiasis, in addition to common causes.

CASE 29 | Pseudomembranous Colitis (*Clostridioides Difficile*)

A 60-year-old man with type 2 diabetes and hypertension presents with crampy abdominal pain, numerous watery stools, and lightheadedness for 3 days. He was recently treated for pneumonia with levofloxacin. He has had no unusual food intake or any sick contacts. On exam, he has a temperature of 36.8, pulse 118/min, respirations 14/min, and blood pressure 110/84 mmHg. His systolic blood pressure drops by 30 mmHg when he goes from lying to standing. He has mild, diffuse tenderness on abdominal exam.

Evaluation/Tests	Basic metabolic panel is notable for hypokalemia, and his CBC is notable for a WBC count of 25,000/mm³. *C. difficile* stool PCR is positive.
Treatment	Oral vancomycin is first-line treatment. Alternative therapy includes fidaxomicin and metronidazole. Volume resuscitation with IV fluids and electrolyte repletion. Recurrent cases can be treated with fecal microbiota transplant (FMT).
Discussion	***Clostridioides* (formerly *Clostridium*) difficile** (*C. diff*) can be relatively indistinct from other causes of acute diarrhea, but the diagnosis should be considered in patients with a recent hospitalization or antibiotic exposure (especially with certain antibiotics such as clindamycin, ceftriaxone, or fluoroquinolones). In severe cases, *C. diff* can cause ileus with toxic megacolon (distended colon with systemic toxicity) and even death. On colonoscopy, yellowish, exudative plaques may be seen, which is the classic "**pseudomembranous colitis.**" *Clostridia* species are gram positive, spore-forming, obligate anaerobic rods that produce several exotoxins that drive virulence and pathogenicity. Specifically, *C. diff* produces toxin A (enterotoxin that damages intestinal enterocytes driving watery diarrhea) and toxin B (cytotoxin that drives epithelial necrosis and pseudomembrane formation). Despite appropriate treatment, recurrence is common and patients may need prolonged antibiotic therapy or a fecal microbiota transplant. **Norovirus** is strongly associated with cruise travel, shellfish consumption, and day care exposure. **Rotavirus** is a reovirus that commonly affects young children in the winter. It can cause secretory diarrhea. This is also commonly seen in patients with sick contacts or day care exposure.

CASE 30 | *Campylobacter Jejuni* Enteritis

A 45-year-old man presents with 3 days of fever, abdominal pain, and bloody diarrhea. He ate some chicken a few days ago, which may have been undercooked. He has had no sick contacts. On exam, the patient has a temperature of 38.4°C, pulse 100/min, respirations 16/min, and blood pressure 110/70 mmHg. Mild diffuse tenderness is noted on abdominal exam. He has no rash.

Evaluation/Tests	BMP is normal, and CBC shows Hgb 11 g/dL, hematocrit 33%, WBCs 14,000/mm³ (85% neutrophils), platelets 350,000/mm³. Peripheral blood smear is normal with no evidence of schistocytes. Stool culture and PCR are pending.
Treatment	Mild cases do not require antibiotics, and treatment is supportive with IV fluids and electrolyte replacement. Patients with moderate to severe symptoms can be empirically treated with a fluoroquinolone or azithromycin.

CASE 30 | *Campylobacter Jejuni* **Enteritis** *(continued)*

Discussion	*Campylobacter jejuni* **enteritis** presents as fever and bloody diarrhea, suggestive of an invasive bacterial pathogen, often after eating undercooked chicken. *C. jejuni* is a gram negative, oxidase positive comma- or S-shaped rod that causes bloody diarrhea, most commonly in children. Transmission is fecal-oral and occurs with ingestion of undercooked or contaminated poultry and meat. Unpasteurized milk and exposure to dogs, cats, and pigs can be a risk factor for acquiring this infection. It can be the inciting event in either Guillain-Barre syndrome (ascending paralysis) or reactive arthritis, which are significant potential complications of *C. jejuni* enteritis
	The main other pathogens to consider include **Shigella**, **EHEC**, and **Salmonella**, which all present very similarly and can be associated with undercooked foods. **Shigella** (due to Shiga toxin) and **EHEC** (due to Shiga-like toxin) can cause hemolytic uremic syndrome (HUS), which presents with a triad of diarrhea, thrombocytopenia, and acute renal failure. EHEC serotype O157:H7 is a common cause of food poisoning outbreaks in the United States.
	Salmonella exposure can also be transmitted by undercooked poultry, eggs, or pet exposure. Salmonella enteritis requires a high inoculum of organisms because it is acid labile, and individuals with normal stomach acid production are less likely to be susceptible to infection. Individuals with reduced acid production (e.g., patients on PPIs) are more susceptible to *Salmonella* infection. **Viral gastroenteritis** is less likely if the diarrhea is bloody.

CASE 31 | Norovirus Gastroenteritis

A 28-year-old woman develops "explosive," watery diarrhea and emesis for 1 day while on a spring break cruise. She has no fever. Other cruise patrons have experienced a similar illness during the trip. She does not think any food she has eaten was improperly prepared. On exam, the patient has a temperature of 36.6°C, with pulse 95/min, respirations 14/min, and blood pressure 110/78 mmHg. She is not in acute distress. Her abdomen is nondistended, and there is mild tenderness to palpation in the lower quadrants bilaterally. She has hyperactive bowel sounds.

Evaluation/Tests	Clinical diagnosis. Stool pathogen PCR, if sent, would return positive for norovirus.
Treatment	Treatment is supportive with fluids and electrolyte replacement.
Discussion	**Norovirus gastroenteritis** classically presents with "explosive" diarrhea as well as nausea and emesis. Norovirus is a positive sense, single-stranded RNA virus with an icosahedral capsid and no envelope (naked). Other viruses can present similarly, but norovirus is very transmissible from person to person (low inoculum of virus required to cause infection), so it is particularly effective at causing disease outbreaks.
	Bacterial diarrhea is less likely; this patient does not have exposures to undercooked meat, eggs, or unpasteurized milk, and she does not have bloody diarrhea.
	Rotavirus is a double-stranded, segmented RNA virus that typically causes nonbloody diarrhea in infants and children.
	Noninfectious colitis secondary to inflammatory bowel disease is highly unlikely given this patient's timeline of symptoms, lack of weight loss, and systemic findings.
Additional Considerations	Sudden onset of nausea and vomiting (in the absence of diarrhea) can be due to ingestion of a preformed toxin such as **S. aureus** or **B. cereus toxins**. The hallmark of the disease is the rapid nature of symptom onset and resolution, with symptoms typically beginning within 1–6 hours from ingestion of the toxin and resolving within a day.
	S. aureus enterotoxin is often found in foods such as dairy, produce, meats, eggs, and salads.
	B. cereus is strongly associated with starchy foods, such as rice, and is strongly associated with eating reheated rice. Symptoms resolve without need for treatment, and management is supportive.

CASE 32 | Giardiasis (*Giardia Lamblia*)

A 22-year-old man presents with 1 month of watery diarrhea, abdominal cramping, weight loss, and increased flatulence. He recently vacationed in Colorado to go hiking, and he drank from a lake during his trip. He has had no sexual activity recently, and no sick contacts. He describes the diarrhea as foul-smelling but nonbloody. On exam, the patient has a temperature of 37.1°C, has a pulse of 75/min, respirations 12/min, and blood pressure 110/78 mmHg. He is not in acute distress. His abdomen is nondistended, and there is mild, diffuse tenderness to palpation.

CASE 32 | Giardiasis (*Giardia Lamblia*) *(continued)*

Evaluation/Tests	BMP is normal. <u>Stool ova and parasite (O&P) microscopy is positive for multinucleated pear-shaped trophozoites and cysts.</u> Stool antigen testing for *Giardia lamblia* is positive. 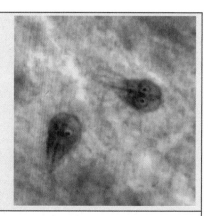 Giardia lamblia trophozoite: Giardia duodenalis trophozoites in Kohn stain. G duodenalis trophozoites are pear-shaped and measure 10–20 mcM in length. In permanent, stained specimens, two large nuclei are usually visible. The sucking disks (used for attaching to the host's mucosal epithelium), median bodies, and flagella (8) may also be seen. (From Global Health, Division of Parasitic Diseases and Malaria, CDC.) Reproduced with permission from Global Health, Division of Parasitic Diseases and Malaria, CDC.
Treatment	Metronidazole.
Discussion	This patient is presenting with **giardiasis** caused by the gastrointestinal pathogen and protozoan ***Giardia lamblia***. *Giardia* is a common enteric parasite within the United States and often presents with <u>chronic diarrhea and malabsorption in otherwise healthy individuals after drinking contaminated water from a freshwater lake.</u> Patients usually have cramping and increased flatulence with a foul-smelling, fatty diarrhea. Giardia can cause a <u>malabsorption syndrome with weight loss.</u> Ova and parasite stool microscopy are less sensitive due to intermittent excretion of cysts, but it is very specific if *Giardia* cysts or trophozoites are seen. If stool O&P is nondiagnostic, colonoscopy can be performed and may show <u>villous atrophy and crypt hyperplasia.</u> Also, patients with underlying primary immunodeficiency conditions, such as <u>common variable immunodeficiency (CVID)</u> or <u>IgA deficiency,</u> are at increased risk of giardiasis, including recurrent disease. ***Cryptosporidium*** is another protozoan that can cause <u>chronic, watery diarrhea, but it is much more common in immunocompromised patients.</u> It is the most common cause of diarrhea in AIDS patients. ***Strongyloides stercoralis*** (threadworm) is a nematode or roundworm that initially burrows from soil into the skin (causing an itchy rash, often on bare feet) and then travels through the blood to the lungs and GI tract. The helminth completes its whole life cycle in the patient, so it can cause chronic infection, which may manifest solely as <u>eosinophilia on labs or include a GI component with abdominal pain and diarrhea.</u> It is unlikely in this patient because he has not traveled to an endemic area like <u>Southeast Asia.</u> ***Entamoeba histolytica*** causes intestinal amebiasis with <u>bloody diarrhea and formation of a liver abscess</u> with characteristic <u>"anchovy paste"</u> exudate. Colonoscopy will reveal <u>flask-shaped ulcers</u> in the lining of the colon. **Inflammatory bowel disease (IBD)** is an important noninfectious cause of chronic diarrhea and weight loss. Crohn's disease could present in this fashion, but infection must be ruled out first.

4

Pathology

Amy Lin, MD

CELLULAR ADAPTATIONS, INJURY, AND DEATH

Cellular adaptations are reversible changes in the structure and function of cells in response to physiologic stresses or pathologic stimuli. These changes include the following:

Cellular Adaptation	Definition	Example
Hypertrophy	Increase in cell size and functional activity	Smooth muscle cells of the uterine myometrium during pregnancy
Hyperplasia	Increase in number of cells	Proliferation of endometrial glands with estrogen excess
Atrophy	Decreased size and activity of cells	Seen in skeletal muscle of an immobilized fractured limb
Metaplasia	Change in cell phenotype	As a result of cigarette smoking, squamous epithelium replaces pseudostratified columnar bronchial epithelium. Metaplasia is usually reversible when the irritant is removed.
Dysplasia	Disordered, precancerous epithelial cell growth	Common in the uterine cervix. Severe dysplasia is a premalignant lesion, while mild dysplasia is reversible.

Cell injury occurs when the capacity of the cell to adapt is exceeded. Causes of cell injury include hypoxia, ischemia, toxins, infectious agents, immunologic reactions, genetic abnormalities, nutritional imbalances, physical agents, and aging.

If the cell is irreversibly injured, it undergoes cell death. There are two major pathways of cell death: necrosis and apoptosis. Necrosis is a pathologic process that occurs with severe, irreversible cell injury that is associated with a host inflammatory reaction. Apoptosis, on the other hand, is a regulated mechanism of cell death that eliminates irreparably damaged and unwanted cells with the least possible host reaction.

CASE 1 Hyperplasia	
A 27-year-old obese woman with no significant past medical history presents with abnormal vaginal bleeding. Her menses started at age 14 and have been irregular since then. They occur every 2–3 months, are heavy, and last 5–7 days. Her last menstrual period was 1 week ago. She is not sexually active and is not taking any medications.	
Evaluation/Tests	Hemoglobin 10 g/dL. Pelvic ultrasound shows thickened endometrial lining and an incidental 3.5-cm right ovarian mass consistent with a follicular cyst. Endometrial curettage was performed, and histologic examination of the endometrium shows an increase in gland-to-stroma ratio, consistent with endometrial hyperplasia, without evidence of atypia.
Treatment	Endometrial curettage and/or progestin therapy. Weight loss may also decrease estrogen stimulation.
Discussion	**Endometrial hyperplasia** is the abnormal proliferation of endometrial glands secondary to increased number of cells and glands with different sizes and shapes. It usually occurs after the unopposed stimulation of estrogen. It is not a premalignant lesion, but it may be a risk factor for future malignancies. In this case, the presence of a follicular cyst (distension of an unruptured Graafian follicle, the most common ovarian mass in young women) caused unopposed estrogen stimulation, resulting in the hyperplastic endometrium. Definitive diagnosis is made by biopsy. Irregular appearance of the lining on imaging may provide clues as well. **Atypical hyperplasia/endometrial intraepithelial neoplasia (AH/EIN)** is analogous to **dysplasia** in the cervix or in a tubular adenoma of the colon. AH/EIN is a premalignant lesion associated with an increased risk of endometrial carcinoma. It is characterized by complex patterns of proliferating glands that show nuclear atypia. Atypical cells have rounded nuclei with open, vesicular chromatin and conspicuous nucleoli. They lose the normal perpendicular orientation to the basement membrane. The histologic features of AH/EIN and well-differentiated endometrial carcinoma often overlap; however, **endometrial carcinoma** shows invasion into the myometrium. Endometrial carcinoma is broadly divided into two categories. Type 1 is endometrioid carcinomas, which are stimulated by estrogen. Type 2 is not stimulated by estrogen and includes serous or clear cell carcinomas.

CASE 2 | Red Infarct, Coagulative Necrosis

A 75-year-old woman with a history of coronary artery disease, hypertension, and diabetes presents with sudden onset excruciating abdominal pain after eating dinner. The pain was generalized to her whole abdomen, and she also noted two episodes of bloody, "currant jelly"–like stools. Exam was notable for an irregular rhythm and distended, nontender abdomen with hyperactive bowel sounds.

Evaluation/Tests	Laboratory results show mild leukocytosis and a normal lipase and liver function. ECG shows atrial fibrillation. Abdominal X-ray is negative for intraperitoneal free air or obstruction. CT angiography of the abdomen demonstrates occlusion of the superior mesenteric artery and bowel wall edema. Patient is taken to the OR for surgical removal of the bowel segment. Gross examination shows a segment of the small intestine that is dusky and red (see image). Microscopic examination shows coagulative necrosis of the intestinal mucosa. Reproduced with permission from Van De Winkel N, Cheragwandi A, Nieboer K, et al: Superior mesenteric arterial branch occlusion causing partial jejunal ischemia: a case report, J Med Case Rep 2012 Feb 6;6;48. 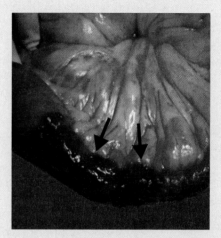
Treatment	Ischemic bowel requires surgical removal. Medical management includes pain control, broad-spectrum antibiotics, and anticoagulation in the setting of atrial fibrillation.
Discussion	**Bowel ischemia/infarctions** cause coagulative necrosis. Infarcts are classified according to color: either red (hemorrhagic) or pale (anemic). **Bowel infarcts** are **red** because blood can flow into infarcted, necrotic tissue by way of unobstructed collateral circulation. Red infarcts can occur because of venous occlusion (e.g., testicular torsion); vascular occlusion of an organ with dual circulation or multiple collaterals (e.g., lung, liver, intestines), or reperfusion (e.g., following angioplasty of an arterial occlusion). **Pale infarct** occurs in solid organs with single (end-arterial) blood supply (e.g., heart, spleen, kidney). Occlusion of a single blood supply prevents reperfusion of the injured area, giving it its characteristic pale color (e.g., occlusion of the left anterior descending coronary artery causing a massive cardiac infarct). The different categories of **necrosis** (coagulative, liquefactive, gangrenous, caseous, fat, and fibrinoid) depend on the type of tissue injured. In this case, ischemia/infarction of the bowel activates a cascade of enzymatic reactions, causing coagulative necrosis. Structural proteins and lysosomal enzymes are denatured due to the injury. This, blocks proteolysis and the lack of lysosomal enzymes allows the damaged cells to maintain a "coagulated" morphology for some time. Histologically, cell outlines are preserved and nuclei disappear. This results in increased cytoplasmic binding of eosin dye and "ghost cells" seen on H&E (hematoxylin and eosin stain). Normal lipase, LFTs, abdominal imaging and presence of bloody stools makes other causes of acute abdominal pain such as acute pancreatitis, small bowel obstruction, and acute cholecystitis less likely.
Additional Considerations	**Liquefactive necrosis** occurs when dead cells are digested into a liquid mass. Examples include an abscess from a focal bacterial infection or infarction within the central nervous system (see image). Compared to coagulative necrosis, liquefactive necrosis involves loss of native tissue architecture and is common in tissue with low protein content (e.g., brain, as shown in image) and/or high concentration of proteolytic enzymes (e.g., pancreas). Within the brain histology image shown, macrophages can be observed engulfing lipid-rich myelin and cellular debris. 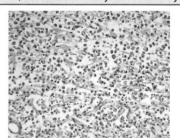 Reproduced with permission from Kemp WL, Burns DK, Brow TG: Pathology: The Big Picture. New York, NY: McGraw Hill; 2008.

CASE 2 | Red Infarct, Coagulative Necrosis *(continued)*

Additional Considerations	
	Gangrenous necrosis is a clinical term that typically refers to necrosis of a limb due to ischemia/infarction. Gangrenous necrosis is classified as follows: • *Dry gangrene*: This is a coagulative necrosis. • *Wet gangrene*: This consists of coagulative necrosis *and* liquefactive necrosis. Wet gangrene typically occurs in the setting of a superimposed bacterial infection. Used with permission from William Archibald, Public Health Image Library, Centers for Disease Control and Prevention. 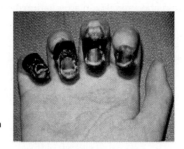
	Caseous necrosis refers to the friable, cheese-like gross appearance that is most frequently seen in tuberculosis infection. Microscopically, caseous necrosis consists of fragmented cells and amorphous granular debris surrounded by granulomatous inflammation. Used with permission from Dr. Yale Rosen/Creative Commons Attribution. 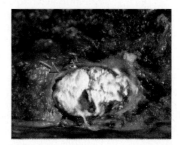
	Fat necrosis refers to areas of fat destruction, which occur as a result of acute pancreatitis or trauma (e.g., injury to breast tissue). Damaged cells release lipases causing fat saponification (necrosis of fat cells with calcium soap formation). Enzymatic fat necrosis. The image shows an area of saponified pancreatic fat (outline) surrounded by an inflammatory reaction and damaged pancreatic acini (arrows). Reproduced with permission from Reisner H. Pathology: A Modern Case Study, 2nd ed. New York, NY: McGraw Hill; 2020. 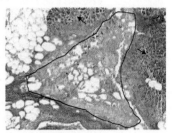
	Fibrinoid necrosis is typically seen in immune reactions involving blood vessels (e.g., vasculitis), resulting in bright pink amorphous material in the vessel wall. Used with permission from Dr. Yale Rosen/Creative Commons Attribution. 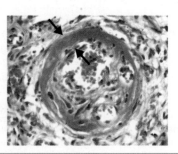

INFLAMMATION

Inflammation is the cellular and molecular response coordinated by the body's defense systems in response to damage, infection, or other causes of cellular injury. The prominent cells involved are those of the immune system. Activation of immune cells and the subsequent release of inflammatory mediators (cytokines, chemokines, complement proteins) can lead to both local and systemic manifestations. Local signs of inflammation include warmness, redness, pain, swelling, and loss of function. Systemic signs of inflammation include fever, leukocytosis, and changes in serum levels of acute phase reactants (e.g., C-reactive protein). This chapter will explore further various key points of the inflammatory response:

- The inflammatory response is a **highly coordinated** mechanism that allows circulating white blood cells to cross endothelia at damage or infection sites, exiting blood vessels and entering tissue. This process of **leukocyte extravasation** has several key steps.

- It is important to differentiate between **acute and chronic inflammatory** responses, as the timing of inflammatory signs and symptoms may provide insight into the etiology and pathogenesis of a particular condition.

- In cases where the immune system is unable to completely eliminate an invader or toxin, formation of a granuloma effectively "walls off" these agents to prevent further damage.

CASE 3 | Leukocyte Extravasation (Leukocyte Adhesion Deficiency Type I)

A 20-day-old boy is brought in for evaluation of fever and fussiness. Past medical history is notable for a previous skin infection, which was treated with antibiotics. His mother has no medical problems, and the delivery was normal. On exam, the child is febrile, and the umbilical stump is still attached and has surrounding erythema consistent with cellulitis.

Evaluation/Tests	CBC shows leukocytosis with neutrophilia. Flow cytometry shows leukocytes with low CD18/LFA-1.
Treatment	Depending on severity, treatment may range from prophylactic antibiotics to stem cell transplant.
Discussion	The patient in this case suffers from leukocyte adhesion deficiency (LAD) type 1, an autosomal recessive disorder with a defect in LFA-1 integrin (CD18) protein on leukocytes. Leukocytes are thus unable to adhere to and migrate out of the blood vessel. As a result, leukocytes cannot travel to the site of infection. Delayed separation of the umbilical cord is a characteristic feature as neutrophil extravasation is required to phagocytose debris from the degenerating cord. Neutrophils are considered the "first responders" in an acute inflammatory reaction and are often among the first cells to arrive at the injury site.

Leukocyte emigration from the vessel to the site of injury involves four important steps:

1. **Margination and Rolling**—E-selectin and P-selectin (on endothelial cells) mediate loose adherence of leukocytes to the vascular wall, which bind to sialyl-Lewis^x (on leukocytes)
2. **Adhesion**—Firm adherence to the vascular wall mediated by ICAM-1 and VCAM-1 (on endothelial cells), which bind to integrins (e.g., CD11/18 or LFA-1) on leukocytes
3. **Diapedesis**—Transmigration across the vascular wall between endothelial cells, which is mediated by PECAM-1/CD31 signaling
4. **Migration**—Guided by chemokines and other signals, leukocytes traveling through tissue interstitium to the injury or infection site

The five steps of leukocyte extravasation. (1) Capillary endothelial cells increase their surface selectins in response to inflammatory mediators such as tumor necrosis factor (TNF) and interleukin-1 (IL-1). (2) Leukocytes (e.g., neutrophils) patrolling the bloodstream slow down and roll along the luminal surface of the endothelial cells when their selectin ligands bind to the selectins. (3) Local inflammatory chemokines bind to the leukocyte's chemokine receptors, triggering a conformational change in their surface integrins from a state that is low affinity to high affinity. (4) The high-affinity integrins interact with endothelial cell adhesion molecules, causing the leukocyte to stop rolling and adhere along the surface of the vessel wall. (5) Using cell adhesion molecules, the leukocytes change shape and transmigrate between the gaps between endothelial cells and into the inflamed tissue, following the chemokine gradient.

Reproduced with permission from Mescher AL. Junqueira's Basic Histology: Text and Atlas, 15th ed. New York, NY: McGraw Hill; 2018.

CASE 3 | Leukocyte Extravasation (Leukocyte Adhesion Deficiency Type I) *(continued)*

Discussion	Any defect on leukocyte adhesion molecules will interfere with the adhesion cascade, resulting in an inefficient leukocyte extravasation and phagocytosis. This predisposes patients to recurrent infections and impaired wound healing.
	Severe combined immunodeficiency (SCID) is a serious immunodeficiency characterized by failure to thrive and recurrent viral, bacterial, fungal, and protozoal infections. In SCID, B- and T-cells are dysfunctional due to defective IL-2R gamma chain or due to adenosine deaminase deficiency.
	Chronic granulomatous disease is the result of NADPH oxidase defect. Patients often present with infections with catalase positive organisms (e.g., *Staph aureus* and *Pseudomonas aeruginosa*).

CASE 4 | Chronic Inflammation (Ruptured Epidermoid Cyst)

A 28-year-old woman presents with a red nodule on her posterior neck. She said it has been present for some time, but it only became red and somewhat painful about 10 days ago. On exam, there is a well-circumscribed, tender, mobile red nodule on the back of her neck without surrounding erythema or fluctuance.

Evaluation/Tests	Excision of the nodule is performed. Histologic examination shows a cyst lined by squamous epithelium filled with keratin debris. There are also areas of infiltrating mononuclear cells, tissue destruction, and granulation tissue with foreign body giant cells.
Treatment	Excision with removal of the cyst lining to prevent recurrence.
Discussion	In this case, the **rupture of an epidermoid inclusion cyst** initiates a cascade of reactions that cause a chronic inflammatory response. The histology shows foreign body giant cells with macrophages surrounded by diffuse chronic inflammation (lymphocytes).
	Symptoms of inflammation are secondary to increased vascular permeability, vasodilation, and endothelial injury. Depending on the duration of the inflammation, the cellular component may vary. Chronic inflammation involves a prolonged inflammatory response with tissue infiltration by mononuclear cells (macrophages, B- and T-lymphocytes and plasma cells). These cells coordinate the prolonged immune response in attempts to repair tissue, resulting in angiogenesis, fibrosis, and scar formation. If left unchecked, chronic inflammation can also cause tissue destruction.
	Chronic inflammation can be seen in multiple contexts, including persistent infections (e.g., tuberculosis), scarring, amyloidosis, neoplasia, and chronic inflammatory conditions (e.g., rheumatoid arthritis or systemic lupus erythematosus). Chronic inflammation can also promote neoplastic transformation, as in the case of chronic HCV infection resulting in hepatocellular carcinoma. Epidermoid cysts can become infected.
	Abscesses will be red, tender, and fluctuant and will present more acutely than epidermoid cyst. Treatment includes incision and drainage (I&D) and antibiotics.
	Angiolipoma is a benign tumor of adipocytes and generally presents as a nontender and nonerythematous subcutaneous nodule.

CASE 5 | Granulomatous Disease (Tuberculosis)

A 56-year-old man, who recently immigrated from rural India, presents with a dry cough and intermittent, mild hemoptysis. He reports significant weight loss and night sweats. He does not smoke. Patient's temperature is 38.2°C, pulse is 96/min, respirations are 22/min, and blood pressure is 132/89 mmHg. On exam, he has bilateral cervical lymphadenopathy and crackles in the upper left lung field.

Evaluation/Tests	Chest X-ray reveals left upper lobe infiltrate. Sputum is positive for acid-fast bacilli. Although not routinely performed, an excisional wedge biopsy with subsequent H&E stain (image) shows multiple foci consisting of groups of histiocytes surrounded by lymphocytes, multinucleated giant cells, and a central area of necrosis. Ziehl-Neelsen stain reveals acid-fast bacilli. 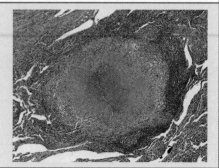
	UIC Virtual Microscope Used with permission from Microscope, University of Illinois College of Medicine.

CASE 5 | Granulomatous Disease (Tuberculosis) *(continued)*

Treatment	Antibiotic regimen for tuberculosis: rifampin, isoniazid, pyrazinamide, and ethambutol (RIPE).
Discussion	Granulomatous inflammation is a subtype of chronic inflammation characterized by the presence of granulomas. Granulomas are structures composed of aggregates of epithelioid macrophages surrounded by a rim of lymphocytes. Activated macrophages can fuse to form multinucleated giant cells. Granuloma formation typically occurs in response to an antigen that cannot be removed by typical immune mechanisms. IFN-γ secreted by Th1-lymphocytes activates macrophages, which then secrete TNF-α. TNF-alpha causes a cycle of further macrophage activation and granuloma formation. Further differentiation is based on whether or not the granuloma has a central area of necrosis. Caseating granulomas have a central area of necrosis, and they often present in granulomas that arise due to an infectious etiology. The next step would be to perform special stains for acid-fast bacilli for *Mycobacterium* or fungal stains (e.g., Gomori methenamine silver stain). Given the presence of caseous necrosis and acid-fast bacilli, the diagnosis is ***Mycobacterium tuberculosis***. Many conditions can lead to granulomatous inflammation, including bacterial (e.g., *Mycobacteria*), fungal (e.g., endemic mycoses), parasitic (e.g., schistosomiasis), autoinflammatory (e.g., sarcoidosis), or foreign-body disease (e.g., berylliosis). Therefore, these conditions should be considered in the differential of a lung biopsy showing granulomatous disease. **Fungal pneumonia** would also present with similar clinical features and caseating granuloma on histology. However, Ziehl-Nieelsen stain would not be positive. Fungal stains such as Gomori methenamine silver stain would reveal a fungal etiology. **Foreign-body granulomatosis** is classically associated with occupational beryllium exposure in the aerospace or manufacturing industry. While berylliosis also tends to affect the upper lobes, histology would reveal noncaseating granulomas. **Sarcoidosis** is often asymptomatic except for lymphadenopathy and is more common in African American women. When symptoms are present, they can affect many organ systems, and chest X-ray findings include bilateral hilar adenopathy and reticular opacities. If done, bronchoalveolar lavage would show an elevated T-lymphocyte CD4+/CD8+ ratio, and lung biopsy with H&E stain would show multiple foci consisting of groups of histiocytes surrounded by lymphocytes, multinucleated giant cells containing star-shaped inclusions, and no central area of necrosis (**noncaseating granulomas**). **Lung cancer** can present similarly, but it would not show granulomatous disease on histology. Sarcoidosis: The hallmark histopathologic feature of sarcoidosis is presence of granulomas (as are apparent numerously in the low-powered image and more closely visualized in the higher-powered inset image). Typically these are referred to as noncaseating which suggests the absence of necrosis. Caseating granulomas are rare in sarcoid and should prompt additional evaluation for an underlying infection. Because malignancy can result in a granulomatous reaction it is important to closely survey biopsy specimens with granulomatous involvement for additional signs of malignancy. Reproduced with permission from Jameson JL, Fauci AS, Kasper DL, et al: Harrison's Principles of Internal Medicine, 20th ed. New York, NY: McGraw Hill; 2018. 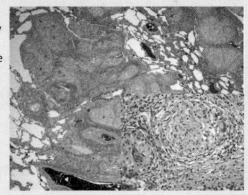

WOUND HEALING

In the aftermath of tissue damage and a subsequent inflammatory response, the next step is promotion of wound healing. Wound healing occurs in three stages: inflammatory, proliferative, and remodeling.

Inflammatory phase—Acute inflammatory response leads to innate immune cell infiltration and increased vessel permeability to clear debris.

Proliferative phase—This begins within days to weeks after a wound occurs. The proliferative phase includes proliferation of fibroblasts, myofibroblasts, endothelial cells (which promotes deposition of granulation tissue and type III collagen), wound contraction, and angiogenesis.

Remodeling phase—Fibroblasts gradually replace granulation tissue with stronger type I collagen, leading to tissue healing or scar formation.

This process is mediated by many effector molecules, including cytokines, FGF, VEGF, PDGF, metalloproteinase, and more. Additional cofactors such as vitamin C, copper, and zinc are required for wound healing; deficiencies in these cofactors can delay repair. Scars form when tissue cannot regenerate (e.g., cardiac myocytes) or when tissue has limited ability for repair (e.g., severe or chronic injury).

CASE 6	Hypertrophic Scar Formation
A 30-year-old woman presents for a 1-month follow-up after a thyroidectomy for a multinodular goiter. She is worried about the appearance of the scar on her neck. On exam, there is a linear, red-pink lesion, measuring 7.5 cm in length and 0.5 cm in diameter on the left lateral neck (see image) that is confined to the borders of the original incision site.	
Evaluations/Tests	Histologic examination shows type III collagen fibers that are parallel to the dermis with some vascular proliferation.
Treatment	The lesion is removed surgically, and there was no recurrence after the removal of the lesion.
Discussion	When tissue repair cannot be accomplished by cell regeneration alone, scar formation ensues. Abnormal and excessive scar formation can result in hypertrophic scars or keloids secondary to overproliferation of collagen fibers during the repair process. Hypertrophic scars are characterized by a raised pink to dark brown (depending on the underlying skin tone) scar with *smooth borders limited to the area of initial skin injury*. Histology shows type III collagen fibers arranged in parallel to the dermis. There is no genetic predisposition, and recurrence is infrequent. **Keloid** formation is more common in ethnic groups with darker skin. Keloids are raised, thickened with irregular borders, and grow *beyond the area of skin injury* (image). Histology shows disorganized proliferation of collagen fibers types I and III. Recurrence is common, and keloids tend to extend beyond the original wound with "claw-like" projections. They frequently present in earlobes, face, and upper extremities.

INTRACELLULAR ACCUMULATIONS AND PATHOLOGIC CALCIFICATION

Cells and tissues may acquire abnormal amounts of different substances, which can be nontoxic (e.g., lipofuscin) or cause varying degrees of injury (e.g., neurofibrillary tangles in Alzheimer's disease). The major pathways of abnormal accumulations are:

1. Inadequate removal of a substance removal (e.g., liver steatosis);
2. Defect in folding, packaging, transport, or secretion of a substance (e.g., alpha1-antitrypsin, amyloidosis);
3. Lack of an enzyme to degrade a metabolite (e.g., lysosomal storage diseases); and
4. Ingestion of indigestible materials (e.g., anthracosis, silicosis).

Pathologic calcification refers to the abnormal deposition of calcium salts into tissue. The two forms of pathologic calcification—dystrophic calcification and metastatic calcification—can be distinguished by the affected tissue type (necrotic or normal, respectively) and whether there are abnormalities in calcium metabolism.

CASE 7	Amyloid Deposition – Primary AL Amyloidosis
A 69-year-old man presents with progressively worsening weakness, weight loss, leg swelling and numbness, and tingling in the hands and feet over the past few months. He does not smoke or use illicit drugs. On exam, he is cachectic, has pale conjunctiva, periorbital edema, and an enlarged tongue with scalloping of the lateral borders. He has jugular venous distention, an S3, and bilateral lower extremity pitting edema, multiple bruises, and hepatomegaly.	
Evaluation/Tests	CBC is notable for anemia and low platelets. BMP is notable for normal glucose and calcium and slightly elevated creatine with a decreased calculated serum anion gap. LFTs are notable for mildly elevated AST and ALT and serum total protein of 6.8 g/dL, as well as serum albumin of 1.8 g/dL. He has nephrotic range proteinuria, and serum protein electrophoresis (SPEP) shows a monoclonal spike (M spike). HIV is negative. Echocardiogram shows thick ventricular walls with a restrictive pattern. Renal ultrasound demonstrates enlarged kidneys with diffusely echogenic parenchyma. Renal biopsy: H&E stain shows glomeruli with mesangial expansion and pink acellular amorphous material depositing around the tubules. Congo red stain under polarized light (see image, right) demonstrates apple green birefringence.

CASE 7 | Amyloid Deposition – Primary AL Amyloidosis *(continued)*

Evaluation/Tests	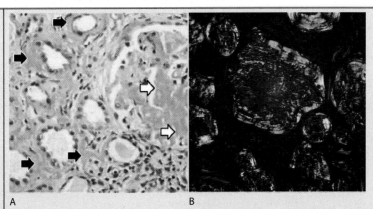A. Reproduced with permission from Mendoza JM, Peev V, Ponce MA, Thomas DB, Nayer A. Amyloid A amyloidosis with subcutaneous drug abuse, J Renal Inj Prev 2013 Nov 2;3(1):11–16. B. Used with permission from Ed Uthman MD. Houston, Texas. WebPathology.
Treatment	The treatment of amyloidosis can include chemotherapy and possible autologous hematopoietic cell transplantation.
Discussion	Amyloidosis is a multisystem disorder, secondary to extracellular deposition of structurally abnormal proteins that form beta-pleated sheets. These misfolded proteins aggregate and form insoluble fibrils that can deposit in tissue and cause cellular injury and impairment without evoking an inflammatory response. **Amyloidosis** can be **primary** or **secondary** to plasma cell dyscrasia such as multiple myeloma, plasmacytoma, monoclonal gammopathy of unknown significance, and other B-cell-lineage hematologic malignancies (Waldenstrom's, Hodgkin's lymphoma, plasmacytoma). Multiple myeloma is characterized by abnormal cells in the bone marrow and amyloid by light chain buildup. Thus there may be an overlap, and an individual can have both diagnoses. Bone marrow biopsy is required to rule out secondary amyloidosis due to malignancy. Clonal proliferation of plasma cells causes AL (light chain or primary) amyloidosis, which is usually systemic. Classic findings include: • An M spike on serum protein electrophoresis (SPEP) due to monoclonal gammopathy; • Free urine light chains (Bence-Jones protein); • Patients with renal involvement may have nephrotic range proteinuria and generalized edema (anasarca); • Macroglossia with indentation of the lateral sides by teeth due to amyloid deposition; • Restrictive cardiomyopathy and symptoms of heart failure; • Sudden death or syncope can occur as a result of arrhythmia or heart block; • Hepatomegaly due to amyloid deposition in the liver. Other manifestations may include peripheral neuropathy, purpura, or other skin manifestations and bleeding diathesis. Other forms of amyloid are AA (amyloid-associated) and β-amyloid protein (Aβ). Other proteins that can form amyloid deposits include transthyretin (TTR) and β2-microglobulin. Diagnose amyloidosis with a histologic examination of tissue under H&E stain and Congo red with polarized light (apple-green birefringence). Special stains can be performed to determine the type of amyloid protein (i.e., AL, AA, TTR). **AA amyloidosis** (also called secondary amyloidosis or reactive systemic amyloidosis) is also systemic, and it is associated with inflammatory conditions such as rheumatoid arthritis, chronic infections or Familial Mediterranean fever or with certain cancers—most commonly renal cell carcinoma and Hodgkin's lymphoma. **β-amyloid protein (Aβ)** is a localized form of amyloidosis in the brain that causes Alzheimer's disease. Localized amyloidosis may also present in medullary thyroid carcinoma, where the deposits are composed of calcitonin. **Transthyretin (TTR) amyloidosis** is a group of disorders that may be hereditary (such as familial amyloid polyneuropathy, familial amyloid cardiomyopathy), or nonhereditary (senile systemic amyloidosis). **Hemodialysis-related amyloidosis** is due to β2-microglobulin deposition, which may occur in patients on long-term hemodialysis. **Fabry's disease** is a rare inherited disorder caused by deficiency of the lysosomal enzyme alpha-galactosidase. It causes abnormal glycolipids accumulations in the cells and can present with proteinuria, renal failure, and neuropathy; it presents in younger patients and does not cause organomegaly.

CASE 8 | Dystrophic Calcification (Psammoma Bodies) in Papillary Thyroid Carcinoma

A 45-year-old woman with no significant past medical history presents with difficulty swallowing, fatigue, and weight loss of approximately 10 pounds over the last 2 months. Physical examination is notable for a right-sided, nontender, firm thyroid nodule.

Evaluation/Tests	Thyroid function tests are normal. Ultrasound of the neck reveals a dominant nodule of the right thyroid lobe with multiple calcifications. Biopsy and histologic examination show multiple papillary structures formed by pleomorphic, overlapping cells with clear intranuclear inclusions ("orphan Annie" nuclei) and grooving. Psammoma bodies are also identified.
Treatment	Hemithyroidectomy.
Discussion	Psammoma bodies are basophilic, laminated, concentric acellular spherules of dystrophic calcification that are common in papillary carcinomas of the thyroid, papillary serous carcinomas of the ovary and endometrium, meningiomas, and malignant mesotheliomas. In addition to the presence of psammoma bodies, histologic exam shows papillary structures formed by cells with clear nuclei ("orphan Annie nuclei"). Grooving is typical of papillary thyroid carcinoma. Psammoma bodies and orphan Annie nuclei are specific for papillar carcinoma in a thyroid neoplasm. **Follicular carcinoma** histology includes uniform follicles that invade the thyroid capsule and vasculature. **Medullary carcinoma** develops from parafollicular cells; histology includes sheets of cells that stain with Congo red. Medullary carcinoma produces calcitonin. Medullar carcinoma is often associated with MEN2A and 2B, so a patient with medullary carcinoma should also be evaluated for pheochromocytoma and parathyroid hyperplasia. **Anaplastic carcinom**a is a locally invasive and undifferentiated neoplasm that confers a poor prognosis. 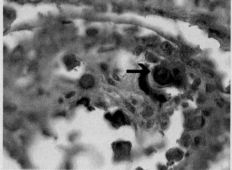 Papillary thyroid carcinomas are one of several tumors associated with psammoma bodies (arrow). Reproduced with permission from Kemp WL, Burns DK, Travis Brown TG. Pathology: The Big Picture. New York, NY: McGraw Hill; 2008.
Additional Discussion	**Dystrophic calcification** occurs in injured or dead tissue. It is common in atherosclerosis and in aging or damaged heart valves, where it may cause organ dysfunction. It is also common in areas of caseous necrosis secondary to tuberculosis. Calcium deposits may be intracellular, extracellular, or both. Serum calcium level is normal. **Metastatic calcification** refers to abnormal calcification in normal tissues that is associated with hypercalcemia. It may occur anywhere in the body but predominantly affects the interstitial tissues of the vasculature, kidney, lung, and gastric mucosa because these tissues excrete acid, and the acidic environment is predisposed to calcium deposition. Morphologically, the deposits look similar to those in dystrophic calcification. In contrast to dystrophic calcification, serum Ca^{2+}, serum phosphate, and parathyroid hormone levels will be elevated. **Calciphylaxis** is an example of metastatic calcification and is a serious complication of end-stage renal disease. Patients may present with multiple dry, black lesions that show medium-sized vessels within subcutaneous fibroadipose tissue with significant calcifications on biopsy. The calcifications cause occlusion and ischemia, which leads to necrosis of the surface epithelium.

NEOPLASIA

Cancer is the second leading cause of death in the United States. Cancers begin with the process of neoplasia, in which the normal regulation of cell proliferation goes awry and cells begin proliferating uncontrollably. Neoplastic progression begins with dysplasia, a pathologic cellular adaptation characterized by loss of tissue orientation, pleomorphism, and nuclear changes. Certain tumor types eventually may progress to form an invasive carcinoma, whereby they degrade the basement membrane, invade surrounding tissues, and can metastasize to distant organs and tissues.

One of the first steps in assessing neoplastic transformation of tissue is to determine whether a tumor is benign or malignant. Benign tumors are well circumscribed and well differentiated, and they show low mitotic activity without evidence of tissue necrosis or metastasis. Malignant tumors, on the other hand, are poorly differentiated, locally invasive, show erratic growth, and have a propensity to metastasize.

Genes related to cancer are categorized as proto-oncogenes (that typically promote cellular proliferation under homeostatic conditions) or tumor suppressor genes (that prevent cellular proliferation under homeostatic conditions). Gain-of-function mutations convert proto-oncogenes to oncogenes, which promote cellular proliferation, which evades normal checkpoint mechanisms. Loss-of-function mutations in tumor suppressor genes result in loss of normal checkpoint mechanisms that regulate cellular proliferation, causing tumor development.

Serum tumor markers are proteins or molecules expressed or secreted by the actively proliferating neoplastic cells. However, they are not used for screening purposes and do not provide a definitive diagnosis; they are *sensitive* but not specific. Instead, they are used for monitoring tumor recurrence and response to therapy. Elevated serum tumor markers present in non-neoplastic conditions and, therefore, obtain a biopsy to make a definitive diagnosis.

In addition to use as tumor markers, proteins secreted by tumor cells can also exert pathologic effects on distant tissues, which is called a paraneoplastic syndrome. Paraneoplastic syndromes have a wide range of presentations depending on the source of the tumor and the substance secreted.

Another systemic effect of cancer, particularly once it has metastasized, is cachexia. Cachexia is characterized by weight loss, muscle atrophy, and fatigue. TNF-α, IFN-γ, IL-1, and IL-6 are all responsible for this phenomenon, but TNF-α in particular leads to appetite suppression and increased basal metabolic rate, which contributes to this weight loss.

CASE 9 | Tumor Suppressor Genes (MEN1)

A 29-year-old man with a history of peptic ulcer disease presents for follow-up. He was put on medications for his peptic ulcer disease, but his pain did not improve, and he now reports worsening headaches and vision loss. His family history is significant for his father and brother with peptic ulcer disease, as well as an uncle with acromegaly who died of gastrointestinal bleeding complications. On exam, he has bitemporal hemianopsia and epigastric tenderness.

Evaluations/Tests	Blood tests reveal elevated serum calcium and gastrin levels. Head CT scan with contrast shows a 0.9-cm solid, enhancing pituitary mass. Endoscopy shows multiple gastric and duodenal ulcers. Because of the strong family history, genetic testing was performed and shows a mutation of the menin (MEN1) gene.
Treatment	Treat with proton pump inhibitors and surgical resection of tumors. Family members should also be referred for further evaluation.
Discussion	Multiple endocrine neoplasia type 1 (MEN1) is an autosomal dominant syndrome resulting from the loss of function of the 2 alleles of the *MEN1* gene located on chromosome 11. *MEN1* is a tumor suppressor gene (TSG) that encodes the protein menin. TSGs encode proteins involved in the regulation of cell growth and DNA repair mechanisms, preventing excess cellular proliferation and accumulation of mutations. Often, one allele of a TSG is still sufficient to serve as a checkpoint; therefore, for a TSG mutation to cause neoplasia, both copies must mutate ("two-hit hypothesis"). Patients who inherit a single mutated copy from their parents are at a higher risk of developing tumors earlier in life given that they need to develop only one mutation to knock out the sole remaining allele. In contrast to TSGs, other cancers are caused by mutations in proto-oncogenes, converting them into an oncogene. These genes often encode proteins involved in cell cycle progression, signal transduction, or production of growth factors. These mutations typically only need to affect a *single* allele.
	MEN1 syndrome affects the 3 Ps—pituitary, parathyroid, and pancreas. This results in pituitary tumors (prolactinomas, growth hormone-secreting tumors, etc.), parathyroid adenomas (hyperparathyroidism), and pancreatic neuroendocrine tumors (gastrinomas, insulinomas, etc.). A strong family history should bring this entity to mind.
	Peptic ulcer disease and **pituitary adenoma** alone do not explain the full constellation of signs/symptoms this patient is experiencing.
	MEN 2A results in parathyroid hyperplasia, medullary thyroid carcinoma, and pheochromocytoma. It is due to a mutation in the RET oncogene and affects cells of neural crest origin.
	MEN 2B classically presents with medullary thyroid carcinoma, pheochromocytoma, mucosal neuromas, and marfanoid habitus. As with MEN 2A, it is also related to RET oncogene mutation. Patients should be evaluated for all tumor types associated with the syndrome.

CASE 10 | Carcinogens (Nitrosamines)

A 53-year-old man who immigrated from Japan presents with significant abdominal pain, weight loss, and black tarry stools. Since arriving to the United States, he has continued his same diet that mainly consists of smoked meats and fish. The patient's BMI is 18. On exam, he has epigastric tenderness, multiple pigmented skin lesions with "stuck on" appearance (seborrheic keratosis), and an enlarged supraclavicular lymph node (Virchow node).

Evaluation/Tests	CBC reveals anemia. Upper endoscopy shows an ulcerative gastric lesion, with the stomach wall appearing grossly thickened and leathery. Biopsy shows mucin-filled cells with peripheral nuclei.
Treatment	Chemotherapy and possible gastrectomy.
Discussion	Diffuse gastric adenocarcinoma, a common form of gastric cancer, presents in patients with exposure to diet-based carcinogens that promote malignant transformation. Nitrosamines are carcinogens that can damage cells, resulting in mutations in TSGs (such as *TP53*), which then promote neoplastic change. Suggest moderation when talking about consuming smoked foods and other foods with increased nitrosamines in order to lower the risk of gastric adenocarcinoma. Characteristic features of this case that suggest gastric cancer include abdominal pain, weight loss, black tarry stools (suggestive of upper GI damage and bleeding), multiple seborrheic keratoses (Leser-Trélat sign), an enlarged supraclavicular node (Virchow node), linitis plastica (thickened stomach), and the appearance of signet ring cells on biopsy. While **GERD** and **acute gastritis** can cause substernal abdominal pain, the patient's weight loss, melena, Virchow node, and Leser-Trélat sign all point to malignancy.

CASE 11 | Oncogenic Microbes (Kaposi's Sarcoma)

A 36-year-old man with HIV presents with multiple flat painless purple-red spots on the bilateral lower extremities. He recently had to stop taking his antiretroviral medication because of a loss of his insurance. He indicates the rash is not painful or itchy.

Evaluation/Tests	CBC: hemoglobin 13.5 g/dL, hematocrit 42%, WBC 3000/mm^3, platelets 200,000/mm^3. CD4+ cell count is 184/mm^3. HIV serology is positive. Biopsy of the skin lesion reveals spindle-shaped cells and positive staining for the DNA virus human herpes virus-8 (HHV-8).
Treatment	Restart antiretroviral medication.
Discussion	This patient presents with Kaposi's sarcoma, a malignancy of lymphatic endothelial cells caused by the oncogenic microbe HHV-8. Kaposi's sarcoma from HHV-8 is commonly seen as an opportunistic infection in immunocompromised patients, especially in HIV patients with CD4+ cell count below 500/mm^3. While lesions are classically found on the skin, they can also present in the mouth, GI tract, and respiratory tract. Several other oncogenic microbes are associated with various cancers including EBV (lymphomas, nasopharyngeal carcinomas), HBV and HCV (hepatocellular carcinoma), HPV (cervical cancer), *H. pylori* (gastric cancer), *Schistosoma haematobium* (bladder cancer), and more. Mechanisms of these microbes vary, with some having proteins and virulence factors that directly promote neoplasia while others more indirectly result in neoplasm by promoting a chronic inflammatory state. **Atopic dermatitis**, or eczema, is not likely in this patient because of the absence of pruritis and a history of atopy. **Stasis dermatitis** is the result of insufficient venous return from the lower extremities, often associated with varicose veins. Lesions are classically hyperpigmented and may result in ulceration. **Contact dermatitis** is a type IV hypersensitivity reaction mediated by T-cells. Lesions will be pruritic, and they may develop as an erythematous rash, blisters, wheals, or urticaria.

CASE 12 | Serum Tumor Markers (CA 125)

A 49-year-old woman presents with intermittent left lower quadrant abdominal pain, weight loss, and constipation. A left adnexal mass is noted on exam.

Evaluation/Tests	Transvaginal ultrasound reveals a 5-cm left adnexal mass. CA 125 is elevated at 2145 U/mL (reference range: 0–35 U/mL).
Treatment	Oophorectomy with staging and possible chemotherapy.

CASE 12 | Serum Tumor Markers (CA 125) *(continued)*

Discussion	This patient presents with ovarian cancer. Elevated serum CA 125 is suggestive of ovarian carcinoma of epithelial origin, most commonly serous adenocarcinoma. However, note that CA 125 levels are more important for monitoring response to treatment (here, an oophorectomy) rather than for initial screening. Diagnosis is suggested by imaging and made by pathology.
	Dermoid cyst would present with an ovarian mass, but CA 125 would not be elevated. Dermoid cysts may contain various tissues from all three germ cell layers (such as hair, teeth, bone, and thyroid). These tumors may result in ovarian torsion due to their size. *Struma ovarii* may arise if the tumor contains thyroid tissue, causing derangements of thyroid hormone levels.
	Endometriotic (chocolate) cyst is an ovarian mass consisting of old menstrual blood and tissue. Endometriosis would present with abnormal uterine bleeding, infertility, and bowel and bladder irregularities along with lower abdominal pain.
	Ovarian torsion would present with acute onset of severe lower abdominal pain along with nausea and vomiting. Large ovarian tumors may cause torsion. Transvaginal ultrasound would show low blood flow to the affected ovary rather than a mass.

CASE 13 | Paraneoplastic Syndromes (Cushing Syndrome) in Small Cell Lung Cancer

A 71-year-old woman with a 40-pack-a-year history of smoking presents with shortness of breath, chronic cough with light hemoptysis, weight gain, and general weakness. Temperature is 37°C, pulse is 88/min, respirations are 23/min, and blood pressure is 152/102 mmHg. On exam, she has crackles in the right upper lobe, lower extremity edema, purple abdominal striae, truncal obesity, and a hump between her shoulders.

Evaluation/Tests	Chest CT reveals a mass in the right upper lung. Serum tests reveal neutrophilia, hyperglycemia, and elevated adrenocorticotropic hormone (ACTH). High-dose dexamethasone suppression test fails to suppress the elevated ACTH levels.
Treatment	Chemotherapy and possible resection of lung tumor.
Discussion	Many tumors may cause paraneoplastic syndromes due to various mechanisms, including excess secretion of normal hormones, secretion of proteins that interact with normal receptors, and production of autoantibodies. Given the ectopic nature of their secretion, these hormones typically are produced without regulation from normal homeostatic mechanisms; hence the failure of the high-dose dexamethasone suppression test in this example.
	Small cell lung carcinoma is notorious for causing paraneoplastic syndromes. An older smoker with other signs of malignancy should raise suspicion for small cell lung carcinoma, causing the secondary findings of Cushing syndrome (hypercortisolism). Other paraneoplastic syndromes in the setting of small cell lung cancer include syndrome of inappropriate antidiuretic hormone (SIADH), cerebellar degeneration, encephalomyelitis, and Lambert-Eaton myasthenic syndrome.
	Adrenal adenoma, pituitary adenoma, and **exogenous use of glucocorticoids** can all cause Cushing syndrome but would not present with the pulmonary symptoms seen in this case, and imaging is consistent with lung cancer.

5

Pharmacology

Christopher Schriever, PharmD
Annette Hays, PharmD

PHARMACOKINETICS

The principles of pharmacokinetics are centered on the absorption (A), distribution (D), metabolism (M), and elimination (E) of a medication administered for a pharmacologic effect. These principles describe the events occurring when a medication is administered, where it is concentrated, and how it is eliminated from the body. Naturally, different medications behave differently, producing their desired pharmacologic effect at a range of concentrations. The *therapeutic window* for a medication describes the concentration range at which a desired pharmacologic effect is produced without increasing toxicity. If these variations or changes in drug levels continue to produce the desired pharmacologic effect without any untoward side effects, this may be considered acceptable. Deviations outside the medication's *therapeutic window* lead to reduced efficacy or increased toxicity. This section describes the effects of medications, foods, or other xenobiotics on the components of ADME and how it can affect medication concentration.

CASE 1 | Zero-Order Kinetics

A 19-year-old man is brought to the emergency room for evaluation of syncope. The friend indicates that the patient was drinking heavily at a fraternity party and then lost consciousness. The patient is difficult to arouse for physical exam; however, he is afebrile, his vital signs are normal, and there are no visible signs of trauma.

Evaluation/Tests	CBC, BMP, and blood glucose are within normal limits. Blood alcohol concentration (BAC) is 320 mg/dL, and urine toxicology screen is negative.
Treatment	Supportive care including hydration, airway protection, and oxygen.
Discussion	The patient's objective findings and witnessed heavy consumption of alcohol suggest that he is suffering from **ethanol intoxication**. Given normal blood glucose and other electrolytes values and negative toxicology screen, hypo- or hyperglycemia, metabolic derangements, or other ingestions are unlikely. Ethanol displays **zero-order elimination kinetics**, meaning that the elimination rate is constant per unit time regardless of the concentration of ethanol in the system. Other examples that follow zero-order elimination are high-dose aspirin and phenytoin. Most other drugs follow first-order elimination kinetics, whereby the elimination rate is directly proportional to the concentration of drug in the system; therefore, concentration decreases exponentially with time as a constant fraction of the drug is eliminated with time.

Comparison of first-order and zero-order elimination. For drugs with first-order kinetics (left), rate of elimination (units per hour) is proportional to concentration; this is the more common process. In the case of zero-order elimination (right), the rate is constant and independent of concentration.
Reproduced with permission from Katzung BG, Kruidering-Hall M, Trevor AJ: Katzung & Trevor's Basic & Clinical Pharmacology Examination & Board Review, 12th ed. New York, NY: McGraw Hill; 2019.

CASE 2 | Loading vs. Maintenance Dose

An 87-year-old woman was transferred to the emergency room from a nursing home after becoming acutely ill. The nursing home aide reported that the patient was confused and had a fever. On exam, the patient is disoriented, appears acutely ill, and is not able to answer questions. The patient's temperature is 39.5°C, blood pressure is 98/48 mmHg, pulse is 122/min, and respirations are 22/min. Her oxygen saturation is 93% on room air, and crackles are noted in the left lung. She is not following commands, but she is moving all extremities.

Evaluation/Tests	ECG shows sinus tachycardia. Chest X-ray shows left lobar pneumonia. CBC is notable for an elevated WBC count. Urinalysis is normal. Blood and cultures are pending.
Treatment	Start broad-spectrum antibiotics.
Discussion	The constellation of signs, symptoms, and lab and CXR findings are consistent with a case of **sepsis secondary to pneumonia**. In this case, vancomycin and piperacillin-tazobactam are selected for Gram positive and Gram negative coverage, respectively. Once an organism is identified, broad-spectrum antimicrobials should be de-escalated. Vancomycin is a bactericidal antimicrobial that inhibits bacterial cell wall synthesis and displays activity against aerobic and anaerobic Gram positive bacteria. Rapid attainment of target serum

CASE 2 | Loading vs. Maintenance Dose *(continued)*

Discussion	concentrations is appropriate for patients that have serious or life-threatening infections. This may be obtained by giving a single vancomycin **loading dose**. Following the loading dose, maintenance dosing with therapeutic trough monitoring suffices as a marker to predict therapeutic efficacy. The loading dose can be calculated for oral or intravenous drugs using the bioavailability (F), target plasma concentration at steady state (C_p), and volume of distribution (V_d).

$$\text{Loading dose} = \frac{C_p \times V_d}{F}$$

Maintenance dose is calculated using the bioavailability (F), target plasma concentration at steady state (C_p), clearance rate (CL), and dosing interval (τ). In renal or liver disease, loading dose is typically unchanged; however, maintenance dose often decreases as a smaller dose is required to maintain steady-state plasma concentrations.

$$\text{Maintenance dose} = \frac{C_p \times CL \times \tau}{F}$$

CASE 3 | Volume of Distribution (Vd) and Clearance

A 38-year-old man is admitted to the hospital for acute liver failure as well as lethargy and moderate confusion consistent with hepatic encephalopathy. On exam, his temperature is 39.0°C, blood pressure is 110/76 mmHg, and pulse is 106/min. He has abdominal distension and hepatomegaly. During examination, the patient suffers a seizure and is given a phenytoin loading dose with maintenance dosing every 8 hours. The next day, the patient is noted to have nystagmus, ataxia, and slurred speech.

Evaluation/Tests	Total bilirubin is 174 µmol/L, ALT is 1305 U/L, AST is 669 U/L, and serum albumin is 1.4 g/dL.
Treatment	Discontinue phenytoin and initiate an antiepileptic with insignificant hepatic metabolism and less protein binding, such as levetiracetam.
Discussion	**Phenytoin toxicity** symptoms include ataxia, nystagmus, dizziness, drowsiness, and fatigue. Based on the patient's profile and symptoms in relationship to administration of the drug, presentation is most consistent with drug toxicity. If symptoms do not improve after discontinuation of the drug, then other possibilities, such as worsening of hepatic encephalopathy, sepsis, or stroke, should be considered. **Volume of distribution (Vd)** is the volume occupied by the total amount of drug in the body in relation to measured plasma concentration. A large Vd indicates that the drug has spread to tissues throughout the body, whereas a small Vd indicates the drug is contained within the circulatory system. Plasma protein-bound drugs, such as phenytoin, may have increased Vd in patients with liver and kidney disease due to decreased protein binding. Phenytoin is an antiepileptic that binds to voltage-dependent sodium channels, resulting in their inhibition. This ultimately increases the membrane threshold for depolarization and lowers neuronal vulnerability to epileptogenic stimuli. In cases of toxicity, excessive inhibition may result in cerebral dysfunction, altered mental status, and incoordination. Patients with acute hepatitis, liver cirrhosis, or liver failure have decreased phenytoin clearance due to liver cell damage. The decrease in functional liver cells reduces existing CYP450 enzymes for phenytoin metabolism. In addition, the Vd is larger because there is decreased plasma protein binding, leading to an increase in unbound phenytoin. Reductions in protein binding are caused by the hypoalbuminemia and hyperbilirubinemia commonly seen in liver disease. $$V_d = \frac{\text{amount of drug in the body}}{\text{plasma drug concentration}}$$

CASE 4 | Half-Life

A 27-year-old woman presents with fatigue and sore throat for the past week. She is sexually active with multiple male partners who do not use condoms consistently. Though she was prescribed birth control pills, she admits to inconsistent use. Her last menstrual period was 2 weeks ago and was normal. Her physical exam is normal.

Evaluation/Tests	CBC, TSH are normal. Monospot, Strep, and gonorrhea tests are negative. CD4+ 300 cells/µL, HIV RNA 28,000 copies/mL.
Treatment	Antiretroviral therapy containing two nucleoside/-tide reverse transcriptase inhibitors (NRTIs) and an Integrase inhibitor is the preferred regimen for treatment-naïve HIV patients.

CASE 4 | Half-Life *(continued)*

Discussion	Patients with acute HIV infections often present with vague symptoms such as sore throat, sweats, fatigue, and fever. Some of these symptoms may be seen in patients with infectious mononucleosis, pharyngitis, thyroid disease, or anemia from various causes. Labs are important to confirm the diagnosis and to rule out other possibilities. Due to the ease of once-daily dosing and lack of contraindications, treatment with single-pill highly active antiretroviral therapy (HAART) consisting of elvitegravir, cobicistat, emtricitabine, and tenofovir is initiated. HAART generally consists of two NRTIs (here, tenofovir and emtricitabine), plus an additional drug (here, the integrase inhibitor elvitegravir). Cobicistat, while not directly active against HIV, is added to inhibit CYP3A4, the enzyme that metabolizes elvitegravir. By adding cobicistat, there is reduced metabolism of elvitegravir, thus improving its bioavailability and half-life. This pharmacokinetic boosting is seen frequently when low-dose ritonavir or cobicistat is added to antiretroviral regimens containing protease inhibitors or the integrase inhibitor, elvitegravir, to increase half-lives and plasma concentrations. The outcomes of the boosting allow less frequent dosing of the affected drugs due to increased half-life. The **half-life** is the time required to decrease the amount of drug in the body by half during elimination. Drugs that follow first-order kinetics and constant infusion take four to five half-lives before they reach steady state. Half-life ($t_{1/2}$) can be calculated using the elimination rate constant, volume of distribution (V_d), and clearance (CL). $$t_{1/2} = \frac{0.7 \times V_d}{CL} \text{ in first-order elimination}$$

CASE 5 | Elimination and Urine pH

A 68-year-old woman is brought to the hospital for confusion. Her son states she is generally healthy except for severe arthritis. She has recently noted that acetaminophen was not helping her pain, and she had started taking large doses of aspirin. On exam, she has labored breathing, and she is confused. She has the following vital signs: temperature 39°C, blood pressure 105/50 mmHg, pulse 101/min, and respirations 30/min. Her oxygen saturation is 98% on room air, and the rest of her exam is normal, with the exception that she is not following commands.

Evaluation/Tests	Serum glucose and CBC are normal. Metabolic panel is notable for anion-gap metabolic acidosis, and serum salicylate concentration is elevated. Urine toxicology screen is negative.
Treatment	Treat with oral activated charcoal, IV fluids, and alkalinization of serum and urine with sodium bicarbonate. Correct hypokalemia.
Discussion	Patients with **salicylate toxicity** may present with vomiting, abdominal pain, fever, confusion, tinnitus, seizures, or coma. Sepsis, diabetic ketoacidosis (DKA), acetaminophen toxicity, and other ingestions should be considered in this type of presentation, but the objective findings and elevated serum salicylate levels are consistent with salicylate toxicity. For medications that are weak acids or bases, nonionized species are more lipophilic and can be reabsorbed by the renal tubules, but the hydrophilic ionized species become trapped in the urine and excreted. $RCOOH \leftrightarrow RCOO^- + H^+$ (e.g., salicylates, pentobarbital, methotrexate) Aspirin (salicylic acid) is a weak acid and toxicity is treated by increasing the pH of urine to shift the equilibrium to the right towards the charged species. Toxic salicylate levels stimulate respiratory drive directly in the CNS, which causes altered mentation and disrupts mitochondrial function. Alkalinizing the serum shifts the equation to the right, creating a concentration gradient for nonionized salicylate to diffuse out of affected tissues (e.g., CNS) and into the extracellular space, where they become trapped as $RCOO^-$. Bicarbonate excreted in the urine creates an environment more basic than serum, and this causes a similar shift in the equilibrium, leading to ionized salicylates trapped in the urine and increased overall excretion. This both decreases the symptoms of salicylate toxicity by drawing it out of affected cells and increases excretion of the salicylates by preventing their reabsorption into somatic cell and the renal tubules. Altering the urinary pH to promote urinary elimination may work similarly for weak bases—using ammonium chloride or ascorbic acid to acidify the urine—this, however, is uncommonly practiced due to iatrogenic toxicity (acidemia). Alterations of urinary pH also change the solubility of some compounds, which may lead to precipitation and nephrolithiasis.

AUTONOMIC DRUGS—CHOLINOMIMETICS

Autonomic drugs (cholinomimetics, muscarinic antagonists, sympathomimetics, and sympatholytics) are used to inhibit or imitate sympathetic and parasympathetic nervous system activity. This drug class is useful for treating various gastrointestinal, cardiovascular, respiratory, and urinary tract disorders. Acetylcholine and norepinephrine are the main neurotransmitters that evoke parasympathetic and sympathetic effects on target tissues, respectively. Drugs targeting these systems often act as physiological antagonists—blockade of the sympathetic nervous system leads to overactivation of the parasympathetic system and vice versa.

Cholinomimetics, or drugs that mimic acetylcholine, are most often used for urinary retention or their miotic effects in glaucoma. These drugs are divided into two categories: direct and indirect. Direct agonists directly stimulate muscarinic and/or nicotinic receptors to elicit a physiological response identical to that of acetylcholine. Indirect agonists increase acetylcholine levels in the synaptic cleft by inhibiting acetylcholinesterase (AChE), the enzyme responsible for acetylcholine degradation. Cholinesterase inhibitors are used frequently to stimulate skeletal muscle and to reverse neuromuscular blockade in patients with myasthenia gravis. Patients with Alzheimer's disease may also benefit from AChE inhibitors (i.e., donepezil) because patients with this disease demonstrate diminished cholinergic transmission in the brain.

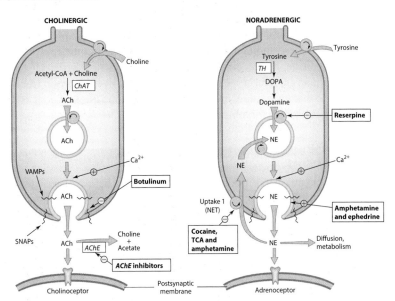

Characteristics of transmitter synthesis, storage, release, and termination of action at cholinergic and noradrenergic nerve terminals are shown from the top downward. Circles represent transporters; ACh, acetylcholine; AChE, acetylcholinesterase; ChAT, choline acety-ltransferase; DOPA, dihydroxyphenylalanine; NE, norepinephrine; NET, norepinephrine transporter; TCA, tricyclic antidepressant; TH, tyrosine hydroxylase.

CASE 6	Indirect Cholinomimetic Agonist

An 87-year-old man with a history of HTN, hyperlipidemia, and recently diagnosed Alzheimer's disease presents with diarrhea and new fecal incontinence for the past month. His medications were changed approximately 1 month ago. Lisinopril was decreased, simvastatin was stopped, and rivastigmine was started. On exam, he is afebrile, and his abdominal exam is notable for hyperactive bowel sounds.

Evaluation/Tests	Stool cultures are negative.
Treatment	Stop rivastigmine.
Discussion	The patient is experiencing a medication side effect: diarrhea and fecal incontinence from rivastigmine. The timing of symptom onset and medication alterations make inflammatory bowel disease and irritable bowel syndrome unlikely diagnoses, and lack of fever and negative stool cultures make infectious causes less likely. Rivastigmine is an acetylcholinesterase inhibitor prescribed to increase the actions of acetylcholine in the setting of Alzheimer's disease, which involves a pathological loss of acetylcholine in the nervous system. However, the procholinergic actions of rivastigmine (and other acetylcholinesterase inhibitors) are not limited to the central nervous system. Increased cholinergic actions systemically may yield the following effects: diarrhea, urinary urgency, incontinence of urine or feces, increased salivation and gastric acid secretion, miosis, bradycardia, and bronchoconstriction (all due to overactivation of parasympathetic responses). This is due to stimulation of nicotinic acetylcholine receptors (N_N and N_M) in the autonomic ganglia, adrenal medulla, and skeletal muscle, and muscarinic receptors (M_{1-5}) located in the heart, smooth muscle, brain, exocrine glands, and sweat glands.

AUTONOMIC DRUGS—MUSCARINIC ANTAGONISTS

Muscarinic antagonists are also known as anticholinergic agents. They inhibit parasympathetic responses due to their antagonistic activity at muscarinic receptors. An abundance of cholinergic synapses in the brain produce excitatory impulses. The antagonism of these cholinergic receptors may cause antiemetic and sedative side effects. When used in conjunction with dopamine agonists, muscarinic antagonists are therapeutic for Parkinson's disease due to more effective balancing of diminished dopaminergic neurotransmission with excessive cholinergic transmission. Muscarinic antagonists should be avoided in patients with constipation and/or urinary retention issues, as well as patients with dementia because anticholinergics can lead to worsening of symptoms.

CASE 7	Muscarinic Antagonists (Ipratropium)
An 11-year-old boy with a history of asthma is brought to the emergency department with acute onset of shortness of breath and wheezing. He had been playing with kittens at his friend's house earlier in the day. Previously, his asthma was well controlled without daily medications. On exam, he is tachycardic and tachypneic with labored breathing and audible wheezes. He is initially treated with albuterol nebulizers and IV corticosteroid. He shows some improvement, but oxygen saturation remains at 90%.	
Evaluation/Tests	Chest X-ray is negative.
Treatment	Add ipratropium.
Discussion	This presentation is consistent with an acute asthma exacerbation secondary to exposure to cat dander. The acute symptoms are inconsistent with a upper respiratory tract infection (URI) or pneumonia. Asthma exacerbation is caused by bronchoconstriction due to inflammation. Reducing inflammation acutely with corticosteroids and bronchodilation are hallmarks of acute therapy. **Short-acting beta agonists**, like albuterol, are primary treatment but are often augmented with ipratropium. Ipratropium is a **rapid-acting muscarinic antagonist** available as a single product or in combination with albuterol in nebulized and inhaler forms. Acetylcholine stimulation at M1 and M3 muscarinic receptors of bronchial smooth muscle cells results in bronchoconstriction. Antagonism at pulmonary muscarinic receptors blocks this constriction, thereby improving airflow.

AUTONOMIC DRUGS—SYMPATHOMIMETICS

Sympathomimetics are drugs that behave agonistically at adrenergic receptors to produce sympathetic responses. Sympathetic nerves release norepinephrine, which bind to adrenergic receptors—α_1, β_1, β_2, and/or prejunctional α_2 receptors. The circulatory system may also carry adrenergic ligands, including norepinephrine, epinephrine, and adrenergic drugs, to the synapse. Termination of the response to norepinephrine occurs following reuptake into the nerve endings. Termination of epinephrine and adrenergic drugs occurs through metabolism by monoamine oxidase and catechol-O-methyltransferase in tissues or the liver following absorption. Similar to cholinomimetics, sympathomimetics can be described as direct or indirect. Direct sympathomimetics act directly on adrenergic receptors, are commonly used in the clinical setting, and include albuterol, epinephrine, norepinephrine, dopamine, mirabegron, dobutamine, phenylephrine, and others. Indirect sympathomimetics do not act directly on the adrenergic receptors, and some such as amphetamine and cocaine work by preventing reuptake of catecholamines or dopamine within the synaptic cleft.

Sympathetic Receptors and Responses in Target Organs

Target	Receptor	Response
Heart	Beta-1 (β_1)	Increased heart rate, contractility, and conduction
Bronchioles	Beta-2 (β_2)	Bronchodilation
Systemic vessels	α_1, β_2	β_2—Vasodilation α_1—Vasoconstriction
Submucosal vessels	Alpha-1 (α_1)	Vasoconstriction
Neuronal endings	Alpha-2 (α_2)	Neurotransmitter inhibition via decreased sympathetic outflow
Renal vascular	Dopamine-1	Vasodilation
Blood vessels	Vasopressin-1	Vasoconstriction

Actions, Effects, and Use of Common Direct Sympathomimetics

Vasopressor	Action on Receptors	Effect	Use
Norepinephrine	Alpha-1 > Alpha-2 > Beta-1	Peripheral vasoconstriction, positive inotropy	Septic shock, hypotension
Epinephrine	Beta > Alpha	Peripheral vasoconstriction, positive inotropy	Anaphylaxis, septic shock
Phenylephrine	Alpha-1 > Alpha-2	Peripheral vasoconstriction	Septic shock
Dopamine	Dopamine > Beta > Alpha	Low dose (dopamine and predominant beta effects): Positive inotropy and chronotropy High dose (increased alpha effects): Peripheral vasoconstriction	Low dose: Bradycardia, heart failure High dose: Septic shock
Vasopressin	Vasopressin	Peripheral vasoconstriction	Septic shock
Dobutamine	Beta-1 > Beta-2 > Alpha	Inotropy, vasodilation	Cardiogenic shock, severe heart failure, cardiac stress testing

CASE 8 | Mirabegron

A 58-year-old woman with a history of Sjögren syndrome presents with urinary urgency, nocturia, and incontinence. The patient states that the symptoms have been worsening over time and that they are not alleviated with reductions in fluid intake. On physical exam, she has dry eyes, dry mouth, and mild vaginal atrophy.

Evaluation/Tests	Urinalysis shows no bacteria, no WBCs, and no leukocyte esterase.
Treatment	Mirabegron.
Discussion	This patient's symptoms are consistent with an **overactive bladder** and inconsistent with a UTI. Mirabegron is the most reasonable treatment option for this patient because it acts as a direct sympathomimetic and β3 receptor agonist, and it relaxes the detrusor smooth muscle in the bladder to increase storage capacity. Patients with overactive bladder have urgency and may have incontinence. This condition can be treated with two different medication classes: antimuscarinic agents or beta-adrenergic agents. While **antimuscarinic agents**, such as tolterodine, oxybutynin, or solifenacin, are most commonly prescribed for overactive bladder, they are not appropriate for this patient due to the xerostomia and keratitis sicca caused by her Sjögren syndrome. In addition to causing urinary retention for treatment of overactive bladder, the inhibition of acetylcholine caused by antimuscarinics produces additional adverse effects such as tachycardia, xerostomia, anhidrosis, blurry vision, keratitis sicca, and constipation. Since mirabegron is not an antimuscarinic, it will not worsen the xerostomia or keratitis sicca.

CASE 9 | Dobutamine

A 64-year-old woman with a history of congestive heart failure is brought to the emergency department with acute chest pain. She collapses on arrival and is emergently intubated. Her vital signs are notable for hypotension, tachycardia, and tachypnea.

Evaluation/Tests	ECG shows anterolateral ST elevation. Troponin level is elevated.
Treatment	Initiate vasopressor and inotropic therapy with dobutamine and potentially norepinephrine. Emergent cardiac catheterization and revascularization.
Discussion	The patient has low tissue perfusion from **cardiogenic shock** secondary to a STEMI. Therefore, she needs emergent revascularization. Vasopressors and inotropic agents can improve cardiac function. Dobutamine is the inotrope of choice in patients with heart failure and cardiogenic shock. Dobutamine binds to both β_1 and β_2 in the sympathetic nervous system, with greater stimulation of the β_1 receptors. Due to this mechanism, dobutamine is a potent inotrope with weaker chronotropic activity. Mild vasodilation may occur at lower doses. Norepinephrine can be given with the dobutamine to maintain the peripheral vascular resistance at lower doses.

CASE 10 | Epinephrine

A 26-year-old woman recently diagnosed with syphilis develops acute shortness of breath and sensation that her throat is closing after receiving a penicillin G benzathine injection in clinic. On exam, she is tachycardic, tachypneic, hypotensive, and has tongue and lip swelling and wheezing.

Evaluation/Tests	Clinical diagnosis.
Treatment	Intramuscular epinephrine, fluids. If the patient cannot protect her airway, she should be intubated.
Discussion	This presentation is consistent with anaphylaxis secondary to penicillin allergy. Anaphylaxis is a life-threatening clinical syndrome caused by sudden release of mast-cell mediators into the blood. It is an IgE-mediated response to certain allergens, including food (peanuts), medications, and insect stings. A small percentage of cases are biphasic, with initial resolution but symptom recurrence after an hour. The most common symptoms involve the skin or mucosa. However, angioedema of the bowel (signaled by abdominal pain, diarrhea, nausea, or vomiting) can cause visceral organ congestion with resultant hypotension. The penicillin administration was a likely trigger of an **IgE-mediated anaphylactic reaction**. A **direct sympathomimetic**, intramuscular epinephrine injection should be given immediately. Epinephrine has a high affinity for β_1 and β_2 receptors, and milder affinity for α_1 receptors in smooth muscle and vascular tissues. The α adrenergic activity causes vasoconstriction that reverses the peripheral vasodilation that occurs during anaphylaxis. This vasoconstriction alleviates angioedema, urticaria, and hypotension. The β adrenergic activity causes bronchodilation, increased cardiac contractility and output, and decreases further mediator release from basophils and mast cells. Epinephrine also increases coronary blood flow.

CASE 11 | Phenylephrine and Norepinephrine

A 74-year-old man with a history of diabetes is brought to the emergency room for altered mental status. The patient lives alone and the family does not know when his symptoms began. On exam, he is unresponsive and appears acutely ill. His temperature is 39.1°C, blood pressure is 70/40 mmHg, pulse is 121/min, respirations are 29/min, and O_2 saturation is 84%. He has bilateral crackles at the bases of the lung fields and a distended, rigid abdomen.

Evaluation/Tests	Blood glucose is 150 mg/dL, WBC count is 21,000 cells/mm³, lactic acid is 8 mmol/L, and blood cultures ×2 are pending. ECG shows sinus tachycardia, and CT abdomen shows an intra-abdominal abscess.
Treatment	Treatment should include empiric IV antibiotics, IV fluids, and a direct sympathomimetic such as norepinephrine or phenylephrine.
Discussion	The patient has **septic shock** due to an intra-abdominal infection. The constellation of signs, symptoms, and normal glucose values are inconsistent with hypoglycemia or DKA. In addition to IV fluids and antibiotics, vasopressors are warranted to maintain appropriate mean arterial pressure of ≥65 mmHg. **Norepinephrine** is often the vasopressor of choice in septic shock. It is a potent α_1 adrenergic agonist, and it has more modest agonistic activity at β_1 receptors. There is a minimal effect on cardiac output with norepinephrine, but it does cause an increase in systolic and diastolic pressures. Due to the less potent ionotropic and chronotropic effects, norepinephrine is useful in patients with elevated heart rates. **Phenylephrine** may also be used as an alternative to norepinephrine in septic shock patients with severe tachycardia or arrhythmias in which an agent that has no β_1 activity may be preferred. Phenylephrine is a pure α adrenergic agonist, causing an increase in systemic vascular resistance due to vasoconstriction with little to no effect on inotropy and chronotropy.

AUTONOMIC DRUGS—SYMPATHOLYTICS

Sympatholytics oppose the effects of the sympathetic nervous system by inhibiting signals produced by epinephrine and norepinephrine. The postsynaptic adrenergic receptor antagonists inhibit cellular signaling pathways via α- and β-receptors. Agonistic activity at presynaptic α_2-receptors inhibits the release of epinephrine and norepinephrine into the presynaptic cleft, thus preventing postsynaptic activation of α- and β-receptors. Sympatholytics are most commonly used for hypertension but have a variety of clinical indications, such as depression, benign prostatic hypertrophy, urinary symptom relief, and post-traumatic stress disorder.

CASE 12 | Alpha-2 Agonist (α-Methyldopa)

A 29-year-old G1P0 woman presents for follow-up blood pressure check. A week ago, at her 24-week OB visit, her blood pressure was noted to be elevated at 166/100 mmHg. She has no medical problems and denies headache, abdominal pain, or blurred vision. She also reports normal fetal movement. On exam, her blood pressure is 168/100 mmHg, pulse is 80, and her lung and cardiovascular exam are normal.

Evaluation/Tests	CBC, CMP, and urinalysis are normal.
Treatment	α-methyldopa.
Discussion	This patient's presentation is consistent with **gestational hypertension**. The absence of proteinuria rules out pre-eclampsia. She should be started on blood pressure–lowering therapy to reduce the risk of stroke and maternal complications. Methyldopa is commonly used for gestational hypertensive treatment. It is a **central α-2 adrenergic agonist**, which causes a decrease in peripheral resistance, blood pressure, and heart rate due to reduced sympathetic outflow. Studies demonstrate fetal safety and mild antihypertensive effects in pregnant patients. Clonidine may also be used, but it often causes more adverse effects.

CASE 13 | Alpha-1 Antagonist (Doxazosin/Tamsulosin)

A 61-year-old man, with a history of hypertension and recently diagnosed benign prostatic hyperplasia (BPH), presents with continued urinary urgency, difficulty initiating urination, and dribbling at the end of urination. Last month, he was started and titrated up on doxazosin from 1 to 4 mg daily. Since the increase 2 weeks ago, he is reporting lightheadedness and dizziness upon standing. His only other medication is hydrochlorothiazide for hypertension. On exam, his mucous membranes are moist, and he has normal skin turgor, but his blood pressure drops from 110/70 mmHg (supine) to 85/58 mmHg (standing).

Evaluation/Tests	Clinical diagnosis. CBC is normal.
Treatment	Switch from doxazosin to tamsulosin. Given low blood pressure, temporarily hold thiazide diuretic.
Discussion	The patient is still suffering typical symptoms of BPH despite a dose increase of doxazosin. He is also likely experiencing **medication-induced orthostatic hypotension** due to increased doxazosin dose. Given moist mucous membranes on exam and no evidence of decreased oral intake or diarrhea, dehydration or GI bleed is not likely. **Doxazosin** reduces the sympathetic tone-induced urethral stricture causing BPH symptoms by competitively inhibiting postsynaptic α_1-adrenergic receptors in prostatic stromal and bladder neck tissues. This **α-1 antagonism** also vasodilates veins and arterioles systemically, decreasing peripheral vascular resistance and blood pressure. Doxazosin could be decreased, but this would not improve the symptoms of BPH. **Tamsulosin** is also an α-1 antagonist with less severe hypotension side effects, so doxazosin should be switched to tamsulosin.

CASE 14 | Nonselective Alpha-Antagonist (Phentolamine)

A 32-year-old man is brought to the emergency room for increased agitation after snorting cocaine 1 hour ago. He typically does not use cocaine and does not take any prescription or over-the-counter medications. On exam, he is notably agitated, tachycardic, and hypertensive. He was given diazepam for agitation and labetalol for elevated blood pressure. However, his blood pressure increased further from 190/100 to 215/130.

Evaluation/Tests	Urine toxicology screen is positive for cocaine only.
Treatment	Treatment for hypertension should include IV phentolamine.
Discussion	This patient is experiencing typical symptoms of **cocaine intoxication**, including agitation, tachycardia, and hypertension due to adrenergic (alpha and beta) hyperstimulation. He has no evidence of any end-organ damage (CNS, cardiac, pulmonary, kidney, or liver injury). If the history was unknown or urine toxicology was negative, other drug ingestions, thyroid storm, alcohol withdrawal, or acute mania should be included in the differential. In general, beta-blockers should be avoided in acute cocaine toxicity due to risk of unopposed alpha-1 activation resulting in worsening hypertension and subsequent tissue ischemia. Labetalol is a mixed alpha/beta blocker that is sometimes used; however, this can also result in unopposed alpha stimulation in rare instances. Phentolamine is **a nonselective alpha blocker**, which causes vasodilation and lower blood pressure. Phentolamine is often used as a second-line therapy for cocaine-induced hypertension.

CASE 15 | Nonselective Beta-Blocker (Propranolol)

A 58-year-old woman with a history of cirrhosis and esophageal varices presents after vomiting bright red blood 10 minutes ago. She typically takes omeprazole, furosemide, spironolactone, and propranolol but has been without her medications for 2 weeks. On physical exam, temperature is 37°C, blood pressure is 100/60 mmHg, pulse is 110/min, and respirations are 16/min. She has jaundice, and her abdomen is distended with a positive fluid wave, suggesting ascites.

Evaluation/Tests	CBC shows Hgb of 8 g/dL. Esophagogastroduodenoscopy (EGD) shows 3 actively bleeding esophageal varices.
Treatment	Treatment should include endoscopically banding varices and restarting propranolol (as well as her other medications).
Discussion	This is a case of **esophageal varices secondary to liver disease**. Liver scarring in cirrhosis leads to increased pressure in the portal venous system. Increased pressure results in formation of varices in the esophagus. Up to 1/3 of patients with varices will develop variceal hemorrhage. **Nonselective β-blockers (propranolol, nadolol)** acting on beta-1 and beta-2 receptors block adrenergic dilation in mesenteric arterioles, resulting in unopposed α-stimulation (and constriction) and decrease in portal blood inflow. Decreased blood flow to mesenteric arterioles decreases portal pressure and reduces pressure in esophageal vessels, which are meant to be a low-pressure environment. The patient discontinuing propranolol likely resulted in increased mesenteric blood flow, increased portal pressure, and variceal hemorrhage.

DRUG REACTIONS

Drug reactions constitute a variety of adverse events associated with the use of certain medications and they are often hard to categorize or identify based solely on presentation. Reactions can be loosely categorized as medication-specific or immune-mediated. Medication-specific reactions are reactions to a specific class or type of medication. Medications exhibiting similar structure or pharmacologic activities may exhibit similar adverse reaction profiles. These reactions may be associated with certain organ systems (such as cardiovascular QT prolongation) or physiologic disturbances (such as diarrhea associated with antimicrobial use). Immune-mediated adverse effects, while exhibiting some pharmacologic class similarities (such as with the antistaphylococcal penicillins causing interstitial nephritis), are typically patient specific and largely mediated by genetic predispositions.

CASE 16 | Drug-Induced Hemolytic Anemia

A 32-year-old man who was recently diagnosed with HIV/AIDS presents with abdominal pain and dark urine. Approximately 2 days ago, dapsone was started for *Pneumocystis* pneumonia prophylaxis instead of trimethoprim/sulfamethoxazole because the patient has a sulfonamide allergy. He denies history of kidney stones or muscles aches or pains. On exam, he was afebrile, tachycardic, and had mild abdominal tenderness.

Evaluation/Tests	CBC shows hemoglobin of 10.7 g/dL, and urinalysis is positive for urobilinogen. Glucose-6-phosphate dehydrogenase (G6PD) level is low.
Treatment	Discontinue dapsone.
Discussion	This presentation is consistent with **medication- (dapsone-) induced hemolytic anemia**. Patients with UTI would have dysuria and urinalysis positive for nitrites or leukesterase, and patients with myoglobinuria typically present with diffuse muscle aches and elevated CPK. Specific medications can precipitate hemolytic reactions, especially in those with G6PD deficiency. Common offending agents include dapsone, primaquine, nitrofurantoin, and methylene blue. For patients from high incident regions or in those receiving medications known to induce hemolytic anemia, screening for enzyme activity may be warranted. Drug-induced hemolytic anemia secondary to G6PD deficiency is observed throughout the world in regions where the incidence of malaria is high.

CASE 17 | Vancomycin Flushing Syndrome

A 68-year-old woman with a history of diabetes mellitus is brought to the emergency department with acute mental status changes. She has no known drug allergies. Her temperature is 39.5°C, blood pressure is 169/103 mmHg, pulse is 120/min, respirations are 28/min, and O_2 saturation is 87% on room air. Lung exam is notable for bilateral crackles. She is empirically started on broad-spectrum antimicrobials for presumed sepsis with cefepime followed by a vancomycin infusion, both over 30 minutes. During the vancomycin infusion, the patient develops a pruritic erythematous rash over her face, arms, and chest.

CASE 17 | **Vancomycin Flushing Syndrome** *(continued)*

Evaluation/Tests	Clinical diagnosis.
Treatment	Stop vancomycin or decrease infusion rate.
Discussion	The onset of symptoms and timing of medication administration are consistent with vancomycin flushing syndrome, previously known as "red man syndrome." This condition is an infusion-related reaction caused by the release of histamine that typically occurs with rapid infusion rates of vancomycin. While it may initially appear as an allergic reaction, it is not considered an allergic reaction. Stopping or slowing the infusion rate, along with administration of antihistamines such as diphenhydramine, will typically bring about resolution of the rash. As is common with a number of other antimicrobials, such as beta-lactams and sulfonamides, allergic reactions can manifest with erythema and itching. Allergic reactions with vancomycin are rare. Disrupting or extending infusion times will help determine if the reaction is allergic or infusion related.

CASE 18 | ACE-Inhibitor Dry Cough

A 57-year-old man with seasonal allergies and hypertension presents with a dry cough. The patient takes antihistamines for his allergies, and he recently started lisinopril for his blood pressure. He does not smoke and reports that his allergies are well controlled. His exam is normal.

Evaluation/Tests	Clinical diagnosis.
Treatment	Discontinue ACE-inhibitor (lisinopril) and switch to angiotensin II receptor blocker (ARB; e.g., losartan).
Discussion	This is a case of **ACE-inhibitor-induced dry cough**. The patient does not have a history of asthma or GERD, and scheduled administration of antihistamines decreases the likelihood that the cough is related to his allergies. The mechanism of action of ACE-I-induced cough is that the medication blocks the enzymatic cleavage of angiotensin I to angiotensin II by angiotensin converting enzyme (ACE). ACE-inhibitors also inhibit the breakdown of some inflammatory cytokines (e.g., bradykinin, thromboxane), which can accumulate in the lung parenchyma and upper airways, causing a dry, nonproductive cough. ARBs do not cause this side effect. This adverse effect is harmless, but it can be bothersome. Angioedema, on the other hand, is a serious side effect of ACE-inhibitors, and they should be avoided in patients with hereditary angioedema.

CASE 19 | Medication-Induced Myopathy (Statins)

A 45-year-old woman with a history of hypertension and hyperlipidemia presents with muscle aches for the past 3–4 weeks. She has been on amlodipine for many years and was started on simvastatin a month ago for her elevated cholesterol. She denies trauma or any recent changes in her activities. Physical exam is unremarkable.

Evaluation/Tests	Creatinine kinase (CK) is elevated at 502 IU/mL.
Treatment	Discontinue simvastatin. Consider alternative treatment.
Discussion	This is a case of **statin-induced myopathy**. The patient's denial of activity alterations and timing of statin initiation make exercise-induced muscle injury less likely. Statin-induced myalgias are well described, typically occurring at higher statin doses and when used in conjunction with other medications such as fibrates, niacin, and other medications known to increase serum levels of statins. The exact mechanism of injury has not been fully elucidated. Initial presentation may occur weeks to months after initiation of a statin. Typically, elevation in CK levels are noted; however, normal CK levels have been reported. In more severe cases, elevated CK over 10 times the upper limit of normal, along with increases in serum creatinine, support a diagnosis of rhabdomyolysis. In cases such as these, aggressive hydration, as well as discontinuing the statin, are required.

CASE 20 | Medication-Induced Hepatitis (Isoniazid)

A 56-year-old man with a history of latent tuberculosis presents with abdominal pain and lethargy. Three months ago, he was started on isoniazid (INH) for a positive PPD result. His exam is notable for RUQ tenderness.

Evaluation/Tests	AST is 475, ALT is 358, INR is 1.3. Alkaline phosphatase is 178, bilirubin (total) is 1.9. Hepatitis A, B, and C panels are negative.

CASE 20 | Medication-Induced Hepatitis (Isoniazid) *(continued)*

Treatment	Discontinue INH, as well as other potentially hepatotoxic agents (ethanol, acetaminophen, etc.).
Discussion	**INH-induced hepatotoxicity** generally occurs after the first 2 months of therapy, and it occurs more prominently in the older population and in those with underlying liver disease. Hepatic metabolism of INH produces toxic metabolites and numerous toxic free radicals within the liver, which are suspected to play a role in the hepatotoxicity. The use of alcohol, acetaminophen, or other hepatically eliminated agents may potentiate the development of INH-induced hepatotoxicity. Once INH is discontinued, serial transaminases are assessed until normalization occurs. **INH-induced peripheral neuropathy** is another side effect that may be encountered due to the depletion of **pyridoxine**. The peripheral neuropathy can be prevented by concomitant administration with exogenous pyridoxine to prevent depletion.

CASE 21 | Agranulocytosis

A 26-year-old man with a history of schizophrenia presents for a follow-up appointment. A month earlier, he was started on clozapine for treatment-resistant schizophrenia. His exam is unremarkable. His labs are notable for a decrease in absolute neutrophil count (ANC) now 400/µL (previously 2400/µL).

Evaluation/Tests	This is a clinical diagnosis, but bone marrow biopsy should be considered if there is no improvement with discontinuation of medication.
Treatment	Discontinuation of offending agent (clozapine). Consider alternative treatment.
Discussion	This is a case of **clozapine-induced agranulocytosis**. Clozapine is a second-generation "atypical" antipsychotic medication used in the treatment of schizophrenia, especially treatment-resistant schizophrenia and schizophrenia with suicidality. One of the major adverse effects is reduction in neutrophils (neutropenia) which can lead to agranulocytosis and be life-threatening. While the mechanism of clozapine-induced neutropenia remains unknown, it appears to be dose independent. The onset is generally during the first 2 weeks of therapy; however, it can present after weeks to months of therapy, thus requiring frequent monitoring. Patients are typically enrolled in a monitoring program whereby they obtain weekly white blood cell counts to monitor for neutropenia.

CASE 22 | Torsade De Pointes

A 33-year-old woman with a history of schizophrenia was admitted to the hospital for aggressive behavior. She was started and titrated up on haloperidol due to continued aggression and delirium. Two days later, she had a syncopal episode. On exam, her blood pressure is normal, but she is tachycardic.

Evaluation/Tests	BMP is within normal limits. ECG shows prolonged QT interval, polymorphic ventricular tachycardia (VT) with change in the amplitude and twisting of the QRS complexes around the isoelectric line (torsade de pointes).
Treatment	Discontinue haloperidol, initiate IV magnesium and isoproterenol to stabilize rhythm. Cardiovert if hemodynamically unstable. Once patient is stable, consider alternative treatment for schizophrenia.
Discussion	**QT prolongation** and **torsade de pointes** caused by haloperidol have been reported following intravenous administration and at oral or intramuscular doses greater than recommended. Patients with underlying cardiac abnormalities, electrolyte imbalances, hypothyroidism, and family history of prolonged QT syndrome are at a greater risk of developing life-threatening arrhythmias with haloperidol administration. A baseline ECG and electrolytes should be obtained and monitored during haloperidol treatment. Other medications that can cause QT prolongation are certain antiarrhythmics (Class IA, III), antibiotics (macrolides), other antipsychotics, antidepressants (TCAs), antiemetics (ondansetron), etc. The mechanisms by which these medication classes cause QT prolongation differ, but most are attributable to blockade of cardiac potassium or calcium channels.

CASE 23 | Tardive Dyskinesia

A 58-year-old man with schizophrenia presents with abnormal movements of his lips and extremities. His schizophrenia symptoms were well managed on risperidone for the past year. His exam is remarkable for involuntary movements of his lips, tongue, and hands.

CASE 23 | **Tardive Dyskinesia** *(continued)*

Evaluation/Tests	Clinical diagnosis
Treatment	Discontinue risperidone. Consider dose-adjustments or alternative treatment.
Discussion	**Tardive dyskinesia** is an involuntary movement disorder most often associated with prolonged use of dopaminergic antagonists. Tardive dyskinesia may be irreversible, and it may evoke lifelong consequences. While first- and second-generation antipsychotics are most commonly implicated in tardive dyskinesia, antiemetics such as metoclopramide are also known to cause this condition. Patients should be monitored for extrapyramidal symptoms, such as dystonia and akathisia, as these findings indicate the patient is at an increased risk of developing tardive dyskinesia. If tardive dyskinesia occurs, the offending drug should be discontinued and an alternative initiated. Can consider switching to clozapine (weaker dopamine-blocking effects) and/or providing a vesicular monoamine transporter (VMAT) inhibitor such as tetrabenazine. Benzodiazepines can be used to treat symptoms.

CASE 24 | Drug-Induced Seizure

A 20-year-old man presents to the emergency room after suffering a witnessed seizure. He denies any previous history of epilepsy or neurologic illness. He has no other medical problems, but he states that he has been trying to quit smoking and started taking bupropion 1 week ago. Additionally, he admits to taking his roommate's tramadol due to an ankle sprain. His exam is unremarkable.

Evaluation/Tests	Clinical diagnosis.
Treatment	Discontinue both bupropion and tramadol.
Discussion	As the patient denies a history of epilepsy and neurologic illness, this presentation is consistent with a **drug-induced seizure**. Both bupropion and tramadol have the potential to lower the seizure threshold and provoke seizures. Bupropion inhibits the reuptake of norepinephrine and dopamine, whereas tramadol is a centrally acting opioid analgesic that binds to mu-opioid receptors and inhibits norepinephrine and serotonin reuptake. Each patient has a different tolerance or threshold for such medications prior to suffering these adverse events. In this patient, both medications should be permanently discontinued and relevant alternative treatments provided. **Varenicline** produces smoking cessation effects by binding to neuronal nicotinic receptors, preventing central nervous dopaminergic stimulation and reducing the rewarding feeling associated with smoking. NSAIDs are appropriate for symptomatic management of a mild sprain.
Additional considerations	While bupropion has no serotonergic activity, it can inhibit the metabolism of other serotonergic medications, including many antidepressants. Classic signs of **serotonin syndrome** include hyperthermia and hyperreflexia. In addition, bulimic patients are at an increased risk of drug-induced seizure secondary to bupropion administration, so it should be avoided in that population.

CASE 25 | Antibiotic Neurotoxicity

A 48-year-old man with ESRD and on dialysis was emergently taken for surgical debridement and started on intravenous imipenem-cilastatin, vancomycin, and clindamycin for necrotizing fasciitis of his left upper extremity. The following day, he had a witnessed seizure. He was given IV lorazepam, and the seizure stopped. His temperature is 38.7°C, blood pressure is 135/79 mmHg, pulse is 80/min, and respirations are 18/min. He is oriented, but he has mild postictal confusion. He has no focal deficits on neurologic exam, and his cranial nerves are intact. He has no nuchal rigidity and negative Kernig's and Brudzinski's signs. His skin is tender and erythematous over the LLE, but the surgical site appears clean.

Evaluation/Tests	BMP, urine output, and vancomycin levels are all normal. EEG is normal.
Treatment	Dialysis and switch imipenem-cilastatin to dose-adjusted meropenem or piperacillin-tazobactam.
Discussion	This is a case of **β-lactam neurotoxicity** causing a seizure. Nearly all β-lactam antibiotics, including carbapenems, have been implicated in some degree of neurotoxicity at high doses, which is usually characterized by altered mentation, hyperreflexia, myoclonus, and, rarely, seizure. Seizures are rare, except when very high doses are used in patients with epilepsy or with renal dysfunction as in this case of a patient with necrotizing fasciitis (toxigenic *Streptococcus pyogenes*) and end-stage renal disease. One of the most common antibiotics to cause seizures is imipenem. Mechanistically, β-lactams competitively inhibit GABA in the brain in a concentration-dependent manner, lowering

CASE 25 | Antibiotic Neurotoxicity *(continued)*

Discussion	the seizure threshold. As β-lactam penetration into the CNS is generally poor without inflamed meninges, neurotoxicity is usually limited to altered mental states that are challenging to differentiate from other causes, such as clinical worsening or ICU psychosis. In this patient for whom aggressive treatment is warranted, it is important to utilize alternative agents with less risk of seizure (e.g., meropenem, piperacillin-tazobactam) while taking care to use appropriate dose adjustments in those with renal dysfunction.

CASE 26 | Photosensitivity

A 16-year-old girl presents with second-degree burns on her face and shoulders. She states that she was sunbathing at the beach as she always does during spring break. Her only mediations include doxycycline, which was started a few months ago to control her acne. On exam, sun-exposed skin is warm, erythematous and blanching, and sensitive to touch.

Evaluation/Tests	Clinical diagnosis.
Treatment	Sunscreen rated at least SPF-30. Oral ibuprofen may be used to manage skin pain and inflammation.
Discussion	The timing of drug administration and onset of symptoms are consistent with **drug-induced photosensitivity**. Many medications, including tetracyclines (here, doxycycline) and sulfonamides, are known to increase photosensitivity, which leads to increased incidence and severity of sunburn. Tetracyclines are often used in addition to topical therapies to treat acne, for both their antimicrobial effects and their anti-inflammatory properties. It is important to discuss the increased risk of sunburn with patients when prescribing tetracyclines, in addition to the risk of esophagitis when taken with inadequate water. Although this scenario has a clear timeline and cause, developing a timeline of medication or other exposure helps to rule out contact dermatitis or autoimmune conditions that also present with exaggerated sunburn. Other drugs that commonly cause photosensitivity include amiodarone and 5-fluorouracil.

TOXICITIES

Drug poisonings and toxicities are a common cause of mortality, and they occur as a result of intentional or unintentional ingestion of drugs. The most common therapeutic classes implicated in drug toxicity cases are antidepressants, sedatives, and antipsychotics. To reduce mortality, it is imperative to understand how different drug toxicities present so that specific treatments may be initiated in a timely manner. Certain drugs have specifically manufactured antidotes to be administered in the case of an overdose (e.g., anti-dig Fab fragments for digoxin toxicity), while others have antidotes with multiple indications (e.g., atropine and glucagon for β-blocker toxicity).

CASE 27 | Toxic Alcohol Ingestion (Methanol/Propylene Glycol/Ethylene Glycol)

An 18-year-old man presents with blurry vision, labored breathing, and sedation after being dared to ingest various car fluids in his friend's garage. His temperature is 37°C, blood pressure is 98/55 mmHg, pulse is 65/min, and respirations are 25/min. On exam, he is alert and oriented to person, place, time, and situation. He has dilated pupils and retinal edema. His lung exam shows Kussmaul respirations, and he has flank tenderness and hematuria.

Evaluation/Tests	BMP and ABG reveal an anion gap metabolic acidosis. Urine toxicology screen is negative. Aspirin and acetaminophen levels are below detectable limits. CBC and glucose are normal. Serum osmolal gap is 4 mOsm/kg.
Treatment	Maintain airway, breathing, and circulation, and start IV sodium bicarbonate to maintain goal pH >7.3 and an alcohol dehydrogenase inhibitor (fomepizole or ethanol). For severe cases such as this, hemodialysis is indicated.
Discussion	This is a case of **toxic alcohol ingestion** (methanol/propylene glycol toxicity). Ingestion of toxic alcohols produces a similar effect as ethanol, but the metabolic by-products can lead to lethal toxicities. Profound anion gap metabolic acidosis and elevated serum osmolality are often seen, depending on the amount ingested and timing of presentation. Metabolic by-products of **methanol toxicity** classically cause ophthalmologic toxicity, while metabolites of **propylene glycol toxicity** commonly cause renal toxicity.

CASE 27 | Toxic Alcohol Ingestion (Methanol/Propylene Glycol/Ethylene Glycol) *(continued)*

Discussion	Patients with **ethylene glycol ingestion** may present with anion gap metabolic acidosis with a high osmolar gap, along with hematuria, acute renal failure, and oxalate crystals in the urine. Ethylene glycol is ultimately metabolized by alcohol dehydrogenase and aldehyde dehydrogenase to oxalate, which can lead to CNS metabolic encephalopathy and renal toxicity. Outside of supportive care, treatment involves inhibiting the metabolism of the toxic alcohols using a competitive inhibitor of alcohol dehydrogenase, fomepizole (preferred), or ethanol. Severe cases also require the use of hemodialysis to rapidly clear both the toxic alcohols and their toxic metabolites.

CASE 28 | Cyanide Poisoning

A 35-year-old man is found at home apneic and unresponsive. Emergency personnel note that no drugs were found at the scene, but there was a half-empty bottle of chemicals found near the patient. The patient was intubated and transferred to the emergency department with the bottle. Family reports that the patient is a jeweler. Exam is notable for sluggishly reactive pupils bilaterally, and temperature is 36.5°C, blood pressure is 90/47 mmHg, and pulse is 130/min.

Evaluation/Tests	Blood alcohol level is normal. Urine toxicology screen is negative. Arterial blood gas indicates profound metabolic acidosis. EKG shows sinus tachycardia with nonspecific ST-T changes. Analysis of the bottle contents reveals the presence of cyanide. CBC and glucose are normal.
Treatment	Treatment should include supportive care and administration of hydroxocobalamin (or sodium nitrite) and sodium thiosulfate.
Discussion	**Cyanide toxicity** is rapidly fatal if not treated with an antidote immediately. While the most common cause of cyanide toxicity occurs due to smoke inhalation, it can also occur due to ingestion or absorption through mucous membranes. Cyanide binds to the ferric ion of cytochrome oxidase, which inhibits the mitochondrial cytochrome complex and terminates oxidative phosphorylation. Cells must then use anaerobic metabolism to generate ATP, which produces lactic acid and leads to metabolic acidosis. The most common symptoms of cyanide toxicity consist of cyanosis, dyspnea, and unconsciousness. These symptoms are similar to some other toxic ingestions. Due to the lack of characteristic symptoms, cyanide toxicity should be treated with an antidote immediately if suspected. This patient is a jeweler, and cyanide is a chemical used frequently for jewelry creation, making this a suspected poison in this case. If available, hydroxocobalamin should be administered. As a vitamin B12 precursor, the cobalt moiety binds to intracellular cyanide to form cyanocobalamin, which is then excreted in the urine. Administration of sodium nitrite induces methemoglobinemia, which occurs following the oxidation of the ferrous moiety in hemoglobin to the ferric form. The methemoglobin acts as a competitive binding site for cyanide to decrease binding to cytochrome oxidase. Sodium thiosulfate is another antidotal option, which donates a sulfur moiety to transform cyanide to thiocyanate that is then renally excreted.
Additional considerations	**Arsenic poisoning** can occur due to acute or chronic exposure. Sources of exposure can be natural, such as volcanic eruptions or drinking water, or they may be due to manufactured products, such as pesticides or pressure-treated wood. Inorganic arsenic is rapidly eliminated from the bloodstream, but it can be detected as metabolites monomethylarsonic acid (MMA) and dimethylarsinic acid (DMA) in the urine during acute toxicity. As a metalloid, arsenic complexes with metals. Treatment is supportive care and includes dimercaprol or DMSA/succimer to chelate the circulating arsenic. **Organophosphates** are cholinesterase inhibitors that cause cholinergic toxicity in patients that consume them. Organophosphates are found in several insecticides, and they are readily absorbed through the skin, gastrointestinal, and respiratory tract. They bind to and inhibit acetylcholinesterase, which leads to accumulation of acetylcholine at neuronal synapses, leading to overactivation of the parasympathetic nervous system. Common signs and symptoms of acute intoxication are salivation, miosis, bradycardia, emesis, and diarrhea. There are no available diagnostic tests to confirm organophosphate poisoning, so clinical signs and symptoms, as well as investigation of potential ingestions must be considered. If organophosphate poisoning is suspected, atropine and/or pralidoxime should be administered. Atropine acts as a competitive antagonist of acetylcholine by binding to muscarinic receptors, and pralidoxime causes reactivation of acetylcholinesterase to help breakdown acetylcholine.

BEERS CRITERIA®

The American Geriatrics Society (AGS) Beers Criteria® for Potentially Inappropriate Medication (PIM) Use in Older Adults provides a list of drugs that should be avoided in patients 65 years and older. The intent is to reduce adverse drug events, improve drug selection, and educate clinicians and patients. It also serves as a tool for evaluating cost, quality, and drug use patterns. It is updated every 3 years.

CASE 29	Beers List—Avoid Benzodiazepines and Hydroxyzine
A 70-year-old man with a past medical history significant for chronic kidney disease, depression, type 2 diabetes mellitus, and hypertension presents with worsening anxiety for the past month. He has had anxiety for years, but his symptoms have progressed, and he is having increasing difficulty sleeping, is unable to relax, and is more fatigued. His wife states that he is constantly worried about minor issues and reports that he gets so worried sometimes that his heart races and he sweats. They deny any recent changes or stressful events in their lives or illicit drug use. He appears anxious, but his vital signs and the rest of the exam is normal.	
Evaluation/Tests	Clinical diagnosis.
Treatment	The patient should be started on an SSRI, buspirone, or pregabalin, but benzodiazepines and hydroxyzine should be avoided because of the Beers criteria.
Discussion	This patient has **generalized anxiety disorder**. **Benzodiazepines** are not recommended for elderly patients because they increase the risk of cognitive impairment, delirium, falls, fractures, and motor vehicle crashes. Metabolism of long-acting benzodiazepines is decreased, and sensitivity is increased in older adults. While hydroxyzine may be used in patients with anxiety, particularly in those suffering from insomnia, it should also be avoided in older adults due to the anticholinergic side effects. SSRI, buspirone, and pregabalin are reasonable options because they are not on AGS's Beers List.
Additional considerations	**Opioids** should be avoided in older adults outside of the setting of severe pain, such as fractures or surgical procedures. Opioids can cause an impairment in psychomotor function that may lead to increased falls and syncope. If opioids must be used for severe pain, proper counseling regarding the sedating effect must be provided to both the patient and caregivers. In addition, efforts should be made to reduce the use of other CNS-active agents concomitantly with opioids. Specifically, Beers criteria recommend against concomitant use of opioids with benzodiazepines due to increased risks of overdose, respiratory depression, and adverse events due to increased sedation. **NSAIDs** are included on Beers List due to their potential to increase the risk of developing gastrointestinal bleeding and peptic ulcer disease. Most NSAIDs inhibit COX-1 and COX-2. COX-1 is utilized by the gastrointestinal mucosa to produce prostaglandins that protect the lining of the mucosa. They may also increase blood pressure and increase the risk of kidney injury in older adults. Chronic NSAID therapy should be avoided in older adults due to these risks.

6
Public Health Sciences

Radhika Sreedhar, MD, MS
Anna Marie Gramelspacher, MD

EPIDEMIOLOGY AND BIOSTATISTICS

Evidence-based medicine involves employing the current best evidence in making decisions regarding patient care. This section will enable students to develop the skills needed to review the evidence and decide if they would like to apply the results of studies to their patients' care. The explanations go over the topic and provide key features that will help students understand how to answer any question that may arise around this topic. The following foundational areas of epidemiology and biostatistics are important to understand:

1. Types of studies and how to interpret their findings appropriately
2. Types of biases present in these studies and how to identify the source of these biases
3. Reliability and validity of a given finding
4. Interpretation of test results, including calculation of sensitivity, specificity, positive predictive value, and negative predictive value
5. Interpretation of study results, including relative risk, odds ratio, and number needed to treat

STUDY DESIGN

The approach to determining the type of study is best done by looking at the starting point of the study and assessing the exposure (risk factor, drug treatment, procedure, etc.) and the outcome or frequency of a particular event (disease, adverse effect, cure, etc.). If both frequency of events in study subjects and exposures were determined at the same point in time, it is a *cross-sectional study*. If exposure occurs first and the frequency of events in study subjects is done at a later point in time, it is a *cohort study*. If the subjects are randomized to experimental treatment or placebo and frequency of events in the study subjects is assessed at a later point in time in a controlled setting, it is an *experimental study*. The gold standard of experimental studies is a *randomized control trial*. If the study starts with cases and controls and the presence or absence of exposure is determined in them, then it is a *case-control study*. These are typical examples of study designs that are often tested on USMLE Step 1.

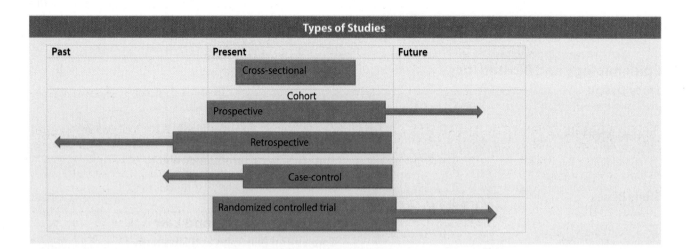

CASE 1	Case Series
A general surgeon observes that 15 of his patients who came for cholecystectomy surgery had pink gallstones. On further questioning, each of these patients reported that they took a pink multivitamin, "pinkamin," for about 3 months before surgery. He plans to publish a report of these patients.	
Discussion	A case series is a collection or review of common features of a small number of cases. Often, the cases present a unique or novel presentation of a disease, and they are accompanied by review of the literature.
Strengths	**Case series** are simple to design, cost-efficient, and easy to conduct. They can also lead to generation of hypotheses for more formal testing or more rigorous study designs.

CASE 1 | Case Series *(continued)*

Weaknesses	No comparison or control group; there is no specific research question; and the results are solely based on interesting observations.

CASE 2 | Cross-Sectional Study

A 47-year-old woman presents to clinic with a flare of eczema. She reports a recent change in diet to include more local fruits and vegetables, and she wants to know if they may be contributing to her symptoms. To answer her question, an article on the topic is reviewed, in which 75 individuals were surveyed on their current dietary habits and whether or not they are experiencing symptoms of eczema.

Discussion	This is an example of a cross-sectional study. Cross-sectional studies are observational studies that examine the frequency of an event in a population at one point in time. Subjects are selected, and there is no particular direction of inquiry as exposures and outcomes are assessed at the same time. This study examines fruit and vegetable consumption, and the symptoms of eczema at one point in time in a survey. These study types are helpful in providing prevalence ratios of an outcome and exposure in a given population. A **prevalence ratio** is the proportion of patients with the outcome divided by the proportion of patients with the exposure.
Strengths	**Cross-sectional studies** are cost-efficient and easy to conduct and implement.
Weaknesses	It is not possible to distinguish cause and effect; inferences are limited to the specific time and are not generalizable to other times; and sampling bias is present (not everyone agrees to participate).
Diagram	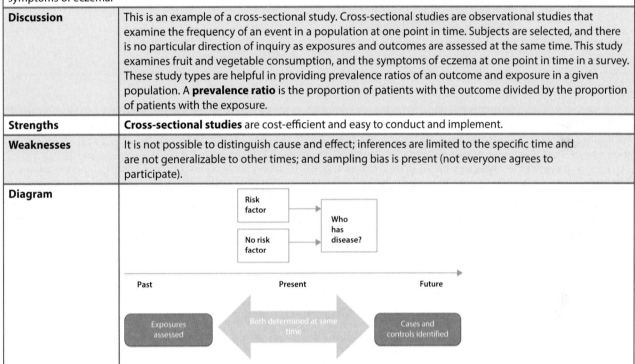

CASE 3 | Case-Control Study

An investigator reviewed the medical records of 600 men between the ages of 40 and 60 who were seen for care at the hospital. The investigator identified 100 with and 100 without chronic obstructive pulmonary disease (COPD). Each patient was interviewed to assess whether there might be mold exposure at home. The purpose of the study was to see if there was an association between mold exposure and development of COPD.

Discussion	This is a typical case-control study where individuals with the outcome of interest are identified first. In this case, the outcome of interest is the incidence of those with COPD (cases) and those without COPD (controls). These patients are then compared to see if there is a difference in the proportion of people with a particular exposure (in this case, mold) in the two groups with the aim of determining if there is an association between the exposure (mold) and the outcome (COPD). This information can be used to determine the odds ratio. The **odds ratio (OR)** indicates the odds of a disease or event occurring in an exposed population compared to the unexposed population.
Strengths	**Case-control studies** are cost- and time-efficient. They can study significant numbers of cases, which is useful for rare conditions.
Weaknesses	Study is retrospective; potential sources of bias include confounding factors, selection bias, and recall bias; over-/underestimation of association since sampling relies heavily on outcome; both exposure and disease have already occurred, making it difficult to establish a temporal relationship.

CASE 3 | Case-Control Study *(continued)*

Diagram	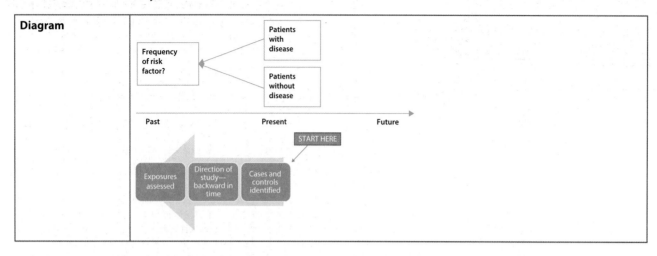

CASE 4 | Cohort Study

An investigator wants to assess whether the use of a novel anesthetic agent given during surgery is associated with interstitial lung disease. The investigator reviewed records and identified 50 patients who were given the novel anesthetic and 50 comparison patients who were given the standard anesthetic agent. All patients underwent annual pulmonary function tests, high-resolution CT scan, and clinical follow-up for 5 years to determine if there was a difference in the number of patients who developed interstitial lung disease between these two groups.

Discussion	This is an example of a **prospective cohort study**, where a group of people with similar baseline characteristics except for exposure are followed in time to determine if there is a difference in the incidence of outcome between the exposed and unexposed groups. The exposure of interest is the novel anesthetic gas, and the outcome of interest is interstitial lung disease. Another type of cohort study is a retrospective cohort study. In a **retrospective cohort study**, researchers use data that has already been collected on a defined group of people to identify their exposure status and then determine if the outcome occurred because of their exposure. This is a cohort study because the exposure and outcome are defined at the beginning of the study.
Strengths	**Cohort studies** can assess temporal relationship, and the data can be used to calculate incidence rate or relative risks (RR), as well as the differences/ratios.
Weaknesses	Large sample sizes are needed; potential confounding factors exist; and they are expensive to conduct.
Diagram	

CASE 5 | Randomized Clinical Trial

A study compares two medications' efficacy in lowering blood pressure: The first is a novel drug, and the second is an ACE inhibitor that is the current standard of care. The study randomly assigns 2000 participants at 15 research sites across the United States to each medication and follows these participants for 5 years. Over the 5-year study period, participants will be monitored for blood pressure reduction, all-cause mortality, and the major sequela of elevated blood pressure (i.e., stroke and MI). Participants will not be informed as to which drug they are taking. Additionally, the individual responsible for collecting all outcome measures will not be informed as to the type of medication the patient is taking. The average reduction in blood pressure, mortality, and risk of major sequela will be compared between the medications at the end of the 5-year study.

Discussion	This is a typical double-blinded randomized controlled trial, where two groups of people with similar baseline characteristics are randomized to receive one of several comparison treatments. The goal of randomization is to minimize sampling bias in order to create study groups that are as similar as possible in terms of their baseline characteristics. The success of randomization efforts is often tested by looking for no statistical difference between study groups by each baseline characteristic.
Strengths	**Randomized clinical trials** minimize bias and confounding variables.
Weaknesses	They are expensive to conduct, and inclusion criteria may limit generalizability.
Diagram	

START HERE

Study starts with randomization to minimize bias → Direction of study---forward in time → Study ends with determination of outcomes

CASE 6 | Phases of Clinical Trials

Discussion	**Phase I clinical trials** often involve a small number of healthy volunteers or disease patients to assess safety, toxicity, and drug pharmacology.
	Phase II clinical trials are also used to assess optimal dosing and adverse effects.
	In **Phase III clinical trials**, the goal is to establish how the novel treatment compares to the current treatment or standard of care among a larger, more generalizable population.
	Phase IV clinical trials involve postmarketing surveillance (after FDA-approval) to monitor for rare or long-term adverse effects.

STUDY BIASES

The outcome of a study can be affected by many factors in the study design. It is important to assess if there are flaws in the design of a study that would explain the relationship seen between the exposure and outcome at the end of the study. Flaws in studies are more common in studies that are observational, have small sample size, and stray from rigorous methodology. When looking at studies for biases, look for a systematic way that cases and controls were treated differently. The way that cases and controls were treated differently helps identify the type of bias. While there are many different types of potential biases within studies, some key biases are outlined here.

CASE 7 | Selection Bias

A 55-year-old woman with a past medical history of ovarian cancer who is currently in remission presents for follow-up. She brings an article she recently found on the relationship between the use of talcum powder and ovarian cancer. She has been using talcum powder since she was a child and would like to know if this could have contributed to her cancer. On review, it is noted that the cases were recruited from hospital records and that controls were recruited by random digit dialing between 9 a.m. and 5 p.m. on weekdays.

CASE 7 | Selection Bias *(continued)*

Discussion	Calling between 9 a.m. and 5 p.m. likely resulted in overrepresentation of individuals who work from home or who are unemployed. Thus they may not represent the study base in terms of use of talcum powder. This is an explanation of selection bias.
	Selection bias is a systematic error in which participants selected in a study group all have a similar characteristic that is unintended by the researchers. This may limit generalizability of findings beyond the specific population selected. The groups in the study differ in the baseline characteristics because of the method of selection of participants and this can distort the results of the study.

CASE 8 | Recall Bias

A 36-year-old woman who recently delivered a baby with Down syndrome brings in a study showing a link between the use of chlorine-based cleaning products and Down syndrome. She wishes to know if she should stop using these products as she plans to conceive again, and she wants to reduce her risk of having another child with Down syndrome. A case-control study was done to determine if there was a link between the use of chlorine-based cleaning products during pregnancy and Down syndrome. The cases were women who had children with Down syndrome and the controls were women who had children without any congenital anomalies. They were asked whether they used chlorine-based cleaning products when they were pregnant, with the intention of determining whether chlorine-based cleaning products were associated with Down syndrome.

Discussion	When someone experiences a disease or adverse event, they are more likely to think about possible reasons for the adverse event and remember previous exposures to potential causative agents. This can lead to **differential recall**, or recall bias. In this example, mothers of children with Down syndrome may be more likely to distinctly remember their exposures (cleaning products) during pregnancy when compared to mothers whose children were born without a congenital anomaly.

CASE 9 | Measurement Bias

A local teaching hospital hopes to decrease its rates of hospital-acquired infections. As a part of this initiative, it completes an observational study on medical student handwashing on an inpatient ward. A researcher is stationed in each hallway and records how many students enter and leave each patient room and whether or not the students used hand sanitizer or washed their hands when entering or leaving the room.

Discussion	Measurement bias is a form of bias in which there is a systemic issue in the collection of the data such that it does not capture the information accurately. The preceding example represents a particular type of measurement bias called **Hawthorne effect**, in which subjects of a study are likely to change their actions if they know they are being observed. In this example, we would not expect to get an accurate measure of the number of students who wash their hands with each patient encounter because the students are aware they are being observed.

CASE 10 | Lead-Time Bias

A 74-year-old man with bladder cancer diagnosed on cystoscopy 2 months ago presents for a second opinion. He brings an advertisement for a new urine cytology test with him, and the advertisement states that it detects bladder cancer earlier than cystoscopy. He asks if his life expectancy would have been better had he done the urine cytology test rather than the standard cystoscopy. The following is an abstract:

A new test for urinary cytology for bladder cancer detection is developed. The survival duration of patients detected by the urinary test is 20 years when compared to the 15-year survival of patients detected by cystoscopy done for evaluation of hematuria. There is no difference in the quality of life measures annually between the two groups. At autopsy, the extent of progression of disease is the same in both groups of patients despite treatment.

Discussion	Because survival is measured from the time of diagnosis, early diagnosis as the result of early screening may result in an overestimation of survival duration. This is called lead-time bias. This is not a true increase in survival but rather an artifact caused by an earlier diagnosis. The overall survival time of the patient is the same regardless of whether the screening test was done or not.

CASE 10 | Lead-Time Bias (continued)

Diagram	
	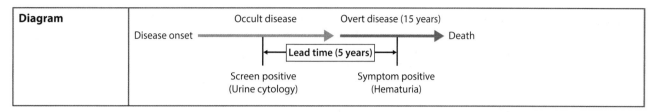

CASE 11 | Length-Time Bias

A 54-year-old male smoker comes into the clinic and inquires about a new salivary test for lung cancer advertised on TV. The following information is noted:

> A new saliva-based screening test for lung cancer is instituted among asymptomatic people. The survival of patients with lung cancer detected by the salivary screening test is compared to survival of patients with lung cancer who were detected by CT scan when they presented with cough and weight loss. It is found that the patients whose lung cancer was detected by the salivary test lived longer than those detected by CT scan when they presented with symptoms. Autopsy results showed that the salivary test–positive lung cancers were less aggressive and slow growing when compared to the CT scan–detected lung cancer.

Discussion	Length-time bias refers to the overestimation of survival duration caused by the relative excess of slowly progressive cases among screen-detected cases. This is because the screening test disproportionately detects cases that are slow growing. The patients with aggressive or rapidly growing tumors tend to die early and therefore are not detected by the screening test as indicated in the accompanying figure. All of the red arrows depict patients who have slow-growing tumors, and the blue represent patients with rapidly growing tumors. The vertical line represents the time the screening test is administered. As shown, only 1 rapidly growing tumor and 4 slowly progressing tumors are detected by the screening test. This represents the length-time bias.
Diagram	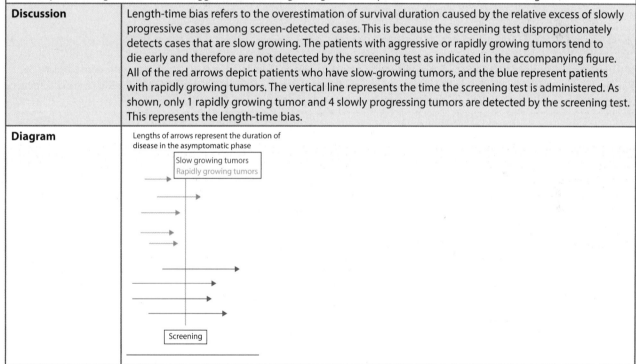

EVALUATION OF TEST RESULTS

When deciding what tests to use on a patient, it is important to consider whether the test is appropriate. The characteristics of the test, such as its sensitivity and specificity, help inform if the test will reveal the necessary information. In general, there are two types of questions:

1. Amongst patients with and without disease, how many have or do not have a positive test result? These types of questions are on the **sensitivity and specificity** of the test. They are stable properties of the test that do not change with the prevalence of disease.
2. Among patients with positive or negative test results, how many have or do not have the disease? These types of questions are on the **positive predictive value (PPV)** and **negative predictive value (NPV)** of the test, which will change with disease prevalence. As prevalence or pretest probability increases, PPV increases and NPV decreases.

A necessary skill is the ability to take data about a given test and use it to determine the sensitivity, specificity, PPV, and NPV of the given test.

Picture the following scenario: A patient brings in an abstract about the use of magnetic resonance imaging (MRI) for screening for breast cancer. She has dense breasts on previous mammography, and she was informed that MRI may be a superior screening test.

Purpose

Breast density can impact the sensitivity of mammography. Women with dense breasts often have to undergo diagnostic mammography and ultrasonography for further evaluation, exposing them to increased radiation risks. We wish to determine the diagnostic characteristics of breast MRI in breast cancer detection in women with dense breast tissue.

Materials and Methods

One hundred seventy-three women with dense breast tissue who underwent mammography/ultrasonography and had been scheduled for biopsy underwent breast MRI exams prior to biopsy. Images were evaluated by three independently blinded radiologists.

Results

Cancer was confirmed histologically in 145 women, and the MRI was positive in 120 of these women. Among the 28 patients without cancer, the MRI was negative in 21. The results of testing are provided in the table here. Among women with dense breast tissue, 94% of patients with a positive MRI were found to have breast cancer.

Conclusion

MRI has good diagnostic characteristics in detecting breast cancer in a selected group of patients with dense breast tissue. Further studies should be done in patients presenting for screening mammography to determine if it will be a good screening test for breast cancer in women with dense breasts.

	Disease + Breast Cancer	Disease—No Breast Cancer	Total
Screen positive test result MRI positive	120 TP True positive	7 FP False positive	127 All screen positive
Screen negative test result MRI negative	25 FN False negative	21 TN True negative	46 All screen negative
Total	145 All disease positive	28 All disease negative	173

CASE 12 | Sensitivity

Based on the preceding scenario and abstract, one would like to know how many patients will have a positive MRI among all patients with breast cancer.

Equation	$$\text{Sensitivity} = \frac{\text{True positives}}{\text{True positives} + \text{False negatives}}$$
Discussion	This question is asking about sensitivity, or the true positive rate. Among all patients with the disease, sensitivity reveals how many patients will have a positive test result ("Positive in disease"). This is 120/145 = 83%.
Diagram	(see table below)

		Disease +	Disease –	Total
	Screen positive test result	TP True positive	FP False positive	All screen positive
	Screen negative test result	FN False negative	TN True negative	All screen negative
	Total	All disease positive	All disease negative	Total population

CASE 13 | Specificity

Based on the scenario and abstract, one would like to know how many patients will have a negative MRI among all patients without breast cancer.

Equation	$$\text{Specificity} = \frac{\text{True negatives}}{\text{True negatives} + \text{False positives}}$$
Discussion	This question is asking about specificity (true negative rate). Among all patients without disease, specificity reveals how many will have a negative test result ("Negative in health")? This is 21/28 = 75%.

Diagram

	Disease +	Disease −	Total
Screen positive test result	TP True positive	FP False positive	All screen positive
Screen negative test result	FN False negative	TN True negative	All screen negative
Total	All disease positive	All disease negative	Total population

CASE 14 | Positive Predictive Value (PPV)

Based on the abstract, the patient would like to know the number of patients that truly have breast cancer among all patients with positive MRI results.

Equation	$$\text{PPV} = \frac{\text{True positives}}{\text{True positives} + \text{False positives}}$$
Discussion	This question is asking about positive predictive value. Among all patients with a positive test result, how many will truly have the disease? This is 120/127 = 94%.

Diagram

	Disease +	Disease −	Total
Screen positive test result	TP True positive	FP False positive	All screen positive
Screen negative test result	FN False negative	TN True negative	All screen negative
Total	All disease positive	All disease negative	Total population

CASE 15 | Negative Predictive Value (PPV)

Based on the abstract, the patient would like to know the number of patients that truly do not have breast cancer among all patients with negative MRI results.

Equation	$$\text{NPV} = \frac{\text{True negatives}}{\text{True negatives} + \text{False negatives}}$$
Discussion	The patient is asking about the negative predictive value of the test. Among all patients with a negative test result, how many will truly not have the disease? This is 21/46 = 45%.

Diagram

	Disease +	Disease −	Total
Screen positive test result	TP True positive	FP False positive	All screen positive
Screen negative test result	FN False negative	TN True negative	All screen negative
Total	All disease positive	All disease negative	Total population

CASE 16 | Prevalence

The patient states that there is no history of any cancer in her family, and she wonders how many people in the study had breast cancer.

Equation	$$\text{Prevalence} = \frac{\#\,\text{new cases}}{\text{Total}\,\#\,\text{people}} \text{ at a point in time}$$
Discussion	The total number of cases of a disease in a population divided by the total population gives the prevalence rate. This will help answer the patients question on how many people in the study had breast cancer. $$\text{Prevalence} = \frac{(TP + FN)}{(TP + FN + FN + TN)} = \frac{145}{173} = 83\%$$

Diagram		Disease +	Disease −	Total
	Screen positive test result	TP True positive	FP False positive	All screen positive
	Screen negative test result	FN False negative	TN True negative	All screen negative
	Total	All disease positive	All disease negative	Total population

CASE 17 | Incidence

The patient is reassured that, although the study had a high prevalence, the study population was only women with an abnormal mammograms who were selected to undergo biopsy. She asks how many new cases of breast cancer occur every year in women with dense breasts.

Equation	$$\text{Incidence rate} = \frac{\#\,\text{new cases}}{\#\,\text{people at risk}} \text{ during specific time period}$$
Discussion	The number of new cases of a disease divided by the number of persons at risk for the disease gives us the incidence rate. In a study of 500 women with dense breasts, 25 were diagnosed with new breast cancer. Based on these study results, the incidence rate of breast cancer in this population of women with dense breasts was $(25/500) \times 100 = 5\%$.
Diagram	

AFTER A PERIOD OF TIME

Additional considerations	**Incidence vs. prevalence** The natural history of disease greatly impacts the relationship between incidence and prevalence. Because incidence is a measure of new cases, and prevalence is a matter of current cases, the rate of recovery affects these measurements. Diseases that have a quick recovery time have a higher incidence and lower prevalence, while chronic diseases have a lower incidence and higher prevalence. Due to the high rate of spontaneous disease resolution and relatively few deaths in influenza, increased incidence may not contribute to much to the growth of prevalence. Conversely, in the case of a more chronic disease such as diabetes, the prevalence is likely higher than the incidence. The proportion of new cases of diabetes in a given time period (incidence) is small, but those patients continue to have the disease for a long time, so the total patients with the disease at any time (prevalence) is higher.

CASE 18 | Likelihood Ratios

Likelihood ratios are a useful tool to determine if doing a test will help change the management of a patient. It is also helpful to compare tests. A 67-year-old man with a history of prior CVA is brought to the ER in a wheelchair by his wife for evaluation of new-onset left leg swelling and redness. His exam is notable for left hemiplegia, mild left leg edema, and erythema. You are not sure whether he has cellulitis or a deep venous thrombus. Your senior resident asks you whether a venous Doppler ultrasound of the leg would give additional information based on your suspicion of a deep venous thrombus as a cause of his symptoms. You review the abstract to help you decide if you should do the ultrasound of the leg or not.

Abstract	**Background** The clinical diagnosis of deep-vein thrombosis is generally thought to be unreliable. We evaluated venous Doppler ultrasonography to determine the potential for an improved and simplified diagnostic approach in patients with suspected deep-vein thrombosis. All patients were clinically assessed with Wells Score to determine the probability for deep-vein thrombosis before they had ultrasonography and venography. All tests were performed and interpreted by independent observers. In all 529 patients, the clinical model predicted prevalence of deep-vein thrombosis in the three categories: 85% in the high pretest probability category, 33% in the moderate category, and 5% in the low category. The sensitivity and specificity of ultrasonogram for patients with low pretest probability of disease is 67% and 98%, respectively (modified from *Lancet* 1995; 345: 1326–30). Based on Wells Score, our patient has a low pretest probability of having a deep venous thrombus with a prevalence of 5% in this population. Should we do an ultrasonogram for him?
Discussion	Pretest probability is the probability of disease based on the patient's presentation before a test is done. The likelihood ratio (LR) of a test provides information about how much the probability of disease will change if we do the test and helps us decide if it is worthwhile to do the test or not. (It is best to do a test only if it significantly changes the probability of disease). Posttest probability is the probability of disease based on the test result. The posttest probability helps us determine if further tests need to be done to confirm the diagnosis or if we are so confident about the presence or absence of disease based on this test result that either the patient can start treatment or be sent home without further tests. Likelihood ratios are also used in clinical practice to quickly compare different strategies and tests that may help with clinical decision making. The likelihood of a test result in a patient with the target disorder compared to the likelihood of the same result in a patient without the target disorder is the likelihood ratio or LR. The formula for +LR and its interpretation is: $$\textbf{Positive LR} = \frac{\text{Sensitivity}}{1 - \text{sensitivity}}$$ $$= \frac{\text{TP rate}}{\text{FP rate}}$$ $$= \frac{\text{Likelihood of a + result in those with the disease}}{\text{Likelihood of a + result in those without the disease}}$$ Values of +LR • >10 very useful as it increases the post-test probability by 45% • 5 moderately useful as it increases the post-test probability by 30% • 2 less useful as it increases the post-test probability by 15% • 1 useless as it does not change the post-test probability In this study, +LR for venous Doppler ultrasound is $0.78/(1 - 0.98) = 39$. This +LR is much greater than 10. This means that a positive ultrasound will increase the post-test probability of DVT from 5% to 50% and will help change the management of the patient. $$\textbf{Negative LR} = (1 - \text{sensitivity})/\text{specificity}$$ $$= \text{FN rate/TN rate}$$ $$= \frac{\text{likelihood of a} - \text{result in those with the disease}}{\text{likelihood of a} - \text{result without the disease}}$$

CASE 18 | Likelihood Ratios *(continued)*

Discussion	Values of −LR
	• <0.1 very useful as it decreases the post-test probability by 45% • 0.2 moderately useful as it decreases the post-test probability by 30% • 0.5 less useful as it decreases the post-test probability by 15% In this study: • −LR for venous Doppler ultrasound is (1 − 0.78)/0.98 = 0.22. • This −LR is close to 0.2. This means that a negative ultrasound will decrease the post-test probability of DVT from 5% to −25% and will help change the management of the patient.

TEST CUTOFFS

The cutoffs for a test result are chosen usually at a point that maximizes the diagnostic characteristics of the test and take into account the cost of the test and its consequences. Changes in the cutoff of tests can impact how many people will be classified as having the disease or not.

CASE 19 | Lowering a Test Cutoff

Based on new epidemiologic data, the cutoff for hypertension was moved from 140/90 to 130/80 mmHg. Based on this change, what will happen to the sensitivity, specificity, and predictive values of a blood pressure reading to diagnose hypertension?

Diagram	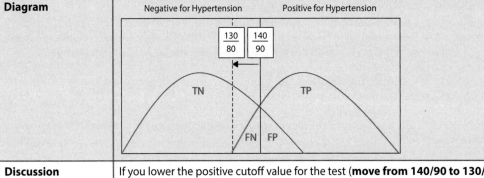
Discussion	If you lower the positive cutoff value for the test (**move from 140/90 to 130/80**), you will increase the number of positive tests (both TP and FP), and decrease the number of negative tests (both TN and FN). This **increases the sensitivity** (by decreasing FN in the denominator) and **decreases the specificity** (by increasing FP in the denominator). The **PPV will decrease** because FP (only in the denominator) has increased, and the **NPV will increase** because FN (only in the denominator) has decreased.

CASE 20 | Raising a Test Cutoff

Based on new epidemiologic data, the cutoff for hypertension for patients over age 80 was moved from 140/90 to 150/95. What will happen to the sensitivity, specificity, and predictive values of a blood pressure reading to diagnose hypertension based on this change?

Diagram	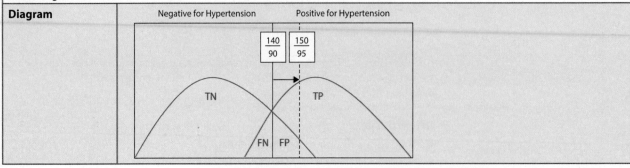

CASE 20 | Raising a Test Cutoff *(continued)*

Discussion	If you increase the positive cutoff value for the test (**move 140/90 to 150/95**), you will increase the number of negative tests (both TN and FN). This **decreases the sensitivity** (by increasing FN in the denominator) and **increases the specificity** (by decreasing FP in the denominator). The **PPV will increase** because FP (only in the denominator) has decreased, and the **NPV will decrease** because FN (only in the denominator) has increased.

RECEIVER OPERATING CHARACTERISTIC (ROC) CURVE

A plot of the true positive rate (sensitivity) against the false positive rate (1 – specificity) of a diagnostic test is called a receiver operating characteristic (ROC) curve. ROC curves are used to help assess the tradeoff between sensitivity and specificity and the accuracy of the test. The accuracy of a test increases as the curve gets closer to the upper left-hand border and is less accurate as it gets closer to the 45° diagonal of the ROC space with the area under the curve providing a direct measure of test accuracy.

CASE 21 | ROC Curve

A new screening test for COPD using lung elastase levels in saliva is studied. For each of the lung elastase enzyme values obtained from saliva, the GOLD criterion that is the standard in diagnosing COPD was used to determine if the patient had COPD.

Data				
	Enzyme Value	**COPD**	**No COPD**	
	5 or less	18	1	
	5.1–7	7	17	
	7.1–9	4	36	
	9 or more	3	39	
	Totals	32	93	

		True Positive Rate	**True Negative Rate**	**False Positive Rate**
	CutOff	**Sensitivity**	**Specificity**	**(1 – specificity)**
	5	0.56	0.99	0.01
	7	0.78	0.81	0.19
	9	0.91	0.42	0.58

Considerations	If we selected a level of 5 as our "cutoff point" (the point at which we called the test positive or negative), the test would have had only 1 false positive and thus would be very specific (99%). However, it would have missed 14 of 32 cases of lung cancer, making it not very sensitive (56%). Therefore, for this cut point, the test's sensitivity is low (missing lots of people with disease), but its specificity is high (few false positives). If we instead selected a cut point of 9, then we would have diagnosed 29 of the 32 people so the sensitivity is high (91%). However, we would have had 54 false positives, so the specificity is low (42%).
Diagram	An ROC curve plots true positive rate (sensitivity) on the *y*-axis against false positive rate (1 – specificity) on the *x*-axis for different cut points of a diagnostic test. For the preceding example, this is the data that would be plotted. The blue line in the figure is the actual plot of the sensitivity of lung elastase against the false positive rate of lung elastase for COPD. The dotted line represents the curve where the true positive rate and the false positive rate of lung elastase for COPD are the same.

CASE 21 | ROC Curve *(continued)*

Diagram	Receiver operating characteristic curve of lung elastase for COPD
	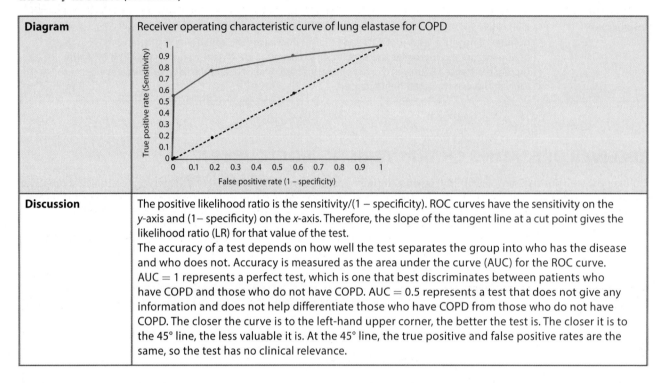

Discussion	The positive likelihood ratio is the sensitivity/(1 − specificity). ROC curves have the sensitivity on the *y*-axis and (1− specificity) on the *x*-axis. Therefore, the slope of the tangent line at a cut point gives the likelihood ratio (LR) for that value of the test. The accuracy of a test depends on how well the test separates the group into who has the disease and who does not. Accuracy is measured as the area under the curve (AUC) for the ROC curve. AUC = 1 represents a perfect test, which is one that best discriminates between patients who have COPD and those who do not have COPD. AUC = 0.5 represents a test that does not give any information and does not help differentiate those who have COPD from those who do not have COPD. The closer the curve is to the left-hand upper corner, the better the test is. The closer it is to the 45° line, the less valuable it is. At the 45° line, the true positive and false positive rates are the same, so the test has no clinical relevance.

QUANTIFYING RISK

When discussing the efficacy of a treatment, it is important to understand the concepts of absolute and relative risks to convey information in simple terms. Using the number needed to treat (NNT) and absolute risk reduction (ARR) or increase is a good way to do so. Interpreting confidence intervals is also important. Recognize that the width of a confidence interval gives information about the sample size adequacy.

Picture the following scenario: A patient is admitted with a myocardial infarction and, upon discharge, inquires if aspirin will benefit him. The following article is reviewed: Randomized trial of intravenous streptokinase, oral aspirin, both, or neither among 17,187 cases of suspected acute myocardial infarction: ISIS-2. ISIS-2 (Second International Study of Infarct Survival) Collaborative Group. *Lancet.* 1988 Aug 13;2(8607):349–60. PMID: 2899772.

Background

Vascular and cardiac injury is a leading cause of morbidity and mortality. The objective of this study is to examine the protective benefits of aspirin use in patients with a recent myocardial infarction in regard to vascular death within 1-month postincident.

Methods

Patients who presented to the emergency room with a myocardial infarction were randomized to placebo or 160 mg/day aspirin, and they were monitored for 1 month after initial presentation for any vascular outcome and death. This study was conducted in 417 hospitals. Both patients and researchers were blinded to the research group of the study participant.

Results

A total of 17,187 patients were randomized to placebo or 160 mg/day enteric-coated aspirin. 804/8587 (9.4%) vascular deaths occurred among patients allocated aspirin tablets vs. 1016/8600 (11.8%) among those allocated placebo tablets (OR: 23%; $p < 0.0001$). The relative risk (RR) for all deaths with aspirin at 160 mg once daily vs. placebo was 0.80 (95% confidence interval: 0.75–1.21).

Conclusions

Daily aspirin at 160 mg appears to be associated with decreased vascular-related death in the month following hospitalization among patients with presentation suspected for myocardial infarction compared to controls.

In this example, we can use the data provided to make a **2 × 2 contingency table**. These tables are useful for assessing disease rates (those with and without) and comparing to those who were given a particular intervention (e.g., drug vs. placebo) or those exposed to a risk factor (e.g., smoking vs. no smoking).

	Vascular Death	No Death	Totals
Aspirin (ASA) experimental group	804	8587 − 804 = 7783	8587
Placebo control group	1016	8600 − 1016 = 7584	8600
Totals	804 + 1016 = 1820	7783 + 7584 = 15,367	17,187

CASE 22 | Event Rates (ER)

Explanation	Event rates (ER) are measures of how often a particular event, typically the outcome or end point of a study, occurs within a groRup of people, typically the patients in that experimental group. In this case, the event is vascular death, and the two experimental groups are the aspirin- (ASA-) treated or placebo-controlled groups. Event rates can subsequently be used to calculate other measurements such as relative risk that are more useful when interpreting a study.
Calculation(s)	**Experimental event rate (EER)** = Absolute risk of vascular death in ASA group $= \dfrac{\text{Risk of vascular death in ASA group}}{\text{Total number of patients in ASA group}}$ = 804/8587 = 9.4% **Control event rate (CER)** = Absolute risk of vascular death in placebo group $= \dfrac{\text{Risk of vascular death in placebo group}}{\text{Total number of patients in placebo group}}$ = 1016/8600 = 11.8%

CASE 23 | Relative Risk (RR)

Explanation	The relative risk (RR) is a ratio of probabilities that compares rates in two populations: the risk of developing disease or an event in the exposed group vs. the risk in the unexposed group. It is based on the incidence of an event or disease, and therefore knowledge of participant exposure is required. In this case, the exposed group are post-MI patients who were given ASA, and the unexposed group is the post-MI patients who were given placebo.
Calculation(s)	**Relative risk (RR)** = EER/CER
Discussion	An RR < 1 indicates that the exposure is associated with decreased disease occurrence (often the case in drug treatment studies). An RR > 1 indicates exposure is associated with increased disease occurrence, which is often the case with harmful exposures or side effects of medications. An RR = 1 indicates no association between exposure and disease. RR is typically used in cohort studies. The relative risk of vascular death among those given aspirin as compared to placebo is 9.4/11.8 = 0.796. This represents aspirin as a **protective** factor as the RR is <1, or the exposure associated with a decrease in disease occurrence. An additional factor that can be calculated from RR is the **relative risk reduction (RRR)**, which is the proportion of RR attributable to the intervention (ASA) compared to control (placebo). RRR = 1 − RR. In this study, the relative risk reduction of vascular death among those given aspirin is 1 − 0.796 = 0.2. In other words, aspirin reduces the risk of vascular death by 20% when compared to the placebo.

CASE 24 | Odds Ratio (OR)

Explanation	Odds compares events with nonevents. The odds ratio (OR) indicates the odds of a disease or event occurring in an exposed population compared to the unexposed population. Odds ratio is typically used in case-control studies where the incidence of disease cannot be obtained as the cases are selected by the investigator.

CASE 24 | Odds Ratio (OR) *(continued)*

Calculation(s)	$OR = \dfrac{\text{Outcome/No outcome in exposed group}}{\text{Outcome/No outcome in unexposed group}}$
Discussion	In this example, if it were a case-control study, the odds of vascular death among those in the aspirin experimental group would be compared to the odds of vascular death among those in the control group. This is calculated as: $OR = \dfrac{804/7783}{1016/7584}$ $\quad = \dfrac{804*7584}{7783*1016}$ $\quad = 0.77$ An OR < 1 indicates a decreased frequency of exposure in someone with the disease, an OR > 1 indicates an increased frequency of exposure in someone with the disease, while an OR = 1 indicates no changes in frequency of exposure in patients with and without the disease. For diseases that have a low prevalence and are considered "rare," OR is similar to RR. Therefore, those in the ASA group had lower odds of vascular death compared to those in the placebo group.

CASE 25 | Absolute Risk Reduction (ARR)

Explanation	Absolute risk reduction (ARR) is the number of percentage points by which actual risk decreases if an intervention is protective compared to a control. The magnitude of absolute risk reduction depends on baseline risk.
Calculation(s)	Absolute risk reduction (ARR) = (EER − CER)
Discussion	The absolute reduction in vascular deaths among those given aspirin was 11.8% − 9.4% = 2.4%. Conversely, if the study had found that aspirin was detrimental to patients and that it increased the risk of vascular death, the **attributable risk** would be relevant. The **attributable risk** is similar to ARR, but it is used for a detrimental intervention. It is the number of percentage points the actual risk goes up due to the detrimental factor. It is calculated by: **Attributable risk (AR) = (CER − EER)**

CASE 26 | Number Needed to Treat (NNT)

Explanation	The number needed to treat (NNT) is a direct measure of intervention effect. Therefore, it is considered more clinically useful. This is the number of people you need to treat in order to find one for whom the treatment worked. Lower NNT corresponds to a better treatment, with the ideal NNT being 1, meaning that everyone in the treatment group shows improvement and that no one in the control group does.
Calculation(s)	NNT = 1/ARR × 100
Discussion	The number of patients with acute myocardial infarction who needed to be treated with aspirin at 160 mg for 1 month to prevent 1 additional vascular death is (1/2.4) × 100 = 41. Therefore, in order to find 1 patient where ASA reduces vascular death, 41 patients must be treated. Conversely, if the study found that aspirin was detrimental to patients and that it increased the risk of vascular death, then the intervention effect is measured in terms of the **number needed to harm (NNH)**. The NNH is similar to NNT but for a detrimental intervention. It represents the number of people who need to be exposed to the detrimental factor to harm 1 person. It is calculated by **NNH = 1/(AR) × 100** Higher numbers generally indicate a safer exposure or treatment. All treatments have benefits and harms. The NNT and NNH are useful measures to help determine the balance of benefits vs. harms. It helps patients better understand the risks and benefits of treatment when information is presented in this manner.

STATISTICAL TESTS, ERRORS, AND VALIDITY

When conducting a research study, it is important to consider the appropriate methods of analysis, including statistical tests that address one's experimental hypothesis accurately. Most statistical tests are designed to test whether a true difference or relationship exists between two or more groups.

Examples of commonly encountered statistical tests include:

- **T-test**—The **T-test** is used to analyze the difference in means of two groups, each with continuous variables. It can be unpaired, independent samples (e.g., mean blood pressure between men and women) or paired, dependent samples (e.g., blood pressure before and after administering a new drug).
- **Analysis of variance (ANOVA)**—**ANOVA** is used to analyze the difference in means between three or more groups of continuous variables (e.g., blood glucose in type 1 diabetics, type 2 diabetics, and healthy controls).
- **Chi-square test**—**Chi-square tests** are used to analyze the difference in percentage of categorical variables in two or more groups (e.g., percentage of males and females who develop subarachnoid hemorrhage).
- **Correlation**—**Correlation** is used to compare the relationship between two continuous variables measured from the same subject (e.g., relationship between height and weight). The correlation coefficient, r, can be between -1 (negative correlation) and $+1$ (positive correlation).

Each of these statistical tests will provide an outcome that can be used to reject or fail to reject the **null hypothesis (H$_0$)**, or the hypothesis of no difference or relationship between two or more groups of data. When a difference or relationship does exist, this is referred to as the **alternative hypothesis (H$_1$)**.

Output of statistical tests can provide useful data in assessing whether there is a statistically significant relationship between two or more groups. Typical outputs of statistical tests include:

- **P-value**—The probability of obtaining results similar to your observed results given that the null hypothesis is true and there is in fact no relationship or difference. Typically, p-values < 0.05 are set to be the threshold of statistical significance. Therefore, if your statistical test gives you a p-value < 0.05, the probability of observing those same results if the null hypothesis was true would be less than 5%.
- **Confidence intervals (CIs)**—Provide a range of values likely to contain a given mean measurement of interest. The level of the CI is determined by the user but is often chosen to be 95%. A 95% CI is used to demonstrate that if the same population were sampled 100 times, the resulting output would be within this range 95 times (95%). The CI is statistically significant when it doesn't cross the **point of no difference** for a given measurement. For ratios or odds (RR, OR, etc.), the point of no difference $= 1$. For absolute measurements (ARR, AR, etc.), the point of no difference $= 0$.

As interpreting the results of clinical studies can have important consequences on the health and well-being of your patients, it is important to ensure correct results from your statistical tests. If no true difference exists, you want your statistical test to fail to reject the null hypothesis. If a true difference does exist, you want your statistical test to reject the null hypothesis. To help envision these possibilities, a common 2×2 contingency table is shown here. Statistical errors can result when the study rejects the null hypothesis despite it being true, or when the study does not reject the null hypothesis despite the alternative hypothesis being true.

	Reality Based on the Entire Population or TRUTH	
Decision based on the **study**	**There is a difference between groups.** H$_A$ or alternate hypothesis	**There is no difference between groups.** H$_0$ or null hypothesis
Reject null hypothesis **(study finds there is a difference between groups).**	**Power = (1 − β)** Alternative hypothesis is true. *Good decision*	**Type 1 error** (false positive) **(probability = α)**
Fail to reject null hypothesis **(study finds no difference between groups).**	**Type 2 error** (false negative) **(probability = β)**	Alternative hypothesis is false. (Probability = 1 − α) *Good decision*

CASE 27 | Type I Error

In a published study of 120 children, those who lived within 1 mile of the expressway had increased odds of requiring hospitalization for an asthma exacerbation in the past year when compared to those who lived over 1 mile away. However, when this odds ratio was adjusted for mold in the home, the p-value was greater than 0.05 (α level chosen for this study), so there was no difference in the number of hospitalizations for asthma between children living within a mile or greater than a mile of the expressway. If the data was not adjusted for mold in the home, the investigators would have incorrectly rejected the null hypothesis.

CASE 27 | Type I Error *(continued)*

Discussion	This is an example of a **type I error**. A type I error occurs when the null hypothesis is true, but the data in the study leads us to reject H_0. This is denoted by the symbol α which is the level of significance of a test. A result is considered statistically significant if the *p*-value is less than α, indicating that the role of chance in explaining the results of the study is less than the value of α (very small), and so the study result is likely to be true. A *p*-value that is greater than α suggests that the result is not statistically significant and that the null hypothesis is true. Typically, an α-value of 0.05 is used in scientific studies.

CASE 28 | Type II Error

A trial of 38 patients with COVID-19 is planned to compare hydroxychloroquine and remdesivir with the null hypothesis that there is no difference in reducing death from COVID-19 between the two drugs. The significance level alpha is set at 0.05, which means that they are willing to accept a 5% chance that they will reject the null hypothesis when it is true. The beta is calculated at 0.025, or 2.5%. This is the probability of committing a type II error. If remdesivir is truly more effective in reducing death rate than hydroxychloroquine and we fail to reject the null hypothesis, we have committed a type II error. When the authors do not reject the null hypothesis in the setting of a difference in death rates between hydroxychloroquine and remdesivir in COVID-19 patients, a type II error occurs. This is likely due to a small sample size, and it can also occur due to a small difference between the two groups.

Discussion	This is an example of a **type II error**. In hypothesis testing, a type II error occurs when the null hypothesis is not rejected when it should be rejected, and the alternative hypothesis is actually true (H_0 is false). This is denoted by the symbol β. When a study has a small sample size, it may not produce a significant result even if there is a true difference between the groups. Similarly, when the difference between the two group is very small, a study may not produce a significant result. These are both examples of type II errors.

CASE 29 | Power

When designing the preceding study, the investigators appropriately required a minimum of 100 children to be enrolled in the study prior to analysis. Their goal in reaching this large a sample size was to be able to correctly reject their null hypothesis if indeed it is false.

Discussion	This example demonstrates the importance of considering the **power** of a study. Power is the ability of the study to correctly reject the null hypothesis when it is incorrect. It can be determined by using the formula $(1 − β)$. By convention, the power of most studies is set at 80%, or $(1 − 20\%)$. Power of a study is increased with a larger sample size, increased expected effect size, and better precision of measurement of the data.

Even when the results of a statistical test are correct, it is still important to consider the validity of a given study, or the accuracy of the findings. Two broad types of validity are internal and external validity. **Internal validity** describes whether a study is free of bias and if its conclusions accurately reflect the actual or true relationship between the variables in the study. A study is considered internally valid if it uses appropriate techniques or methodology, if it is adequately powered to detect differences between groups, and if there are no biases. **External validity** (or **generalizability**) describes whether the results of a study can be applied to the general population. A study is considered generalizable if it has a spectrum of patients similar to the general population, if the treatment is feasible in most similar settings, and if the potential benefits of treatment should outweigh potential harms for most patients.

Validity can be thought of as **accuracy**, for example, how accurate is a study testing/measuring what it intends to test or measure; as just described, this is related to bias and generalizability. **Reliability** can be thought of as **precision**, or how often would the researchers be able to find the same results for the study. You can increase the precision in a study by decreasing the random error or by increasing the statistical power. These concepts, while similar, do not occur simultaneously. One can have a finding with both a high validity and low reliability and vice versa.

HEALTH CARE ETHICS AND LAW

It's important to understand the fundamentals of medical ethics and how to apply them in common situations. When working through these scenarios, think about the ethical principles at play in the situation at hand. If the concern is over autonomy, pick the option that allows for the most patient autonomy possible while considering their decision-making capacity.

Remember that a provider's personal beliefs should not interfere with the patient's desires. Several core ethical principles and situations, along with their legal background, are highlighted here to help guide one to the right decision. The correct decision is often the most patient-centered one.

CORE ETHICAL PRINCIPLES AND SITUATIONS

CASE 30 | Autonomy

A 42-year-old woman with heavy menstrual bleeding due to fibroids presents with fatigue, shortness of breath, and continued vaginal bleeding. She is alert and oriented to person, place, time, and the current situation. Her hemoglobin on presentation is 5.8 g/dL (baseline Hgb is 8 g/dL). It is recommended that she receive a blood transfusion. The patient is a practicing Jehovah's Witness and refuses to accept the blood transfusion.

Considerations and Next Steps	The patient should demonstrate a clear understanding of the risks of refusing treatment. It should be confirmed that she has decision-making capacity, that the decision is her own, and that she is not being influenced by others.
Clinical Decision	The patient has a right to refuse the blood transfusion. Her wishes should be respected by her treating physician, and she should not be given a blood transfusion.
Discussion	Autonomy is the obligation to respect patients as individuals and to honor their preference in accepting or refusing medical care. This patient demonstrates a desire to not accept a recommended blood transfusion based on her religious beliefs, which must be respected. This patient has decision-making capacity; if the patient lacked decision-making capacity and her wishes were not recorded, there would be no basis to deny her a blood transfusion. Furthermore, this patient is able to communicate her preferred option; she understands the information provided and potential consequences; and she provides a clear rationale behind her decision. Some Jehovah's Witnesses may carry a blood refusal card to signify desire to refuse blood transfusions. However, if they do not have this card and present in a medical emergency, the physician can give a life-saving blood transfusion. If the patient is a minor, the physician should provide life-saving treatment regardless of parental wishes.

CASE 31 | Beneficence

A 28-year-old man is brought into the emergency room unconscious after being the unrestrained driver in a motor vehicle accident. His cervical spine was stabilized in the field, and he has two large-bore IVs established. During evaluation by the trauma team, abdominal ultrasound demonstrates significant free fluid in the abdomen. Lab tests indicate a low hemoglobin. The patient is hemodynamically unstable with hypotension and tachycardia despite aggressive IV fluid resuscitation. The trauma team decides a blood transfusion is necessary.

Considerations and Next Steps	The patient is unconscious and therefore unable to communicate. The medical indications for blood transfusion are clear.
Clinical Decision	The patient should receive the blood transfusion.
Discussion	Beneficence refers to a physician's duty to act in a patient's best interest. This patient demonstrates the need for a blood transfusion, and there is no indication that he is a Jehovah's Witness. Under the principle of beneficence, this patient should receive the transfusion as it is in the best interest of saving his life.

CASE 32 | Nonmaleficence

A 45-year-old woman with a history of liver cirrhosis seeks treatment for toenail fungus. Topical agents were not effective, and the oral agent had to be discontinued because her liver function tests had worsened on treatment. She returns to the clinic, demanding a retrial of the oral agent as she had noted some improvement in her nails.

Considerations and Next Steps	The patient should be informed of the risks and benefits of the treatment and possible alternatives.
Clinical Decision	The patient should not be given the oral agent that had caused worsening of her liver function tests.

CASE 32 | Nonmaleficence (continued)

Discussion	Nonmaleficence means "do no harm" and refers to a physician's obligation to balance the risks and benefits of action in order to best treat the patient. In this case, the oral agent may improve her toenail fungus but potentially cause a much more serious problem such as liver failure. Therefore, safer alternatives, if any, should be explored with the patient.

CASE 33 | Justice

Two patients are brought into the emergency room at the same time. One is an elderly man brought in from a nursing home with an elevated temperature, low blood pressure, and concern for sepsis. The second patient is a young adult man complaining of upper respiratory symptoms with normal vital signs. There is only one provider to see patients, and the physician must decide whom to evaluate first.

Considerations and Next Steps	Obtain vital signs for each patient. Vital signs demonstrate that the elderly gentleman is more acutely sick and in need of more expedited medical treatment.
Treatment	The physician should first attend to the more unstable patient. In this case, the elderly patient should be treated first.
Discussion	Justice is the principle of treating patients fairly and equitably. This does not imply that patients will be seen at the same time. Some patients may need to wait a longer time for care if the medical condition of another patient demands the physician's attention. Both patients will receive medical care (fairness). This situation illustrates the importance of triage.

CASE 34 | Confidentiality

A 34-year-old man requests testing for sexually transmitted infections. He has had 4 female sexual partners in the last 6 months and uses condoms occasionally. He has entered a monogamous relationship with one female partner, and he states that he wants the test results to remain confidential.

Considerations and Next Steps	The patient has requested that the test results not be shared with anyone else. Confidentiality must be maintained unless there is risk of harm or death to the patient or others.
Clinical Decision	The patient should be offered testing for STIs, including HIV, gonorrhea, and chlamydia.
Discussion	In this case, the course of action depends on the results of the STI testing. If the tests are negative, then confidentiality should be maintained based on the principles of patient privacy and autonomy. If the patient tests positive for an STI, then any current or recent sexual partners must be informed so they can receive the appropriate medical testing and care. The physician should encourage the patient to initiate this communication, but under mandatory reporting laws, physicians have the legal duty to report statutorily defined reportable illnesses to public health officials regardless of the patient's actions. If the patient refuses to contact his sexual partners, public health officials will notify the people at risk, but without mentioning the patient's name. This would constitute an exception to patient confidentiality. Other exceptions to patient confidentiality can include harm to self (suicide) or others (homicide, abuse), epileptic patients, and other causes of impaired driving.

HEALTH CARE LAW

While slight variations in health care laws exist from state to state, some guiding principles are true across the nation. It is important to recognize these situations and the appropriate courses of action.

CASE 35 | Informed Consent

Prior to undergoing elective surgery for gallstones, a 26-year-old woman patient is asked to sign a document that she has been informed of the procedure and agrees to undergo the procedure.

Considerations and Next Steps	The process of obtaining informed consent requires that the procedural information be disclosed to the patient, the patient is able to understand and has decision-making capacity (the ability to reason and make decisions), and that there is no coercion or manipulation of the patient.
Clinical Decision	Informed consent must be obtained from the patient.

CASE 35 | Informed Consent *(continued)*

Discussion	Obtaining informed consent involves a discussion of the nature of the proposed treatment/procedure, reasonable alternatives to the proposed treatment, the risks/benefits of each option and of obtaining no treatment, and an evaluation of patient understanding and preference. Patients can revoke consent at any time, as long as they have maintained their decision-making capacity. Ideally, informed consent is performed by the physician who will perform the procedure, but at a minimum the provider must have in-depth understanding of the procedure and be able to answer patient questions. Informed consent can be waived by patients, if the patient lacks decision-making capacity, or in emergency situations.

CASE 36 | Consent for Minors

A 16-year-old woman is requesting contraception and testing for STIs at a routine office visit. She is consensually sexually active with one male partner who is 16 years old. She does not want her parents to be informed of her requests.

Considerations and Next Steps	Although the patient is a minor (less than 18 years old; there are exceptions), parental consent is usually not required in the context of STIs, contraception, and pregnancy.
Clinical Decision	The patient should be provided STI testing, pregnancy testing, and contraceptive information/medication without the physician informing her parents.
Discussion	A minor is any person <18 years of age. Parental consent should be obtained for most medical procedures and treatments except for issues related to sex (contraception, STIs, pregnancy), drugs (substance abuse treatment), emergency situations (life-saving treatments such as blood transfusions or emergency surgeries), or if the minor is legally emancipated from guardians. In these situations, the provider is not required to obtain parental consent and can honor the patient's wishes of confidentiality. Even when the minor's assent is not required and parents or guardians have given consent, the physician should still seek assent from the minor. In cases where a child is put in significant risk for harm due to parental refusal, physicians can obtain a court injunction or involve child protective services to proceed with life-saving medical treatment of a minor. Involvement of hospital ethics committees should be sought when there is not a clear response.

CASE 37 | Decision-Making Capacity

A 29-year-old man is brought into the emergency department after being assaulted at a bar. Paramedics state there was loss of consciousness, and the trauma team has a suspicion for an acute intracranial process. The patient wakes up and becomes combative and actively resists treatment. Urine toxicology screen is positive for amphetamines.

Considerations and Next Steps	Urine toxicology has confirmed that the patient is intoxicated, which explains his combativeness. There is a concern for an acute intracranial process, which would necessitate imaging and likely treatment. The patient does not currently have decision-making capacity as he is intoxicated, he does not appear to understand his situation, and he is in an unstable condition.
Clinical Decision	The patient should be treated for suspected intracranial injury in addition to any other injuries he has.
Discussion	Decision-making capacity refers to the real-time determination, made by health care professionals, that dictates whether or not a patient is capable of making a medical decision. Capacity is something that can change throughout a patient's care (e.g., they become unconscious, delirious, or sober). This patient should be treated on the basis that he would likely accept care if he were not intoxicated. Decision-making capacity is determined by the treating physician, and it is done in relation to a specific health care–related decision. This is different from competency which is determined by a judge and relates to whether an individual is able to make any health care–related decisions at all. A common scenario is one in which a patient has some degree of cognitive decline but is able to understand and explain back the risks and benefits of a medical procedure fully. If patients are able to do this and understand the consequences of their decision, they are considered decisional despite their cognitive decline and regardless of whether the physician agrees with the patient's choice.

CASE 38 | Advance Directives

An 82-year-old woman in the surgical ICU is in critical condition status post multiple neurosurgical procedures. She is delirious, tachypneic, tachycardic, and her blood pressure is gradually trending down. The care team is concerned that the patient is approaching cardiopulmonary arrest and must make preparations for further intervention. The patient's husband and two children are present.

Considerations and Next Steps	The care team should determine if the patient has some form of official advance directive on file. This could include a written (living will) or oral advance directive, a designated medical power of attorney (health care proxy), or documentation of a do-not-resuscitate (DNR) or do-not-intubate (DNI) order.
Clinical Decision	If there is an official advance directive on file, then this should guide any pertinent medical decisions. If there is no official advance directive available, a surrogate decision maker must be consulted.

CASE 39 | Power of Attorney/Surrogate Decision Maker

A 64-year-old man with stage 4 lung adenocarcinoma with metastasis to the brain has become unconscious and is intubated. Attempts at weaning the patient off the ventilator over subsequent days are unsuccessful, and the patient has no official advance directive on file. Numerous family members, including the patient's wife, sister, and two children, are present.

Considerations and Next Steps	The patient is unconscious and does not have an official advance directive on file; thus the patient's own preferences regarding treatment cannot be ascertained.
Clinical Decision	The patient's family must be consulted in order to decide on what treatment will be pursued. Priority of the surrogate decision maker is, from highest to lowest: spouse, adult children, parents, siblings, other relatives.
Discussion	The purpose of a surrogate decision maker is to have someone make medical decisions on behalf of the patient if the patient has become incapacitated. Decisions should be made based on what the patient would have wanted. In this case, the patient's wife is the primary decision maker, but the physician should encourage an open dialogue among the family. If the patient has no family, then a substitute may be someone who clearly knows the patient's wishes and cares about the patient.

CASE 40 | Elder Abuse

An 80-year-old woman with dementia presents to clinic for routine checkup. The patient is accompanied by her 60-year-old daughter. On exam, the patient is pleasant but only answers basic questions, which are her baseline mental status. The patient does not appear to have bathed for many days, and her clothes are dirty and smell of urine. She has lost 10 pounds since her last visit 3 months ago.

Considerations and Next Steps	The physician suspects that the patient is being neglected and is concerned that she is in an unsafe living environment. The patient is unable to provide much history due to her dementia. The patient's daughter tells the physician that they are managing fine at home and don't need any assistance.
Clinical Decision	The physician should file a report with Adult Protective Services to investigate the living situation.
Discussion	Based on the patient's physical appearance, there is concern for neglect, which is a form of elder abuse. The patient is especially vulnerable to abuse because of her inability to provide an adequate history and to relay information to the physician. Other risk factors for elder abuse include financial dependence, caretaker perception of the elderly patient as a burden, and caretaker substance abuse. Potential signs to look out for include poor hygiene, injuries (fractures, lacerations, burns, etc.) without appropriate or consistent explanations, or changes in behavior especially when the caretaker is in the room vs. outside the room. While detailed laws vary state by state within the United States, physicians should generally report suspected elder abuse to the appropriate government agency for follow-up investigation. If the patient is in immediate danger, they should be admitted to the hospital.

CASE 41 | Child Abuse

A 3-year-old boy is brought into the emergency room for a broken arm. The mother and father tell different stories about how the injury happened. On exam, the physician notices various bruises on the boy's body.

Considerations and Next Steps	The inconsistencies in the parents' stories, as well as the bruising on the boy's body, are concerns for child abuse.

CASE 41 | Child Abuse (continued)

Clinical Decision	Child Protective Services (CPS) should be contacted to ensure that the child is in a safe environment at home.
Discussion	Child abuse is unfortunately common. The most common form of child maltreatment is neglect, or failure of a parent or guardian to provide a child with adequate food, shelter, supervision, education, and/or affection. Physical abuse can be seen at any age, but it occurs more frequently in young children. Child abuse should be suspected in cases where the history does not match the physical findings or in children with repeated hospitalizations. In infants, abuse may present as failure to thrive, irritability, somnolence, seizures, or apnea. Children may exhibit poor hygiene or behavioral abnormalities. On exam, look for bruises in different stages of healing, immersion burns (buttock or stocking glove distribution without splash marks), or spiral fractures. Noncontrast CT may show subdural hematomas, while MRI can visualize white matter changes associated with violent shaking. Ophthalmologic exams are useful to examine for retinal hemorrhages. Parent or guardian stories are often inconsistent with the type of injury sustained by the child and are delayed from the time of injury. Sexual abuse involves genital, anal, or oral trauma, and victims may present with sexually transmitted or urinary tract infections. This occurs more frequently in children ages 9–12 years old. Sexual abuse should be suspected if a child has genital trauma, bleeding/discharge, or an excessive preoccupation or knowledge of adult sexual behaviors. If sexual abuse is suspected, testing for gonorrhea, syphilis, chlamydia, and HIV is warranted. Physicians are required by law to report any and all reasonable suspicions of child abuse or endangerment. Even if the physician is wrong in his or her assumptions, child protective services must be contacted to open a formal investigation into the child's safety. The child abuse reporting system for doctors is designed to be *sensitive*, not *specific*, which means that it is acceptable if some false positive reports are filed. It is very important to consider child abuse in the differential diagnosis when a child presents with an injury and to report any suspected cases.

CASE 42 | Intimate Partner Violence/Domestic Violence

A 45-year-old woman presents to a physician in the primary care setting after a head injury. She tells the physician that her husband threw a plate at her head and that he has been physically and verbally abusive to her for many years.

Considerations and Next Steps	The patient is describing a situation of domestic abuse. The physician listens to the patient's story and confirms that at this time she is safe while her husband is traveling for work and she is staying with a relative.
Clinical Decision	The physician should not pressure the patient to leave her partner. The physician is not legally obligated to report the incident to authorities.
Discussion	Intimate partner violence is an unfortunately common occurrence. Risk is highest in younger females, including pregnant women. Injuries (fractures, lacerations, burns, etc.) typically lack appropriate or consistent explanations; they may be repetitive in nature; or they may present with signs of both acute and chronic injury. Other signs include changes in behavior, especially when the partner is in the room vs. outside the room. Signs to look out for in a potential abuser include refusal to leave the patient alone with a provider or let the patient answer provider questions. Physicians are not required by federal law to report incidents of domestic violence. The physician should support the patient, ensure the patient's safety, and provide resources the patient may need such as contact information for a social worker, a domestic abuse hotline number, etc. This should also include discussion of an emergency plan of what the patient can do in the event of an emergency.

7

Cardiovascular

Noreen T. Nazir, MD
Amer K. Ardati, MD
George T. Kondos, MD
Jonathan D. Meyer, MD

CHEST PAIN—CARDIAC

Chest pain is a common and important presenting symptom with a broad range of cardiac and noncardiac causes. Chest pain can be caused by cardiac, pulmonary, gastrointestinal, musculoskeletal, psychiatric conditions or drugs. Associated symptoms are usually helpful in determining the cause, and the scope can often be narrowed to just a few diagnoses by history alone. A focused physical exam helps further narrow the differential diagnosis.

Differential Diagnosis for Chest Pain

Cardiac	Pulmonary	Gastrointestinal	Other
Angina (stable and unstable) Myocardial infarction (MI) Pericarditis Heart failure (HF) Myocarditis Vasospasm Aortic dissection Valvular heart disease (e.g., MVP, aortic stenosis) Arrhythmia	Pneumothorax Pulmonary embolus (PE) Pleuritis Pneumonia/bronchitis Chronic obstructive pulmonary disease (COPD) Asthma	Gastro-esophageal reflux (GERD) Esophageal spasm Boerhaave syndrome Peptic ulcer disease (PUD) Gastritis Pancreatitis Cholecystitis Mallory-Weiss syndrome	Panic attack Takayasu arteritis Acute chest syndrome (sickle cell disease) Trauma Breast disorders Referred pain
Musculoskeletal (MSK)	**Skin**	**Malignancy**	**Drugs**
Costochondritis Tietze syndrome Muscle strain	Herpes zoster (Varicella zoster virus)	Lymphoma Thymoma Lung cancer Breast cancer	Cocaine Amphetamines Sumatriptan Ergot alkaloids

Key History Findings and Chest Pain Differential Diagnosis
(see "Chest Pain—Pulmonary" in "Respiratory" chapter for additional details)

Chest Pain with Key Associated History Findings	Diagnoses
Associated with SOB	Consider cardiac or pulmonary causes
Sudden onset, nonexertional chest pain	MI, vasospasm, unstable angina, pneumothorax, PE
Exertional pressure or pain Radiation to neck and/or left shoulder/arm Relieved with rest or nitrates	Angina
Tearing chest pain, radiation to back	Aortic dissection
Pain relieved sitting and leaning forward Worse lying down	Pericarditis
Fever	Pericarditis, myocarditis, pneumonia, pleuritis
Worse after meals Sour taste in mouth, hoarseness Worse when lying down at night Improved with PPI/H2-blockers or antacids	Consider GI causes (GERD, PUD, gastritis)
Radiation to the shoulder or trapezius ridge	Diaphragmatic irritation (e.g., due to cholecystitis, pneumonia/effusion)
Associated with wheezing	Asthma/COPD, HF
Associated with hemoptysis	PE, pneumonia, bronchitis, cancer
Worse with deep inspiration (pleuritic pain)	PE, pericarditis, pleuritis, pneumonia
Acute pain after prolonged immobilization On estrogen (e.g., oral contraceptive pills)	PE
Chest pain, dyspnea after violent vomiting	Boerhaave syndrome, Mallory Weiss syndrome
Chest pain, ~2 weeks after viral infection associated with dilated cardiomyopathy	Myocarditis

(continued)

Key History Findings and Chest Pain Differential Diagnosis
(see "Chest Pain—Pulmonary" in "Respiratory" chapter for additional details) (*continued*)

Chest Pain with Key Associated History Findings	Diagnoses
Improved with NSAIDS	MSK causes, pericarditis
History of anxiety or panic attacks	Anxiety, panic attack
Woman with atypical symptoms ("burning" sensation in chest, dyspnea, sweating, vomiting, fatigue, lightheadedness, or panicky feelings)	Angina or MI, coronary vasospasm or mitral valve prolapse
Young adult without cardiovascular risk factors presenting with intermittent nonexertional chest pain, anxiety, and palpitations	Mitral valve prolapse, panic attacks
Children, adolescents, and young adults	Consider: Kawasaki syndrome, vasospastic angina due to cocaine, congenital heart disease, premature coronary artery disease due to familial hyperlipidemia, bicuspid aortic valve, or anomalous coronary arteries
Young adult with Marfan's and chest pain	Aortic dissection, spontaneous pneumothorax
Shoulder pain with radiation to ipsilateral ulnar nerve distribution	Pancoast tumor
Sickle cell and chest pain	Acute chest syndrome

Key Physical Exam Findings and Chest Pain Differential Diagnosis
(see "Chest Pain—Pulmonary" in "Respiratory" chapter for additional details)

Chest Pain with Key Associated Exam Findings	Diagnoses
Acute distress that is positional (worse lying back)	Pericarditis
Pulse and BP discrepancy in upper extremities Crescendo-decrescendo (diamond-shape) murmur radiating to carotids Weak and delayed pulse (pulsus parvus et tardus)	Aortic dissection
Coarse rales	Pulmonary edema
Elevated JVP (>7–8 cm or 3 cm above the sternal angle)	Right-sided heart failure (due to left-sided failure or pulmonary hypertension), constriction, restrictive cardiomyopathy, or tamponade
S3	Severe left ventricular systolic dysfunction due to acute MI with decompensated heart failure
S4	Underlying ventricular hypertrophy (due to chronic hypertension or hypertrophic cardiomyopathy)
Decrease systolic BP with inspiration (pulsus paradoxus)	Cardiac tamponade, COPD, or pneumothorax
Alternating ECG amplitude between beats (electrical alternans)	Pericardial effusion
Asymmetric absent breath sounds	Pneumothorax or pleural effusion
Tympany upon percussion of chest wall	Pneumothorax
Dullness to percussion of chest wall	Pleural effusion
Focal abnormal lung sounds (bronchophony, egophony)	Pneumonia or lung cancer
Wheezing	Asthma, COPD, or HF
Epigastric tenderness	GI causes: GERD, pancreatitis, or PUD
Reproducible Chest wall tenderness	MSK or costochondritis
Rash in dermatomal distribution	Herpes zoster

The history and focused physical exam are the foundation of developing concise and pragmatic differential diagnoses. Diagnostic testing and trials of therapeutic interventions can help refine, refute, and confirm the ultimate diagnosis. Selective use of the following tests and interventions are often helpful:

- *Labs*: Cardiac biomarkers (troponin, high sensitivity troponin), BNP, D-dimer, ABG
- *Studies*: Pulse oximetry, electrocardiogram (ECG), chest X-ray, chest CT, echocardiogram
- *Interventions*: Nitroglycerin, antacids, bronchodilators, diuretics

	Acute Coronary Syndrome (ACS)			
	Stable Angina	**Unstable Angina**	**NSTEMI**	**STEMI**
ECG	Normal (NL)	NL, ST depression or T wave inversions	NL, ST depression or T wave inversions	ST elevations
Cardiac biomarkers	NL	NL	Elevated	Elevated
Pathophysiology	Stable plaque, but vessel not able to dilate adequately to meet demand	Plaque rupture, thrombus causing new partial occlusion (no infarct)	Plaque rupture, thrombus causing subendocardial infarct	Plaque rupture, thrombus causing transmural infarct
Typical presentation	Stable, predictable symptoms; relieved with rest	New angina, occurs at rest, or change in stable symptoms	Sudden, persistent chest pain	Sudden, persistent chest pain

CASE 1 | Stable Angina

A 65-year-old man with a history of hypertension, type 2 diabetes, hyperlipidemia, and tobacco use presents with intermittent chest pain for the past 2 months. He describes it as a squeezing pressure sensation in his left parasternal to midclavicular area with radiation down his left arm that is associated with mild shortness of breath. The symptoms occur each time he climbs more than two flights of stairs, and it improves after he rests for a few minutes. His vital signs as well as his cardiovascular, pulmonary, and abdominal exams are normal. There is no reproducible chest wall tenderness or lower extremity edema.

Evaluation/Tests	Clinical diagnosis. If ordered, exercise ECG would show ≥1 mm ST depression in more than one contiguous lead. A stress echo would show induced regional wall motion abnormalities consistent with ischemia.
Treatment	Treat with aspirin, statin, and anti-anginal medications (beta blockers, calcium channel blockers, and/or nitroglycerin). Optimize risk factors (i.e., diabetes, hypertension) and encourage lifestyle modifications (i.e., diet, exercise, smoking cessation). Patients that have persistent symptoms despite optimal medical therapy can safely be offered revascularization.
Discussion	Stable angina typically occurs when there is an obstructive atherosclerotic lesion in the coronary arteries that is over 70% occlusive. Cardiac risk factors include age (male patients >45, female patients >55), male sex, HTN, DM, dyslipidemia, family history of premature coronary artery disease (CAD) (males <55, females <65), smoking, and abdominal obesity. At times, the chest pain is described as a discomfort or pressure sensation rather than pain. Additional symptoms can include dyspnea, nausea, diaphoresis, lightheadedness, dizziness, and easy fatigability. Typical angina is provoked by exertion and relieved with rest or nitroglycerin. Physical exam findings are often normal. If a patient has atypical or vague symptoms, an exercise test stress test can confirm the diagnosis.
	The relatively short duration of pain and association with exertion makes **acute coronary syndrome (ACS)** (unstable angina, NSTEMI, and STEMI) less likely. New onset angina, chest pain at rest, or change in previous predictable angina in a patient with known CAD or cardiac risk factors are characteristic features of ACS. Physical exam findings are often normal.
	Unstable angina (UA) occurs secondary to coronary atherosclerosis plaque rupture and subsequent thrombus formation, without complete occlusion of the coronary artery. The pain associated with UA tends to be more severe and typically lasts for 15 minutes or more. Patients with UA should be hospitalized on a telemetry unit to be stabilized, monitored for arrhythmias, and initiated on a protocol to rule out an MI, which includes checking serial ECGs and cardiac biomarkers. ECG may show ST depression and T wave inversions, and cardiac biomarkers would be normal. Once stabilized and asymptomatic, the patient may either undergo stress testing or proceed to coronary angiogram if there is high risk of ischemia.

CASE 1 | Stable Angina *(continued)*

Additional Considerations	**Vasospastic (aka variant or prinzmetal) angina** is a condition in which chest pain results from transient vasospasm in the coronary arteries, limiting blood flow and causing transient ischemia. The chest pain typically occurs at rest and may be triggered by drugs or substances such as triptans (e.g., sumatriptan), cocaine, cannabis, ephedrine-based products, or alcohol. It is a diagnosis of exclusion, and it is important to rule out a fixed obstructive coronary artery lesion.

CASE 2 | Acute Coronary Syndrome (ACS): STEMI (ST-Segment Elevation Myocardial Infarction)

A 65-year-old man with a history of hypertension, diabetes, and hyperlipidemia presents with severe chest pain and shortness of breath for 1 hour. His symptoms began when he woke up in the morning and have been increasing in severity. The pain radiates down his left arm, and he feels light-headed, dizzy, and nauseous. On exam, he appears anxious, distressed, and diaphoretic. Vitals signs are temperature is 99.3°F, pulse is 110/min, blood pressure is 150/76 mmHg, respirations are 24/min, pulse ox is 98% RA. Blood pressure and pulse are equal in both arms. Cardiovascular exam is notable for an S4 heart sound. Pulmonary and abdominal exams are normal, and there is no reproducible chest wall tenderness or lower extremity edema.

Evaluation/Tests	ECG shows ST segment elevations in two or more contiguous leads along with reciprocal ST segment depressions. Troponin levels are elevated (may not be present until 6 hours after symptom onset). CBC, BMP, and CXR are all normal. 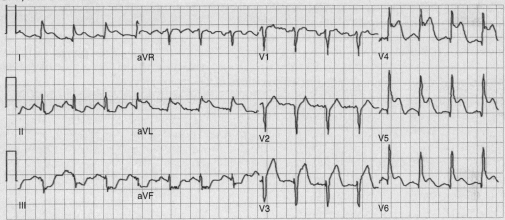 ECG shows ST-segment elevation in the precordial leads, as well as I and aVL, indicative of acute anterolateral STEMI due to proximal left anterior descending (LAD) coronary artery occlusion. Note the reciprocal ST depression in the inferior leads.
Treatment	Cardiac catheterization and primary percutaneous coronary intervention (PCI). If PCI is not available, treat with thrombolytics. Also administer platelet inhibitors (aspirin, clopidogrel), anticoagulation, and nitroglycerin, and/or morphine.
Discussion	**ACS: STEMI** (ST-segment elevation myocardial infarction), is a transmural infarct. The patient has significant cardiac risk factors, characteristic chest pain, ECG changes showing ST elevations in two contiguous leads, and there are elevations in cardiac biomarkers. The typical findings for transmural or full thickness myocardial wall infarcts are ST elevations. Q waves may also develop as the infarct evolves. Cardiac biomarker positivity lags symptoms by hours. **ACS: NSTEMI (non-ST-segment elevation myocardial infarction) or NSTE ACS (non-ST-segment elevation acute coronary syndrome)** will present similarly, and cardiac biomarkers will be elevated, but ECG will not show ST elevations. During an NSTEMI, the subendocardium (inner 1/3 of myocardium) is especially vulnerable to ischemia. When infarcts occur in this area, the typical ECG may show ST segment depression, T wave inversions, or may be normal. **Unstable angina** may present similarly to myocardial infarction but has no elevation in cardiac biomarkers.
Additional Considerations	**Complications of myocardial infarction (MI):** MIs are most often caused by coronary artery atherosclerotic plaque rupture, and complications include death, arrhythmias, heart failure, ventricular septal rupture, free wall rupture, aneurysm, or pseudoaneurysm formation, mitral regurgitation due to papillary muscle rupture, fibrinous pericarditis, and Dressler syndrome. Risk factors for developing complications include no reperfusion or delayed presentation. **Free wall rupture** can result in either pseudoaneurysm or cardiac tamponade.

CASE 2 | Acute Coronary Syndrome (ACS): STEMI (ST-Segment Elevation Myocardial Infarction) *(continued)*

Additional Considerations	A **pseudoaneurysm** occurs when the ventricular free wall rupture is contained by the pericardium and presents with recurrence of chest pain and tachycardia. CXR would show an enlarged cardiac silhouette with a bulge at the left heart border. The murmur may be continuous or only systolic, mimicking the murmur of mitral regurgitation. Occasionally, there may be no murmur. The distinction between a true LV aneurysm (caused by thinning of the scarred myocardium) and pseudoaneurysm is important due to the lower likelihood of rupture from a true LV aneurysm. If the rupture is not contained, rapid blood accumulation in the pericardial space results in **cardiac tamponade** with hypotension, pulsus paradoxus, jugular venous distension, and shock. If the rupture from an infarcted myocardium happens at the ventricular septum, an **acquired ventricular septal defect** can occur. This results in a left-to-right shunt and associated murmur (holo- or pansystolic murmur is best heard at the sternal border on physical exam). Patients present with right and left ventricular failure from volume overload created by the shunt. **Systolic heart failure** is related to the size of infarction and is typically associated with a proximal left anterior descending artery occlusion. Patients present either early or late after infarction with typical signs and symptoms of congestive heart failure. **Dressler syndrome** is acute pericarditis following a transmural MI and is thought to be an autoimmune phenomenon resulting in fibrinous pericarditis. It typically occurs a few weeks after MI or heart surgery.

CASE 3 | Acute Pericarditis

A 27-year-old woman presents with chest pain for the past 3 days. The pain is sharp and worsens with deep breaths and when lying flat and improves by sitting and leaning forward. One week ago, she had flu-like symptoms. On exam, she is in mild distress, but her vital signs and pulse oximetry are normal. Cardiac exam is notable for a left substernal three-component friction rub that is louder in the left sternal border. She has no reproducible chest wall tenderness or lower extremity edema, and the rest of her exam is unremarkable.

Evaluation/Tests	ECG shows nonterritorial ST elevation (concave up) without the presence of reciprocal changes and diffuse PR depression. 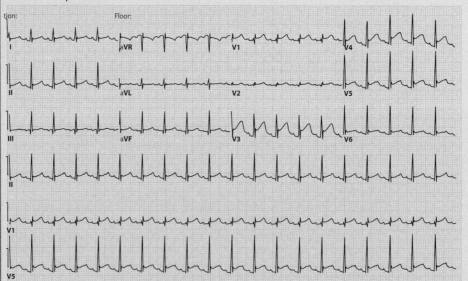 Reproduced with permission from Jameson J, Fauci AS, Kasper DL, et al: Harrison's Principles of Internal Medicine, 20th ed. New York, NY: McGraw Hill; 2018.
Treatment	Treat underlying cause and use NSAIDS to reduce pain and inflammation. Colchicine also has been shown to reduce symptoms and recurrence.
Discussion	This clinical presentation is consistent with pericarditis, which is inflammation of the pericardial sac surrounding the heart. The pleuritic pain is often described as improving with sitting and leaning forward and worsening with lying flat or taking a deep breath. The most common cause is idiopathic (presumed viral). Other causes include post-MI (such as Dressler syndrome), postoperative (after open-heart surgery), aortic dissection, systemic lupus erythematosus, rheumatoid arthritis, tuberculosis (TB), uremia, drugs, cancers, and radiation therapy. Diagnosis is made by the characteristic ECG findings just noted. Chest X-ray is helpful to rule out other causes. White blood cell count and inflammatory markers such as

CASE 3 | Acute Pericarditis *(continued)*

Discussion	CRP and ESR can be elevated. Cardiac biomarkers are usually normal but may be mildly elevated in cases with concomitant myocarditis. Echocardiogram may show pericardial effusion or thickening but is not required to make the diagnosis. Patients with **pleuritis** or **pleurisy** may present with chest pain that is worse with deep inspiration and improved with NSAIDS. Causes of pleurisy include infections, pulmonary embolus, ACS, collagen vascular diseases, or medications. Inflammation of the pleura may cause a friction rub, but the ECG would be normal.

CASE 4 | Aortic Dissection

A 36-year-old man with a history of dislocated lens as a child presents with chest pain over the past 6 hours. The chest pain is substernal, severe, and tearing in quality with radiation to his back. He feels short of breath and lightheaded. He was involved in a motor vehicle accident earlier in the day. On exam, he is afebrile and tachycardic, and his oxygen saturation is 93% on room air. Blood pressure is 200/100 mmHg in his right arm and 150/90 mmHg in his left arm. He is tall, thin, and in moderate distress. His chest is sunken in (pectus excavatum), and he has a decrescendo diastolic murmur in the aortic area that is loudest at the lower left sternal border (aortic regurgitation).

Evaluation/Tests	Chest CT scan with contrast shows a false lumen caused by an intimal tear (indicated by red arrow). Used with permission from Dr. James Heilman/Wikimedia Commons.
Treatment	Emergent surgery may be indicated, especially with an ascending aortic dissection.
Discussion	This presentation is most concerning for acute aortic dissection in a patient with **Marfan syndrome**. Aortic dissections are associated with rapid-deceleration chest trauma, aortic aneurysms, connective tissue disorders, Marfan syndrome, and cocaine use. Blood pressure disparity of 20 mmHg or greater between the arms occurs when the false lumen that forms prevents appropriate blood flow to one arm. A widened mediastinum on chest X-ray or CT scan or aortic wall tear on transesophageal echocardiogram or MR angiogram would confirm the diagnosis. Ascending aortic dissections (Stanford A) can cause aortic regurgitation, myocardial infarction, or tamponade. For Stanford B (below ligamentum arteriosum), initial medical management is reasonable though surgery may be required with end-organ malperfusion. Patients with Marfan syndrome can present with a **pneumothorax**. Patients with pneumothorax would have diminished breath sounds in the affected lung and no blood pressure disparities in the arms.

DYSPNEA—CARDIAC

Dyspnea is more commonly known as a subjective feeling of shortness of breath. It can be a normal sensation after heavy exercise, but it becomes abnormal when it is associated with mild exertion or at rest. It usually stems from an abnormality in ventilation or oxygenation and is commonly due to cardiac, pulmonary, or hematologic conditions.

Differential Diagnosis for Dyspnea (see "Respiratory" chapter for additional etiologies)

Cardiovascular	Pulmonary	Rheumatologic	Musculoskeletal

<u>Pump problems</u>
Heart Failure (HF)
  Heart failure with reduced ejection fraction (HFrEF)
  Heart failure with preserved ejection fraction (HFpEF)
  Cor pulmonale
	COPD/Emphysema
	Asthma
	Bronchitis
	Bronchiectasis
	Aspiration
	Pneumothorax
	Obstructive sleep apnea (OSA)
		Rheumatic heart disease
		<u>Vasculitides</u>
		  Granulomatous Polyangiitis (GPA)
		  Eosinophilic granulomatosis with polyangiitis (EGPA)
			Rib fracture
			Muscle strain
			Muscular dystrophies
			Poliomyelitis
			Scoliosis
			Kyphosis

(continued)

Dyspnea Differential Diagnoses (see "Respiratory" chapter for additional etiologies) (*continued*)

Cardiovascular	Pulmonary	Neurologic	Hematology

Cardiovascular
Cardiomyopathy (CM)
  Ischemic CM, nonischemic
  CM, dilated CM, hypertrophic
  obstructive CM (HCM), restrictive/
  infiltrative CM
  Myocarditis (dilated CM)
Ischemia
  Angina
  ACS
Pericardium
  Pericardial effusion
  Cardiac tamponade
  Pericarditis
Valvular
  Aortic stenosis
  Mitral stenosis
  Mitral regurgitation (MR)
Aortic
  Aortic dissection
Rhythm
  Arrhythmias (e.g., atrial fibrillation)
Congenital Heart Disease (e.g., ASD, VSD)
	Pulmonary
	Pneumonia
	Atelectasis
	Acute respiratory Distress
	syndrome (ARDS)
	Neonatal respiratory Distress
	syndrome (NRDS)
	Pleural effusion
	Interstitial lung disease (ILD)
	Lung cancer
	Cystic fibrosis
	
	Pulmonary-Vascular
	Pulmonary hypertension
	Pulmonary embolus
	Hereditary hemorrhagic
	telangiectasia
	Alveolar hemorrhage
	Vasculitides
		Neurologic
		Central sleep apnea
		Neuromuscular weakness
		(ALS, myasthenia gravis)
		Phrenic nerve palsy
		
		Gastrointestinal
		Gastrointestinal bleeding
		Ascites
		
		Endocrine
		Hypothyroidism
		Hyperthyroidism
		Carcinoid syndrome
			Hematology
			Anemia
			Leukemia
			Methemoglobinemia
			Acute chest syndrome
			(sickle cell disease)
			
			Miscellaneous
			Sarcoidosis
			Obesity hypoventilation
			Pregnancy
			Panic attack/anxiety
			Altitude sickness
			Inhalation injuries
			
			Drugs
			(e.g., daptomycin,
			cocaine)

The chronicity, quality of symptoms, triggers, environmental and occupational exposures, and important associated symptoms such as cough, chest pain, wheezing or stridor, fevers or edema will help narrow down the DDx. Important cardiac-related information includes previous history of congenital heart problems, coronary artery disease, hypertension, dyspnea on exertion, or symptoms of orthopnea or paroxysmal nocturnal dyspnea (PND). Focused pulmonary and cardiac exam in addition to assessment for edema and weakness will help further narrow the DDx. For instance, physical exam findings pointing toward heart failure or volume overload include elevated (>8 cm) jugular venous pressure (JVP), murmurs or abnormal heart sounds (S3 suggestive of advanced systolic left-sided heart failure, S4 hypertensive heart disease, loud P2—pulmonary hypertension, fixed split S2–ASD), or displaced point of maximal impulse (PMI), bibasilar crackles on lung exam or dullness to percussion (pleural effusion), ascites, and bilateral lower extremity edema. Initial useful labs and tests include assessing oxygen saturation (SPO$_2$) with pulse oximetry, CBC to check for anemia, basic metabolic panel (BMP), and TSH to check for hyper- or hypothyroidism. Arterial blood gas (ABG) can quantify the oxygenation of the blood and can indicate respiratory acidosis. Cardiac biomarkers, brain (B-type) natriuretic peptide (BNP), and D-dimer can also be useful in assessing for ischemia, heart failure, and pulmonary embolus, respectively. Imaging can show parenchymal pulmonary and cardiac abnormalities. Other testing may include chest X-ray, CT scan, ECG, and echocardiography. Pulmonary-focused testing may also be warranted (refer to "Respiratory" chapter). For example, pulmonary function tests can identify obstructive or restrictive lung disease.

Key History Findings and Dyspnea Differential Diagnosis
(see "Dyspnea—Pulmonary Causes" in "Respiratory" chapter for more details)

Dyspnea with Key Associated History Findings	Diagnoses
Acute onset	Pneumothorax, pulmonary embolus (PE), MI, flash pulmonary edema due to MI, HF, or mitral regurgitation (MR)
Dyspnea with exertion, relieved with rest	Angina
Chest pain or pressure	Acute coronary syndrome, PE, pneumothorax
Palpitations	Arrhythmias
Swelling or fluid retention	Heart failure, ascites (liver disease), nephropathy
Nocturnal or early morning dyspnea	Asthma, heart failure (HF)

(continued)

Key History Findings and Dyspnea Differential Diagnosis
(see "Dyspnea—Pulmonary Causes" in "Respiratory" chapter for more details) (*continued*)

Dyspnea with Key Associated History Findings	Diagnoses
Orthopnea, paroxysmal nocturnal dyspnea, lower extremity edema	Heart failure, pericardial effusion with or without cardiac tamponade, constrictive pericarditis
Smoking history	COPD, lung cancer, MI
Cough with purulent sputum	Pneumonia, cystic fibrosis, chronic bronchitis
Occupational exposure (coal miner, metal worker, sand blaster, construction or shipping)	Pneumoconiosis
Birdkeeper or farmer	Hypersensitivity pneumonitis
History of bleeding	Anemia

Key Physical Exam Findings and Dyspnea Differential Diagnosis
(see "Dyspnea—Pulmonary Causes" in "Respiratory" chapter for more details)

Dyspnea with Key Associated Exam Findings	Diagnoses
Pale conjunctiva	Anemia
Clubbing	Chronic hypoxia
Obesity, large neck	OSA or obesity hypoventilation syndrome
Stridor	Foreign body aspiration, epiglottitis, or angioedema
Wheezes	Asthma, COPD, or HF
Diffuse expiratory and inspiratory wheezing	Asthma
Irregular heartbeat	Arrhythmias
Decrease breath sounds and dullness to percussion (*usually unilateral*)	Pleural effusion
Bilateral: hyperresonant to percussion and decreased breath sounds, wheezing	COPD
Absent breath sounds on affected side, tracheal deviation away from affected side	Tension pneumothorax
Asymmetric chest expansion, diminished breath sounds, inspiratory crackles, bronchophony, egophony, increased tactile fremitus, dullness to percussion, whispered pectoriloquy on affected side	Pneumonia or pleural effusion
Inspiratory crackles bilaterally, clubbing	Pulmonary fibrosis
Bilateral inspiratory crackles	Pulmonary edema
Elevated jugular venous pressure (JVP) or jugular venous distension (JVD), hepatojugular reflex, displaced apical impulse, S3, lung crackles, lower extremity edema	Heart failure (HF)
Muffled heart sounds	Pericardial Effusion
Hypotension, muffled heart sounds, elevated JVP (Beck's triad)	Cardiac tamponade
Elevated JVP (normal X and rapid Y descent), Kussmaul's sign, pulsus paradoxus, pericardial knock, friction rub, ascites, hepatomegaly, peripheral edema	Constrictive pericarditis
Crescendo-decrescendo systolic murmur heard best in the aortic area radiating to the carotids and left ventricular apex.	Aortic stenosis
Loud S1 with opening snap (sound), low pitched diastolic rumble with presystolic accentuation heard best in the left ventricular apical area	Mitral stenosis
Holosystolic murmur heard best at the apex in the left lateral decubitus position radiating to the axilla	Mitral regurgitation
Lung crackles and new holosystolic murmur heard best at apex	Flash pulmonary edema from mitral chordae rupture
Muscular weakness	Neuromuscular disorder (e.g., ALS, myasthenia gravis)

CASE 5 | Heart Failure with Reduced Ejection Fraction (HFrEF), Ischemic

A 68-year-old man with a history of coronary artery disease with 3 vessel CABG and hypertension presents with worsening cough, fatigue, and shortness of breath for the past 2 weeks. He denies chest pain but notes mild leg swelling. He recently started sleeping on 4 pillows instead of 2 (orthopnea) and gasps for breath when trying to sleep (PND). On exam, his vital signs are as follows: temperature 37.0°C, pulse is 80/min, blood pressure is 100/60 mmHg, respirations are 22/min, and SpO_2 is 90% on RA. He has an elevated JVP (>8 cm), a laterally displaced cardiac left ventricular impulse, an S3, bibasilar crackles, hepatomegaly with a positive hepatojugular reflex, and bilateral pitting edema of his legs.

Evaluation/Tests	Transthoracic echocardiogram (TTE) shows a reduced left ventricular ejection fraction of 40% (normal range 55–65%). CBC, BMP, TSH, and urinalysis (UA) are all normal. BNP is elevated, and CXR shows an enlarged cardiac silhouette, interstitial edema, cephalization, and Kerley B lines (consistent with pulmonary edema).
Treatment	Medications to treat HFrEF include loop diuretics, ACE-inhibitor, ARB, ARB with neprilysin inhibitor (ARNI), beta blocker (BB), spironolactone, and/or hydralazine/nitrates.
Discussion	This presentation and echocardiogram results are consistent with acute decompensated heart failure secondary to reduced ejection fraction (HFrEF). Usual symptoms of HFrEF include shortness of breath, dyspnea on exertion, fatigue, orthopnea, paroxysmal nocturnal dyspnea (PND), weight gain, hepatomegaly, and lower extremity swelling. The most common cause of HFrEF is ischemic cardiomyopathy. Blunting of the pathologic neurohormonal response to heart failure is the cornerstone of contemporary therapy. Treatment is tailored at achieving euvolemia, improving/maintaining systolic function, slowing progression of atherosclerosis, and preventing cardiac arrhythmias. Aggressive evaluation and control of cardiac disease risk factors and underlying cardiac disease are imperative. The combination of S3 and crackles makes pneumonia, liver failure, and nephrotic syndrome unlikely.

CASE 6 | Heart Failure with Reduced Ejection Fraction, Nonischemic

A 46-year-old woman with chronic alcohol abuse presents with dyspnea on exertion for 3 weeks. She notes associated lightheadedness and intermittent leg swelling but denies chest pain. She does not have any other cardiac risk factors. On exam, she is thin, and her vital signs are as follows: temperature is 37°C, pulse is 108/minute, blood pressure is 94/58 mm/Hg, respirations are 14/minute, and SpO_2 is 93% on RA. She has an elevated JVP, laterally displaced PMI, a 2/6 holosystolic murmur best heard at apex (mitral regurgitation), bibasilar crackles, and bilateral 1+ pitting edema to mid-shins.

Evaluation/Tests	Transthoracic echocardiogram (TTE) shows reduced ejection fraction with an enlarged left ventricle. CBC, BMP, TSH, UA, and troponin levels are normal. BNP is elevated, and CXR shows an enlarged cardiac silhouette and pulmonary edema.
Treatment	Advise alcohol cessation. Medications to treat HFrEF include loop diuretics, ACE-inhibitor/ARB or ARNI, beta blocker, spironolactone, and/or hydralazine/nitrates.
Discussion	This presentation is consistent with **HFrEF secondary to chronic alcohol use**. Presentation can range from insidious and slowly progressing to sudden onset and immediately life-threatening. Depending on severity, patients may present with a new mitral regurgitation murmur caused by severe dilation of the left ventricle (termed functional mitral regurgitation). If the offending agent is identified and removed, certain cardiomyopathies can be reversed. While this patient's etiology is from alcohol abuse, other causes of HFrEF include hereditary disorders or acquired conditions such as ischemia, thyroid disease, peripartum cardiomyopathy, thiamine deficiency, Chagas disease, anthracycline toxicity (e.g., doxorubicin), autoimmune disorders, myocarditis, or infiltrative processes such as hemochromatosis (which can present either as HFrEF or as restrictive cardiomyopathy).

CASE 7 | Heart Failure with Preserved Ejection Fraction (HFpEF)

A 73-year-old man being followed for monoclonal gammopathy of unknown significance (MGUS) presents with dyspnea on exertion and leg swelling for 8 days. He denies chest pain but endorses paroxysmal nocturnal dyspnea. He also reports pain and tingling in his hands, specifically in the first 2 digits. His wife notes that his tongue seems to be enlarged. Physical exam is significant for an elevated JVP that increases with inspiration, an S4 loudest at the left lower sternal border, bilateral bibasilar crackles in the lower lung fields, hepatomegaly, and 2+ pitting edema.

Evaluation/Tests	Transthoracic echocardiogram (TTE) shows impaired filling (diastolic dysfunction) and normal ejection fraction (EF). BNP is elevated, and CXR shows pulmonary edema. ECG shows low voltage. Fat pad or cardiac biopsy shows apple green birefringence with Congo red staining (pale pink deposits).

CASE 7 | Heart Failure with Preserved Ejection Fraction (HFpEF) *(continued)*

Treatment	Volume overload can be managed with loop diuretics. Unlike, HFrEF, this condition does not respond to beta blockers or renin angiotensin antagonists. Advanced heart failure therapies such as transplant or left-ventricular assist devices can be considered in select patients.
Discussion	This presentation is consistent with **HFpEF secondary to amyloid**. This type of cardiomyopathy is broken into two categories: restrictive and infiltrative. **Restrictive** factors affect myocardial relaxation and include postradiation fibrosis, endocardial fibroelastosis, and Loffler endocarditis. **Infiltrative** factors deposit in the myocardium and include amyloidosis, hemochromatosis, and sarcoidosis. Any of these factors can lead to decreased filling and diastolic dysfunction. Signs and symptoms of infiltrative disease include low-voltage of QRS amplitude on ECG and Kussmaul's sign (jugular venous engorgement with inspiration). **Amyloidosis** may also be associated with carpal tunnel syndrome, nephrotic syndrome, liver infiltration, and macroglossia. AL amyloidosis (as in this case) is due to deposition of immunoglobulin light chains originating from plasma cell dyscrasia. Amyloidosis may also result from deposition of transthyretin (ATTR), which may be hereditary or wild-type (previously referred to as senile amyloidosis). ATTR may be treated with tafimidis, which has been shown to reduce mortality. Hereditary ATTR can be treated with liver transplant. Other helpful tests to establish baseline or rule out other causes include TSH, BMP, and CBC. Biopsy is needed to confirm the diagnosis. **Severe anemia** can cause dyspnea and high output failure but not JVD and crackles. **Pulmonary hypertension** may cause crackles if there is left heart failure but would not typically have an S4.

CASE 8 | Cor Pulmonale

A 62-year-old woman with severe COPD presents with bilateral lower leg swelling for several months. Initially, her swelling would resolve with elevation of her legs, but it has been persistent recently. She has chronic shortness of breath that is stable. On exam, her vital signs are temperature is 37.5°C, pulse is 87/min, blood pressure is 132/74 mmHg, respirations are 18/min, SPO_2 sat is 89% on RA. She has JVD, a loud palpable S2, an S4, and a sustained left parasternal impulse, distant lung sounds, hepatomegaly, hepatojugular reflex, and bilateral pitting edema to her thighs.

Evaluation/Tests	TTE shows enlarged RV and elevation of the pulmonary artery systolic pressure. Right heart catheterization shows elevated pressures in the pulmonary artery and a normal wedge pressure. Left heart catheterization is without any significant coronary artery blockage. ECG shows right atrial enlargement, RVH, and right axis deviation. CXR shows right ventriculomegaly with enlarged pulmonary arteries and hyperinflated lungs with flattened diaphragms.
Treatment	Treat severe COPD with triple therapy (long-acting muscarinic agents, long-acting beta-agonists, and inhaled steroids). Hypoxia, which is a potent pulmonary vasoconstrictor, must be avoided. Supplemental oxygen should be titrated to avoid SPO_2 <89%. Diuretics can help manage volume overload created by RV failure.
Discussion	Right-sided HF due to pulmonary disease is referred to as cor pulmonale, or **Group 3 pulmonary hypertension**. Chronic hypoxia secondary to lung disease (e.g., chronic COPD) results in pulmonary arterial vasoconstriction resulting in pulmonary hypertension and eventual right ventricular failure. The physical exam findings include elevated JVP, sustained parasternal impulse, hepatomegaly, bilateral pitting edema, and lack of pulmonary crackles. Patients may also have a loud P2, narrow splitting of second heart sound, and a palpable pulmonary impulse (felt in the left 2nd intercostal space and caused by closure of the pulmonic valve) consistent with pulmonary hypertension. Treatment is tailored toward treating the underlying cause such as COPD, avoiding hypoxia, and limiting hypervolemia. Pulmonary hypertension due to lung disease (Group 3 pulmonary hypertension) is distinguished from **Group 1 pulmonary arterial hypertension PAH** by the presence of an underlying lung pathology. PAH is often idiopathic but may be associated with drug toxicity, connective tissue disease, congenital heart disease, or HIV infection. Pulmonary hypertension may also be due to chronic thromboembolic disease **(Group 4)**, or due to left heart disease **(Group 2)** (e.g., HFrEF, HFpEF, valvular heart disease), or due to blood or other rare disorders causing pulmonary HTN **(Group 5)** (e.g., myeloproliferative disorders, sarcoidosis, thyroid disease). Treatments designed for Group 1 pulmonary hypertension (prostacycline agonists, nitric oxide-cyclic guanosine monophosphate enhancers and phosphodiesterase-5 inhibitors) have not been found to be efficacious in Group 3 disease.

CASE 9 | Atrial Septal Defect (ASD)

A 30-year-old man presents with worsening exertional dyspnea for the past year. He was previously very active and participated in sports regularly, but over the last year he has had progressive dyspnea on exertion with modest activity. On exam, vital signs are temperature is 37.0°C , pulse 90/min, blood pressure 120/70 mmHg, respirations are 18/min, SPO$_2$ is 97%. He has an elevated JVP, hyper dynamic left lower sternal border impulse (this reflects a volume overloaded RV from the L → R shunt), fixed split S2, and a 2/6 crescendo-decrescendo midpeaking systolic murmur loudest at the left upper sternal border. His lungs are clear, and his abdomen is distended but nontender, and he has bilateral lower extremity edema.

Evaluation/Tests	Transthoracic echocardiogram can allow visualization of ASD (Doppler or bubble study shows a shunt through an ASD). Cardiac MRI can be used for further imaging detail. ECG shows an incomplete right bundle branch block, and a CXR shows cardiomegaly, right atrial enlargement, and enlarged pulmonary arteries.
Treatment	Surgical or percutaneous closure of ASD. The pulmonary hypertension associated with an ASD can be managed with medications like diuretics, prostacyclins, endothelin receptor blockers, and phosphodiesterase inhibitors.
Discussion	This presentation is concerning for an **ASD with associated pulmonary hypertension**. The presence of signs of right-sided volume overload such as elevated JVD, abdominal distension, and lower extremity edema are consistent with pulmonary hypertension with right ventricular failure.
	Patients with an ASD maybe asymptomatic or have dyspnea due to decreased lung compliance from the left to right shunt, causing an increased pulmonary blood volume, or present with a paradoxical embolic stroke from a venous thrombus. If the left-to-right shunt is large, some may develop pulmonary hypertension (as in our patient) due to the increased blood flow and pressures in pulmonary vasculature. Patients with untreated ASD are at an increased lifetime risk of developing atrial fibrillation.
	Severe pulmonary hypertension with advanced RV failure may eventually lead to right-to-left intracardiac shunting, known as **Eisenmenger's syndrome**. Deoxygenated blood flows from the right side of the heart to the left side, bypassing the lungs, resulting in hypoxemia and cyanosis.
	Symptoms of Eisenmenger's syndrome include dyspnea with exertion. Signs include cyanosis, clubbing, and polycythemia. Various types of intracardiac shunts such as ASD, ventricular septal defect (VSD), and patent ductus arteriosis (PDA) may cause Eisenmenger syndrome. Right-sided heart pressures decrease in the first few seconds after birth as the lungs expand and fill with air. Blood preferentially flows down a pressure gradient from the left side of the heart to the right side across the ASD, VSD, or PDA. This increases blood flow to the right heart and subsequently to the lungs. If persistent, the left-to-right shunt can result in the development of pulmonary arterial hypertension. As pulmonary hypertension progresses, the blood flow across the cardiac defect will decrease as the pressure gradient decreases. Murmurs that had been more pronounced in childhood may decrease despite the defect still being present (a pulmonic regurgitant murmur is likely to become more pronounced). If pulmonary blood pressure exceeds systemic blood pressure, then the blood flow across the cardiac defect will reverse and preferentially flow right to left, causing Eisenmenger physiology.
	The murmur associated with an ASD results from increased flow across the pulmonic valve. The location and quality of the murmur will be similar to **pulmonary stenosis**; however, unlike in pulmonary stenosis, ASD will have a fixed-split S2 heart sound. The fixed splitting of the second heart sound is caused by the increased volume from the left-to-right atrial shunt. The increased volume goes across the pulmonic valve. The pulmonic valve therefore stays open longer and closes later. The venous return to the right heart cannot be further augmented by inspiration.

CASE 10 | Myocarditis

A 23-year-old man with no medical problems presents with chest pain and shortness of breath for 1 week. He recently recovered from a cough, nasal congestion, fevers, and myalgias. On exam, he is in mild respiratory distress and is sitting upright. His vital signs are as follows: temperature is 37.8°C, pulse is 105/min, blood pressure is 85/52 mmHg, RR is 24/min, and SPO$_2$ is 90%. He has an elevated JVP, S3, bibasilar crackles, and bilateral pitting edema to the knees. His extremities are cool.

Evaluation/Tests	BNP, troponin, ESR, and CK are elevated. A leukocytosis may be present. ECG shows AV block, and CXR shows vascular congestion, pulmonary edema, and cardiomegaly. Echo shows dilated chambers and globally reduced left ventricular ejection fraction. Cardiac MRI confirms myocarditis by the presence of myocardial edema and late gadolinium enhancement uptake.
Treatment	If patients present with mild heart failure symptoms without evidence of end-organ malperfusion or shock,treat as HFrEF. If patients have signs and symptoms of cardiogenic shock, they may require inotropic or mechanical circulatory support. Immunosuppression has not been found to be beneficial in myocarditis but may have a role in patients with giant cell myocarditis.

CASE 10 | Myocarditis *(continued)*

Discussion	Myocarditis is an inflammatory disease of the myocardium, which can be secondary to multiple causes. The most common causes are viral infections such as Coxsackie B, parvovirus B19, adenovirus, HIV, and hepatitis C virus. *Borrelia burgdorferi* (Lyme disease) and *Trypanosoma cruzi* (Chagas disease) can cause myocarditis in endemic areas (such as Northeastern US for Lyme disease and Mexico for Chagas disease). Noninfectious causes include autoimmune diseases (giant cell myocarditis, systemic lupus erythematosus). Endomyocardial biopsy is the gold standard for making the diagnosis but is not frequently done due to its invasive nature. On biopsy, the presence of lymphocytic infiltration associated with injury to myocytes in the absence of ischemia suggests myocarditis. Depending on the etiology, some patients may require immunosuppressive therapy, colchicine, or high-dose aspirin treatment. Avoiding physical activity in the acute phase is key due to an increased risk of arrhythmias and sudden cardiac death. Patients with **acute rheumatic fever** may present similarly after a sore throat due to a strep infection, but other signs and symptoms include joint pains, rash, and cardiac murmur. Patients with **pericarditis** would have diffuse ST elevations on ECG, and patients with **glomerulonephritis** would have an abnormal urinalysis.

CASE 11 | Cardiac Tamponade

A 32-year-old woman with systemic lupus erythematosus (SLE) presents with chest pain, fever, and shortness of breath for the past 3 days. She came to clinic because of worsening lightheadedness and near fainting. On exam, she appears ill, lethargic, and has a dry oral mucosa. Her vital signs are as follows: temperature is 38°C, respirations are 24/min, SPO_2 is 95%, pulse is 118/min, and blood pressure is 96/60mmHg. A 10-mm drop in the systolic pressure is found with inspiration (pulsus paradoxus). She has an elevated JVP, muffled heart sounds, and weak pulses are noted on inspiration that return to normal during expiration.

Evaluation/Tests	ECG shows sinus tachycardia, low-amplitude QRS complexes, and electrical alternans. Chest XR shows a large cardiac silhouette with a "water bottle" appearance. Echocardiogram shows a large pericardial effusion with collapse of right cardiac chambers during diastole, respiratory variations of volume and flow, and a dilated inferior vena cava dilation without collapse.
Treatment	Pericardiocentesis to drain the pericardial fluid.
Discussion	This patient has cardiac tamponade, a syndrome in which the heart becomes compressed by fluid accumulating in the pericardial sac. Tamponade classically presents with Beck's triad: hypotension, muffled heart sounds, and jugular venous distension. Causes of pericardial effusions include autoimmune disorders, malignancy, infections (TB, viral, and, rarely, bacterial), advanced kidney disease, trauma, or association with aortic dissection. Pericardial effusion can progress to cardiac tamponade. The finding of **pulsus paradoxus** should strongly signal that cardiac tamponade may be present. The finding of an exaggerated decrease in systolic blood pressure with inspiration occurs due to the hemodynamics associated with the drop in intrathoracic pressure. This decrease of pressure during inspiration increases the filling of the right ventricle. In the case of tamponade, the pericardial fluid does not allow the heart to fully expand, and this increased filling of the right ventricle expands across the interventricular septum (as opposed to the pericardium), causing systemic hypotension because the left ventricle is unable to completely fill. The large amount of fluid in the pericardium causes the heart to swing in place and is seen on the ECG as **electrical alternans** as the heart moves towards and away from the chest wall. A patient with cardiac tamponade needs emergent pericardiocentesis to remove the fluid in the pericardium to reduce the pressure surrounding the heart. Studies on the fluid should include tests for infections including tuberculosis.

MURMURS

Cardiac murmurs are a common physical exam finding, and they are caused by turbulent blood flow. Normal blood flow through the heart is laminar and does not cause an abnormal sound. Murmurs may be classified as pathologic due to a leaky or stenotic cardiac valve, an abnormal communication between cardiac chambers (e.g., VSD), or a communication between the great vessels (e.g., PDA). A murmur may also be described as physiologic/functional, meaning that the murmur is caused by a physiologic condition outside of the heart. Once the underlying condition is treated, the murmur resolves. Examples of physiological/functional murmurs include hypervolemic state of pregnancy, severe anemia, and hyperthyroidism.

Occasionally a murmur may be described as "innocent" when it is due to a hyperdynamic cardiac circulation. Innocent murmurs are commonly heard in infancy and childhood and disappear by adulthood.

In order to appreciate heart murmurs, it is essential to perform a thorough cardiac examination. This may require placing the patient in different positions such as supine, lateral decubitus, sitting, or standing. Additional maneuvers that decrease preload (asking the patient to hold their breath, Valsalva, or stand) or increase afterload (rapid squatting/sustained hand grip) may be necessary to further distinguish the murmur. The bell of the stethoscope is used for low-intensity sounds such as mid-diastolic murmur of mitral stenosis. A diaphragm is used for high-pitched sounds such as ejection clicks or systolic murmurs.

Heart murmurs may be characterized by location (e.g., apical), by intensity (grades I–VI), by time of occurrence (systolic vs. diastolic), duration (early or late), radiation, and quality (e.g., blowing). As a rule, any murmur that is systolic of a high-grade intensity (grades IV–VI) or pansystolic is considered pathologic. All diastolic murmurs are considered pathologic.

In order to further assess murmurs, a resting 12-lead ECG, chest X-ray, and echocardiography can be used to further refine the diagnosis heard on physical exam.

Key History Findings and Murmur Differential Diagnosis

Murmurs with Key Associated History Finding	Diagnoses
History of (H/O) rheumatic fever	Mitral valve regurgitation (earlier) or stenosis (later), aortic stenosis (later)
Fever and new murmur	Infective endocarditis (IE), acute rheumatic fever
H/O IV drug use	Tricuspid valve regurgitation from IE
Recent MI with a late presentation and new systolic murmur	Mitral regurgitation from a papillary muscle rupture or dysfunction, or VSD from a septal rupture
H/O bicuspid aortic valve	Aortic stenosis, aortic insufficiency
Turner's disease	Aortic stenosis
Athlete passing out or dying during an athletic event	Hypertrophic cardiomyopathy (HCM)
H/O chest pain, heart failure, and/or syncope	Severe aortic stenosis
Children, adolescents, and young adults	Consider congenital heart defects: ASD, VSD, PDA, or pulmonic stenosis

Key Physical Exam Findings and Murmur Differential Diagnosis

Murmurs with Key Associated Exam Findings		Diagnoses
Increased with inspiration		Right-sided murmurs, particularly tricuspid regurgitation
Systolic Murmurs		
High pitched blowing plateau holosystolic murmur, radiating to axilla. Best heard at apex.	S_1 S_2 S_1	Mitral regurgitation
Plateau holosystolic murmur, increases with inspiration. Best heard at left lower sternal border (LLSB)	S_1 S_2 S_1	Tricuspid regurgitation
High-pitched, holosystolic murmur. The smaller the VSD, the louder the murmur. Best heard at 3rd left intercostal space (ICS).	S_1 S_2 S_1	Ventricular septal defect (left to right shunt)

(continued)

Key Physical Exam Findings and Murmur Differential Diagnosis (*continued*)

Murmurs with Key Associated Exam Findings		Diagnoses
Harsh, crescendo-decrescendo, ejection murmur, radiating to carotids (in severe cases: decreased A2 and a late peaking murmur), increases with squatting and decreases with Valsalva or standing. Best heard at right 2nd ICS	S_1 ◆ S_2 S_1	Aortic stenosis
Midsystolic, crescendo-decrescendo murmur (in severe cases: wide split S2 and decreased P2). Best heard at left 2nd-3rd ICS	S_1 ◆ S_2 S_1	Pulmonic stenosis
Harsh/mid to late systolic murmur, increases with Valsalva or standing (decrease preload) and decreases with squatting or sustained hand grip. S3, S4 may be present. Best heard at left 3rd-4th ICS	S_1 ◆ S_2 S_1	Hypertrophic cardiomyopathy (HCM)
Mid systolic click (C) with late systolic murmur "click-murmur syndrome." Standing/Valsalva moves the systolic click and murmur earlier and increases loudness. Squatting or sustained hand grip moves the click and murmur later and decreases the loudness. Best heard at apex	S_1 C S_2 S_1	Mitral valve prolapse
Systolic ejection murmur, crescendo-decrescendo, at the left upper sternal border (LUSB). Wide fixed S2. Best heard at LUSB	A_2 P_2 S_1 ◆ S_2 S_1	Atrial septal defect
Diastolic Murmurs		
High pitched, blowing, diastolic, decrescendo murmur, best heard sitting/leaning forward in end-exhalation. Best heard at left 3rd ICS	S_1 S_2 ◀ S_1	Aortic regurgitation
Decrescendo murmur. Best heard at LLSB	S_1 S_2 ◀ S_1	Pulmonic regurgitation
Opening snap (OS), high pitched sound, after S2 (heard best with the diaphragm) accompanied by a decrescendo diastolic rumble with pre-systolic accentuation. Murmur best heard with a bell in left lateral decubitus position at apex	S_1 S_2 OS ◀▶ S_1	Mitral stenosis
OS may be heard. Decrescendo diastolic murmur with pre-systolic accentuation increased with inspiration and other maneuvers which increase venous return and blood flow across the tricuspid valve. Best heard at LLSB	S_1 S_2 OS ◀▶ S_1	Tricuspid stenosis

(continued)

Key Physical Exam Findings and Murmur Differential Diagnosis (*continued*)

Murmurs with Key Associated Exam Findings		Diagnoses
	Systolic and Diastolic Murmur	
Harsh, continuous, crescendo-decrescendo, machinery-like murmur, radiates toward clavicle. Best heard at left 2nd ICS	S_1 S_2 S_1	Patent ductus arteriosus (PDA)

CASE 12 | Rheumatic Heart Disease (Mitral Stenosis)

A 20-year-old woman presents with acute shortness of breath 1 hour after giving birth. She emigrated from another country in her second trimester. Her pregnancy was uncomplicated, but her prenatal care was limited. Her only known medical history is that she was told she had a heart murmur as a teenager. She recalls frequent sore throats as a child and an episode of prolonged illness as a teen with fever, migratory arthritis, and chest pains. On exam, her vital signs are as follows: temperature is 36.2°C, pulse is 90/min, blood pressure is 95/60, respirations are 26, and SpO$_2$ is 88%. She has a diastolic rumble following an opening snap, best heard at the apex, diffuse bilateral crackles, and edema in her lower extremities.

Evaluation/Tests	Echo: left atrial enlargement, thickened mitral valve leaflets with elevated transmitral gradient. D dimer is negative.
Treatment	Diuretics to reduce preload, beta-blockers, possible percutaneous balloon mitral valvuloplasty. Rheumatic heart disease also requires prophylactic antibiotic prior to dental procedures to prevent endocarditis
Discussion	This patient is presenting with **mitral stenosis from rheumatic heart disease**. Rheumatic fever and subsequent rheumatic heart disease are the consequences of an untreated pharyngeal infection with group A beta-hemolytic streptococci (GAS). Rheumatic heart disease typically affects the mitral valve, but the aortic and tricuspid valves can be involved as well. Rheumatic heart disease is a late manifestation due to inflammation and scarring of the valve during acute rheumatic fever. Pregnancy, specifically the postpartum period, can cause decompensation due to rapid fluid shifts in a previously asymptomatic woman. Diagnosis of acute rheumatic fever is based on Jones criteria (requires 2 major or 1 major + 2 minor findings). Major: migratory polyarthritis, cardiac involvement (carditis, pericarditis, valvulitis), subcutaneous nodules, erythema marginatum, Syndenham chorea. Minor: fever, elevated ESR, h/o rheumatic fever, history of untreated GAS pharyngitis, polyarthralgias, prolonged PR interval. Rheumatic fever with cardiac involvement requires lifelong penicillin prophylaxis to prevent progression to rheumatic heart disease. Mitral stenosis is most commonly caused by rheumatic fever. Early in the course of the disease, patients are asymptomatic. Symptoms then usually present in the 3rd or 4th decade of life due to pulmonary HTN and RV failure and include dyspnea on exertion, palpitations, chest pain, hemoptysis, orthopnea, and edema. Cardiac exam shows accentuated first heart sound and an opening snap after S2 followed by a mid-diastolic rumbling murmur. Surgical interventions such as percutaneous mitral balloon valvotomy or valve replacement are indicated in patients with severe symptomatic mitral stenosis. Patients with **amniotic fluid embolism** or **pulmonary embolus** can present with acute shortness of breath and hypoxia; however, they would not typically have the characteristic MS murmur and signs of volume overload. Patients with **peripartum cardiomyopathy** typically present more gradually with signs and symptoms of volume overload, an S3, and, if present, a murmur consistent with mitral regurgitation.

CASE 13 | Aortic Stenosis

A 75-year-old man with hypertension presents with progressively worsening fatigue and dyspnea on exertion. He also reports chest discomfort with exertion, and he passed out for a few minutes last week when he was rushing to catch the bus. On exam, his vital signs are as follows: temperature is 36.4°C, pulse is 78/min, blood pressure is 140/110 mmHg, respirations are 16/min, and SPO$_2$ is 96% on RA. The carotid pulses are delayed and diminished (parvus et tardus), and the point of maximal impulse (PMI) is sustained. Auscultation reveals a 2/6 harsh systolic late peaking crescendo-decrescendo murmur at the right upper sternal border with radiation to the carotids, and his lungs are clear to auscultation.

CASE 13 | Aortic Stenosis *(continued)*

Evaluation/Tests	Transthoracic echocardiogram (TTE): thickened, calcified aortic valve, dilated aortic root, and left ventricular hypertrophy. CBC, troponin, and BNP are normal. ECG shows left ventricular hypertrophy and left atrial abnormalities
Treatment	Aortic valve replacement (surgical vs. transcatheter).
Discussion	Aortic stenosis (AS) can be due to a senile calcific valve disease, calcified bicuspid valves (Turner's syndrome, congenital abnormalities), or rheumatic disease. Many patients are asymptomatic until the stenosis is severe, and then they present with a triad of dyspnea on exertion, angina, and syncope. Left ventricular failure is a common result of severe aortic stenosis. Aortic valve replacement via TAVR (catheter-based transaortic valve replacement) or via open heart surgery is indicated for severe, symptomatic aortic stenosis. The AS murmur must be differentiated frequently from the murmur of **hypertrophic cardiomyopathy (HCM)**. Maneuvers that increase LV preload will increase the intensity of the AS murmur (standing to sitting) but decrease the murmur associated with HCM. Acute MI, COPD, and HF may present with dyspnea on exertion and chest discomfort; however, the murmur and tests in this case are all consistent with aortic stenosis.

CASE 14 | Aortic Regurgitation

A 63-year-old woman with hypertension presents with worsening dyspnea on exertion, angina, orthopnea, and palpitations. On exam, her vital signs are as follows: temperature is 36.2°C, pulse is 101/min, blood pressure is 150/50 mmHg (widened pulse pressure), respirations are 28/min, and SPO_2 is 98%. She has elevated JVP, her carotid pulse appears to be collapsing, her point of maximal impulse (PMI) is laterally displaced, and there is a grade 3/6 diastolic decrescendo murmur in the third left intercostal space. The lungs have bibasilar crackles, and there is 2+ edema in the lower extremities.

Evaluation/Tests	ECHO shows aortic regurgitation, dilated left ventricle, LV dysfunction, dilated aortic root, and early closure of mitral valve. BNP is elevated, and CXR shows LVH, a dilated aorta, and pulmonary edema. Troponins are normal.
Treatment	Treatment includes diuresis for congestive symptoms and afterload reduction with agents such as ACEi or ARBs to help with forward flow. Severe symptomatic aortic regurgitation often requires aortic valve replacement.
Discussion	Aortic regurgitation can be acute (e.g., infective endocarditis or acute rheumatic fever) or chronic (congenital diseases such as Marfan syndrome or associated with senile calcification) in nature. Chronic aortic regurgitation is often asymptomatic for years before it manifests with symptoms or left ventricular dysfunction. Symptoms can include palpitations, shortness of breath, or chest pain. Acute, severe aortic regurgitation is hardly ever tolerated and presents with acute pulmonary edema and other signs of heart failure. Exam findings may include a diastolic decrescendo murmur, a displaced PMI, S3, or wide pulse pressure (large difference between systolic and diastolic BP). Other findings include water-hammer or Corrigan's pulse (rapidly increasing pulse that collapses suddenly) noted by raising and lowering the patient's arm or an Austin-Flint murmur. Patients often have a widened pulse pressure (difference between systolic and diastolic pressure). The chronic effect of the recirculating blood in the left ventricle results in ventricular dilation and hypertrophy, which can be eccentric or concentric. Patients with ischemic heart disease, mitral stenosis, or HF can present with similar symptoms, but the murmur and tests in this case are consistent with aortic regurgitation.

CASE 15 | Mitral Regurgitation

A 55-year-old man with coronary artery disease presents with worsening shortness of breath for 3 months. On exam, there is a soft S1 followed by a high-pitched plateau holosystolic murmur at the apex that radiates to the axilla. Auscultation of the lungs reveals bibasilar crackles.

Evaluation/Tests	TTE is the imaging of choice for diagnosis and will show mitral regurgitation, dilated LA and LV, and decreased ejection fraction. ECG and troponin are normal. BNP is elevated, and CXR is consistent with pulmonary congestion.

CASE 15 | **Mitral Regurgitation** (continued)

Treatment	Diuresis for congestive symptoms, afterload reduction with vasodilators (ACEI/ARB or alpha-blockers) to aid in forward flow, optimize blood pressure, and treat CAD. Mitral valve surgery is indicated in severe or acute cases of mitral regurgitation.
Discussion	Mitral regurgitation is a common valvular heart abnormality. Acute causes include papillary muscle rupture, dysfunction from ACS, or endocarditis. Chronic causes include rheumatic heart disease and cardiomyopathy. In chronic mitral regurgitation, symptoms can be insidious, and patients may be asymptomatic until they develop left ventricular dysfunction. Symptoms include shortness of breath and fatigue. Physical exam reveals the holosystolic, harsh murmur of mitral regurgitation. This is often associated with signs of heart failure such as pulmonary crackles, pitting edema, and an S3. Treatment of acute mitral regurgitation often requires surgical repair or replacement. Chronic mitral regurgitation due to LV dilation is termed functional mitral regurgitation, as this is a function of the dilation of the mitral valve annulus, and not underlying pathology of the valve. Patients with HF, ACS, AS may present similarly; however, the exam and imaging in this case are consistent with mitral regurgitation.
Additional Considerations	Patients with **tricuspid regurgitation** often present with signs and symptoms of right heart failure with elevated JVP, lower extremity edema, ascites, elevated liver transaminases, and holosystolic murmur at the LLSB that increases with inspiration due to the negative intrathoracic pressure causing increased preload. Causes of tricuspid regurgitation are similar to mitral regurgitation, including ischemia/infarction, endocarditis (consider if fever and h/o IV drug abuse), rheumatic heart disease, or RV failure with dilation of the tricuspid annulus.

CARDIAC TUMORS

Cardiac tumors are rare. Most adult patients present in their 4th to 6th decade of life. About 10% are associated with genetic/familial conditions. Symptoms are related to the location of the tumor. Right-sided tumors present with right heart failure symptoms (e.g., peripheral edema) and pulmonary emboli. Left-sided tumors present with left heart failure, systemic emboli, and obstruction resulting in syncope. Intramural tumors often present with arrhythmias and other conduction abnormalities. As such, even benign tumors can be dangerous and warrant resection.

CASE 16	**Cardiac Tumor (Myxoma)**
	A 43-year-old woman presents with chronic progressive shortness of breath over the past several months. She also notes low-grade fevers, fatigue, paroxysmal nocturnal dyspnea, and intermittent chest pain. On cardiac auscultation, a diastolic murmur is heard at her left sternal border with an extra "plopping" heart sound heard immediately after S2.
Evaluation/Tests	Echo shows large atrial pedunculated mass with a "ball valve" obstruction in the left atrium.
Treatment	Surgical resection.
Discussion	A left atrial myxoma is the most common primary tumor of the heart. Patients may present with constitutional symptoms (fever, weight loss, arthralgias) and symptoms of mitral stenosis (shortness of breath, dyspnea on exertion). The fever from myxoma is related to the tumor causing elevations in a pro-inflammatory cytokine IL-6. A myxoma is free floating with a long stalk and can have a "wrecking ball" effect by intermittently obstructing the mitral valve. The gelatinous nature of the myxoma can result in thrombo-embolization, causing ischemic strokes, so anticoagulation is often indicated. Auscultation classically reveals a "tumor plop" in early diastole when the tumor is forced into the mitral valve. Definitive treatment is surgical resection; pathology reveals myxoma cells in a glycosaminoglycan matrix and hence the gelatinous nature. **Endocarditis** may present similarly but the echo in this case is diagnostic for a tumor. Benign tumors should be at the top of the differential given the location of the mass and pedunculated appearance on echo; however, a **malignant tumor** cannot be completely ruled out until pathology is done.

CYANOSIS

Cyanosis is a bluish skin discoloration representing tissue hypoxia, which stems from deoxygenated hemoglobin in the blood. Cyanosis can be difficult to assess; thus a thorough exam of lips, nail beds, earlobes, and mucous membranes is helpful. It is a rare but alarming physical exam finding and requires immediate treatment of the underlying cause. Cyanosis can be separated into central and peripheral etiologies. Peripheral cyanosis is caused by decreased peripheral circulation. Central cyanosis indicates systemically deoxygenated hemoglobin, which can be a result of cardiac abnormalities, hypoventilation, pulmonary disease (see "Respiratory" chapter), hemoglobin abnormalities, or cellular toxins. Patent ductus arteriosis can cause differential cyanosis, with the lower extremities cyanotic and sparing the upper extremities because the upper extremities are perfused prior to the lesion.

Initial workup of cyanosis should include a complete blood count, basic metabolic panel, arterial blood gas, and chest radiograph. If congenital heart disease is suspected, an echocardiogram is warranted.

Careful history and exam can be very helpful in determining the causes of cyanosis. Associated symptoms of edema or orthopnea may be suggestive of a cardiac or pulmonary vascular cause. Rapid deterioration can point to respiratory distress syndrome (ARDS or NRDS). It is also important to explore medication use and new medications. Cardiac causes are often congenital. (See Respiratory chapter for additional discussion.)

Clues for Special Populations

	Diagnosis
Infants	Cyanosis, which begins in the first hours to days of life, is concerning for right-to-left shunt congenital heart diseases. These include transposition of great arteries, persistent truncus arteriosus, tetralogy of Fallot, total anomalous venous return, Ebstein anomaly, hypoplastic left heart syndrome, and tricuspid atresia. Congenital heart disease can have variable presentation and can become more evident once the PDA begins to close because the PDA allows for left-to-right circulation and can provide compensation while it remains open.
Toddlers	If tetralogy of Fallot does not present as cyanosis in infancy, it may present later in toddlers. It may be described as a toddler who cannot keep up with his classmates at recess and has to squat when catching their breath. "Tet" spells may be noted.
Young adults	Difficult-to-control hypertension in young adults should raise suspicion for coarctation of aorta. They may also have claudication on exertion and lower extremity cyanosis secondary to the often associated PDA.
Any age	Right ventricular failure symptoms may indicate untreated congenital heart disease that has progressed to Eisenmenger syndrome. Individuals with surgical corrections of congenital heart disease who have been lost to follow-up may present with symptoms of right- and left-sided heart failure later in life.

Key Findings and Cyanosis Differential Diagnosis

Cyanosis with Key Associated Findings	Diagnoses
Progressive cyanosis in the first 2 weeks of life	As the PDA closes the symptoms start. Tricuspid atresia (may hear PDA or VSD murmurs), total anomalous pulmonary venous return, hypoplastic left heart syndrome, coarctation of aorta
Cyanosis, hypoxia, tachypnea, failure to thrive within the first hours or days. CXR with an oval- or egg-shaped cardiac silhouette with a narrow superior mediastinum.	Transposition of great arteries (murmurs may be absent or a faint systolic murmur may be present)
Cyanosis, hypoxia, tachypnea, failure to thrive in the first week with prominent neck veins. "Figure of eight" or "snowman" on CXR	Total anomalous pulmonary venous return. "Figure of eight" or "snow man" on CXR refers to small cardiac silhouette with large pulmonary vascularity.
Dyspnea with feeding, poor growth, and sudden hypercyanotic "tet" spells. Cyanosis improves with squatting. Harsh systolic murmur at the left upper sternal border with a single heart sound (S2); prominent right ventricular impulse and systolic thrill may be noted. Boot-shaped heart on CXR.	Tetralogy of Fallot

(continued)

Key Findings and Cyanosis Differential Diagnosis (*continued*)

Cyanosis with Key Associated Findings	Diagnoses
Wide pulse pressure and bounding arterial pulses, harsh systolic murmur with a thrill audible along left sternal border, loud and single S2	Truncus arteriosus
Ejection systolic murmur at the left upper sternal border; widely fixed S2	Atrial septal defect (murmur is secondary to increased flow across the pulmonic valve)
High-pitched, holosystolic murmur. Best heard in 3rd, 4th, and 5th left intercostal space	Ventricular septal defect (cyanosis a late finding secondary to Eisenmenger physiology)
History of childhood murmur or known VSD/ASD, now with new onset JVP, hepatomegaly, lower extremity edema, left parasternal heave (RVH) pulmonary congestion, cyanosis, clubbing, loud P2, holosystolic murmur at left sternal border (TR)	Eisenmenger syndrome
Intermittent claudication on exercise in older children; prominent pulsation in the neck. Hypertension, reduced lower extremity pulses, brachial-femoral delay, lower blood pressure in lower limb compared to upper, ejection systolic murmur in back or can be continuous.	Coarctation of aorta
Bilateral pulmonary infiltrates	Cardiogenic pulmonary edema, pneumonia, ARDS, NRDS
Snoring, Nocturnal oxygen desaturation, large tonsils	Obstructive sleep apnea
Old heating system or early winter	Carbon monoxide poisoning
Sodium nitroprusside use	Cyanide poisoning
Exposure to nitrates, benzocaine	Methemoglobin
Worsening extremity cyanosis in cold weather	Raynaud's, scleroderma

CASE 17 | Tetralogy of Fallot (ToF)

An 8-month-old boy with Down syndrome is brought to the clinic for evaluation as he turns blue when he cries or feeds ("tet" spells). His mother has a history of alcohol use during the pregnancy.

On exam, he is underweight and turns blue with crying; clubbing is noted in upper extremities. A systolic thrill along the left sternal border, and a sustained right ventricular impulse along the left sternal border is noted. On auscultation, there is a loud and harsh systolic ejection murmur radiating to the pulmonary and aortic areas, with a single S2. His lungs are clear to auscultation bilaterally.

Evaluation/Tests	Echo shows an overriding aorta, VSD, pulmonary infundibular stenosis, and RVH. ECG with right axis deviation and RVH, and CXR shows a "boot"-shaped heart due to RV enlargement.
Treatment	Surgical repair.
Discussion	ToF is the most common cyanotic congenital cardiac defect and is characterized by a tetrad of pulmonary infundibular stenosis, RVH, an overriding aorta, and a VSD. The degree of pulmonary infundibular stenosis predicts prognosis and the severity of symptoms. Children will often "learn" the behavior of suddenly stopping during activity and squatting. This maneuver increases afterload, which decreases the right-to-left shunt and improves hypoxia. The single S2 is caused by the inaudible P2 because of low pulmonary pressures. ToF can be associated with Down syndrome and DiGeorge syndrome (thymic aplasia, 22q11 deletion) and fetal alcohol syndrome. In **transposition of the great arteries**, imaging would show aorta connected to RV and pulmonary trunk connected to LV. Prenatal screening with fetal ultrasound can often identify this abnormality, but occasionally it can be missed. CXR would show an enlarged, globular, egg-shaped heart (a finding known as "egg on a string"). This condition needs to be surgically repaired. Until the baby can receive surgery, the PDA patency should be maintained with PGE1 (e.g., alprostadil) to allow for some mixing of blood and thus some oxygenation.

CASE 18 | Ventricular Septal Defect (VSD)

A 15-year-old boy with a past medical history of an unrepaired "hole in his heart" as a child presents with worsening exertional dyspnea for the last several months. On exam, his vital signs are as follows: temperature is 37.0°C, pulse is 90/min, blood pressure is 120/70 mmHg, respirations are 18/min, and SPO_2 is 97%. There is elevated JVP, sternal lift (RV enlargement), and a laterally displaced PMI. On auscultation, there is a harsh, holosystolic murmur and palpable thrill at LLSB and bibasilar crackles in the lungs.

Evaluation/Tests	Echo reveals an intracardiac shunt thru VSD and RVH (from elevated pulmonary vascular resistance (PVR)). CXR shows cardiomegaly and increased pulmonary vascular markings (enlarged pulmonary artery)
Treatment	Percutaneous closure device or surgical repair.
Discussion	VSDs are the most common congenital cardiac defects, and they usually occur in the membranous septum. There are many variations of VSDs in terms of size, shape, and location. The murmur is typically described as a harsh murmur best heard at the left lower sternal border. It is also associated with fixed splitting of S2 due to increased flow through the pulmonary circulation from left to right shunting. Patients with small congenital shunts are often asymptomatic, and they may close spontaneously in childhood, but some can persist into adulthood. VSDs can cause pulmonary hypertension (Eisenmenger's), and heart failure as in this patient. Acquired VSDs can occur postmyocardial infarction. Treatment is either surgical or transcatheter closure of the symptomatic defect.
Additional Considerations	**ASD** is characterized by a widely fixed S2 with a systolic ejection murmur at the left upper sternal border. ASD is classically associated with stroke from venous thromboembolism "paradoxical embolism." They can also result in Eisenmenger's syndrome. Treatment is transcatheter septal occlusion. ASD is also associated with many other congenital heart defects, such as tricuspid atresia and anomalous pulmonary venous return, or seen as part of fetal alcohol or Down syndrome. PFO results from failure of closure of the foramen ovale. They can rarely be associated with cryptogenic strokes, similar to an ASD. **Ebstein anomaly** is a congenital heart abnormality that is associated with in utero lithium exposure. The hallmark of the Ebstein anomaly is inferior displacement of the tricuspid valve, artificially "atrializing" the ventricle. It is associated with right-sided HF, tricuspid regurgitation, and arrhythmias arising from accessory conduction pathways. It can also be associated with mild-severe intra-atrial shunt, which can cause cyanosis. Echo would show a dilated right atrium and right ventricle and tricuspid regurgitation with delayed closure of the valve and significant apical displacement of the valve into the RV ("atrializing" the ventricle).

PALPITATIONS

Palpitations, or the sensation of strong, rapid, or irregular heartbeats, is a common medical concern and a frequent cause of health care visits in both the adolescent and adult populations. Palpitations can be due to excessive caffeine intake, smoking, stress/anxiety, or arrhythmias. Arrhythmias are abnormal or irregular heartbeats. In the initial assessment, the first step is to identify if the palpitations are due to an underlying cardiac or a noncardiac cause. A thorough history, including the timing of the palpitations, associated symptoms, and any lifestyle changes, is often critical to deduce the appropriate diagnosis and guide subsequent treatment. Further information may be provided to help narrow the differential, including information about recent stressors, social history, previous medical history, and family history (FHx). Clues that point to a cardiac cause include a history of cardiovascular diseases that may predispose patients to arrhythmias. The causes can be acquired (e.g., ischemic heart disease) or familial (HCM, long QT syndrome). Mitral valve prolapse (MVP) and myocarditis can also present with palpitations. MVP can be appreciated on physical exam, and myocarditis can be elicited by taking a detailed history. Noncardiogenic causes of arrhythmias include medications (such as amphotericin), hyperthyroidism, lung disease, and anemia.

Differential Diagnoses for Palpitations

Cardiac	Neuro/Psych
Sinus tachycardia	Panic attack
Premature atrial contractions	Generalized anxiety disorder
Atrial tachycardia	Somatization
Multifocal atrial tachycardia (MAT)	Depression
Atrial fibrillation	Postural orthostatic tachycardia syndrome (POTS)
Atrial flutter	
Atrioventricular reentrant tachycardia (AVRT)	**Other**
AV nodal reentrant tachycardia (AVNRT)	Stimulant use/ingestion (cocaine, caffeine)
Premature ventricular contractions (PVC)	Toxin ingestion
Ventricular tachycardia	Drug-induced
Ventricular fibrillation	Acute rheumatic fever
Mitral valve prolapse	Anemia
Myocarditis	Hyperthyroid
Hypertrophic cardiomyopathy (HCM)	Pheochromocytoma
Congenital heart disease	Paragangliomas
Ebstein's anomaly	Hypoglycemia
Long QT syndrome	Pregnancy
Brugada syndrome	
Wolf-Parkinson-White (WPW) syndrome	
Torsade de pointes	

If a patient's palpitations are determined to be from an arrhythmia, it is important to identify the type of arrhythmia. Arrhythmias can be divided into supraventricular and ventricular arrhythmias. Supraventricular tachycardias (SVTs) arise in the AV node (AVNRT, AVRT) or atrium (atrial fibrillation, atrial flutter or MAT) and therefore typically have a narrow QRS complex. Ventricular arrhythmias include ventricular tachycardia and ventricular fibrillation, have a wide QRS, and are fatal if not defibrillated. On initial assessment, all patients should receive an ECG. Further testing may include measurement of basic electrolytes, thyroid function studies, and ambulatory ECG monitoring. High-risk features associated with palpitations include syncope, cardiac arrest, dyspnea, lightheadedness, angina, or signs of heart failure.

Key Findings and Palpitations Differential Diagnosis

Palpitations with Key Associated Findings	Diagnoses
FHx of sudden cardiac death or ventricular tachycardia	Long QT syndrome, hypertrophic cardiomyopathy, Brugada syndrome
Young athlete, syncope during sports	Hypertrophic cardiomyopathy
Preceding uncontrollable fear of certain situations or events	Generalized anxiety disorder, panic attacks
Excessive exercise, active sports, strong focus on body image	Stimulant use, eating disorder
Short, sudden onset, rapid palpitations, no other symptoms relieved with Valsalva	AVNRT, AVRT
Sweating, flushing, headaches, high blood pressure	Pheochromocytoma
Wheezing, history of COPD/asthma	Multifocal atrial tachycardia, atrial fibrillation, atrial flutter
Diarrhea, heat intolerance, weight loss, sweating, puffy eyes, hair loss	Hyperthyroid
Recent viral illness, fevers, elevated JVP, leg swelling	Myocarditis
Diarrhea, QT prolonging medications (antiemetics, antifungal medications, etc.)	Torsades de pointes

Key Electrocardiogram Findings and Palpitations Differential Diagnosis

ECG Findings		Diagnosis
QTc >450–470 ms		Long QT syndrome
PR interval prolonged > 200 msec		First-degree AV block
PR progressively gets longer, then QRS "dropped"		Second-degree AV block (Mobitz I/Wenckebach)
Dropped QRS not preceded by PR lengthening		Second-degree AV block (Mobitz II)
P and QRS not in rhythm, more Ps than QRS		Third-degree AV block/ complete heart block
P waves preceding each QRS complex with rates >100 BPM		Sinus tachycardia
Inverted P wave after QRS		AVNRT, AVRT
Initial broad upsloping of QRS complex (delta wave)		Wolf-Parkinson-White syndrome (AVRT)
Multiple P wave morphologies, usually with different PR intervals		Multifocal atrial tachycardia (MAT)
Coarse or no P waves, irregularly irregular QRS rhythm		Atrial fibrillation
Regular, typically broad P wave at 300–350 BPM (flutter (F) waves)		Atrial flutter
Usually regular, wide complex QRS; no discernible P waves or QRS-P wave dissociation		Ventricular tachycardia
Wide complex QRS with rhythmic variations in QRS amplitude; no discernible P waves or QRS-P wave dissociation		Torsades de pointes
Coved ST segment elevation in V1–V3		Brugada syndrome

CASE 19 | Atrial Fibrillation (AFib)

A 56-year-old obese woman with hypertension, diabetes, and sleep apnea presents with palpitations, fatigue, and shortness of breath for the last 2 weeks. Initially, her palpitations were intermittent, but today they have been persistent, and she is more short of breath. On exam, her vital signs are normal except for a heart rate of 136/min. Her rhythm is irregularly irregular, the lungs are clear bilaterally, and there is no edema in the lower extremities.

Evaluation/Tests	ECG: R to R irregular interval, an absence of P waves; CBC, troponin, BNP, TSH are normal.
Treatment	Rate control, anticoagulation, cardiovert.
Discussion	Risk factors for the development of atrial fibrillation (AFib) include advanced age, hypertension, sleep apnea, alcohol consumption, diabetes, heart failure, valvular disease, hyperthyroidism, and pulmonary embolism. If a patient is hemodynamically unstable (hypotensive, chest pain, altered mental status, or congestive heart failure), cardioversion is indicated to convert the patient to sinus rhythm. If the patient is stable, medically manage with rate control medications such as beta-blockers or calcium channel blockers to slow conduction through the AV node. Patients with high risk of stroke should be anticoagulated, and this risk is based on their comorbidities including heart failure, hypertension, age >65, diabetes, previous history of stroke, or atherosclerotic vascular disease (the Chads2Vasc score). Antiarrhythmics or cardioversion may be considered after achieving rate control and stability.
Additional Considerations	**Atrial flutter:** ECG will show a sawtooth pattern of P waves with rate ~300 and ventricular rate ~150. Patients can be asymptomatic or present similarly to patients with AFib, with palpitations, fatigue, lightheadedness, or syncope. Treatment is similar to AFib.

CASE 20 | Wolf-Parkinson-White Syndrome (WPW)

A 29-year-old healthy man presents with intermittent palpitations and lightheadedness for years. His general health has been good, and he denies any other problems. His vital signs and exam are normal.

Evaluation/Tests	ECG: sinus rhythm with a short PR interval with a slurring of the upstroke of the QRS complex or a delta wave; CBC and TSH is normal.
Treatment	Catheter-guided ablation of the accessory pathway.
Discussion	The patient has electrocardiographic changes suggestive of pre-excitation or Wolff-Parkinson-White (WPW). This entity is characterized by the presence of tachycardia due to an accessory pathway. Patients may be asymptomatic or present with tachycardia, dizziness, dyspnea, or syncope. If the patient is hemodynamically unstable, urgent electrical cardioversion is necessary. If the patient is hemodynamically stable and WPW is known, the use of procainamide (class Ia) or ibutilide (class III) can be given to terminate the arrhythmia. Avoid using AV nodal blocker agents (beta-blockers and calcium channel blockers) because they might worsen the tachycardia by blocking the AV node, thus favoring conduction down through the accessory pathway. Definitive treatment of the symptomatic patient is catheter-guided ablation of the accessory pathway. Patients with PAC/PVC, other arrhythmias, panic attacks, or hyperthyroidism may present similarly but would not have the characteristic ECG findings.

CASE 21 | Supraventricular Tachycardia (AV-Nodal Re-Entrant Tachycardia)

A previously healthy 22-year-old woman presents with several episodes of intermittent palpitations and shortness of breath for the past 3 weeks. Previously, she was able to control these episodes with deep breathing exercises. The current episode started 15 minutes ago. On exam, she appears anxious, but the rest of her physical exam is normal except for a pulse of 160/min.

Evaluation/Tests	ECG shows arrow complex tachycardia, rate 140 with P wave following the QRS deflection, "buried" inside the T wave.
Treatment	Initially treat with vagal maneuvers such as Valsalva or carotid massage. If SVT continues, then adenosine can be given to transiently block the AV node. If recurrent and problematic, prophylaxis can be initiated with AV nodal blocking agents such as beta blockers or calcium channel blockers.
Discussion	This patient is presenting with **supraventricular tachycardia (SVT)**. SVT can arise in either the AV node (AVNRT, AVRT) or atrium (AFib/flutter or MAT) and therefore typically has a narrow QRS complex. This is the most common arrhythmia in younger patients without comorbid conditions. Possible triggers for SVT include infection, anemia, hypo- or hyperthyroidism, electrolyte disturbance, ischemia, and anxiety/pain. In hemodynamically unstable patients, electrical cardioversion is indicated. Catheter ablation is the definitive treatment.

CASE 21 | Supraventricular Tachycardia (AV-Nodal Re-Entrant Tachycardia) *(continued)*

Discussion	Patients with **panic attacks** would not have the characteristic ECG abnormalities.
	In **sinus tachycardia**, each QRS is preceded by a P wave. The most common causes of sinus tachycardia (HR > 100) are infection, dehydration, bleeding, hyperthyroidism, pulmonary embolism, and decompensated heart failure. Fever increases heart rate 10 bpm for every 1°C above normal temperature.

SYNCOPE

Syncope is defined as transient and abrupt loss of consciousness and postural tone secondary to decreased blood flow to the brain. The episodes typically last for a few seconds, and there is spontaneous recovery. The etiology can be cardiac, neurological, neural-mediated (reflex), and psychiatric. Reflex (neural-mediated) syncope is the most common type, especially in young adults; this includes vasovagal syncope, situation syncope (e.g., micturition), and carotid sinus hypersensitivity syndrome.

The etiology of syncope can be difficult to determine in up to 50% of individuals. A thorough history and physical exam is key when evaluating syncope. It is important to ask about prodromal (warning) symptoms such as palpitations, chest pain, dyspnea, lightheadedness, dizziness, weakness, diaphoresis, nausea, and epigastric discomfort preceding the event. Also ask about any postictal (after seizure) symptoms such as confusion, drowsiness, headache, tongue biting, and loss of bowel or bladder function noted after recovery. Inquire about personal history of heart disease, seizures, and family history of sudden cardiac death, and obtain any eyewitness accounts of the sequence of events and if seizure activity was noted. Initial evaluation should involve checking vital signs, including orthostatic blood pressure and heart rate, and a thorough cardiac and neurologic exam. Initial important tests include checking blood glucose, electrolytes, CBC, and ECG. If cardiac causes are suspected, patients should be placed on continuous telemetry monitoring or followed up with an outpatient Holter or event monitor and echocardiogram. Reflex syncope may need further evaluation with tilt-table testing. If neurological causes of syncope are suspected, consider EEG and brain imaging with MRI or CT scan.

Differential Diagnoses for Syncope

Cardiovascular	Neurologic	Reflex syncope	Other
Arrhythmias	Seizures	Vasovagal	Dehydration (orthostatic hypotension)
Structural heart disease	Cerebrovascular accident (CVA)	Situational syncope (e.g., cough, micturition, defecation)	Pulmonary embolus (PE)
Severe aortic stenosis	Transient ischemic attack (TIA)		Bleed (e.g., trauma, GI bleed)
Hypertrophic cardiomyopathy	Autonomic dysfunction	Carotid sinus hypersensitivity	Pseudoseizures
Severe pulmonic stenosis	Subclavian steal syndrome		Metabolic (e.g., hypoglycemia)
Coronary artery anomalies	Vertebrobasilar insufficiency		Drugs/medication (e.g., alcohol, anti-HTN meds, tricyclic antidepressants, anti-arrhythmics)
Cardiomyopathy			
Cardiac tumors			
Primary pulmonary hypertension			
Myocardial infarction			
Aortic dissection			
Cardiac tamponade			

Key History Findings and Syncope Differential Diagnosis

Syncope with Key Associated History Findings	Diagnoses
History of heart disease	Arrhythmias, acute MI, decompensated HF
Family history of sudden cardiac death	Malignant arrhythmias, HCM, long QT syndrome
History of palpitations	Arrhythmias
Chest pain or chest pressure	Acute MI, aortic dissection, PE, AS
Occurs with exercise No prodrome, short duration (seconds)	Arrhythmias, AS, HCM
Dyspnea on exertion or at rest, paroxysmal nocturnal dyspnea, orthopnea	Decompensated HF, pulmonary hypertension
Malignancy or recent travel with prolonged immobilization	PE

(continued)

Key History Findings and Syncope Differential Diagnosis (continued)

Syncope with Key Associated History Findings	Diagnoses
Associated with strong emotional trigger, upright posture with features of diaphoresis, warmth, nausea, pallor, fatigue	Vasovagal syncope
Occurs with tying a tie or buttoning top buttons of a dress shirt	Carotid sinus hypersensitivity
H/O diarrhea, poor appetite, GI bleed or new medications (antihypertensives)	Orthostatic hypotension
Focal weakness, paresthesias, slurred speech	CVA/TIA
H/O seizure disorder, post-ictal (confusion, tongue biting, incontinence of bowel or bladder), witnessed seizure activity	Seizure
H/O DM or uremia or Parkinson's and lightheadedness with standing	Autonomic insufficiency
Taking insulin or oral hypoglycemic medications for DM	Hypoglycemia
Associated with specific activity (micturition, defecation)	Situational syncope
New medications or up titration of previous medications (diuretics, alpha-blockers, vasodilators, nitrates, TCA, antiarrhythmics)	Medication induced
Children or young adults with family history of sudden cardiac death	Arrhythmias, WPW, Brugada, Long QT syndrome, supraventricular tachycardia, HCM
H/O anxiety, depression, or other psychiatric disorders	Consider psychiatric causes

Key Physical Exam Findings and Syncope Differential Diagnosis

Syncope with Key Associated Exam Findings	Diagnoses
Decrease in systolic blood pressure of >20 mmHg or a decrease in diastolic blood pressure >10 mmHg from supine to standing position (often associated increase in postural heart rate)	Orthostatic hypotension
Hypoxia, tachypnea, tachycardia	Pulmonary embolus
Interarm blood pressure differential greater than 20 mm Hg	Aortic dissection
Harsh, crescendo-decrescendo, systolic ejection murmur best heard in right 2nd intercostal space (sitting/leaning forward), radiating to carotids (Decreased A2 in severe cases)	Aortic stenosis
Harsh/midsystolic murmur best heard in left 3rd–4th intercostal space. Murmur increases with Valsalva/ standing (decrease preload) and decreases with rapid squatting/sustained hand grip (increase afterload), +S4	Hypertrophic cardiomyopathy (HCM)
Midsystolic: crescendo-decrescendo murmur best heard LUSB (in left 2nd–3rd intercostal space) (in severe cases, wide split S2 and decreased P2)	Pulmonic stenosis
Crackles, JVP, lower extremity edema, cold, clammy, S3	Decompensated heart failure
JVD, hypotension, decreased heart sounds (Beck's triad), tachycardia, pulsus paradoxus	Cardiac tamponade
Focal neurologic deficits	CVA, neurologic causes

CASE 22 | Hypertrophic Cardiomyopathy

A 18-year-old man presents after a syncopal episode during exercise. He also reports occasional exertional chest pain, lightheadedness, and palpitations. On exam, there is a prominent, sustained PMI (LV impulse) and a harsh/midsystolic murmur best heard in left 3rd–4th intercostal space. The murmur increases with Valsalva/standing and decreases with rapid squatting/sustained hand grip. An S4 can be heard.

Evaluation/Tests	Echocardiography shows severe, asymmetric ventricular septal myocardial hypertrophy. ECG shows LVH and nonspecific ST changes. CBC, BMP, and glucose levels are normal.
Treatment	Avoid high-intensity sports. Beta-blockers are first-line agents. Nondihydropyridine calcium channel blockers are second line, followed by disopyramide as third line. The goal of treatment is to reduce ionotropy ("the squeeze" of the heart) to limit left ventricular outflow obstruction.
Discussion	Hypertrophic cardiomyopathy (HCM) or hypertrophic obstructive cardiomyopathy (HOCM) is the end result of cardiac myocytes hypertrophy to the point of impairment of the LV outflow tract. This can result in reduced cardiac output and subsequent syncope. The disorganized myocyte array also predisposes these patients to ventricular arrhythmias and sudden death. Most cases are familial with autosomal dominant inheritance and mutations in genes encoding sarcomeric proteins (myosin binding protein C and β-myosin heavy chain). HOCM is differentiated from HCM by an increased gradient of the left ventricular outflow tract (LVOT) and systolic anterior motion of the mitral valve. HCM is concentric LVH that results from conditions such as from chronic hypertension, Pompe disease (a glycogen storage disorder), and Friedreich ataxia. Classically, the systolic murmur of HOCM decreases when the patient goes from standing to sitting, which is the opposite effect of aortic stenosis. Diagnosis of HCOM is primarily made by imaging, which will show the asymmetric septal hypertrophy, particularly in a patient without hypertension. While competitive sports should be avoided, moderate-intensity exercise training has been shown to be safe and associated with an improvement in exertional capacity. Surgery or septal ablation is aimed to treat syncope, and an implantable cardioverter defibrillator (ICD) may be indicated in high risk patients.
	Congenital long QT syndrome is a group of inheritable (most often autosomal dominant) channelopathies that cause prolongation of the QT interval by alterations in the cardiac potassium, sodium, or calcium channels. These patients often present with aborted sudden cardiac death during sporting events (similar to HOCM).
	A long QT increases the potential for polymorphic ventricular tachycardia (**torsades de pointes**) and can result in sudden cardiac death. Characteristic ECG findings for torsades include prolonged QTc and polymorphic ventricular tachycardia with twisting QRS ("twisting of peaks"). Prolonged QT can also be acquired due to medications (e.g., macrolide/fluoroquinolone antibiotics and psychiatric medications), electrolyte abnormalities, or structural heart disease. Family screening is warranted to evaluate risk of sudden cardiac death in relatives.
	Brugada syndrome is an autosomal dominant genetic disorder with variable expression affecting sodium channels and is characterized by an abnormal ECG pattern in conjunction with an increased risk of ventricular arrhythmias and sudden cardiac death. It is more common in male than in female patients, especially of Asian descent. The abnormal rhythms may occur in the setting of fever or rest. The diagnosis is typically made in adulthood. ECG shows a pseudo-right-bundle branch block with "coved" ST segment elevation in V1–V3.

CASE 23 | Heart Block (Third-Degree AV Block)

A 70-year-old man with coronary artery disease presents for evaluation after experiencing sudden loss of consciousness. He feels very lightheaded and fatigued. He reports that the last thing he remembered was standing up and then waking up on the floor. He did not bite his tongue or lose control of his bladder or bowel. The episode was witnessed by his son, who did not notice any abnormal motor movements. On exam, his vital signs are as follows: temperature is 37.0°C, pulse is 30/min, blood pressure is 85/65 mmHg, and respirations are 16/min. Cardiac exam is notable for bradycardia. His neurologic exam is normal.

Evaluation/Tests	ECG shows bradycardia and complete atrial and ventricular dissociation (no correspondence between P waves and QRS complexes). Labs including BMP, CBC, LFTs, TSH, troponin were normal. CXR and echocardiogram were normal.
Treatment	Treatment is aimed at restoring cardiac output by increasing the heart rate with either atropine or electrical cardiac pacing. Discontinue any medications that may cause bradycardia and treat any underlying etiology.

CASE 23 | Heart Block (Third-Degree AV Block) *(continued)*

Discussion	Complete heart block or third-degree atrioventricular (AV) block indicates that there is no conduction between the atria and the ventricles. When this occurs, the atria and ventricles beat independently and cause decreased cardiac output, which can lead to syncope and cardiogenic shock. Complete heart block can occur following MI with infarction of the AV node (supplied by the posterior descending artery), in advanced cardiomyopathy, infiltrative disease affecting the conduction system such as sarcoidosis and amyloidosis, myocarditis (especially Lyme disease), electrolyte abnormalities such as hyperkalemia, hypothyroidism, or unopposed high vagal tone. **Sinus node dysfunction** is a common disorder in the elderly and is caused by normal aging of the sinus node or surrounding tissue, causing delayed conduction to the ventricles. It typically presents with fatigue, syncope/presyncope, or intermittent palpitations. Severity of symptoms correlates with the rate of the underlying escape rhythm (junctional or ventricular). ECG would show sinus bradycardia with intermittent pauses. Treat with a permanent pacemaker. Individuals with **first-degree AV block** and **second-degree AV block (Mobitz I/Wenkebach)** are usually asymptomatic and require no treatment. **Second degree-Mobitz II** may progress to third-degree block and therefore should be treated with a pacemaker.

Key Electrocardiogram Findings and AV Blocks

ECG Findings	AV Blocks
PR interval prolonged > 200 msec	First-degree AV block
PR progressively gets longer, then QRS "dropped"	Second-degree AV block (Mobitz I/Wenckebach)
Dropped QRS not preceded by PR lengthening	Second-degree AV block (Mobitz II)
P and QRS not in rhythm, more Ps than QRS	Third-degree AV block/complete heart block

SHOCK

Shock occurs when there is organ underperfusion from circulatory failure; it is an emergent condition and can lead to death without immediate treatment. At a cellular level, shock induces a state of tissue hypoxia due to either decreased oxygen delivery and/or increased oxygen consumption. The effects of shock are initially reversible but can become irreversible and, if untreated, can lead to multiorgan failure and death. Types of shock include hypovolemic, cardiogenic, obstructive, and distributive. Clinical features suggestive of shock include hypotension, tachycardia, oliguria, altered mental status, tachypnea, cool clammy skin, metabolic acidosis, and lactic acidosis. Treatments vary for each type of shock, so a correct diagnosis is important. For example, fluids are detrimental to cardiogenic shock but are the most important initial treatment in hypovolemic shock. (See the "Pharmacology" chapter for additional cases.)

History and exam help to differentiate between the different types of shock.

In cardiogenic shock, cardiac output (CO) decreases, and systemic vascular resistance increases (SVR). Due to pump failure, fluid backup occurs, and preload and left end diastolic volume are increased. An echocardiogram can reveal poor cardiac function. Invasive testing for diagnosis is not routinely done, but a right heart catheterization can help distinguish between different types of shock. A high pulmonary capillary wedge pressure (PCWP) correlating with elevated preload would suggest cardiogenic shock, while a low/normal PCWP would suggest hypovolemic/septic shock. A low mixed venous blood (MVO_2 or SvO_2) and central venous ($ScvO_2$) measurements suggest cardiogenic shock, while high levels suggest septic shock. Due to leaky vessels and swelling, the tissue is not able to extract oxygen as well in the periphery, so mixed venous blood is higher in sepsis and anaphylaxis.

Septic shock is a type of vasodilatory/distributive shock. Initially, the systemic vascular resistance is low; in order to compensate, the cardiac output is increased. If not optimally treated, it eventually decreases. The PCWP is initially normal, and there is usually no pulmonary congestion. Obtaining cultures from different sources (blood, urine, sputum) and focused imaging should be done and broad-spectrum antibiotics initiated. Once an organism is identified, treatment can be tailored appropriately. When fluid resuscitation fails to improve the clinical status, vasopressors and inotropic support should be considered. Laboratory values, including a lactic acid level (a surrogate for organ hypoperfusion), CBC, BMP, and inflammatory markers (ESR/CRP), are important initial tests.

Treatment involves managing the underlying cause of shock. For septic shock, antibiotics and volume resuscitation are needed. For cardiogenic shock, treatment involves inotropic support and diuresis. For anaphylactic shock, steroids and epinephrine are used. For certain types of shock, vasopressors or vasoactive agents are used.

Differential Diagnoses for Shock

Cardiogenic Shock	Obstructive Shock	Distributive Shock	Hypovolemic Shock
Acute MI Heart failure Valvular dysfunction Arrhythmia	Cardiac tamponade Cor pulmonale Pulmonary embolus Air embolism Fat embolism Amniotic fluid embolism Tension pneumothorax	Sepsis Anaphylaxis CNS injury	Dehydration Hemorrhage Burns

Types of Shock and Key Findings

Diagnosis	Key Findings	CO	SVR	PCWP (preload)
Septic shock	Fever, infectious symptoms, warm extremities	Increased initially, later decreased	↓	Normal/↓
Cardiogenic shock	Chest pain, edema, cool extremities	↓	↑	↑
Anaphylactic shock	Known allergen exposure, recent medication ingestion, bee stings, facial swelling, hives, wheezing	↑	↓	Normal/↓
Hemorrhagic shock	H/O trauma, bleeding, melena	↓	↑	↓

CASE 24 | Septic Shock

A 64-year-old woman with diabetes is brought to the emergency room with confusion. Ten days ago, she developed a productive cough, fever, and chills. On exam, her vital signs are as follows: temperature is 39°C, blood pressure is 70/40 mmHg, pulse is 120/min, respirations are 24/min, and SPO_2 is 80% on high-flow nasal cannula. She is not oriented to time or place. She has dry mucous membranes and labored breathing with appreciable crackles at the right lung base. Her jugular veins are flat, and the rest of her exam is normal.

Evaluation/Tests	WBC, BUN, creatinine and lactate levels are elevated. Blood sugars and troponin levels are normal. CXR shows a right lobar pneumonia, and ECG shows sinus tachycardia. Blood cultures are pending.
Treatment	Treat with IVFs and broad-spectrum antibiotics until the causative organism is identified. Maintain blood pressure (sometimes requires IV pressor medications, such as norepinephrine, vasopressin, or dopamine) and oxygen saturation levels above 88–92%.
Discussion	Septic shock is a life-threatening condition of circulatory failure from disorganized and hyperacute inflammatory response that most commonly manifests as hypotension and altered mental status. Empiric antibiotics administered within 1 hour improve survival. Efforts to determine and treat the source of infection should be immediately undertaken. In **cardiogenic shock,** expect to see signs and symptoms of heart failure such as JVD, bilateral lung crackles and edema, abnormal ECG, or elevated cardiac enzymes. If tamponade or HF is suspected, an echocardiogram should be obtained.

MISCELLANEOUS CASES

CASE 25 | Primary (Essential) Hypertension (HTN)

A 45-year-old man presents for routine health maintenance. He is feeling well and has no complaints. Three months ago at a walk-in clinic, his blood pressure was noted to be 150/88 mmHg. On exam, his vital signs are temperature 36.2°C, pulse 75/min, blood pressure 150/80 mmHg, and respirations 14/min. The rest of his physical exam is normal.

Evaluation/Tests	Urinalysis (UA), ECG, BMP, lipids, glucose are normal.
Treatment	Initial treatment consists of lifestyle modification that includes exercise, DASH diet (Dietary Approaches to Stop Hypertension), limiting salt and alcohol intake, and medication therapy. First-line medications include thiazide diuretics, dihydropyridine calcium channel blockers, ACEi, or ARBs. Beta-blockers are considered second-line therapy.
Discussion	Essential hypertension is a common disorder. A minimum of two readings over 4 weeks apart of >140/90 mmHg is needed to make the diagnosis. UA, ECG, BMP, lipids, and glucose should be done to assess for end organ damage and to assess overall cardiovascular risk. Further testing may be indicated to evaluate for secondary causes such as pheochromocytoma and hyperaldosteronism. **White coat hypertension** manifests as elevated blood pressure readings in a clinical setting but normal values outside of this setting. It should be confirmed with ambulatory blood pressure monitoring. **Secondary causes of hypertension** should be suspected in patients presenting at a very young or old age or presenting with resistant or accelerating hypertension. Causes include Cushing disease, hyperaldosteronism, pheochromocytoma, obstructive sleep apnea, renal artery stenosis, and coarctaction of the aorta. **Primary hyperaldosteronism** is a common cause of secondary hypertension; clues to look for would be a young patient with hypertension and hypokalemia.
Additional Considerations	**Aortic coarctation** is a severe narrowing of the descending aorta, typically near the insertion of the ductus arteriosus immediately after the left subclavian artery branch. In severe cases, infants can present with severe LV failure and shock after the closure of the ductus arteriosus. In adults, coarctation presents with claudication during exercise, unequal pulses, and difficult–to-control hypertension. It can also present with stroke, aortic dissection, heart failure or endocarditis. Susceptible patients include those with a bicuspid aortic valve and Turner syndrome.

CASE 26 | Peripheral Arterial Disease (PAD)

A 65-year-old man with diabetes, hypertension, tobacco use, and coronary artery disease presents with exertional bilateral calf pain for 9 months. The pain usually resolves with rest. On exam, he has no edema in his legs but has diminished dorsalis pedis pulses bilaterally and hair loss on both legs up to his mid-calf circumferentially.

Evaluation/Tests	Ankle-brachial index (ABI) <0.5.
Treatment	Smoking cessation, antiplatelets, statins, and exercise.
Discussion	The most common manifestation of peripheral arterial disease is claudication, which is described by patients as leg cramping on exertion. It is typically relieved with rest. A noninvasive tool to evaluate a patient with claudication is the ankle-brachial index (ABI). Blood pressure is measured in the ankle (AP) and arm (brachial) (BP) and a ratio AP/BP is calculated. A score >0.9 is normal. A score <0.40 indicates severe obstruction. Angiography is used to guide revascularization strategies. A PDE inhibitor, cilostazol, can increase walking distance and reduce symptoms but is contraindicated in patients with LV dysfunction. PAD is due to longstanding atherosclerotic vascular disease (chronic buildup of cholesterol within the arterial wall). It is accelerated by vascular damage from smoking, hypertension, and diabetes and can occur in any vascular bed from cerebrovascular causing stroke, coronary resulting in MI, intestinal causing mesenteric ischemia, or abdominal aorta causing an aneurysm. Surgical or endovascular revascularization is indicated for patients with lifestyle-limiting symptoms despite medical therapy. Patients with spinal stenosis or osteoarthritis may present with lower extremity pain but would not have diminished pulses.

CASE 27 | Ruptured Abdominal Aortic Aneurysm (AAA)

A 67-year-old man, with diabetes, hypertension, tobacco use, and coronary artery disease, presents with sudden, severe lower abdominal pain radiating to the back and buttocks. On exam, his vital signs are temperature 37.0°C, pulse 125/min, blood pressure 90/50 mmHg, and respirations 16/min. His abdomen is very tender, and a pulsatile mass is palpable in the epigastric area. There is ecchymosis around the umbilicus (Cullen's sign). He has no costovertebral angle tenderness, but there is ecchymoses on his back and abdominal flanks (Grey Turner's sign).

Evaluation/Tests	Abdominal ultrasound shows increased diameter of the abdominal aorta.
Treatment	Surgical or endovascular repair.
Discussion	This patient's triad of abdominal pain, hypotension, and palpable pulsatile mass indicates ruptured AAA and requires emergent surgical repair. Abdominal aortic aneurysm is the expansion of the lumen and dilation of the wall of the aorta (normal diameter of infrarenal aorta is ~2 cm). Risk factors include smoking, increasing age, male sex, and family history (atherosclerotic risk factors). Most AAAs are without symptoms and are found incidentally or during screening of high-risk patients. Symptomatic patients may have impending rupture, which can quickly result in death.

VASCULITIDES

Vasculitis is the inflammation of blood vessels, either as a primary disease or secondary to an underlying condition. Vasculitis should be on the differential when multiple organs are involved and the patient has systemic symptoms such as fevers, malaise, and weight loss. Important history questions to ask include a history of HIV, hepatitis, endocarditis, drug abuse (cocaine), and previous thrombotic events. On physical exam, pay close attention to the organs involved and look for rashes, ulcers, asymmetrical pulses, and/or bruits. Important initial tests include erythrocyte sedimentation rate (ESR), C-reactive protein (CRP), CBC, BMP (renal function), and urinalysis (UA).

Large-vessel vasculitides include giant cell temporal arteritis (GCA) and Takayasu arteritis. Medium-vessel vasculitides include polyarteritis nodosa (PAN), Kawasaki disease, and thromboangiitis obliterans. Small-vessel vasculitides include granulomatosis with polyangiitis (formerly called Wegener's), eosinophilic granulomatosis with polyangiitis, microscopic polyangiitis, Behçet syndrome, and IgA vasculitis. Mimickers of vasculitis include cancers, infections (endocarditis, hepatitis, sepsis), coagulopathies (DIC, TTP, antiphospholipid antibody syndrome), and cholesterol emboli.

ANCA-associated Vasculitides and Lab Tests

Vasculitides	Tests
Granulomatosis with polyangiitis (GPA) (Wegener)	cANCA, antiproteinase 3 (PR3)
Microscopic polyangiitis (MPA)	pANCA, antimyeloperoxidase (MPO)
Eosinophilic granulomatosis with polyangiitis (Churg-Strauss)	pANCA, anti-MPO, elevated IgE, eosinophilia

CASE 28 | Giant Cell (Temporal) Arteritis (GCA)

A 72-year-old woman with polymyalgia rheumatica presents with right-sided headache and blurry vision for 3–4 days. She also reports pain with chewing. She has chronic bilateral shoulder and hip pain with morning stiffness and recent weight loss. On exam, she has a low-grade fever, decreased visual acuity of her right eye, and funduscopic exam shows white pallor and edema of the optic disc. Her right temporal artery is tender with reduced pulsations. She has no dental caries or tenderness over her temporomandibular joint (TMJ).

Evaluation/Tests	ESR > 100 mm/h. Definitive diagnosis is achieved with temporal artery biopsy, which will show focal, segmental granulomatous inflammation.
Treatment	Prednisone.
Discussion	Giant cell arteritis (GCA), also known as temporal arteritis, is the most common primary vasculitis characterized by inflammation of the branches of the carotid artery. Affected arteries may include external carotids, temporal, ciliary, ophthalmic, and subclavian and its branches. GCA is more common in Caucasians and women >50 years old. **Temporal arteritis** should be considered in patients presenting with temporal or other atypical headaches, visual changes, or jaw claudication. Patients with GCA may also report scalp pain, headaches, and tenderness over the temporal artery. These symptoms are usually unilateral. Other complications include forearm ischemia if the brachial artery is involved, aortic

CASE 28 | **Giant Cell (Temporal) Arteritis (GCA)** *(continued)*

Discussion	aneurysm, and aortic dissection. Systemic symptoms are common and include weight loss, malaise, and low-grade fevers. An important lab finding is an elevated ESR or CRP. Thirty to fifty percent of patients with GCA have concurrent **polymyalgia rheumatic (PMR)**. PMR presents with symptoms of symmetric pain and stiffness in shoulder, neck, and hip regions. If PMR is diagnosed, it is important to inquire about GCA symptoms because untreated GCA can cause permanent blindness. Patients with **rheumatoid arthritis** would have symmetric joint swelling/pain. Patients with dental caries or temporomandibular joint syndrome (**TMJ**) or **migraine** headache do not present with visual changes and inflammation.

CASE 29 | Polyarteritis Nodosa (PAN)

A 53-year-old man with hepatitis B and hypertension presents with a 3-month history of abdominal pain, unintentional weight loss of 10 pounds, arthralgia, malaise, headaches, and low-grade fevers. He also notices decreased sensation on the lateral aspect of his right calf. On exam, his vital signs are as follows: temperature 38.4°C, pulse 85/min, blood pressure 160/95 mmHg, and respirations 20/min. He has a reddish-blue lace-like skin discoloration (livedo reticularis) on his forearms, and abdominal exam is nontender, but a bruit is heard in the LUQ. His elbow and knee joints are tender to palpation, but no synovitis or crepitus is noted, and there is decreased sensation over the right calf.

Evaluation/Tests	Abdominal angiogram shows microaneurysms and spasms of the mesenteric and renal arteries. CBC: WBCs at 14, Hgb 10.9, platelets 120,000; ESR: elevated and BMP with elevated BUN; creatinine, ANCA, and hep C are negative. IgA, complement levels, and urinalysis are normal.
Treatment	Steroids and cyclophosphamide.
Discussion	PAN affects medium and small-sized arteries, resulting in arterial inflammation and narrowing that can lead to aneurysms and microaneurysms. There is an association with hepatitis B and other infections, but most cases are idiopathic. The affected organs typically include the kidneys, GI tract (especially mesenteric artery and small intestine), peripheral nervous system, and skin. If the renal arteries are involved, there can be a decrease in GFR and hypertension (diastolic pressures usually above 90 mmHg due to decreased renal artery flow and increased RAAS activation). Renal manifestations are not due to glomerulonephritis. Abdominal manifestations are very common, and a history of chronic or intermittent ischemic pain (pain after eating) is often reported. Neurological manifestations include mononeuritis multiplex (painful, asymmetric peripheral neuropathy). Skin manifestations include livedo reticularis, purpura, and painful subcutaneous nodules. Arteriogram of affected organs show microaneurysm and vascular spasm. Diagnosis often requires pathology; resection showing transmural inflammation of the arterial wall with fibrinoid necrosis. Mortality is high and requires aggressive treatment with IV steroids and cyclophosphamide. The key to differentiating PAN from other vasculitis or **Goodpasture syndrome** is the lack of glomerulonephritis (normal UA). The lungs are unaffected, unlike in Goodpasture syndrome. **Henoch-Schoenlein purpura (HSP)** can present very similarly, but it is an immune complex disease affecting small vessels resulting in low complements and elevated IgA levels, and urine sediment is present.

CASE 30 | Kawasaki Disease

A 3-year-old boy is brought to clinic for evaluation of high fevers, decrease in appetite, malaise, and rash. He had no complications at birth, vaccinations are up to date, and there have been no known sick contacts. On exam, he is very irritable and clings to his mother, and his vital signs are temperature of 39°C, pulse of 148/min, blood pressure of 85/55 mmHg, and SPO$_2$ of 94% on room air. Bilateral conjunctival injection, a strawberry tongue, dry mucous membranes, and cracked red lips are present. He has an extensive erythematous rash with desquamation, involving both palms and soles and his groin. His hands and feet are swollen, and he has nontender anterior cervical lymphadenopathy bilaterally. He is tachycardic, but no murmurs are heard, and the rest of his exam is normal.

Evaluation/Tests	Clinical diagnosis. CBC shows anemia, leukocytosis, and thrombocytosis. Viral panel and blood cultures are negative. AST, ALT, and creatinine are elevated. ECHO may be normal and ECG may show sinus tachycardia
Treatment	IV immunoglobulin and aspirin.

CASE 30 | Kawasaki Disease *(continued)*

Discussion	Kawasaki disease (KD) is a mucocutaneous lymph node syndrome, which presents as acute necrotizing vasculitis of the medium and small-sized vessels. It can cause coronary artery disease in children. Affected patients are usually <5 years old, male, and Asian or black. There is a seasonal predominance with peaks occurring in late winter-spring, suggesting a possible underlying infectious trigger. Diagnosis of KD is clinical, as there are no specific tests. Diagnostic criteria include persistent fever >5 days; oral changes including injected pharynx or lips, cracked or fissured lips, strawberry tongue, conjunctivitis, polymorphous rash; erythema and induration of hands and/or feet seen in acute phase; periungual desquamation; and cervical lymphadenopathy. Coronary artery damage, which can present as aneurysm, calcification, or stenosis, is the most serious complication. Systemic inflammation of other organs can also occur, such as meningitis, myocarditis (resulting in heart failure), pericardial effusions, and pericarditis and valvular vegetations. **Scarlet fever** is caused by *Streptococcus* infection, and patients tend to have tender lymphadenopathy; the rash has tiny papillae ("sandpaper rash"). Potential complications include glomerulonephritis. Measles or other infections are unlikely as viral panel and blood cultures are negative.

CASE 31 | Granulomatosis with Polyangiitis (GPA)

A 55-year-old man with chronic sinusitis presents with hemoptysis for the past 3 days. He has noted some weight loss, generalized arthralgia, epistaxis, and occasional hematuria and difficulty hearing. He has never smoked, he has never traveled outside the US, and he works as an office manager. On exam, he is tachypneic and has a fever and bilateral maxillary sinus tenderness and diffuse crackles on lung exam.

Evaluation/Tests	Lung biopsy shows necrotizing granulomas and focal necrotizing vasculitis. A CBC shows WBC of 13,000/mm³ (<2% eosinophils), Hb of 11.4 g/dL, and a platelet count of 500,000/mm³. ESR is 105 mm/h. Creatinine is elevated. c-ANCA/anti-PR3 is positive. Urine analysis is positive for hematuria and red cell casts and proteinuria. CXR shows diffuse nodular opacities.
Treatment	Treatment consists of high-dose glucocorticoids and cyclophosphamide for 6 months. After 6 months, maintenance therapy includes methotrexate, azathioprine, or mycophenolate mofetil.
Discussion	Granulomatosis with polyangiitis (formerly known as Wegener's granulomatosis) is the most common ANCA-positive vasculitis. It typically affects middle-aged to older patients with northern European predominance. Affected organs include the upper respiratory tract (including nose, sinuses, and ears), lungs, skin, and kidneys. Patients can present with sinus pain, rhinitis, epistaxis, and, from long-term inflammation, cartilage damage and collapse (saddle nose deformity). Eustachian tube dysfunction can lead to hearing loss. Inflammation in the trachea can lead to airway stenosis and obstruction. Ocular inflammation may result in impaired vision. Skin manifestations include painful cutaneous nodules, palpable purpura, and urticarial and ulcerative lesions. Patients with lung involvement may present with lung nodules or infiltrates, as well as hemoptysis from diffuse alveolar hemorrhage. Lung biopsy is the most diagnostic because both vasculitis and necrotizing granulomas will be noted (presence of both is characteristic of GPA). Kidney dysfunction can result from rapidly progressive crescentic glomerulonephritis. Biopsy would show crescent moon–shaped deposits in the glomeruli. Kidney biopsy is high yield if kidney involvement is present but may show only vasculitis; however, in the setting of clinical symptoms (classic upper airway manifestations, pulmonary infiltrates/nodules, and urinary abnormalities consistent with glomerulonephritis) and positive c-ANCA/anti-PR3 serology, the diagnosis can be made. **Microscopic polyangiitis** is associated with p-ANCA and typically does not have nasopharyngeal involvement.

CASE 32 | Eosinophilic Granulomatosis with Polyangiitis (EGPA)

A 51-year-old man with poorly controlled asthma presents with 3 weeks of progressive shortness of breath and new onset hemoptysis. Over the past week, he noted a rash on his extremities and weakness in his left leg. On exam, his vital signs are temperature of 38.3°C, pulse of 94/min, blood pressure of 136/85 mmHg, and respirations 30/min. He has diffuse lung crackles bilaterally and decreased sensation of the left leg. His extremities are covered with raised nonblanching palpable erythematous lesions (palpable purpura) on lower extremities.

CASE 32 | **Eosinophilic Granulomatosis with Polyangiitis (EGPA)** *(continued)*

Evaluation/Tests	Tissue biopsy shows necrotizing vasculitis with eosinophilic infiltrates. CBC shows hypereosinophilia and elevated ESR and CRP. BMP and urinalysis (UA) are normal. CXR shows patchy focal bilateral infiltrates.
Treatment	Treatment of mild or limited EGPA includes glucocorticoids alone. In severe disease, glucocorticoids plus cyclophosphamide is preferred, followed by maintenance therapy with less toxic immunosuppressing agents.
Discussion	Eosinophilic granulomatosis with polyangiitis (formerly known as Churg-Strauss syndrome) is the rarest ANCA-associated vasculitis. Strong association exists with asthma and eosinophilia. Patients with EGPA will often have a history of allergic rhinitis, nasal polyps, or asthma. Lung involvement is common; patients may present with hemoptysis and migratory infiltrates on CXR. Peripheral neuropathy may occur as well. Skin involvement is common and presents with purpuric skin rash due to inflammation of the blood vessels. Typically, ANCA-positive patients will display p-ANCA/anti-MPO patterns. However, 40% of patients will be ANCA negative; thus, a negative ANCA test should not eliminate EGPA diagnosis. Kidney disease is less common than other ANCA vasculitides, so UA and creatinine are typically normal.

8

Endocrinology

Farheen Dojki, MD
Claudia Boucher-Berry, MD

Hypothalamic-Pituitary Disorders
1. Cushing Disease (ACTH-Secreting Pituitary Adenoma)
2. Hyperprolactinemia
3. Pituitary Adenoma (Hypopituitarism)
4. Acromegaly
5. Central Diabetes Insipidus
6. Syndrome of Inappropriate Antidiuretic Hormone

Adrenal Gland Disorders
7. Congenital Adrenal Hyperplasia (21-Hydoxylase Deficiency)
8. Cushing Syndrome (Exogenous Corticosteroids)
9. Primary Hyperaldosteronism (Conn's Syndrome)
10. Primary Adrenal Insufficiency (Addison Disease)
11. Pheochromocytoma
12. Neuroblastoma

Thyroid Disorders
Hyperthyroidism
13. Graves' Disease
Hypothyroidism
14. Hashimoto Thyroiditis

Thyroid Enlargement/Mass
15. Papillary Thyroid Cancer
Parathyroid Disorders
Hyperparathyroidism
16. Primary Hyperparathyroidism
Hypoparathyroidism
17. Hypoparathyroidism
18. Pseudohypoparathyroidism
Pancreatic Endocrine Disorders
19. Hypoglycemia
20. Type 1 Diabetes Mellitus
21. Type 2 Diabetes Mellitus
22. Diabetic Ketoacidosis
23. Hyperosmolar Hyperglycemic State
Neuroendocrine Tumors
24. Carcinoid Syndrome
25. Multiple Endocrine Neoplasia Type 1

The endocrine system consists of multiple organs throughout the body that are connected through hormonal pathways. Disorders of the endocrine system arise from states of excess or deficiency of hormones. The underlying cause of a hormonal excess or deficiency can be multifactorial. For instance, disruption of the hypothalamic-pituitary-adrenal (HPA) axis can occur due to chronic high-dose steroids, infections, brain injury, or cancers. Endocrine tumors can be nonfunctioning, or they can cause an increase or decrease in hormone secretion of the affected gland. They can be caused by spontaneous mutations, or they can be associated with familial syndromes such as multiple endocrine neoplasm (MEN).

Symptoms associated with endocrine disorders are nonspecific and often vague. Additionally, there is significant interaction between the different hormones in the endocrine system such that an excess of one hormone can produce deficiency of another hormone, and, as a result, the patient may experience symptoms of both conditions. Therefore, it is important to obtain a complete, detailed history. On physical exam, it is important to note blood pressure, heart rate, and volume status (mucous membrane, skin turgor, and orthostatic blood pressure). Papilledema on fundoscopic exam and visual field defects such as bitemporal hemianopsia (absence of the outer half of both the right and left visual fields) may indicate a pituitary lesion. The thyroid gland should be assessed for goiter or any masses. Abdominal exam may detect masses; skin exam may reveal hyperpigmentation (reflecting elevated ACTH seen in adrenal insufficiency) or acanthosis nigricans (reflecting elevated insulin levels). A thorough genitourinary exam and assessment for secondary sexual characteristics may provide valuable clues to a diagnosis. Neuromuscular exam assessing for strength and spasm, sensation, and reflexes can also provide important clues to diagnosis.

In real life and in testing situations, note that scenarios will not be presented as a "pituitary" or "adrenal" problem. Instead, a patient will present with a constellation of symptoms, exam findings, and initial lab abnormalities. Based on the information, the first step is to generate a differential diagnosis (DDx) and to determine the next steps in the evaluation to determine the etiology. For example, symptoms and/or signs of elevated cortisol levels may be due to Cushing disease or Cushing syndrome caused by exogenous steroids or ectopic ACTH secretion.

HYPOTHALAMIC-PITUITARY-ADRENAL (HPA) AXIS DISORDERS

Hypothalamus: Hormones include corticotropin-releasing hormone (CRH), thyrotropin-releasing hormone (TRH), growth hormone–releasing hormone (GHRH), gonadotropin-releasing hormone (GnRH), and dopamine (which inhibits prolactin). Disorders of the hypothalamus will negatively affect the function of the pituitary and the downstream end organs. Clinically, it may be difficult to distinguish if a disorder originated in the hypothalamus or the pituitary.

Pituitary: The pituitary gland is the master gland of the endocrine system, and it is divided into two lobes based on embryologic development. The anterior lobe (adenohypophysis) is derived from an invagination (Rathke's pouch) of oral ectoderm. Anterior lobe hormones include adrenocorticotropic hormone (ACTH or corticotropin), thyroid-stimulating hormone (TSH or thyrotropin), growth hormone (GH or somatotropin), follicle-stimulating hormone (FSH), luteinizing hormone (LH), prolactin, and melanocyte-stimulating hormone (MSH). The posterior lobe (neurohypophysis) is derived from neuroectoderm. Posterior lobe hormones include antidiuretic hormone (ADH, vasopressin, or AVP) and oxytocin.

Whenever the pituitary gland is affected, there is a downstream effect that will cause problems in the other endocrine systems. When the disease process begins in the gland itself, the disorder is referred to as "primary" (i.e., primary adrenal insufficiency suggests that the main problem is within the adrenal gland). When the pituitary is the main cause of the hormone deficiency or excess, then it is called "secondary" (i.e., secondary adrenal insufficiency suggests loss of ACTH from the pituitary gland) or tertiary if the problem is due to impaired regulation from the hypothalamus.

Hyperfunction: Excess pituitary hormone production is usually caused by pituitary adenomas, but it can also be a side effect of certain medications such as atypical antipsychotics.

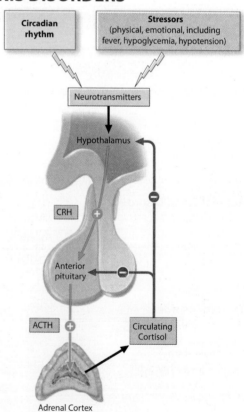

Regulation of the hypothalamic-pituitary-adrenal (HPA) axis. ACTH, adrenocorticotropic hormone; CRH, corticotropin-releasing hormone.
Reproduced with permission from Jameson JL, Fauci AS, Kasper DL, et al: Harrison's Principles of Internal Medicine, 20th ed. New York, NY: McGraw Hill; 2018.

Hypofunction (hypopituitarism): Deficiency of pituitary hormones is usually due to a central nervous system (CNS) tumor (e.g., craniopharyngioma) or a nonfunctional pituitary adenoma that invades and occupies the sella turcica. Acute cases of hypopituitarism can occur in pregnant women who experience postpartum bleeding (Sheehan syndrome) or sudden hemorrhage of the pituitary gland (pituitary apoplexy). Other causes of hypopituitarism include pituitary agenesis or dysgenesis, trauma, surgery, medications, infections, and other cancers.

Adrenal: The adrenal cortex secretes three main categories of steroids: mineralocorticoids, glucocorticoids, and androgens. The adrenal medulla secretes catecholamines.

Hyperfunction: Adrenal hormones may be overproduced due to an adrenal tumor or an error in hormone biosynthesis.

Hypofunction (adrenal insufficiency): In primary adrenal insufficiency, cortisol is low because there is decreased activity of the adrenal gland due to an autoimmune phenomenon (Addison disease), genetic disorder in hormonal biosynthesis, surgery, or infection. As a result of low cortisol levels, ACTH levels will be high; therefore, patients will present with symptoms of adrenal insufficiency and increased skin pigmentation. In secondary adrenal insufficiency, ACTH levels are low, leading to absent or low cortisol secretion. Aldosterone secretion will be normal in secondary adrenal insufficiency because aldosterone secretion is stimulated by renin and potassium, not ACTH.

Hormone Excess or Deficiency and Presenting Signs and Symptoms

Hormone	Excess/Deficiency	Symptoms/Signs	DDx
Cortisol	Excess	Hypertension, hyperglycemia excessive weight gain, truncal obesity, buffalo hump, abdominal striae, bruising, decreased linear growth in children, proximal muscle weakness	Exogenous steroids Pituitary hypersecretion (Cushing disease) Paraneoplastic ACTH secretion (small cell lung cancer, carcinoid) Cushing syndrome
	Deficiency	Hypotension, hypoglycemia, anorexia, weight loss, abdominal pain, fatigue, decreased libido, hyperpigmentation (primary adrenal insufficiency)	Hypopituitarism (craniopharyngioma, pituitary adenoma, infections, Sheehan syndrome, traumatic brain injury, cancers (primary or metastatic) Addison disease Adrenoleukodystrophy Autoimmune polyglandular syndromes Waterhouse-Friderichsen syndrome Abrupt discontinuation of chronic exogenous steroid use
Growth hormone (GH)	Excess	*Gigantism:* Rapid growth *Acromegaly:* Large tongue, jaw prognathism, frontal bossing, diaphoresis, large hands and feet Hyperglycemia	GH secreting pituitary adenoma *Gigantism* (GH excess occurs before growth plates close) *Acromegaly* (GH excess occurs after growth plates close)
	Deficiency	Short stature Hypoglycemia Micropenis in male infants	Hypopituitarism
Prolactin	Excess	Menstrual irregularities, infertility Decreased libido Galactorrhea	Prolactinoma (most common) Drug-induced hyperprolactinemia (e.g., antipsychotics) Breast-feeding (delayed postpartum ovulation to prevent pregnancy) Chronic diseases (e.g., hypothyroidism, liver or kidney disease)
	Deficiency	Impaired lactation	

(continued)

Hormone Excess or Deficiency and Presenting Signs and Symptoms (*continued*)

Hormone	Excess/Deficiency	Symptoms/Signs	DDx
Thyroid	Excess	Sweating, palpitations, tachycardia, arrhythmias, systolic hypertension, Hyperactivity, diarrhea, weight loss, Weakness, fatigue, insomnia, Decreased libido, infertility, Menstrual irregularity	Primary hyperthyroidism: Graves' disease Toxic adenoma Thyroiditis Iodine induced hyperthyroidism Secondary hyperthyroidism: TSH-secreting pituitary adenoma (extremely rare)
	Deficiency	Infants/children: Widened anterior fontanelle, jaundice, macroglossia, hypothermia, umbilical hernia/abdominal distention, developmental delay, poor linear growth, delayed puberty Children/adults: Hair loss, dry skin, brittle nails, cold intolerance, weight gain, bradycardia, fatigue, depression, constipation, decreased libido, irregular menses/ Amenorrhea, puffy face, Proximal muscle weakness, nonpitting edema, Periorbital edema	Primary hypothyroidism: Iodine deficiency Congenital hypothyroidism Autoimmune hypothyroidism (Hashimoto thyroiditis) Postpartum thyroiditis Subacute granulomatous thyroiditis Riedel thyroiditis Secondary hypothyroidism: Hypopituitarism
Vasopressin (ADH)	Excess	Hyponatremia symptoms: Nausea, headache, altered mental status	Syndrome of inappropriate antidiuretic hormone secretion (SIADH) Paraneoplastic ADH secretion (small cell lung cancer)
	Deficiency	Polydipsia, polyuria including nocturia	Central diabetes insipidus (DI) Nephrogenic DI
Androgens	Excess	Females: Increased male pattern body hair (chin, chest, back) and hair loss (central, temporal), acne, early pubic/axillary hair development, clitoromegaly, irregular menses, deepened voice Males: In pediatrics, increased penile length, early pubic/ axillary hair development	Congenital adrenal hyperplasia due to 21-hydroxylase deficiency Premature adrenarche Adrenal tumor Exogenous androgen exposure FSH or LH-secreting pituitary adenomas (rare)
	Deficiency	Delayed puberty Micropenis in male infants Menstrual irregularity Decreased libido, infertility Decreased pubic/axillary hair	Hypogonadotropic hypogonadism (if associated with loss of sense of smell, Kallman syndrome (decreased GnRH from hypothalamus)) Congenital adrenal hyperplasia due to 17-α-hydroxylase deficiency

(*continued*)

Hormone Excess or Deficiency and Presenting Signs and Symptoms (*continued*)

Hormone	Excess/Deficiency	Symptoms/Signs	DDx
Aldosterone	Excess	Hypertension, hypokalemia	Adrenal aldosterone–producing adenoma (Conn's syndrome) Congenital adrenal hyperplasia due to 17-α- or 11β-hydroxylase deficiency Syndrome of apparent mineralocorticoid excess (e.g., black licorice ingestion) Renovascular hypertension Juxtaglomerular cell tumors Edema (from cirrhosis, heart failure, nephrotic syndrome) Bilateral adrenal hyperplasia
	Deficiency	Salt craving, hypotension, hyperkalemia, hyponatremia	Primary adrenal insufficiency Renal tubular acidosis type IV Congenital adrenal hyperplasia due to 21-hydroxylase deficiency
Catecholamines	Excess	Hypertension, heart palpitations, headaches, sweating	Pheochromocytoma/paraganglioma
	Deficiency	Catecholamine deficiency is rarely associated with any clinical syndrome.	

Important diagnostic tests may include imaging such as ultrasound, CT, or MRI to evaluate or look for particular lesions. Often, hormone levels are needed to confirm a diagnosis and exclude other differential diagnoses.

Diagnostic Studies to Help Distinguish Causes of Cortisol Excess

Diagnostic Tests	Pituitary Hypersecretion	Ectopic ACTH Secretion	Adrenal Hypersecretion	Exogenous Steroids
Salivary cortisol or 24 h urinary free cortisol	↑	↑	↑	↑
ACTH	↑	↑	↓	↓
Low-dose dexamethasone suppression test: AM cortisol level	↑	↑		
High-dose dexamethasone suppression test: AM cortisol level	↓	↑		
MRI	Pituitary adenoma			

Diagnostic Studies to Help Distinguish Causes of Cortisol Deficiency

Diagnostic Tests	Na⁺/K⁺	AM Cortisol	AM ACTH	ACTH Stimulation Test	Aldosterone/Renin	Hyperpigmentation	21-Hydroxylase Antibodies
Primary adrenal insufficiency	Na⁺ ↓/K⁺ ↑	↓	↑	Abnormal	↓/↑	Yes	Yes
Secondary adrenal insufficiency	Often normal	↓	↓	Abnormal	Normal	No	No

Key Findings and Diagnoses

Key Findings	Diagnoses and (Key Labs)
Metabolic abnormalities (obesity, DM, hyperlipidemia, HTN), easy bruising and fractures, and weight gain. Central obesity with thin extremities and a rounded, plethoric face. Enlarged posterior cervical (buffalo hump) and supraclavicular fat pads, wide violaceous striae along abdomen and axilla. Decreased proximal muscle strength.	Cushing syndrome/disease Exogenous steroid use
Metabolic abnormalities, heart failure, OSA, painful joints, jaw/dental complaints, excessive sweating, and weight gain. Coarse facial features, enlarged tongue, widely spaced teeth, and deep voice; prominent protruding forehead with broad nasal bridge (frontal bossing). Finger and toe thickening, and large hands and feet.	Acromegaly (high GH)
Lethargy, nausea, vomiting, seizure in afebrile, euvolemic patient with low sodium and normal cortisol and TSH.	SIADH (low sodium and low serum osmolality, elevated urine osmolality)
Short stature, delayed puberty or menstrual irregularities, decreased libido, fatigue, cold intolerance, constipation, headaches, and absence of the outer half of both the right and left visual fields (bitemporal hemianopsia)	Hypopituitarism (low cortisol, GH, LH/FSH, and FT4)
Hypotension, nausea, vomiting, abdominal pain, weight loss (+*hyperpigmentation of face and palmar creases*)	Adrenal insufficiency (primary adrenal insufficiency) (low cortisol)
Complicated delivery with hypotension and now persistent hypotension, vomiting, fatigue, and patient not anemic or septic	Sheehan syndrome (low cortisol)
Hypotensive, febrile patient with headache, nausea, vomiting, abdominal pain, mental status changes, neck stiffness, and rash	Meningitis, sepsis, Waterhouse-Friderichsen syndrome
Polyuria, polydipsia, nocturia, bed wetting, normal blood glucose level	Diabetes insipidus (normal-high sodium)
Heat intolerance, sweating, weight loss, increased appetite, diarrhea, menstrual irregularity, anxiety, palpitations, proximal muscle weakness, brisk reflexes, warm moist skin, onycholysis (separation of nail from nail beds), pretibial myxedema (localized nonpitting edema of shins)	Hyperthyroidism (low TSH, high free T4, and high total T3)
Exophthalmos or proptosis (protrusion of the eyeballs), thyroid bruit, and pretibial myxedema are the pathognomonic findings of Graves' disease. Other symptoms and signs of hyperthyroidism will also be present.	Hyperthyroidism–Graves' disease (low TSH, high free T4, and high total T3)
Weight gain, cold intolerance, fatigue and dyspnea on exertion, constipation, menstrual irregularity. Bradycardia, dry, cool skin, coarse brittle hair and nails, generalized nonpitting edema, periorbital edema, proximal muscle weakness, delayed/slow relaxing reflexes	Secondary (central) hypothyroidism (low or normal TSH, and low FT4) Primary hypothyroidism (high TSH and low FT4)
Poorly controlled HTN and low potassium	Hyperaldosteronism (plasma aldosterone concentration/plasma renin activity (PAC/PRA) ratio >30)
Fluctuating high blood pressures, palpitations, sweating, headaches	Pheochromocytoma (high fractionated catecholamines/metanephrines)
Kidney stones, abdominal pain, and bony pain	Primary hyperparathyroidism (high calcium and PTH)
Joint pain, enlarging skull, hearing loss, and elevated alkaline phosphatase	Paget's disease
Tingling of the hands, feet, and mouth; muscle cramps; positive Trousseau's sign (carpal spasm following occlusion of brachial artery with BP cuff); and Chvostek's sign (contraction of facial muscles when tapped rapidly)	Hypoparathyroidism (low PTH and low calcium)

(continued)

Key Findings and Diagnoses (*continued*)

Key Findings	Diagnoses and (Key Labs)
3Ps (pituitary, parathyroid, pancreatic)	MEN 1
Medullary thyroid cancer, pheochromocytoma, primary hyperparathyroidism	MEN 2A
Medullary thyroid cancer, pheochromocytoma, mucosal neuromas	MEN 2B
Polyuria, polydipsia, polyphagia, and elevated blood sugars	Diabetes
Polyuria, polydipsia, polyphagia, weight loss, blurry vision with abdominal pain, mental status changes, hypotension, Kussmaul respirations, fruity breath, anion gap metabolic acidosis, hyperkalemia, elevated blood glucose	Diabetic ketoacidosis

HYPOTHALAMIC-PITUITARY DISORDERS

Pituitary adenomas account for 10% of all intracranial neoplasms. They are benign tumors that can be functional or non-functional. Functional adenomas can secrete pituitary hormones including prolactin, GH, ACTH, and TSH. If the adenoma secretes prolactin, this may result in inappropriate lactation in both men and women. GH secretion may cause acromegaly or gigantism. Nonfunctional adenomas can be asymptomatic, or they can cause mass effect from compression of the hypothalamic-pituitary axis. Patients may present with headache or bitemporal hemianopsia from compression of the optic chiasm. The diagnosis is made by brain MRI and measurement of pituitary hormones, as well as end-organ hormone levels (prolactin, IGF-1, ACTH and cortisol, TSH and free T4, LH/FSH, and estradiol or testosterone). Treatment of pituitary tumors secreting prolactin includes dopamine agonists, such as bromocriptine and cabergoline. Other functional tumors and nonfunctioning pituitary adenomas that cause mass effect require transsphenoidal surgical resection. Pituitary adenoma may also present as part of the MEN1 syndrome, which includes parathyroid and pancreatic neuroendocrine tumors.

Differential Diagnosis for Pituitary Mass

Prolactin, GH, ACTH, or TSH secreting tumor
Nonfunctioning pituitary adenoma
Other tumors (e.g. germ cell, gliomas, metastatic disease)
Granulomatous disease
Abscess
Vascular lesion

CASE 1 | Cushing Disease (ACTH-Secreting Pituitary Adenoma)

A 36-year-old woman with type 2 diabetes mellitus, hypertension, and obesity presents with difficulty losing weight. Despite calorie restriction and increased activity, she has had a 10-pound weight gain over the last 6 months. Her diabetes has progressively worsened, and she now requires insulin therapy for control. She also reports several vaginal yeast infections and easy skin bruising. On exam, her blood pressure is 160/100 mmHg, and she has central obesity with thin extremities and a rounded plethoric face. Posterior cervical and supraclavicular fat pads are enlarged, and wide violaceous striae are visible along the abdomen and axilla.

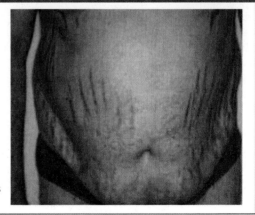

Clinical features of Cushing's syndrome. Note central obesity and abdominal striae.
Reproduced with permission from Jameson JL, Fauci AS, Kasper DL, et al: Harrison's Principles of Internal Medicine, 20th ed. New York, NY: McGraw Hill; 2018.

CASE 1 | Cushing Disease (ACTH-Secreting Pituitary Adenoma) (continued)

Evaluation/Tests	Midnight salivary cortisol levels are elevated. After giving low-dose dexamethasone, AM cortisol remains above 1.8 mcg/dL, and the ACTH level is elevated. MRI brain shows the presence of a mass lesion in the location of the pituitary gland.
Treatment	First line is transsphenoidal pituitary surgery. For refractory cases, bilateral adrenalectomy with lifelong daily glucocorticoid and mineralocorticoid replacement therapy is recommended.
Discussion	This patient is presenting with Cushing disease, which is caused by an ACTH-secreting pituitary adenoma, leading to excess cortisol secretion from the adrenal gland. Cortisol is secreted by the zona fasciculata of the adrenal cortex and plays important roles in the regulation of appetite, blood pressure, insulin resistance, gluconeogenesis, lipolysis, proteolysis, wound healing, inflammatory responses, bone formation, and more. Cortisol secretion from the adrenal cortex is regulated by ACTH from the anterior pituitary, which in turn is regulated by CRH from the hypothalamus. Cushing syndrome is the state of excess cortisol from any cause. Cushing disease is the manifestation of cortisol excess resulting specifically from an ACTH-producing pituitary adenoma. Excess cortisol causes central fat deposition, proximal muscle weakness, metabolic abnormalities (T2DM, HTN, hyperlipidemia), skin thinning, bruising, osteoporosis with fracture, and increased risk of infections. The workup will help differentiate where the excess is coming from. ACTH levels will be high from pituitary hypersecretion or ectopic ACTH secretion. A high-dose dexamethasone suppression test (ACTH will suppress in Cushing disease) can differentiate pituitary ACTH source vs. ectopic source. If the excess cortisol were coming from **exogenous steroids** or a **primary adrenal hypercortisolism**, the patient would have low ACTH levels as feedback loops would go to the brain and inhibit further secretion of ACTH. Because the problem here is within the brain itself (at the level of the pituitary), this level of regulation is lost, so ACTH levels are elevated despite elevated cortisol. Given the patient's lack of history of cancer, lack of other concerning symptoms, and brain MRI showing a lesion in the pituitary, **paraneoplastic ACTH secretion** (such as from small cell lung cancer) is less likely.
Additional Considerations	**Nelson syndrome** is an enlargement of a preexisting ACTH-secreting pituitary adenoma following bilateral adrenalectomy for refractory Cushing disease. Removal of adrenal glands as the source of cortisol production results in lack of feedback on hypothalamic CRH and pituitary ACTH secretion. Continued stimulation from CRH results in pituitary tumor growth and excess release of ACTH. Patients may present with headache, tunnel vision, and hyperpigmentation from mass effect of the tumor on the surrounding structures and from the effects of elevated ACTH on the skin. Hypopituitarism can occur when the normal pituitary tissue is destroyed by the tumor. Regular monitoring of patients with Cushing disease after bilateral adrenalectomy helps identify Nelson syndrome early.

CASE 2 | Hyperprolactinemia

A 26-year-old woman presents with missed periods and galactorrhea. She has had only 3 periods in the last 6 months, and they have been lighter than usual. When waking, she notes fluid on her shirt and inside her bra. She is not sexually active. Physical exam reveals bilateral milky nipple discharge with no breast masses. No visual field defects are noted.

Evaluation/Tests	Serum prolactin levels are elevated (>200 ng/mL). Pregnancy test is negative. TSH and free T4 levels are normal. MRI brain reveals a mass lesion in the region of the pituitary gland.
Treatment	First line is dopamine agonist treatment (cabergoline, bromocriptine). For refractory cases, consider transsphenoidal pituitary surgery.
Discussion	This patient is presenting with elevated prolactin levels due to a prolactin-secreting pituitary adenoma (prolactinomas). Hyperprolactinemia in women occurs most commonly due to pregnancy to support milk production and lactation for breast-feeding, but this patient's pregnancy test was negative. Prolactinomas are another common cause of hyperprolactinemia and occur more commonly in women. Symptoms include galactorrhea, oligomenorrhea, and/or infertility (due to low LH and FSH resulting in anovulation). Men with prolactinomas often present later than women, and they present with symptoms of hypogonadism or pituitary mass effect. Patients with large pituitary tumors should be screened for hypopituitarism. The larger the tumor, the higher the expected prolactin level. Dopamine agonists are first-line therapy. Dopamine is also known as prolactin-inhibiting factor, and it is normally released by the hypothalamus to regulate secretion of prolactin from the pituitary gland. **Hypothyroidism** can cause elevated serum prolactin by the lack of feedback inhibition, causing elevations in upstream TSH and TRH. TRH can directly stimulate prolactin secretion, so checking thyroid levels is an important step when evaluating patients with galactorrhea.

CASE 3 | Pituitary Adenoma (Hypopituitarism)

A 52-year-old man presents with concerns about low libido. He has reduced interest in sexual activity, and he is not experiencing early morning erections for the last year. He also notes lower energy, modest weight gain, constipation, cold intolerance, and headaches. He denies any recent testicular trauma or symptoms of depression. On exam, his blood pressure is 99/58 mmHg, and he has cool and dry skin, central obesity, and a normal genitourinary exam. Visual acuity is normal, but visual field confrontation testing reveals bitemporal hemianopsia.

Evaluation/Tests	Serum TSH, free T4, FSH, and LH are low. Testosterone levels drawn at 8 a.m. are low. Prolactin levels are normal. MRI reveals a mass in the region of the pituitary gland.
Treatment	Transsphenoidal pituitary surgery is indicated given the visual field defects. This patient also requires hormone replacement therapy (e.g., thyroxine and testosterone).
Discussion	This patient is presenting with signs and symptoms concerning for hypopituitarism, a disorder characterized by insufficient production of multiple pituitary hormones. One of the most common causes is a nonfunctional or **nonsecreting pituitary adenoma**, as seen in this patient. Pituitary adenomas arise from anterior pituitary cells. Functional tumors can lead to unique clinical states, including acromegaly and Cushing disease. Most tumors are nonfunctional, and they may be clinically silent. Larger tumors may compress the optic chiasm, resulting in bitemporal hemianopsia. Hypopituitarism results from injury to the normal gland, and it can cause growth hormone deficiency, secondary hypogonadism, secondary hypothyroidism, secondary hypoadrenalism, or, rarely, diabetes insipidus. Hypopituitarism is evaluated by symptomatology along with biochemical testing mostly for end-organ abnormalities (e.g., low free T4, low cortisol). **Prolactinomas** are the most common pituitary adenomas and are characterized by prolactin levels >200. Other causes of hypopituitarism include **craniopharyngioma** (seen in children or elderly), **Sheehan syndrome** (ischemic infarct of pituitary following postpartum bleeding), **empty sella syndrome** (atrophy or compression of pituitary, often seen in obese women or idiopathic), and **pituitary apoplexy** (sudden hemorrhage, usually due to an existing pituitary adenoma with fragile blood vessels). The presence of a mass in the pituitary region on MRI rules out these causes. **Primary hypogonadism** can be associated with decreased libido, but it is not usually associated with constipation, cold intolerance, and visual defects. **Primary hypothyroidism** can lead to the systemic symptoms as well as the loss of libido, but TSH would be elevated.

CASE 4 | Acromegaly

A 45-year-old man with type 2 diabetes mellitus, hypertension, and obstructive sleep apnea presents with concerns about weight gain and painful joints. He reports wrist/hand pain and weakness, along with worsening control of his diabetes. On exam, his blood pressure is 146/92 mmHg, he has coarse facial features, prominent jaw and brow, enlarged tongue, widely spaced teeth, and prominent protruding forehead with broad nasal bridge (frontal bossing). Finger and toe thickening is noted more prominently at joints. When he flexes his wrists for 1 minute, he starts to feel tingling and numbness in his fingers (Phalen's sign). Hepatomegaly is noted on abdominal exam.

Evaluation/Tests	Serum insulin-like growth factor-1 (IGF-1) levels are elevated and are not suppressed with a 75-g oral glucose tolerance test. Serum ferritin is normal. MRI brain reveals a pituitary mass.
Treatment	Surgical resection of pituitary adenoma. Some patients may require treatment with octreotide (somatostatin analog), pegvisomant (GH receptor antagonist), or cabergoline (dopamine agonist). Monitor for hypopituitarism and treat associated conditions (e.g., diabetes, sleep apnea, carpal tunnel syndrome).
Discussion	This patient is presenting with acromegaly, a disease of growth hormone (GH) excess most commonly caused by a GH-producing pituitary adenoma. Patients are at increased risk for heart disease, joint disease (carpal tunnel syndrome, arthropathy, arthritis), T2DM, hypertension, sleep apnea, and jaw or dental problems. Other common features include frontal bossing, large hands and feet, coarse facial features, large tongue, deep voice, and excessive sweating. Other signs may include bitemporal hemianopsia due to compression of the optic chiasm. There is an increased risk of colorectal polyps and cancer. Congestive heart failure is the most common cause of death in patients with acromegaly. GH works to stimulate production of IGF-1, mainly in the liver, which is the primary effector of GH signaling. IGF-1 level is a highly sensitive screening test; it is not specific, and levels may be falsely elevated in various conditions (e.g., pregnancy). Therefore, a confirmatory test (GH suppression test with oral glucose challenge) should be performed. The normal response to an oral glucose challenge is suppression of the GH level. Failure to suppress GH after giving 75 g of glucose confirms the diagnosis of acromegaly.

CASE 4 | Acromegaly (continued)

Discussion	Patients with **hemochromatosis** may present similarly with joint pains and worsening diabetes but will lack the coarse features and other bony/soft tissues changes seen in acromegaly. Hemochromatosis is a disease marked by excess iron absorption and resulting iron overload in tissues (elevated serum ferritin is one hallmark). It primarily affects the liver, but it can also damage the pancreas (causing diabetes), skin (bronze pigmentation), heart (cardiomyopathy), pituitary (hypogonadism), and joints (arthropathy).
Additional Considerations	In children, excess growth hormone manifests as **gigantism** because growth hormone promotes longitudinal growth prior to the closure of epiphyseal growth plates. Epiphyseal plates are made of hyaline cartilage and are found in the metaphysis of long bones. Once closed, excess GH will not promote longitudinal growth and will instead cause symptoms and signs of acromegaly.

CASE 5 | Central Diabetes Insipidus

A 38-year-old man presents with polyuria and polydipsia. Over the last 3 months, he has felt nearly constant thirst and he has had 5–6 episodes of nocturia. He only has relief with consumption of large volumes of cold water. Exam shows dry mucous membranes.

Evaluation/Tests	Plasma osmolality is 295 mOsm/kg, and serum sodium is 145 mEq/L. Serum calcium, glucose, and HbA1c levels are normal. Urine osmolality is 275 mOsm/kg, and specific gravity is 1.005. The patient is instructed to avoid drinking water for several hours, and measurements are taken again every hour. Plasma osmolality increases to 305 mOsm/kg, serum sodium increases to 155 mEq/L, and urine osmolality shows no change. Desmopressin (DDAVP) is given to the patient, and measurements are taken every 30 minutes for 2 hours. There is a large increase in urine osmolality to 700 mOsm/kg. Brain MRI shows no mass lesion; however, there is thickening of the pituitary stalk.
Treatment	Desmopressin (DDAVP) and free access to liquids.
Discussion	This patient is presenting with central diabetes insipidus (central DI). Diabetes insipidus is a disorder related to impaired activity of antidiuretic hormone (ADH), resulting in free water loss and the production of large volumes of dilute urine (polyuria). High-normal or high plasma osmolality triggers thirst that patients are often unable to satisfy (polydipsia). Central DI in particular involves deficient ADH production from the hypothalamus. ADH is normally synthesized in the hypothalamus, transported along neurophysins through the pituitary stalk for storage in the posterior pituitary until needed for its urine-concentrating ability. Most cases of central DI are idiopathic, and they may involve an autoimmune attack on the hypothalamus and pituitary stalk, which may manifest as thickening of the pituitary stalk on brain imaging (as in this patient). Other known causes of central DI include pituitary tumors (e.g., adenoma, craniopharyngioma), metastases, traumatic brain injury, ischemia (e.g., Sheehan syndrome), or as a consequence of neurosurgery. Each of these conditions renders the central nervous system unable to synthesize and secrete ADH. Initial lab findings may reveal mild hypernatremia and a high-normal or slight increase in plasma osmolality. Urine osmolality will be relatively low (<300 mOsm/kg). To help confirm the diagnosis, a water deprivation test is performed. This will cause a rise in serum sodium and plasma osmolality without changing urine osmolality. When the ADH analog desmopressin is subsequently given, the urine osmolality will rise >50% in central DI. **Nephrogenic DI** presents identically and is due to a failure at the level of the kidney to respond to circulating ADH. It can occur as a side effect to medications such as lithium or ADH antagonist (demeclocycline), develop secondary to hypercalcemia or hypokalemia, in the setting of renal disease, or be inherited as a genetic defect in the ADH receptor. Nephrogenic DI will have similar initial lab values and response to the water deprivation test; however, when desmopressin is administered, the plasma osmolality will remain elevated, and, most important, the urine osmolality will remain low. **Primary/psychogenic polydipsia** is a psychological disorder of pathologic water drinking. Thirst is the primary factor driving the polyuria. Initial labs including low urine osmolality will be similar to DI; however, the water deprivation test will result in urine osmolality returning to normal. Desmopressin is not needed for the diagnosis of primary polydipsia.

CASE 6 | Syndrome of Inappropriate Antidiuretic Hormone

A 54-year-old man is brought for evaluation of altered mental status. His family notes the patient has been more confused in the last week, and his spouse found him minimally responsive this morning. She also reports that he recently developed a cough with bloody sputum, and he has lost a lot of weight. He has no known medical conditions, but he has a history of smoking 2 packs of cigarettes daily for the past 30 years. On exam, he is afebrile, respirations are 10/min, pulse is 108/min, blood pressure is 110/80 mmHg. He is somnolent but arousable, and he has moist mucous membranes and no signs of volume overload. Testing for orthostatic hypotension is negative. Labs are notable for a serum sodium of 122 mEq/L.

Evaluation/Tests	Serum osmolality is <275 mOsm/kg. Serum sodium is 124 mmol/L (low). Urine osmolality is >100 mOsm/kg. BUN, uric acid, and creatinine levels are low. TSH and early morning cortisol are normal. Toxicity screen is negative. CT of the chest shows a large hilar mass within the left lung.
Treatment	Treat SIADH with fluid restriction. If the patient is severely symptomatic, carefully administer hypertonic saline with frequent sodium monitoring to ensure that serum Na correction does not exceed 8 mEq/L–10 mEq/L in the first 24 hours. Add a loop diuretic and sodium tablets, as needed, or ADH antagonists, including conivaptan, tolvaptan, or demeclocycline. ADH receptor antagonists (conivaptan, tolvaptan) will bind to the V2 vasopressin receptor in the principal cells of the renal collecting duct preventing ADH action. This causes increased water excretion without the loss of electrolyte and a rise in the serum sodium.
Discussion	This patient is presenting with syndrome of inappropriate antidiuretic hormone secretion (SIADH), a condition of hyponatremia associated with decreased water excretion. As the name implies, this results from excess ADH when serum osmolality is already low. It can be caused by a myriad of conditions: ectopic ADH production (e.g., small cell lung cancer), intracranial tumors or elevated intracranial pressure, pulmonary disease, or medications (e.g., SSRIs, carbamazepine, cyclophosphamide). This particular patient had a finding on CT that was suggestive of small cell carcinoma of the lung, making a paraneoplastic syndrome due to ectopic secretion of ADH most likely. ADH, or vasopressin, is synthesized in the supraoptic and paraventricular nuclei of the hypothalamus and is then transported by neurophysins to the posterior pituitary (neurohypophysis) for storage and secretion. ADH decreases serum osmolality by increasing urine osmolality. ADH binds to V2-receptors within principal cells of the renal collecting duct, promoting insertion of aquaporin water channels into the cell and increased water reabsorption. This contributes to the regulation of blood volume and pressure. The hyponatremia in SIADH must be managed, along with the underlying cause of the increased ADH secretion. Symptoms from SIADH range from lethargy, nausea, or vomiting to coma, seizure, and death. Evaluating the patient's volume status will immediately rule out hyponatremia associated with hypervolemic or hypovolemic states. In this euvolemic patient with hyponatremia and low serum osmolality, the differential includes SIADH, psychogenic polydipsia, tea and toast diet/beer potomania, adrenal insufficiency, and hypothyroidism. In euvolemic hyponatremia, ADH should not be activated because the kidneys should be trying to eliminate excess water in order to normalize serum sodium. In this patient, the urine osmolality is greater than serum osmolality, which means that ADH is present and the kidneys are concentrating urine inappropriately. SIADH is a diagnosis of exclusion; therefore, **hypothyroidism** and **adrenal insufficiency** should be ruled out, as was done in this scenario. In **psychogenic polydipsia**, urine osmolality should be very low, and the patient should have polyuria. In the **tea and toast diet/beer potomania**, individuals are consuming low protein, low solute, and high water intake diets, and their ability to excrete free water becomes impaired and they develop hyponatremia. **Medications** such as antidepressants, antipsychotics, and chemotherapies can also cause hyponatremia, making it important to review patients' medication lists.

ADRENAL GLAND DISORDERS

The adrenal cortex secretes three main categories of steroids: mineralocorticoids, glucocorticoids, and androgens. The adrenal cortex is divided into three zones: the zona glomerulosa (G), zona fasciculata (F), and zona reticularis (R). Zona glomerulosa produces aldosterone (salt), zona fasciculata produces cortisol (sugar), and zona reticularis produces androgens (sex hormones). The adrenal medulla secretes catecholamines.

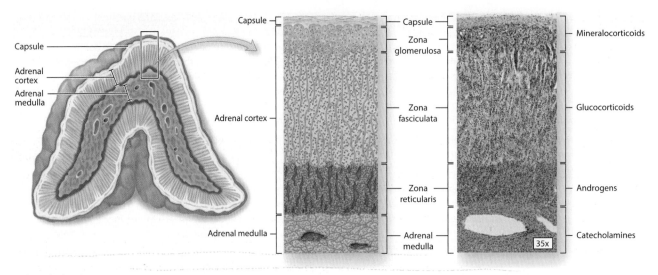

Adrenal gland.
Left Side: Reproduced with permission from McKinley M, O'Loughlin VD. Human Anatomy, 2nd ed. New York, NY: McGraw Hill; 2008; middle and right: Dr. Alvin Telser/McGraw Hill Education.

Congenital adrenal hyperplasia (CAH) is a group of autosomal recessive conditions caused by mutations or defects in enzymes involved in the biosynthesis of steroid hormones within the adrenal cortex. There are three main types of CAH, as illustrated in the following table.

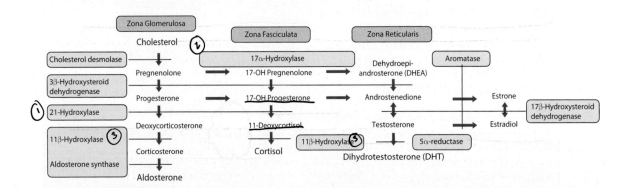

Deficiency	Presentation	Cortisol	Mineralocorticoids	Sex Hormones	Labs
21-hydroxylase	Hyperpigmentation Hypotension/hyperkalemia Infancy: salt wasting Female infants: virilization, clitoromegaly Children: precocious puberty (nonclassic form)	↓	↓ aldosterone	↑	17-hydroxy-progesterone: ↑ Renin: ↑ Cortisol: ↓ Testosterone: ↑ Sodium: ↓ Potassium: ↑
17α-hydroxylase	Hyperpigmentation HTN/hypokalemia Female: primary amenorrhea or delayed puberty Male: ambiguous genitalia or undescended testes	↓	↑ aldosterone	↓	Androstenedione: ↓ Aldosterone: ↑ Renin: ↓

(continued)

Deficiency	Presentation	Cortisol	Mineralocorticoids	Sex Hormones	Labs
11β-hydroxylase	Hyperpigmentation HTN/hypokalemia Female: virilization	↓	↓ aldosterone but ↑ deoxycorticosterone (DOC)	↑	Renin: ↓ DOC: ↑ 11-deoxycortiosol: ↑

CASE 7 | Congenital Adrenal Hyperplasia (21-Hydroxylase Deficiency)

An 8-day-old boy is brought for evaluation of recurrent vomiting, poor feeding, and irritability. His parents are concerned that he has been sleeping more and that he does not wake up to feed on his own. The patient is afebrile, but his heart rate is elevated and blood pressure is low. On physical examination, the newborn appears lethargic and dehydrated with dry mucous membranes and a sunken anterior fontanelle. Hyperpigmentation of the scrotum is seen; otherwise external genitalia appear normal with palpable testes present.

Evaluation/Tests	Serum sodium and chloride are low; potassium is high; and bicarbonate and glucose are low. Serum pH is 7.35. Aldosterone levels are low, and plasma renin activity is elevated. Serum 17-hydroxyprogesterone is >1000 ng/dL (very high).
Treatment	Immediate IV fluids and salt repletion, followed by dextrose; glucocorticoid and mineralocorticoid replacement as needed.
Discussion	This patient presents with the most common form of CAH, known as 21-hydroxylase deficiency. The 21-hydroxylase enzyme is responsible for converting progesterone and 17-hydroxyprogesterone into 11-deoxycorticosterone (precursor to corticosterone and aldosterone) and 11-deoxycortisol (precursor to cortisol), respectively. Defect in this enzyme therefore leads to the accumulation of progesterone and 17-hydroxyprogesterone. Since 21-hydroxylase is not involved in the biosynthesis of sex hormones, excess of these precursors is then shunted toward increased synthesis of sex hormones. The lack of aldosterone and cortisol accompanied by increased sex hormones accounts for the clinical manifestation of this disease. Low aldosterone results in hyponatremia and hyperkalemia (salt wasting in severe cases, as seen here) and low cortisol results in hypotension and hypoglycemia. Excess androgens can result in ambiguous genitalia with virilization in females while boys may have normally appearing external genitalia. Both sexes can have labial or scrotal hyperpigmentation. If not identified by newborn screening, severe cases typically present at 1 to 3 weeks of age with dehydration, poor feeding failure to thrive, lethargy or irritability, hypotension, hyponatremia, and hyperkalemia. If not diagnosed and adequately treated, severe cases of congenital adrenal hyperplasia can be fatal. Mild disease may not present until later in childhood with precocious puberty due to excess sex hormones. Diagnosis is confirmed with very high serum concentration of 17-hydroxyprogesterone (17OHP), usually above 1000 ng/dL.

The two other forms of CAH are 17α-hydroxylase and 11β-hydroxylase deficiencies. 17α-hydroxylase acts early in adrenal steroid biosynthesis at multiple steps. It first converts pregnenolone and progesterone to 17-hydroxypregnenolone and 17-hydroxyprogesterone, respectively. It then further acts on these products to convert them into dehydroepiandrosterone (DHEA) and androstenedione, respectively. Both of these are sex hormone/androgen precursors.

17α-hydroxylase deficiency blocks the formation of both glucocorticoid and sex hormone precursors, resulting in an elevation of mineralocorticoids. The compensatory increase in ACTH, due to the failure of cortisol production, stimulates the overproduction of 11-deoxycorticosterone and corticosterone, which leads to hypertension and hypokalemia. Affected males present with ambiguous genitalia and intra-abdominal undescended testes, while females may present with primary amenorrhea or delayed puberty and hypertension. The treatment is glucocorticoid (hydrocortisone) and sex steroid replacement.

11β-hydroxylase deficiency involves a defect in 11β-hydroxylase, which prevents the conversion of 11-deoxycortisol to cortisol and 11-deoxycorticosterone to corticosterone; this leads to low cortisol and low aldosterone levels. The resulting increase in ACTH secretion causes the accumulation of 11-deoxycortisol and 11-deoxycorticosterone, increased sex steroid synthesis, and adrenocortical hyperplasia. Infants will have elevated androgen levels, which cause the masculinization of the female fetus. Patients may present with hypertension and hypokalemia secondary to increased 11-deoxycorticosterone level. If not diagnosed at birth, this will present with signs of premature adrenarche (body odor and axillary and pubic hair growth).

CASE 8 | Cushing Syndrome (Exogenous Corticosteroids)

A 41-year-old woman with rheumatoid arthritis (RA) presents for evaluation of weight gain. She was diagnosed with RA 6 months ago and has had progressive pain and swelling in multiple joints. Her rheumatologist prescribed several immune-modulating agents, but she continues to take 20 mg of prednisone to control her symptoms. She reports 30-pound weight gain, increased facial hair, and acne, as well as polyuria and polydipsia. Her blood pressure is 150/92 mmHg. Her exam reveals central obesity, preauricular fat pad enlargement, several dark purple abdominal striae, and decreased proximal strength.

Evaluation/Tests	Midnight salivary cortisol is elevated. 24-hour urinary free cortisol levels are elevated. Serum ACTH level is <5 pg/mL (low). Serum hemoglobin A1c is 8.1%. MRI brain is normal, with no evidence of mass lesions.
Treatment	Taper off steroids and treat RA with a steroid-sparing therapy.
Discussion	This patient is presenting with **Cushing syndrome**, and the most common cause is chronic use of **exogenous corticosteroids**. Cushing syndrome is a disease state of excess cortisol that can result from endogenous (e.g., adrenal adenoma or carcinoma) or exogenous (e.g., heavy or chronic corticosteroid use) sources. The presence of autoimmune or inflammatory conditions should signal the possibility of exogenous corticosteroid use because they are often prescribed for these conditions. Clinical manifestations are identical regardless of the underlying cause, and they include weight gain, metabolic syndrome (diabetes, HTN, hyperlipidemia), muscle weakness, easy bruising, and reduced bone mineral density (osteopenia/osteoporosis). In Cushing syndrome, ACTH levels will be low as the endogenous or exogenous cortisol will result in negative feedback on the hypothalamus and anterior pituitary. When an exogenous (iatrogenic) source of steroids is identified, no additional diagnostic test is necessary. If the cause is iatrogenic, efforts should be made to obtain control of the disease being treated with a steroid-sparing therapy. Tapering steroid dosing over weeks to months is necessary to avoid an adrenal crisis or acute adrenal insufficiency given that long-term glucocorticoid therapy results in suppression of the hypothalamic-pituitary-adrenal (HPA) axis. **Obesity** due to excess calories will cause weight gain but not hirsutism, acne, purple abdominal striae, and proximal muscle weakness. **Type 2 diabetes** can present with polyuria and polydipsia but not the other symptoms listed in this case. **Polycystic ovarian syndrome (PCOS)** is associated with glucose intolerance, weight gain, hirsutism, and acne, but it is not associated with proximal muscle weakness and purple abdominal striae. The presence of a normal brain MRI and low ACTH levels rules out **Cushing disease** due to an ACTH-secreting pituitary adenoma. Given the patient's history of rheumatoid arthritis and chronic prednisone treatment, endogenous causes of Cushing syndrome, such as adrenal adenoma, hyperplasia, or carcinoma, are unlikely as these are rare.

CASE 9 | Primary Hyperaldosteronism (Conn's Syndrome)

A 52-year-old man with hypertension, hyperlipidemia, and depression returns to clinic for follow-up of his difficult-to-control blood pressure. His current blood pressure medications are hydrochlorothiazide, amlodipine, lisinopril, and hydralazine. He is compliant with his medications; he has a low-salt diet, and he exercises regularly. He lost 20 pounds intentionally. He checks his blood pressure at home regularly, and it has been consistently elevated. His blood pressure is 175/110 mmHg. Review of the patient's chart shows intermittent hypokalemia for the past 4 years. On physical exam, there are no signs of edema.

Evaluation/Tests	Serum pH is 7.55. Serum potassium is 3.2 mEq/L, bicarbonate is 34 mEq/L. Plasma aldosterone concentration/plasma renin activity (PAC/PRA) ratio is >30. Oral sodium loading test and saline infusion test fail to suppress aldosterone secretion. CT reveals no renal artery stenosis, but it does indicate the presence of a unilateral adrenal mass.
Treatment	For patients with unilateral disease, laparoscopic adrenalectomy is curative. For patients with bilateral adrenal disease or for those who are not candidates for surgery, treat with mineralocorticoid receptor antagonists (spironolactone or eplerenone).
Discussion	This patient presents with primary hyperaldosteronism (Conn's syndrome), a syndrome of increased aldosterone secretion from the adrenal cortex. Primary aldosteronism can be seen in the context of adrenal adenoma, adrenal carcinoma, or bilateral adrenal hyperplasia. It is a common cause of secondary hypertension presenting with hypokalemia, metabolic alkalosis, increased plasma aldosterone, and decreased plasma renin. Aldosterone is a mineralocorticoid hormone secreted by the zona glomerulosa of the adrenal cortex, and it is primarily involved in the regulation of sodium levels and volume status. It is secreted in response to decreased blood volume (via angiotensin II) and increased plasma potassium.

CASE 9 | Primary Hyperaldosteronism (Conn's Syndrome) *(continued)*

Discussion	After secretion into the systemic circulation, aldosterone arrives at the principal cells in the late distal tubule and collecting ducts of the nephron to stimulate reabsorption of sodium and secretion of potassium. It can also act on nephron α-intercalated cells to promote H$^+$ secretion, hence the metabolic alkalosis seen with hyperaldosteronism. High aldosterone increases NaCl delivery to the macula densa, decreasing renin release from nearby juxtaglomerular cells in a negative feedback loop. Patients with primary hyperaldosteronism often present with difficult-to-control blood pressure despite the use of multiple antihypertensive medications and intermittent hypokalemia. PAC will be high, PRA is suppressed (less than 1 ng/mL/hr), and the PAC/PRA ratio is greater than 20. Confirmatory testing is done with a saline suppression test, in which introduction of saline suppresses PAC to less than 5 ng/dL in individuals who do not have the disease. Patients with primary hyperaldosteronism may actually have a normal sodium level, and they may lack significant extracellular fluid volume expansion due to a mechanism known as aldosterone escape. The body is able to compensate for increased sodium reabsorption and blood volume by triggering increases in renal blood flow, glomerular filtration rate, and secretion of atrial natriuretic peptide.
	Patients with **secondary hyperaldosteronism** have excess aldosterone secretion secondary to increased renin. Renin is secreted by juxtaglomerular (JG) cells in the kidney in response to decreased renal blood pressure, increased sympathetic tone, or decreased NaCl delivery to the distal convoluted tubule. Renin acts via the renin-angiotensin-aldosterone system to cause multiple effects, one of which is secretion of aldosterone from the adrenal cortex. Causes of secondary hyperaldosteronism include renovascular hypertension, juxtaglomerular cell tumors (reninomas), and edema secondary to cirrhosis, heart failure, or nephrotic syndrome. As opposed to primary hyperaldosteronism, patients with secondary hyperaldosteronism will have increased plasma renin and edema due to failure of the aldosterone escape mechanism.
	Bartter syndrome is a renal tubular defect that presents with polyuria, polydipsia, metabolic alkalosis, and hypokalemia, but blood pressure is usually normal.
	Liddle syndrome is another renal tubular defect that presents similarly to hyperaldosteronism, but aldosterone levels are usually decreased.
	Licorice ingestion can lead to an acquired **syndrome of apparent mineralocorticoid excess**, which presents with hypertension, hypokalemia, metabolic alkalosis but decreased serum aldosterone levels. Licorice inhibits 11-betahydroxysteroid dehydrogenase type 2, the enzyme that inactivates cortisol. The inhibition of this enzyme allows cortisol to bind to the mineralocorticoid receptor and to cause symptoms of mineralocorticoid excess.

CASE 10 | Primary Adrenal Insufficiency (Addison Disease)

A 45-year-old woman presents with fatigue, lightheadedness, and anorexia with occasional nausea and vomiting for several months. She has unintentional weight loss and cravings for salty/sweet foods. On exam, she is afebrile; respirations are 15/min, pulse is 92/min, blood pressure is 112/78 mmHg supine and 96/58 mmHg standing. She has hyperpigmentation on her face, in her palmar creases, and in the pattern of the bra straps.

Evaluation/Tests	Complete blood count is normal. Serum pH is 7.30, sodium is 130 mEq/L, potassium is 5.4 mEq/L, bicarbonate is 20 mEq/L. Anion gap is 10 mEq/L (normal). Early morning serum cortisol is low; serum ACTH is high.
Treatment	Glucocorticoid (hydrocortisone) and mineralocorticoid (fludrocortisone) replacement therapy.
Discussion	This patient is presenting with **primary adrenal insufficiency**, which occurs due to failure of the adrenal gland and results in low levels of mineralocorticoids and glucocorticoids. It most commonly occurs secondary to chronic autoimmune destruction of the adrenal cortex, known as **Addison disease**. Symptoms include nausea, vomiting, abdominal pain, orthostatic hypotension, hyperpigmentation, weight loss, and salt craving. In response to low cortisol levels, the anterior pituitary increases release of ACTH. One characteristic feature of primary adrenal insufficiency is skin hyperpigmentation. ACTH shares structural similarities to α-melanocyte-stimulating hormone (α-MSH) as they are both derived from the same precursor molecule, pro-opiomelanocortin (POMC). Increased expression of ACTH therefore also drives increased production of α-MSH, which, combined with the ability of ACTH to also stimulate melanocytes, results in hyperpigmentation. Other causes of chronic primary adrenal insufficiency include infection (tuberculosis, HIV, syphilis, and mycoses), infiltrative diseases (e.g., hemochromatosis, sarcoidosis), metastasis, adrenal hemorrhage, thrombosis, or drugs. Typical findings include

CASE 10 | Primary Adrenal Insufficiency (Addison Disease) *(continued)*

Discussion	hyponatremia, hyperkalemia, low AM cortisol, and high ACTH levels. 21-hydroxylase antibodies are usually present in primary adrenal insufficiency. If morning cortisol levels are not diagnostic, an ACTH stimulation test should be performed using the ACTH analog cosyntropin. Patients with primary adrenal insufficiency will not respond adequately to cosyntropin, so serum cortisol levels will not increase substantially. Although rarely used clinically, metyrapone stimulation test is another option to diagnose adrenal insufficiency. Metyrapone inhibits 11β-hydroxylase, which converts 11-deoxycortisol to cortisol. Administration of metyrapone should lead to a rise in serum 11-deoxycortisol; however, this will not occur in adrenal insufficiency. If serum ACTH levels are elevated in this context, this will also confirm primary adrenal insufficiency. **Secondary adrenal insufficiency** is a failure of adrenal hormone release secondary to decreased ACTH production in the pituitary gland. Given the decreased ACTH production, there is no skin/mucosal hyperpigmentation. There is also no hyperkalemia as aldosterone synthesis within the adrenal gland is preserved due to an intact renin-angiotensin-aldosterone system. **Tertiary adrenal insufficiency** occurs with disruption of the hypothalamus input (corticotrophin-releasing hormone/CRH) to the pituitary, such as with suppression of the hypothalamic-pituitary-adrenal axis in chronic steroid use. Decreased CRH will lead to decreased ACTH.
Additional Considerations	**Waterhouse-Friderichsen syndrome** is an acute primary adrenal insufficiency due to bilateral adrenal infarction and/or hemorrhage. It most commonly develops in the setting of septicemia, with gram negative diplococcus *Neisseria meningitides* as the most common pathogen. Other bacterial organisms may also cause this syndrome. *N. meningitidis* causes meningococcal meningitis, and it can induce significant production of inflammatory cytokines and lead to sepsis due to virulence factors such as lipooligosaccharide. Additional risk factors for developing Waterhouse-Friderichsen syndrome include a history of anticoagulant therapy, coagulopathy, or splenectomy. Patients often present in shock, and they have abdominal or flank pain, often preceded by short illness of fever, malaise, and headaches. Rash, coagulopathy (DIC), and cardiovascular collapse also occur.

Adrenal Gland Mass

The differential for an adrenal mass includes adenoma, carcinoma, neuroblastoma, and pheochromocytoma. Diagnosis is made by imaging (CT or MRI), laboratory studies, and biopsy.

Neuroblastomas are the most common malignant tumors of the adrenal gland, specifically in children less than 4 years old. Children typically present with abdominal distension and a palpable, firm, irregular mass that crosses the midline. Diagnostic imaging is supported by measurement of homovanillic acid (HVA) and vanillylmandelic acid (VMA) in the urine. Biopsy of the lesion demonstrates Homer Wright rosettes.

Pheochromocytomas are endocrine tumors that produce and secrete catecholamines. They present with symptoms of severe hypertension, headache, episodic flushing, and tachycardia. The diagnosis is confirmed by measuring urine metanephrines, urine vanillylmandelic acid, and plasma metanephrines. Standard treatment for both tumor types is resection. Prior to resection of pheochromocytomas, the patient should be treated with irreversible alpha blockade (phenoxybenzamine) followed by beta blockade (propranolol). Alpha blockade is required prior to beta blockade in order to prevent hypertensive crisis.

Key Findings and Adrenal Mass Differential Diagnosis

Key Findings	Diagnosis
Palpable abdominal mass that crosses the midline in a child (<4 years old)	Neuroblastoma
Homer Wright rosettes	Neuroblastoma
Hypertension, headache, tachycardia, and flushing	Pheochromocytoma
Marfanoid body habitus and medullary thyroid carcinoma	Pheochromocytoma (MEN type 2B)

CASE 11 | Pheochromocytoma

A 42-year-old man presents with progressively worsening headaches over the last year. His episodic bilateral headaches are associated with palpitations, blurry vision, shortness of breath, and tremor. These episodes initially were sporadic but lately have been occurring more frequently. He is not on any medications and does not use illicit or OTC drugs. On exam, his vitals are temperature is 37.5°C, blood pressure is 220/120 mmHg, respirations are 17/min, and pulse is 102/min. He is diaphoretic and has a fine hand tremor bilaterally.

CASE 11 | Pheochromocytoma *(continued)*

Evaluation/Tests	Urine toxicity screen is negative. Plasma free metanephrines are elevated. Follow-up confirmatory test with 24-hour urine collection shows increased metanephrines, homovanillic acid, and vanillylmanelic acid in urine. Abdominal CT shows a large heterogeneous mass with areas of cystic change within the left adrenal gland.
Treatment	Surgical resection of the adrenal mass. To avoid catecholamine surge and hypertensive crisis during surgery, an α-adrenergic antagonist (phenoxybenzamine) is given first to normalize blood pressure, followed by β-blocker (e.g., propranolol, metoprolol, etc.) later to further control blood pressure and tachycardia.
Discussion	Pheochromocytoma should be considered in patients who have refractory hypertension, episodic headache, palpitations, diaphoresis, flushing, and tremors. Pheochomocytomas are neuroendocrine tumors derived from the chromaffin cells of the adrenal medulla. The tumors secrete catecholamines—norepinephrine, epinephrine, and dopamine—in a pulsatile manner, thus leading to intermittent symptoms correlating with an exaggerated sympathetic response. Several germline mutations can give rise to familial pheochromocytoma. These include mutations associated with multiple endocrine neoplasia type 2, neurofibromatosis, and von Hippel-Lindau disease. Elevated levels of catecholamine breakdown products such as metanephrines, homovanillic acid, and vanillylmandelic acid (at least two- to three-fold the upper limit of normal) in urine or blood suggests pheochromocytoma. Adrenal/abdominal CT or MRI is used to localize the mass. MRI may show marked hyperintensity on T2 images (lightbulb sign). Some pheochromocytomas may also secrete erythropoietin (EPO), contributing to a polycythemia. Extra-adrenal location of a catecholamine-secreting tumor with symptoms resembling those of a pheochromocytoma is referred to as a **paraganglioma**. These tumors can be found in several locations throughout the body, including the wall of the bladder, the organ of Zuckerkandl at the bifurcation of the aorta, or at the level of the carotid body in the neck. Patients presenting with **Serotonin syndrome** would have a history of SSRI and other serotonergic drug use. Classic presentation includes fever, altered mental status, hypertension and tachycardia, diarrhea, and rigidity. The constellation of symptoms exhibited by our patient is more indicative of pheochromocytoma.

CASE 12 | Neuroblastoma

An 18-month-old boy is brought for evaluation of a "lump" in his abdomen. Mom reports that the boy seemed more tired recently but denies any other symptoms. Vital signs are normal. On physical examination, a deep purple coloring is noted around the eyes, and his abdomen is distended with a palpable mass in the right upper quadrant.

Evaluation/Tests	Spot urine homovanillic acid and vanillylmandelic acid (catecholamine metabolite) levels are elevated. Abdominal ultrasound reveals a heterogeneous solid lesion with calcifications that crosses the midline. MRI of the area reveals a heterogeneous mass with cystic and hemorrhagic areas. Biopsy reveals a tumor within the adrenal medulla characterized by small round blue/purple cells and Homer-Wright rosettes. Staining of the tissue is positive for bombesin and neuron-specific enolase (NSE).
Treatment	Surgery ± chemotherapy or radiotherapy.
Discussion	**Neuroblastoma** is the most common tumor of the adrenal medulla in children, originating from neural crest cells (anywhere along the sympathetic chain), and it presents typically in children <4 years of age. The median age of presentation is 17 months. Neuroblastoma presents initially in the adrenal glands in 50% of cases. The most common presentation is abdominal distention and a palpable, firm, irregular mass that crosses the midline. Typical presentation can include opsoclonus-myoclonus (dancing eyes and dancing feet), ataxia, and periorbital ecchymosis (raccoon eyes) due to orbital metastases. Patients can also present with weight loss, anorexia, night sweats, fever, persistent bone or joint pain, or UTI from obstructing abdominal mass. Most patients are normotensive; however, catecholamine release can lead to hypertension, diarrhea, and other symptoms. When neuroblastoma occurs before 12 months of age, the survival rate is high. Neuroblastoma is associated with overexpression of the *N-myc* oncogene. **Wilms tumor** will also present as an abdominal mass in a child <4 years of age, but it usually arises from the kidney and is unilateral, smooth, and does not cross the midline. Wilms tumor will show up on ultrasound as a solid mass in the kidney. **Hepatoblastoma** will also present as an abdominal mass in a child <4 years of age, but it arises from the liver. **Pheochromocytomas** are the most common tumor of the adrenal medulla in adults.

THYROID DISORDERS

Hyperthyroidism

Thyroid hyperfunction can be secondary to autoimmunity (Graves' disease), a hyperfunctioning thyroid nodule, temporary thyroiditis, or a genetic disorder (McCune-Albright syndrome). Regardless of the cause of hyperthyroidism, the symptoms are the same. The workup for hyperthyroidism helps distinguish one cause from another.

Weight loss can be seen in both cortisol deficiency and elevated thyroid hormone levels. However, the weight loss with cortisol deficiency is associated with poor appetite compared to weight loss in hyperthyroidism, which is associated with increased food intake.

Diagnostic Studies to Help Distinguish Causes of Thyroid Excess

Hyperthyroidism	TSH (thyrotropin)	Free T4/T3	Radioactive Iodine Uptake Scan	Thyrotropin Antibodies	Possible Findings
Graves' disease	↓	↑ FT3>>FT4	Diffuse uptake	Positive	Proptosis, goiter with bruit
Toxic adenoma	↓	↑	Focal uptake	Negative	Nodular or asymmetric goiter
Thyroiditis	Often ↓ acutely, followed by possible ↑ in hypothyroid phase	↑ in hyper-thyroid phase, then ↓ in hypothyroid phase	↓	Negative	Smooth goiter, maybe painful in some forms (subacute, infectious, radiation, trauma)
TSH-producing pituitary adenoma	↑	↑	Diffuse uptake	Negative	Headaches, visual field defect, pituitary adenoma on MRI imaging
Iodine-induced hyperthyroid (Jod-Basedow phenomenon)	↓	↑	Variable depending on the preceding exogenous iodine load	Negative	Smooth goiter, history of iodine exposure (e.g., IV contrast, amiodarone)

CASE 13 | Graves' Disease

A 41-year-old woman presents with unintentional weight loss, intermittent palpitations, diarrhea, difficulty concentrating, and trouble sleeping. On exam, she is afebrile, blood pressure is 160/95 mmHg, and pulse is 108/min. She appears anxious, and her skin is warm. Protrusion of both eyeballs is seen (proptosis). She has a nontender, enlarged thyroid with bruit. Her reflexes are brisk, and there is mild tremor on outstretched hands.

Evaluation/Tests	TSH level is low, with elevated levels of both free T3 and T4. Serum testing for thyroid receptor IgG autoantibodies is positive.
Treatment	Symptom control with β-blocker. Treat the hyperthyroidism with antithyroid medications (thionamides). Long-term, definitive treatment with either surgery or radioactive iodine may be required.
Discussion	This is a classic presentation of **Graves' disease**, the most common form of hyperthyroidism. It is an autoimmune disease in which thyroid-stimulating immunoglobulins or thyrotropin receptor antibodies activate the thyrotropin receptor, causing excess thyroid hormone synthesis and secretion. Patients typically present with signs of increased metabolism, including weight loss, heat intolerance, insomnia, diarrhea, anxiety, and menstrual changes. Physical exam can show tachycardia, thinning hair, brisk reflexes, and ophthalmopathy (exophthalmos and periorbital edema) with lid-lag. It is important to note that the ophthalmopathy is specific to Graves' disease and that it does not present in other forms of hyperthyroidism. This infiltrative ophthalmopathy is characterized by lymphocyte infiltration into connective tissue that secrete proinflammatory cytokines, which then stimulate retro-orbital fibroblasts to produce excess glycosaminoglycans. Dermal fibroblasts can also be stimulated, leading to pretibial myxedema. On histology, the thyroid biopsy will show tall, crowded follicular epithelial cells with "scalloped" colloid.

CASE 13 | Graves' Disease (continued)

Discussion	Although Graves' disease is the most common cause of hyperthyroidism, other causes to consider when ophthalmopathy is not present include toxic multinodular goiter, toxic thyroid adenomas, and thyroiditis. **Toxic multinodular goiters** involve focal patches of hyperfunctioning follicular cells that release T3 and T4 independent of TSH regulation. While most **thyroid adenomas** are nonfunctional or "cold," they may be rarely "hot" or "toxic" and secrete thyroid hormones. Inflammation of the thyroid gland (**thyroiditis**) can lead to hyperthyroidism, especially early on due to destruction of cells and release of thyroid hormone. As more of the thyroid is destroyed over time, this may be replaced with chronic hypothyroidism (as can be seen in Hashimoto thyroiditis, a common cause of hypothyroidism). All of these cases would lack thyroid-stimulating immunoglobulins. Toxic thyroid adenomas would show only focal uptake of radioactive iodine, while thyroiditis would show decreased areas of focal uptake. In **pituitary-based hyperthyroidism (central hyperthyroidism)**, TSH will be normal or elevated despite an increase in free T3 and T4 levels.
Additional Considerations	**Thyroid storm** is a severe form of thyrotoxicosis that leads to dysfunction of multiple organs. It constitutes a medical emergency with a mortality rate of 15–20%, making it essential to recognize and initiate treatment as soon as possible. The cardinal features of thyroid storm encompass symptoms from the central nervous system (reduced cognition, agitation, delirium, confusion, coma), GI tract (nausea, vomiting, diarrhea, abdominal pain, jaundice), and cardiovascular system (tachycardia, atrial fibrillation, arrhythmias, lower extremity edema, heart failure, cardiogenic shock). Thermoregulatory dysfunction is common with patients having very high fever. A triggering factor like infection, heart attack, surgery, or trauma is also common. Thyroid storm is most common in individuals with underlying Graves' disease, and it can also be triggered by radioactive iodine therapy in a patient that is in a thyrotoxic state. In addition to treating the underlying trigger, the mainstays of treatment in thyroid storm are to decrease thyroid hormone production with propylthiouracil or methimazole in order to reduce thyroid hormone secretion and inhibit synthesis of new thyroid hormone (Wolff-Chaikoff effect) with potassium iodide solution and to reduce peripheral conversion of T4 to T3 with glucocorticoids. Adrenergic symptoms are controlled with beta blockers. Cooling blankets are used for treating hyperthermia. Once the patient is stable and euthyroid, radioactive iodine or total thyroidectomy is indicated to prevent recurrent severe thyrotoxicosis.

Hypothyroidism

Thyroid gland hypofunction will present differently depending on the age of the patient. Infants with congenital hypothyroidism are at increased risk for developmental delay if not treated appropriately. Similar to hyperthyroidism, the etiology of hypothyroidism can be varied, but the symptomatology is similar.

CASE 14 | Hashimoto Thyroiditis

A 46-year-old woman with no significant history presents with weight gain, decreased appetite, and fatigue for several months. Despite dieting and exercising, she is unable to lose weight. She also reports irregular menses, constipation, and always feeling cold. On exam, blood pressure is 105/70 mmHg, skin appears dry, face and eyes are puffy with loss of lateral 1/3 of her eyebrows, and her reflexes are slowed. The thyroid gland is diffusely enlarged and nontender.

Evaluation/Tests	TSH is elevated, and T3 and T4 levels are decreased. Pregnancy test is negative. Serum ESR is within normal limits. Serum thyroid peroxidase (TPO) antibody test is positive.
Treatment	Levothyroxine (thyroid hormone replacement).
Discussion	This patient is presenting with hypothyroidism due to **Hashimoto thyroiditis (chronic lymphocytic thyroiditis)**, the most common cause of hypothyroidism in iodine-sufficient regions. Symptoms of hypothyroidism can be relatively nonspecific or include fatigue, weight gain, dry skin/hair, menstrual irregularity, cold intolerance, dyspnea on exertion, and depressed mood. Clinical findings may include bradycardia, diffuse alopecia, brittle hair and nails, dry skin, puffy facies and periorbital edema, generalized nonpitting edema (myxedema), proximal muscle weakness, carpal tunnel syndrome, signs of decreased cardiac output, slow return phase of deep tendon reflexes, hyperlipidemia, hyponatremia, and

CASE 14 | Hashimoto Thyroiditis *(continued)*

Discussion	elevated CK. Depending on the cause, the thyroid gland may be small, normal, or large. Typical laboratory findings include an elevated TSH, decreased free T4, and TPO or thyroglobulin antibodies. Characteristic pathologic findings include the presence of lymphocyte aggregates within germinal centers and Hürthle cells around atrophic thyroid follicles. It is important to note that early in the course of the disease, patients may show signs and symptoms of hyperthyroidism as the thyroid follicles are destroyed and thyroid hormones are released. However, over time, the thyroid loses ability to synthesize additional T3 and T4 as more follicles are destroyed, ultimately resulting in hypothyroidism. Thyroid hormone deficiency can occur in a variety of disorders, but it is often due to primary thyroid failure from autoimmune disease, iodine deficiency, drugs (lithium, amiodarone), postpartum or postviral thyroiditis, previous thyroid ablation or resection, or cretinism. **Central hypothyroidism** can be caused by hypopituitarism (secondary) or hypothalamic causes (tertiary) or due to severe illness (functional). **Postpartum thyroiditis** can occur up to 1 year after delivery. **Subacute granulomatous (de Quervain) thyroiditis** can occur after a viral illness, typically presenting with a very tender thyroid and an elevated ESR. **Riedel thyroiditis** presents with a fixed, hard, painless goiter as a result of fibrous tissue replacing thyroid gland, and it may be associated with other IgG4-related systemic diseases. Patients with **iodine deficiency** typically present with a large goiter and no antithyroid antibodies.
Additional Considerations	**Myxedema coma** is a rare form of extreme hypothyroidism that leads to the dysfunction of multiple organs. Findings including mental status changes, hypothermia, bradycardia, hypotension, and reduced respiratory drive, the latter of which can lead to hypoxemia and hypercapnia. It constitutes a medical emergency with a high mortality rate if not recognized and treated early. A triggering factor is common; cold weather (most commonly presents in the winter months), infection, heart attack, stroke, or trauma occurring in a patient with untreated hypothyroidism may precipitate myxedema coma. Patients will have the usual symptoms and signs of hypothyroidism, but they may have more pronounced fluid retention, facial puffiness, tongue enlargement, and skin thickening and discoloration (deposition of glycosaminoglycans in the dermis) due to long-standing hypothyroidism. One should not wait for labs to return prior to initiation of treatment. In addition to ensuring the presence of a patent airway, the ability to breathe, and maintenance of circulation, the mainstay of treatment is to reestablish the euthyroid state by administering IV levothyroxine. Concurrent treatment with an IV glucocorticoid should be initiated as well to prevent adrenal crisis until underlying adrenal insufficiency is ruled out (a cortisol level is drawn just prior to treatment initiation). **Congenital hypothyroidism (cretinism)** results from decreased or absent action of thyroid hormone during development and early infancy. Most cases are not hereditary and result from thyroid dysgenesis. Other causes of congenital hypothyroidism include inborn errors of thyroid hormone synthesis, iodine deficiency, antibody-mediated maternal hypothyroidism, or dyshormonogenetic goiter. Most cases are identified by newborn screening in the first week of life. In areas where screening is not available, the classic presentation includes increased head circumference and fontanelles; feeding difficulties (sluggishness, somnolence); enlarged, protuberant tongue; constipation (unresponsive to treatment); umbilical hernia; pale, puffy face; and poor brain development. Early treatment of congenital hypothyroidism is crucial to attain an optimal neurodevelopmental outcome.

Thyroid Enlargement/Mass

Thyroid enlargement (goiter) may occur without any demonstrable changes in the thyroid hormone levels. Goiters can be seen in cases of hypothyroidism or hyperthyroidism, but a euthyroid patient may also present with a goiter. **Thyroid nodules** can be functional or nonfunctional. The first step in managing these patients is to assess them for any symptoms of hypothyroidism, hyperthyroidism, or mass effect (difficulty swallowing, hoarseness). Baseline laboratory workup and thyroid ultrasound may be necessary to help determine the cause of the thyroid enlargement. Nonfunctioning nodules >1 cm with suspicious features should be considered for biopsy to rule out malignancy.

Thyroid cancer has four main histologies: papillary, follicular, medullary, and anaplastic. Treatment includes resection and/or radioactive iodine; the need for systemic treatment depends on the type of thyroid cancer and the extent of disease.

Papillary thyroid cancer is the most common type of thyroid cancer. It is slow-growing, and it typically spreads locally to the lymphatics in the neck. They are usually driven by either *BRAF* or *RAS* mutations. Risk factors for papillary thyroid cancer include head and neck radiation, as well as Gardner syndrome and Cowden syndrome. Biopsy of the cancer demonstrates Orphan Annie eyes, which are empty-appearing nuclei with central clearing and psammoma bodies.

2. Follicular thyroid cancers frequently spread hematogenously to distant sites, such as brain, bone, lung, and liver. They are often associated with an *RAS* mutation.

Medullary thyroid cancers account for 2–3% of thyroid cancers. Risk factors include head and neck radiation and MEN type 2 syndrome, which is associated with an *RET* mutation. The tumor cells arise from parafollicular cells, or C cells, which produce calcitonin. Pathology demonstrates sheets of cells in an amyloid stroma and positive staining with Congo red.

Anaplastic thyroid cancers typically occur in older patients, and they are highly malignant with a poor prognosis.

Key Findings and Thyroid Cancer Differential Diagnosis

Key Findings	Diagnoses
History of neck radiation	Papillary or medullary
Gardner or Cowden syndrome Psammoma bodies Orphan Annie eyes Papillary carcinoma Reproduced with permission from Ali SZ, Cibas ES: The Bethesda System for Reporting Thyroid Cytopathology. New York: Springer Verlag; 2010.	Papillary
Hematogenous spread (metastatic disease)	Follicular
MEN type 2 Parafollicular cells (calcitonin-producing cells) C cells Positive Congo Red (amyloid) stain	Medullary
Older patients Aggressive and poor prognosis	Anaplastic

CASE 15 | Papillary Thyroid Cancer

A 49-year-old woman who received radiation treatment as a child for Hodgkin's lymphoma presents for a progressively enlarging neck mass. She reports worsening anterior neck discomfort for 6 months, difficulty swallowing solid food for the last 3 months with occasional regurgitation of food, and difficulty breathing when lying flat on her back. She has a visible mass in her right anterior neck that is mildly tender to palpation with associated enlarged cervical lymph nodes.

Evaluation/Tests	TSH and free T4 levels are normal. Thyroid ultrasound shows a 4.5-cm mass in the right thyroid with irregular borders, and it contains internal microcalcifications. Fine needle aspiration shows empty-appearing nuclei with central clearing, laminated calcium deposits (psammoma bodies), and nuclear grooves.
Treatment	Thyroidectomy potentially followed by radioiodine therapy depending on surgical pathology findings and levothyroxine treatment.
Discussion	This is a classic story for **papillary thyroid carcinoma (PTC)**, the most common malignancy of the thyroid gland. Common risk factors include a history of radiation exposure (therapeutic radiation for childhood malignancies, radiation of the head/neck/chest for treatment of medical conditions or extensive medical imaging, or secondhand exposure to nuclear fallout), and a family history of thyroid cancer in a first-degree relative. Genetic associations include mutations in *BRAF* or *RAS*; *RET/PTC* rearrangements are more commonly found after radiation exposure and in childhood PTC. Thyroid cancer is usually asymptomatic and is found on palpation of the thyroid or incidentally on radiologic studies obtained for other purposes. Exam findings include rapid and progressive growth of the thyroid nodule, partial mobility or a fixed nodule to the underlying tissue, increased hoarseness indicating involvement in the recurrent laryngeal nerve, or cervical lymphadenopathy. TSH and T4 levels are usually normal. Ultrasound findings suggesting that a thyroid nodule is malignant include irregular borders, low echogenicity (hypoechoic), taller than wide in the transverse plane, increased vascularity, and internal microcalcifications. Papillary thyroid carcinomas are usually well differentiated with an excellent prognosis. The first-line treatment for papillary thyroid cancer is surgical removal of the thyroid. Potential surgical complications include hoarseness (damage to recurrent laryngeal nerve), hypocalcemia (damage

CASE 15 | Papillary Thyroid Cancer *(continued)*

Discussion	or removal parathyroid gland), and dysphagia or dysphonia (damage to recurrent and superior laryngeal nerves). Postoperatively, radioactive iodine treatment may be administered to those with nodal or distant metastases. Levothyroxine treatment serves two purposes: (1) to replace thyroid hormone after thyroidectomy and (2) to suppress the TSH level so that any remaining thyroid cancer is not stimulated. Biopsy is key in making the diagnosis.

Thyroid adenomas are benign solitary growths that are usually nonfunctional. **Follicular thyroid carcinoma** has a similar appearance, but it shows invasion of the capsule and vasculature. **Medullary thyroid carcinoma** arises from the parafollicular C cells of the thyroid, and it produces calcitonin and histologically appears as a sheet of cells in an amyloid stroma.

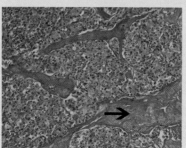

Medullary thyroid carcinoma. Amyloid (arrow) is often associated with these tumors. Medullary thyroid carcinoma can be sporadic, but also has familial forms, as well as being a component of multiple endocrine neoplasia, type 2 (MEN 2). Hematoxylin and eosin, 200×. Reproduced with permission from Kemp WL, Burns DK, Travis Brown TG. Pathology: The Big Picture. New York, NY: McGraw Hill; 2008.

Anaplastic thyroid carcinoma usually presents with extensive invasion of nearby structures, and it is more common in older patients. The remainder of the thyroid malignancies consists of metastases and lymphoma (often associated with Hashimoto thyroiditis).

Additional Considerations	**Nontoxic/nonobstructive multinodular goiters** are usually slow growing, and they can be observed/monitored with ultrasound. Surgery is indicated if a nodule is suspicious for malignancy or if the large goiter is causing compressive symptoms such as dyspnea, hoarseness, or dysphagia. When >2 thyroid nodules are secreting thyroid hormone autonomously, the goiter is referred to as a **toxic multinodular goiter**. Patients can present with signs and symptoms consistent with hyperthyroidism and compressive symptoms such as dyspnea, dysphagia, and/or neck pressure. The diagnosis is confirmed by a thyroid scan showing increased uptake in discrete areas along with low TSH and high T4. The hyperfunctioning follicular cells are distended with colloid, and they release increased thyroid hormones typically due to an activating mutation in the TSH receptor. These hot nodules are typically not malignant, but they can be treated with antithyroid medications, radioactive iodine, or thyroidectomy. **Goiters** secondary to **iodine deficiency**, thyroiditis, Graves' disease, or TSH-secreting pituitary adenoma are usually smooth and diffusely enlarged. **Cancerous nodules** are usually nonfunctioning and "cold" on scans.

PARATHYROID DISORDERS

Hyperparathyroidism

The parathyroid glands are 2 to 6 small endocrine glands (usually two superior and two inferior) located on the posterior aspect of the thyroid gland. They are the endocrine glands responsible for the production of parathyroid hormone (PTH), an essential hormone that responsible for increasing serum calcium and decreasing serum phosphate levels. PTH excess is usually due to a parathyroid mass that may be the result of a genetic disorder. The resulting increase in parathyroid hormone release will cause hypercalcemia and hypophosphatemia. The signs and symptoms patients experience result from biochemical abnormalities. Symptoms of hypercalcemia include polyuria, polydipsia, abdominal pain, constipation, weakness, and neuropsychiatric disturbances. Physiologic causes of PTH elevation include calcium and vitamin D deficiency. It is important to keep in mind that abnormal levels of calcium and vitamin D in the body can negatively affect bone deposition and that patients may present with bone complaints.

Diagnostic Studies to Help Distinguish Causes of High Calcium and/or High PTH

Disorder	Calcium	Phosphorus	Vitamin D	Parathyroid Hormone (PTH)	Manifestations
Primary hyperparathyroidism Parathyroid adenoma Parathyroid hyperplasia Parathyroid carcinoma	↑	↓	Normal or ↓	↑	Kidney stones (hypercalciuria) Osteitis fibrosa cystica
Secondary hyperparathyroidism Chronic kidney disease Hypocalcemia Vitamin D deficiency	↓ or normal	↑ (if renal failure) or ↓ (other causes)	↓	↑	Renal osteodystrophy Osteomalacia
Tertiary hyperparathyroidism Chronic kidney disease	↑	↑	Normal or ↓	Very ↑	Renal osteodystrophy
Ectopic secretion of PTH-related peptide (PTHrp) Tumors (squamous cell carcinoma of lung, head, and neck; renal, bladder, breast, and ovarian carcinoma)	↑	↓	Normal or ↓	↓	
Vitamin D/A/Calcium toxicity Increased Ca intake Increased vitamin D or A	↑	Normal or ↓	↓, normal, or ↑	↓	
Familial hypocalciuric hypercalcemia (FHH)	↑	Normal	Normal	Normal–↑	

CASE 16 | Primary Hyperparathyroidism

A 54-year-old woman with a history of anxiety presents for routine evaluation. She reports increased stress, fatigue, poor concentration, and constipation. She also has a history of recurrent kidney stones. She does not take any vitamins or supplements. Routine labs show an elevated calcium level.

Evaluation/Tests	Basic metabolic panel is notable for elevated calcium, low phosphorus, and PTH > 65 pg/dL (elevated), and 24-hour urine calcium level is elevated. TSH and vitamin D levels are normal. Ultrasound and nuclear Tc99m-sestamibi scan reveal an enlarged right superior parathyroid gland.
Treatment	Parathyroidectomy of one or more parathyroid glands.
Discussion	This patient is presenting with **primary hyperparathyroidism**, the most common cause of which is a **parathyroid adenoma**, a benign PTH-producing tumor of one of the parathyroid glands. PTH is normally released by the chief cells of the parathyroid gland, and it acts on bone and kidney to increase serum calcium and to decrease serum phosphate levels. Excess PTH in the setting of a parathyroid adenoma will result in hypercalcemia and hypophosphatemia. Elevated calcium in the urine can drive the formation of renal stones and polyuria. Most patients are asymptomatic, and the diagnosis is often made incidentally after obtaining routine labs. Skeletal findings can include subperiosteal thinning and erosions within the phalanges, a characteristic "salt and pepper" skull on imaging, and osteitis fibrosa cystica caused by the formation of cystic bone spaces that fill with brown fibrous tissue. While primary hyperparathyroidism is most commonly caused by a single parathyroid adenoma, multigland **parathyroid hyperplasia** can be seen, especially in patients with chronic kidney disease. Presentation of PTH-mediated hypercalcemia in multiple young family members should raise suspicion of **multiple endocrine neoplasia (MEN) type 1 or 2A**. The lack of other endocrine tumors in this patient makes MEN less likely. Rarely, **parathyroid carcinoma can cause primary hyperparathyroidism**. Given its rarity and no evidence of invasion of surrounding tissue, parathyroid carcinoma is unlikely in this case. **Vitamin D toxicity** can cause hypercalcemia and hypercalciuria; however, there would be an elevated vitamin D level.

CASE 16 | **Primary Hyperparathyroidism** *(continued)*

Discussion	**Secondary hyperparathyroidism** involves a problem outside of the parathyroid glands that results in low calcium or high phosphate. This drives a compensatory response from the parathyroid glands to increase secretion of PTH. Secondary hyperparathyroidism is most commonly seen with chronic kidney disease due to hypovitaminosis D and hyperphosphatemia. Given this patient's high serum calcium and low serum phosphate, this is unlikely. **Tertiary hyperparathyroidism** develops in response to refractory or untreated secondary hyperparathyroidism. Chronic hypocalcemia secondary to chronic renal disease results in compensatory hyperplasia of parathyroid cells. Even with treatment of the chronic hypocalcemia in tertiary hyperparathyroidism, the hyperplastic parathyroid glands continue to release PTH. Therefore, PTH levels will be significantly elevated, and serum calcium levels will be high.
Additional Considerations	**Familial hypocalciuric hypercalcemia (FHH)** is an autosomal dominant condition in which a gene mutation in the G-protein-coupled calcium-sensing receptor (CASR) shifts the normal threshold range of calcium required to initiate release of PTH upward, leading to high-normal or mildly high serum calcium and PTH levels. The kidney retains calcium, thus leading to low calcium level in the urine. When the findings of high-normal or mildly high serum calcium and PTH levels are found, diagnosis is made with a 24-hour urine calcium collection, where the collected total 24-hour calcium level is low. A high serum calcium with low urine calcium is diagnostic of FHH. A family history of hypercalcemia is typically present. FHH generally has a benign and asymptomatic course, and it can be managed with observation. For those with severe hypercalcemia, serum calcium levels can be lowered with cinacalcet, which allosterically activates the calcium-sensing receptor on parathyroid chief cells and reduces PTH secretion.

Hypoparathyroidism

Parathyroid hormone deficiency may result from the abnormal development or absence of development of the parathyroid glands. Parathyroid deficiencies can also be seen in autoimmune destruction of the parathyroid glands or surgical excision (usually after a thyroid procedure). Resistance to parathyroid hormone will cause symptoms of parathyroid deficiency, even though there will be high serum levels of PTH. The symptoms associated with hypoparathyroidism are related to the biochemical findings of hypocalcemia and hyperphosphatemia. Symptoms and signs of hypocalcemia include fatigue, seizures, arrhythmias, and Chvostek and Trousseau signs.

Diagnostic Studies to Help Distinguish Causes of Low Calcium and/or Abnormal PTH

Disorder	Serum Calcium	Serum Phosphorus	25-OH Vitamin D	PTH	Manifestations
Hypoparathyroidism Surgical resection Autoimmune destruction DiGeorge syndrome	↓	↑	Normal	↓	Tetany, Chvostek signs (contraction of facial muscles), Trousseau sign (carpal spasm), fatigue, seizures, arrhythmias
Vitamin D deficiency rickets	↓	↓	↓	↑	Pathologic bow legs (genu varum), bead-like costochondral junctions (rachitic rosary), craniotabes (soft skull)
Pseudohypoparathyroidism End-organ resistance to PTH	↓	↑	Normal	↑	Albright hereditary osteodystrophy: shortened 4th/5th digits, short stature, obesity, developmental delay
Pseudopseudohypoparathyroidism Defective G protein (paternal inheritance) but no PTH resistance	Normal	Normal		Normal	Albright hereditary osteodystrophy features on physical exam

CASE 17 | Hypoparathyroidism

A 34-year-old woman with a history of primary hyperparathyroidism undergoes resection of a parathyroid adenoma. Immediately post-op, the patient reports perioral numbness. On exam, vital signs are stable, but on tapping of the facial nerve anterior to the right ear, ipsilateral twitching of the patient's lip is noted (Chvostek's sign). When the blood pressure cuff is inflated for several minutes, spasms in the outstretched hand are observed (Trousseau's sign).

Evaluation/Tests	STAT serum ionized calcium is low.
Treatment	Administer IV calcium. Serum calcium is measured and corrected frequently in the post-op setting of parathyroidectomy. If low, magnesium levels should also be corrected. Hypophosphatemia is usually not corrected as calcium and phosphate can precipitate and lead to worsening of hypocalcemia. Electrolyte abnormalities usually self-regulate once the immediate post-op setting has passed.
Discussion	This patient presents with hypoparathyroidism; she exhibits classic signs and symptoms of hypocalcemia as a result of **hungry bone syndrome**. Hungry bone syndrome can occur upon resection of a parathyroid adenoma or after a subtotal/total parathyroidectomy. Hungry bone syndrome is believed to occur as a result of the sudden drop in PTH that accompanies removal of parathyroid tissue. Prior to removal of parathyroid tissue, elevated PTH levels predominate and result in a net efflux of calcium from the bones. Upon surgical removal of parathyroid tissue, PTH levels are suddenly lowered. Bones become "hungry" and increase their uptake of calcium, phosphate, and magnesium, resulting in hypocalcemia, hypophosphatemia, and hypomagnesemia. The hypocalcemia results in perioral numbness, paresthesia of the hands and feet, muscle cramps, and the positive Trousseau's sign (carpopedal spasm), and Chvostek's sign (lip spasm). Hypoparathyroidism can be due to accidental damage (during thyroidectomy), excision of the parathyroid glands, autoimmune destruction of the parathyroid gland, or parathyroid aplasia (DiGeorge syndrome). The presence of spasms (Trousseau's and Chvostek's signs) is classic for hypocalcemia, making other options less likely. Severe **hypomagnesemia** can cause neuromuscular hyperexcitability (tremor, tetany, convulsions) and cardiovascular manifestations, such as widened PR intervals and atrial and ventricular arrhythmias.

CASE 18 | Pseudohypoparathyroidism

A 6-year-old girl is brought to clinic for evaluation. Her mother is concerned because her daughter is shorter than the rest of the family and has been gaining weight excessively. She noted that her daughter has been on calcium and vitamin D for the past 3 years, which was prescribed by her previous pediatrician. Vital signs are normal, except the girl's hand shows spasms when the cuff is inflated when taking the blood pressure. On physical exam, the patient has short stature, obesity, round facies, shortened 4th/5th digits, and subcutaneous calcifications.

Evaluation/Tests	Labs show low serum calcium, elevated phosphorus, and elevated PTH levels.
Treatment	Calcium supplementation, calcitriol (D_3) supplementation.
Discussion	This patient is presenting with **pseudohypoparathyroidism type 1A**, an autosomal dominant condition with maternal inheritance of an inactivating mutation in the *GNAS1* gene, which encodes a Gs protein α-subunit. Defects in this gene result in end-organ resistance to PTH. Normally, the *GNAS1* gene undergoes genomic imprinting in humans whereby expression of the gene in the kidney and bone is determined only by the maternal allele. Maternal inheritance of a defective gene therefore results in resistance to PTH with ensuing hypocalcemia, hyperphosphatemia, and elevated PTH. This imprinting does not occur in other organs, so inheritance of any defective allele can drive additional findings collectively known as Albright hereditary osteodystrophy. Features of this include shortened 4th/5th digits, short stature, obesity, round face, developmental delay, and subcutaneous calcifications. Genetic testing for the mutation can be performed, although it is not necessary for diagnosis. Given the imprinting that occurs in bone and kidney, inheritance of a defective paternal allele has a different presentation referred to as **pseudopseudohypoparathyroidism**. Because the paternal allele is normally silenced in the kidney and bone in this condition, the PTH, serum calcium, and phosphate are unaffected and therefore will be normal. There is no end-organ resistance to PTH. However, the patient will still display features of Albright hereditary osteodystrophy. In **hypoparathyroidism,** the parathyroid gland is unable to produce and release PTH, so PTH levels will be low.

PANCREATIC ENDOCRINE DISORDERS

The endocrine pancreas is responsible for production of hormones such as insulin, glucagon, and somatostatin. Dysfunction of the pancreas may lead to overproduction of these hormones or decreased production of these hormones. The main pancreatic hormone is insulin, which plays a role in glucose homeostasis. Excess insulin production will produce symptoms of hypoglycemia, while insufficient insulin production will result in hyperglycemia.

CASE 19 | Hypoglycemia

A 55-year-old woman with a past medical history of hypertension and well-controlled diabetes mellitus type 2 is brought to the emergency department for altered mental status. Per the family, the patient had been doing well, but she reported feeling a little lightheaded and sweaty and went to rest this afternoon. She did not wake up for dinner, and when her family went to wake her up, they reported difficulty arousing her. She is currently being treated with the GLP-1 analog exenatide, which is injected subcutaneously twice per day. She lives with her husband, who has poorly controlled diabetes type 1, and he is on large doses of injection insulin glargine and aspart. On exam, her vital signs are afebrile, blood pressure is 128/86 mmHg, pulse is 102/min, respirations are 12/min, and she appears very somnolent.

Evaluation/Tests	Serum glucose is 40 mg/dL. HbA1c is 6.2%. Serum insulin is elevated, and proinsulin and C-peptide are low. Sulfonylurea and meglitinide screens are negative. Urine toxicity screen is negative for illicit drugs.
Treatment	Dextrose.
Discussion	This case is an example of severe **hypoglycemia** caused by use of exogenous insulin, as the patient appears to have confused her injectable glucagon-like peptide-1 (GLP-1) receptor analog exenatide for her husband's injectable insulin glargine or aspart. GLP-1 is an incretin normally secreted by the intestines in response to food ingestion, and it helps to regulate serum glucose levels by controlling gastric emptying and promoting insulin release. GLP-1 receptor analogs such as exenatide or liraglutide work to decrease glucagon release, delay gastric emptying, increase glucose-dependence insulin release, and promote satiety. Her husband is on two injectable insulin preparations: the more rapid-acting aspart and the long-acting glargine. These directly bind the insulin receptor and promote glucose update, which could lead to hypoglycemia. As this patient's diabetes is well controlled (indicated by her normal hemoglobin A1c), she is more sensitive to exogenous insulin and prone to developing hypoglycemia. Symptoms include sweating, tremors, tachycardia, lightheadedness, dizziness, and anxiety. In diabetics, overtreatment with insulin or sulfonylureas (glipizide, glyburide, glimepiride) as well as skipping meals, poor oral intake, or exercise can contribute to hypoglycemia. Reduced renal function decreases the clearance of insulin, which can also trigger hypoglycemia. In nondiabetics, hypoglycemia often presents with **Whipple's triad**: presence of symptoms, documentation of a low glucose level (often below 55 mg/dL), and relief of all symptoms with proper treatment. Common causes of hypoglycemia in nondiabetics include surreptitious or accidental use of sulfonylureas or insulin, insulinoma (tumor of insulin-secreting β-cells), adrenal insufficiency (low cortisol production), critical illnesses, or consumption of alcohol. Laboratory workup begins with measurement of serum insulin and its precursors such as proinsulin and C-peptide. Within the rough endoplasmic reticulum, preproinsulin is cleaved to proinsulin, which is then stored in secretory granules. Proinsulin is cleaved into insulin when glucose enters the β-cell, and the cell releases C-peptide as the secretory granules. Therefore, elevated proinsulin and C-peptide will only be seen with endogenous insulin sources. In the case of accidental or surreptitious **exogenous insulin use**, the insulin levels will be high while proinsulin and C-peptide levels will be low. Insulin levels would be high with **surreptitious use of a sulfonylurea**, but proinsulin and C-peptide levels would also be high due to the endogenous production of insulin. This is not what the patient is experiencing given her negative screen for sulfonylurea drugs. **Insulinomas** are tumors of pancreatic β-cells that overproduce insulin, and they result in recurrent attacks of hypoglycemia. Blood glucose will be low, but proinsulin and C-peptide levels will be high given the endogenous source of insulin production. Treatment of insulinoma involves surgical resection, and it may be associated with multiple endocrine neoplasia type 1.

CASE 20 | Type 1 Diabetes Mellitus

A 12-year-old boy presents for a well child visit with his mother. His mother reports that he has been more tired than usual. Upon questioning, he admits to waking up frequently to urinate and has not been sleeping well. He also reports recent increased thirst and weight loss.

CASE 20 | Type 1 Diabetes Mellitus *(continued)*

Evaluation/Tests	Fasting plasma glucose level is 200 mg/dL; HbA1c is 7.5%.
Treatment	Injectable insulin preparations.
Discussion	This patient is presenting with **type 1 diabetes mellitus (T1DM)** (formerly called insulin-dependent diabetes mellitus or juvenile diabetes). It is the most common form of diabetes in childhood and, is characterized by autoimmune destruction of pancreatic islet β-cells due to a combination of genetic and environmental factors. This results in low or absent levels of endogenously produced insulin and affected individuals depend on exogenous insulin to prevent development of diabetic ketoacidosis (DKA). Presence of autoantibodies such as glutamic acid decarboxylase antibodies is seen. T1DM is associated with other autoimmune diseases such as thyroiditis, celiac disease, and Addison disease. Girls and boys are almost equally affected, and peaks of presentation occur in two age groups: 5–7 years and at the time of puberty. The natural history of the disease includes four distinct stages: (1) preclinical B-cell autoimmunity with progressive defect of insulin secretion, (2) onset of clinical diabetes, (3) transient remission "honeymoon period," and (4) established diabetes. Diagnosis of diabetes is confirmed with fasting (>8 hours) plasma glucose ≥126 mg/dL, 2-hour oral glucose tolerance test ≥200 mg/dL (2 hours after consumption of 75 g of glucose in water), or hemoglobin A1C ≥6.5% (reflects average blood glucose for the past 3 months). T1DM shows severe glucose intolerance, classic symptoms of polyuria, polydipsia, polyphagia, and weight loss. There is no association with obesity, and genetic predisposition is relatively weak as it has a 50% concordance rate in identical twins. Inheritance is polygenic, with an increased risk associated with the HLA-DR4 and HLA-DR3 haplotypes. On histology, pancreatic islet β-cells will show leukocytic infiltrates. **Diabetes insipidus** will also present with polyuria and polydipsia. Sodium levels may be elevated, but glucose is normal. This condition is much more rare than DM. **Type 2 DM** will also present with polyuria and polydipsia, but patients are typically overweight and may have acanthosis nigricans. Sometimes, lab tests are needed to differentiate type 2 from type 1 DM. Autoantibodies to β-cell antigens such as islet cell cytoplasm (ICA), insulin autoantibody (IAA), antibodies to glutamic acid decarboxylase are detected in serum of type 1 patients but are not seen in type 2.

CASE 21 | Type 2 Diabetes Mellitus

A 47-year-old man with a history of hypertension and hyperlipidemia presents with polyuria, polydipsia, and polyphagia for the past few months. He has also noticed some blurry vision and tingling in his feet. On exam, his blood pressure is 128/80 mmHg, and his BMI is 33. His fundoscopic exam is normal. He has velvety hyperpigmentation on the back of his neck (acanthosis nigricans). On foot exam, his dorsalis pedis pulses are normal. He has no skin lesions or breakdown, but his monofilament test is abnormal (indicating neuropathy).

Evaluation/Tests	Serum HbA1c is 8%, fasting plasma glucose is 210 mg/dL.
Treatment	Lifestyle modifications including increased exercise, improved diet, avoidance of sugar-sweetened foods and beverages, diabetes education, and weight reduction. Typical pharmacological therapy includes metformin as monotherapy or in combination with other medications. If symptomatic with significant hyperglycemia, add insulin.
Discussion	This patient is presenting with **type 2 diabetes mellitus (T2DM)**, which can present with hyperglycemic symptoms (polyuria, polydipsia, polyphagia, blurred vision, and weight loss). However, it can also present with little to no symptoms depending on how insulin resistant and how elevated the blood glucose is. Obesity, family history, diet rich in carbohydrates, and sedentary lifestyle are risk factors for developing diabetes. It is more frequent with advancing age, but it is occurring in younger age groups now because of the obesity epidemic. Hypertension and hyperlipidemia are not risk factors, but they tend to coexist in the same patients. Testing for DM includes two consecutive positives tests of any of the following: (1) HbA1c ≥6.5%, (2) fasting plasma glucose ≥126 mg/dL, (3) 2-hour oral glucose tolerance test ≥200 mg/dL, or (4) a single episode of a random plasma glucose ≥200 mg/dL in a patient with hyperglycemic symptoms (polyuria, polydipsia, nocturia). Beyond lifestyle modifications, the most common oral medication is metformin, a biguanide that improves insulin sensitivity among many other actions. Other commonly used classes include sulfonylureas, thiazolidinediones, and DPP-4 inhibitors. Injectable hormone analogue options include daily or weekly GLP-1 agonists and insulins. Diabetics also need an annual dilated eye exam to evaluate for diabetic retinopathy, a foot exam to assess for peripheral neuropathy, and a urine microalbumin level to screen for diabetic nephropathy. It is important to treat hypertension and microalbuminuria with an ACEI or an ARB and to treat hyperlipidemia with lifestyle modifications and statins. The goal is to bring HgA1C below 7% while avoiding hypoglycemia.

CASE 21 | Type 2 Diabetes Mellitus (continued)

Discussion	Compared to **T1DM**, T2DM has a relatively strong genetic predisposition, with a 90% concordance rate in identical twins. There is no association with HLA haplotypes, and glucose tolerance is usually mild to moderate. There are variable numbers of β-cells within islets; however, they display deposits of islet amyloid polypeptide (IAPP).
	Benign prostatic hyperplasia (BPH) will also present with polyuria and nocturia. Additional features of the patient's history may include dysuria and difficulty starting and stopping urine stream.
	Diabetes insipidus will present with increased thirst and polyuria, similar to T2DM. However, other symptoms of T2DM such as blurry vision and unintentional weight loss do not occur.

CASE 22 | Diabetic Ketoacidosis

A 4-year-old boy is brought to the emergency department by his mother for 2 days of abdominal pain and vomiting. When she went to check on him this morning, she noticed he was not easily arousable. Review of systems is positive for increased thirst, increased urination, nocturia, fatigue, and weight loss. On exam, pulse is 145/min, blood pressure is 80/50 mmHg, and respirations are deep at 40/min with a fruity odor. Capillary refill is delayed, and he has dry mucous membranes.

Evaluation/Tests	Serum labs show hyperkalemia and blood glucose >400 mg/dL. The patient has an elevated anion gap metabolic acidosis with pH 7.3, serum bicarbonate 12 mEq/L, and anion gap of 12 mEq/L. Urine and blood tests are notable for the presence of ketones.
Treatment	IV fluids, IV insulin, and potassium (to replete intracellular stores); glucose if necessary to prevent hypoglycemia.
Discussion	This patient is presenting with **diabetic ketoacidosis (DKA),** a potentially life-threatening complication of diabetes mellitus that is the end result of the metabolic abnormalities resulting from a severe deficiency of insulin or from insulin ineffectiveness. This is the second most common form of presentation for T1DM in most populations. DKA is classified as mild, moderate, or severe depending on the degree of metabolic acidosis and clinical presentation. DKA and its complications are the most common cause of hospitalization, mortality, and morbidity in children with type 1 DM. Factors that precipitate DKA include poor metabolic control or missed insulin doses, illness/infection, medications (steroids), and drugs and alcohol. DKA is characterized by hyperglycemia, acidosis, and ketonemia. Due to the lack of insulin, the peripheral tissues are unable to take up glucose. This leads to hyperglycemia, which drives dehydration by causing excessive polyuria. This osmotic diuresis will cause potassium loss through the urine, thus causing total body potassium depletion; however, serum labs will show hyperkalemia because intracellular stores of potassium are depleted. In the absence of insulin, excess fat breakdown occurs. Increased free fatty acids circulate in the bloodstream and are then made into ketone bodies (B-hydroxybutyrate > acetoacetate). The acetoacetate is metabolized into acetone (producing the fruity breath odor). The increased ketone bodies lead to the increased anion gap metabolic acidosis. DKA can further lead to several complications including mucormycosis infection, cerebral edema, cardiac arrhythmias, and heart failure.
	Severe **gastroenteritis** can present with abdominal pain, vomiting, and dehydration. Serum glucose is usually not elevated, so there is no associated polyuria or polydipsia.
	A **hyperosmolar hyperglycemic state** is usually seen in T2DM and not T1DM. It may present with polyuria, polydipsia, hyperglycemia, and altered mental status. Usually, labs will show increased serum osmolality in the absence of acidosis.

CASE 23 | Hyperosmolar Hyperglycemic State

A 71-year-old woman with a history of type 2 diabetes mellitus, hypertension, and chronic kidney disease is brought to the emergency room with lethargy, confusion, vomiting, and generalized weakness progressing over the course of a day. She lives in assisted living, but she takes her own medications. On exam, she is somnolent but arousable, disoriented, and not able to follow many commands. Her vital signs are afebrile, pulse is 122/min, blood pressure is 101/67 mmHg, and respirations are 12/min. She has dry mucous membranes and decreased skin turgor. STAT fingerstick blood glucose is >500.

Evaluation/Tests	Serum pH is 7.4. Complete metabolic panel reveals sodium 127 mg/dL, potassium 3.4 mg/dL, creatinine and BUN elevated to 2.9 and 57 mg/dL respectively, anion gap 10, and glucose 1174 mg/dL. Measured serum osmolality is 331 mOsm/kg, and phosphate is 2.8 mg/dL. CBC shows leukocytosis with WBC count 13,000/mm³. Urinalysis is negative for ketones but positive for WBCs and nitrites. Urine culture is pending. Chest X-ray is normal.

CASE 23 | Hyperosmolar Hyperglycemic State (continued)

Treatment	Intensive fluid resuscitation with normal saline and IV insulin drip. Potassium replacement as needed. Regularly check glucose and serum chemistry to ensure decreasing glucose and improvements in sodium and potassium levels. Once insulin requirements on the drip are low, subcutaneous long-acting insulin is given, and insulin drip is discontinued.
Discussion	This patient is presenting in a **hyperosmolar hyperglycemic state (HHS)**, another serious complication of diabetes mellitus typically associated with T2DM. Patients tend to present after several days of developing polyuria, polydipsia, and weight loss. They are more likely to develop lethargy, focal deficits, and coma—which, if untreated, can progress to death. Events are usually precipitated by a trigger, most commonly infections such as pneumonia or urinary tract infection (as in this patient) or from discontinuation of insulin. Decreased water intake, particularly in older patients, can promote the development of HHS. Although most patients in HHS present with a serum potassium in the normal range, HHS patients usually have a substantial total body potassium deficit, caused by both diuresis and secondary hyperaldosteronism. Hyperosmolarity drives potassium out of cells, leading to normal or near-normal serum concentration levels. Significant hyperglycemia results in excessive osmotic diuresis, leading to severe dehydration. **Diabetic ketoacidosis (DKA)** is most often seen in patients with T1DM, and it is characterized by anion gap acidosis.

NEUROENDOCRINE TUMORS

Neuroendocrine tumors are a large class of epithelial neoplasms that may secrete functional hormones. Neuroendocrine tumor biopsy demonstrates cells with salt and pepper chromatin, organized in prominent rosettes. Cells stain positive for chromogranin A. There are many types of neuroendocrine tumors; four of the most important to recognize include carcinoid tumors, gastrinomas, insulinomas, and glucagonomas.

Carcinoid tumors arise from nests of neuroendocrine cells. These tumors secrete serotonin (5-HT). Patients are usually asymptomatic unless the carcinoid tumor metastasizes to the liver; then the serotonin is directly released into circulation, causing carcinoid syndrome. Carcinoid syndrome consists of diarrhea, cutaneous flushing, wheezing, or right-sided heart disease. Management of carcinoid tumors includes treatment with a somatostatin analog, such as octreotide. Somatostatin analogs inhibit the release of serotonin by binding the somatostatin receptors on the tumor cells and decreasing the symptoms of carcinoid syndrome. In addition to controlling these symptoms, surgical resection of the tumor is often required.

Gastrinomas secrete excess gastrin, which causes parietal cells to hypersecrete gastric acid. This results in Zollinger-Ellison syndrome, which includes peptic ulcer disease, diarrhea, and weight loss. Diagnosis is made by measuring fasting serum gastrin levels; equivocal results can be further evaluated with the secretin stimulation test. Gastrinomas are managed with PPIs, somatostatin analogs, and resection.

An **insulinoma** will present with severe hypoglycemia because this pancreatic beta-cell tumor causes elevated insulin levels. It must be distinguished from excessive exogenous insulin use by quantifying c-peptide levels. An elevated c-peptide is indicative of insulinoma rather than surreptitious insulin use. Insulinoma treatment primarily involves tumor resection.

Glucagonomas are tumors arising from pancreatic alpha cells that present clinically with hyperglycemia and diabetes as might be expected given the function of glucagon. Glucagonomas also present with a characteristic skin disorder called necrolytic migratory erythema, DVTs, and weight loss. Treatment involves surgery and somatostatin analogues.

**CASE 24	Carcinoid Syndrome**	
A 70-year-old woman with a past medical history of hypertension and arthritis presents for evaluation of diarrhea. She reports a 10-month history of watery diarrhea associated with intermittent facial flushing, diffuse-cramping abdominal pain, 10-pound weight loss, and dyspepsia. Her only medication is amlodipine. On exam, she has visible flushing and telangiectasias on her cheeks. Her blood pressure is 132/85 mmHg, and her pulse is 80/min. Abdomen is diffusely tender to palpation without rebound tenderness or guarding. Lungs are clear to auscultation.	
Evaluation/Tests	Electrolytes, blood count, and liver profile are normal. Chromogranin A levels are elevated. 24-hour urinary excretion of 5-hydroxyindoleacetic acid (5-HIAA) (end product of serotonin metabolism) is elevated. CT of the abdomen shows a mass in the small intestine and multiple masses in the liver.

CASE 24 | Carcinoid Syndrome (continued)

Treatment	Treat with octreotide, a somatostatin analog, and antidiarrheal medication such as loperamide. Surgical resection may be used for solitary lesions. Chemotherapy is used in some cases.
Discussion	This is a classic presentation of carcinoid syndrome. **Carcinoid tumors** are the most common tumors of the small intestine, and most of them do not produce symptoms until the tumor has metastasized. Neuroendocrine tumors of the gastrointestinal tract secrete a variety of molecules into the blood, the most common of which is serotonin (5-HT). Serotonin is metabolized in the liver and the lungs. Small bowel venous drainage goes through the liver, and serotonin is metabolized before it can cause serotonin syndrome systemically. When the tumor metastasizes past the liver, it may begin releasing serotonin into the systemic bloodstream and cause symptoms such as diarrhea, facial flushing, wheezing, tricuspid regurgitation or pulmonary stenosis (right-sided valvular heart disease). Depending on tumor location, further symptoms can be specific to a particular organ, such as bowel obstruction from intestinal carcinoid, and right upper quadrant pain and hepatomegaly from liver-based carcinoid. Carcinoid syndrome most commonly involves secretion of serotonin, if there is clinical suspicion of carcinoid syndrome, a 24-hour urine collection for 5-HIAA is the first step in the workup. The breakdown product of serotonin is 5-HIAA, and it will be elevated in carcinoid syndrome. Subsequent workup is focused on tumor localization and staging using CT, MRI, and somatostatin receptor nuclear scans using radiolabeled octreotide or Ga68-dotatate, a synthetic somatostatin analogue. Medical therapy with somatostatin analogs such as octreotide is the mainstay of treatment to curb growth of the tumors because most carcinoid tumors express the somatostatin receptor. Most patients with carcinoid syndrome have metastatic disease at presentation, so surgical removal of the tumor(s) is not the first line in therapy. **VIPomas** and **gastrinomas** can also cause diarrhea, but they wouldn't typically cause flushing. **Serotonin syndrome** would have a clear history of serotonergic drug use, and symptoms would be more acute. **Pheochromocytoma** would not present with diarrhea. In addition, the small bowel is an unlikely location for pheochromocytoma to arise.

CASE 25 | Multiple Endocrine Neoplasia Type 1

A 24-year-old woman presents with irregular menses, galactorrhea, and recurrent abdominal pain. She describes 1 year of menstrual change with cycles every other month, and she also has milky bilateral breast discharge. She has had more marked acid reflux symptoms and midabdominal pain. Medical history includes primary hyperparathyroidism with previous parathyroidectomy.

Evaluation/Tests	Basic metabolic panel is notable for elevated calcium, low phosphorus, and PTH > 65 pg/dL (elevated), and 24-hour urine calcium level is elevated. TSH and vitamin D levels are normal. Prolactin and gastrin levels are elevated. Pregnancy test is negative. MRI of the pituitary shows pituitary adenoma.
Treatment	Prolactinoma is treated with dopamine agonist therapy and surgical resection of gastrinoma. Consider parathyroidectomy.
Discussion	**Multiple endocrine neoplasia type 1 (MEN1)** syndrome is caused by mutations in the *MEN1* tumor suppressor gene that encodes the protein menin. Mutation in *MEN1* leads to tumors in several endocrine organs summarized by the "3 Ps": parathyroid, pancreatic, and pituitary. Patients often present with primary hyperparathyroidism from parathyroid hyperplasia of all glands or a parathyroid adenoma. Patients also develop pancreatic endocrine tumors, including gastrinomas (most common and leading to Zollinger-Ellison syndrome), insulinomas, glucagonomas, or VIPomas. Pituitary tumors are often functional, and they may secrete either prolactin (prolactinoma) or growth hormone. Additional nonendocrine tumors can occur including angiofibromas, meningiomas, and lipomas. Most tumors are benign, but malignancy can occur. Diagnosis is supported by two or more MEN1 manifestations, one MEN1 manifestation, and a first-degree relative with MEN1 syndrome or with genetic testing. Treatment depends on which tumors develop in an individual. Prolactinoma is treated with dopamine agonist therapy. Hyperparathyroidism requires 3.5 gland resection, which lowers the risk of recurrence but ensures some remaining parathyroid tissue. Enteropancreatic tumors require surgical resection. Regular screening is needed for other tumor development in MEN1-identified patients and family. The constellation of symptoms and lab findings is consistent with MEN.

CASE 25 | Multiple Endocrine Neoplasia Type 1 *(continued)*

Discussion	**Pregnancy** can cause elevated prolactin levels and galactorrhea in premenopausal women. **Prolactinoma** can occur independent of MEN syndrome and present with mass effect/visual disturbance (bitemporal hemianopsia), galactorrhea/amenorrhea, and decreased bone density (women) and low libido and infertility (men). **Gastritis** can be acute or chronic. Acute causes of gastritis include NSAIDs, curling ulcers, and brain injury. Chronic gastritis can be caused by *H. pylori* or autoimmunity.
Additional Considerations	**Multiple endocrine neoplasia type 2A (MEN 2A)** is characterized by the triad of primary hyperparathyroidism (usually multiglandular), medullary thyroid cancer (elevated calcitonin levels), and pheochromocytoma. Affected patients will present with symptoms suggestive of these processes, including renal stones, a fast enlarging neck mass, and intermittent severe hypertension accompanied by common symptoms of pheochromocytoma. Germline mutations in the *RET* oncogene are associated with MEN 2A. There is a genotype-phenotype correlation, meaning that the particular RET mutation defines the spectrum of possible clinical presentations and the timing of medullary thyroid cancer presentation, which may allow for planned prophylactic thyroidectomy prior to the onset of disease. Medullary thyroid cancer is treated with total thyroidectomy along with dissection and removal of any local or regional metastases, followed by lifelong thyroid hormone replacement and close monitoring for recurrence. Surgical resection of pheochromocytoma is indicated, following pretreatment with α and β adrenergic blockade to expand blood volume, prevent hypertensive crisis perioperatively, and prevent unopposed β stimulation. Patients with asymptomatic hypercalcemia from primary hyperparathyroidism can be monitored; however, a parathyroid adenoma should be resected. **Multiple endocrine neoplasia type 2B (MEN 2B)** is characterized by the triad of medullary thyroid cancer, pheochromocytoma, and mucosal neuromas. Unlike MEN 2A, hyperparathyroidism is not present. MEN 2B is also caused by germline mutations in the *RET* oncogene. Marfanoid habitus (long limbs, wingspan greater than height, hyperlaxity), and mucosal neuromas are unique to MEN 2B. As in MEN 2A, medullary thyroid cancer and pheochromocytoma are treated with total thyroidectomy and adrenalectomy, respectively. Mucosal neuromas (see figure A) are self-limited, and they are generally monitored and removed for aesthetic purposes. 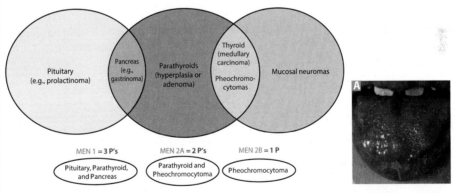 MEN syndromes have autosomal dominant inheritance. There is some overlap between the clinical presentations of the MEN syndromes. This figure depicts the different organ systems involved in each and where that overlap occurs. Reproduced with permission from Martucciello G, Lerone M, Bricco L, et al: Multiple endocrine neoplasias type 2B and RET proto-oncogene, Ital J Pediatr 2012 Mar 19;38:9.

9

Gastrointestinal

Waddah Alrefai, MD
Ryan Bolton, MD
Euna Chi, MD
Robert Carroll, MD

Dysphagia and Odynophagia
1. Gastroesophageal Reflux Disease (GERD)
2. Achalasia
3. Zenker's Diverticulum
4. Esophageal Squamous Cell Carcinoma

Abdominal and Rectal Pain
5. Cholecystitis
6. Acute Pancreatitis
7. Gastric Cancer
8. Appendicitis
9. Diverticulitis
10. Chronic Mesenteric Ischemia
11. Intussusception

GI Bleed
12. Mallory-Weiss Tear
13. Esophageal Varices
14. Peptic Ulcer Disease
15. Crohn's Disease
16. Angiodysplasia
17. Colorectal Cancer
18. Lynch Syndrome
19. Anal Cancer

Nausea and Vomiting
20. Hypertrophic Pyloric Stenosis
21. Small Bowel Obstruction Secondary to Incarcerated Hernia

Diarrhea, Constipation, and Steatorrhea
22. Irritable Bowel Syndrome (IBS)
23. Celiac Disease
24. Chronic Pancreatitis
25. Hirschsprung's Disease

Jaundice
26. Acute Hepatitis A
27. Pancreatic Cancer
28. Primary Sclerosing Cholangitis (PSC)
29. Primary Biliary Cholangitis (PBC)
30. Hemochromatosis
31. Hepatocellular Carcinoma (HCC)

Ascites
32. Alcoholic Cirrhosis
33. Chronic Hepatitis C
34. Budd-Chiari Syndrome
35. Spontaneous Bacterial Peritonitis (SBP)

DYSPHAGIA AND ODYNOPHAGIA

The main function of the esophagus is transmission of food from the mouth to the stomach. Disorders of the esophagus and swallowing present with three types of symptoms. The most common is "heartburn" or epigastric pain radiating into the chest with substernal burning. Gastroesophageal reflux disease (GERD) is the most common cause of noncardiac chest pain. Untreated GERD can cause strictures, resulting in swallowing problems. **Dysphagia** is a more specific symptom and indicates difficult or bad (dys-) swallowing (phagia). The severity can range from forced or multiple swallows to near impaction of food. **Odynophagia** or pain (odyn-) with swallowing is the least common of the three types of swallowing symptomatology and strongly suggests infectious or inflammatory disorder of the esophageal mucosa.

Chest pain (see "Cardiovascular" and "Respiratory" chapters) may arise from cardiopulmonary pathology and/or esophageal diseases. In the acute presentation, cardiopulmonary workup should be prioritized first with esophageal disorders evaluated after these conditions have been excluded. Chest pain associated with either dysphagia and/or odynophagia is typically esophageal in nature.

Dysphagia is often difficult to accurately localize. The sensation of food sticking in the throat or cervical esophagus can range from globus sensation (the feeling of a lump in the throat) to strictures or cancers of the distal esophagus. Pointing to a particular area of the chest as the site of obstruction is often accurate in localizing pathology, suggesting signaling through the somatic rather than visceral (vagus nerve) nervous system.

Intermittent dysphagia to solid foods suggests a mobile obstruction, while persistent solid food dysphagia is more indicative of a fixed obstruction. When it occurs with dysphagia, weight loss is an alarm symptom and merits urgent endoscopic evaluation. Finally, dysphagia for solids and liquids suggest motility disorders of the esophagus. This commonly includes achalasia, scleroderma, or diffuse esophageal spasm.

In an immunocompetent host, odynophagia results most often from pill-induced ulcers, aspirin, bisphosphonates, tetracyclines, and potassium preparations. These ulcers typically occur at the transition point between proximal skeletal muscle (upper 1/3) and distal smooth muscle (distal 2/3). Infectious causes of odynophagia are more common in immunosuppressed hosts (HIV, organ transplant, cancer chemotherapy) and include fungal (candida) esophagitis as well as viral agents such as herpes simplex virus (HSV) and cytomegalovirus (CMV). Candida esophagitis can occur in otherwise immunocompetent patients with diabetes mellitus or recent exposure to steroids or broad spectrum antibiotics, similar to candida pharyngitis or "thrush." Herpes esophagitis is occasionally seen in immunocompetent hosts as well.

Differential Diagnoses for Dysphagia/Odynophagia

Dysphagia	Odynophagia	Nonesophageal Causes
GERD Esophageal web/Plummer-Vinson syndrome Pharyngoesophageal (Zenker) diverticulum Esophageal spasm Achalasia Systemic sclerosis (scleroderma) Eosinophilic esophagitis Cancers Tracheoesophageal anomalies (fistulas, atresia)	Infections (candida, HSV, CMV) Pill-induced (aspirin, bisphosphate, tetracycline or potassium supplements) Caustic ingestion Severe GERD Cancers	Thyromegaly Cervical osteophytes Cricoid webs Neurologic/muscular disorders (stroke, ALS, Parkinson's, dementia, MS, myasthenia gravis, dementia, muscular dystrophy)

Key History Findings and Dysphagia/Odynophagia Differential Diagnosis

Dysphagia with Key Associated History Findings	Diagnoses
Intermittent dysphagia to solids	Esophageal web, ring, strictures
Persistent dysphagia to solids	Fixed obstruction: stricture, ring
Dysphagia solids and liquids	Motility disorders: achalasia, diffuse esophageal spasm, scleroderma
Associated with chest pain	Esophageal spasm
Associated with joint problems, skin tightening	Systemic sclerosis (scleroderma)
Associated with food impactions, atopy	Eosinophilic esophagitis
Regurgitation of foul-smelling food	Pharyngoesophageal (Zenker) diverticulum
Odynophagia in immunocompromised patient	Fungal (candida), viral (HSV, CMV)
Odynophagia and history of aspirin, bisphosphate, tetracycline, or potassium pill use	Ulcers secondary to pills
Dysphagia with alarm symptoms (weight loss, anorexia, progressive symptoms), or associated with chronic GERD/Barret's	Consider cancers

Useful tests and procedures in evaluating esophageal disorders include barium swallow (esophagram), esophageal manometry, and upper endoscopy/Esophagogastroduodenoscopy (EGD). Biopsies and dilation can be performed with an endoscope.

CASE 1 | Gastroesophageal Reflux Disease (GERD)

A 45-year-old obese woman presents with dysphagia, chronic intermittent cough, and chest burning for several months. Her symptoms are worse after large meals or lying down. Her difficulty swallowing has intensified recently, which prompted her to schedule an appointment. Tums helped with the burning sensation in the past, but her symptoms are getting worse. She has not lost weight. She recently started verapamil for hypertension. On physical exam, oropharynx is clear without erythema or exudates, lungs are clear to auscultation, and she has mild tenderness to palpation in the epigastric region.

Evaluation/Tests	Endoscopy is normal.
Treatment	PPI therapy to suppress acid production and lifestyle modifications; eliminate agents that affect the lower esophageal sphincter (LES) tone (i.e., verapamil).
Discussion	Gastroesophageal reflux disease (GERD) occurs when there is an inappropriate decrease in the LES tone. Typical symptoms include burning in the throat or chest, hoarseness, chronic cough, sour taste in mouth, globus sensation, dysphagia, and history of asthma. Typical EGD findings are normal, but they may show esophagitis, strictures, erosions, and Barrett esophagus. Patients without alarm symptoms can be treated with a trial of proton pump inhibitor (PPI) and lifestyle modifications (avoiding alcohol, caffeinated, acidic foods/beverages, not lying down for several hours after a meal, sleeping with the head of the bed elevated, and losing weight). Certain medications (such as calcium channel blockers, nitrates, albuterol, and anticholinergic drugs) should be avoided if possible because they may aggravate symptoms by decreasing LES tone. Upper endoscopy is recommended for alarm symptoms (weight loss, dysphagia, bleeding, treatment unresponsive to PPI, patient >50 years with >5–10 years of heartburn) to rule out **adenocarcinoma** complicating **Barrett's esophagus** (intestinal metaplasia). Barrett's esophagus is associated with an increased risk of esophageal adenocarcinoma. It requires surveillance endoscopies and chronic PPI therapy. Patients with **esophageal strictures**, **peptic ulcer disease** (PUD), or gastritis can present similarly, but the constellation of presenting symptoms is most consistent with GERD. Patients with strictures have a fixed defect, and they report the sensation of food getting stuck. PUD and gastritis typically present with epigastric pain with chronic NSAID use or *Helicobacter pylori* infection.
Additional Considerations	Individuals with **pill-induced esophagitis** typically present with painful swallowing and retrosternal chest pain due to an offending medication such as tetracyclines, NSAIDs, iron, or potassium chloride. Bisphosphonates are especially high risk, and patients should be advised to take with a full glass of water and remain upright for 30 minutes after ingestion.

CASE 2 | Achalasia

A 35-year-old woman presents with progressive difficulty swallowing both solids and liquids. Her symptoms have worsened over the past 5 years. She initially only had symptoms with solids, and she progressively has had symptoms with liquids. She also notes regurgitation of undigested food. She denies weight loss. In the past, she has had multiple trials of PPIs without improvement of her symptoms.

Evaluation/Tests	Barium esophagram shows dilated esophagus with narrow gastroesophageal junction (**"bird's beak" sign**). Manometry shows aperistalsis in the distal 2/3 of the esophagus with associated incomplete LES relaxation. Dilated esophagus Reproduced with permission from Farrokhi F, Vaezi MF. Idiopathic (primary) achalasia, Orphanet J Rare Dis 2007 Sep 26;2:38.
Treatment	Treatment aims to decrease pressure of lower esophageal sphincter with dilation, botox injections, or medications such as calcium channel blockers, nitrates, or sildenafil.

CASE 2 | Achalasia (continued)

Discussion	Achalasia results from loss of normal peristalsis in the distal esophagus and failure of the lower esophageal sphincter to relax. This is due to a decrease in inhibitory neurotransmitters in the myenteric (Auerbach) plexus. It is most commonly diagnosed in middle-aged men and women and characterized by progressive dysphagia to solids and liquids over years. It is classically diagnosed by barium swallow showing a "bird's beak" sign, but manometry is also diagnostic with aperistalsis in the distal 2/3 of the esophagus and associated incomplete lower esophageal sphincter relaxation. EGD is helpful in ruling out other causes. Achalasia is associated with increased risk of cancer. **Pseudoachalasia** can present similarly but is caused by Chagas disease (*Trypanosoma cruzi*) or extraesophageal malignancies causing mass effect. **Esophageal strictures** are secondary to chronic GERD or caustic ingestions or radiation treatment. Affected individuals report solid foods getting stuck. It is typically a fixed defect that is treated with endoscopy with balloon dilation. **Esophageal rings** are associated with **eosinophilic esophagitis**, which is common in patients with food allergies and atopy.
Additional Considerations	**Plummer-Vinson syndrome** is seen typically in middle-aged white women. Dysphagia is generally accompanied by iron deficiency anemia. Diagnosis is confirmed with endoscopic visualization of the upper esophageal web. Plummer-Vinson is associated with an increased risk of squamous cell carcinoma of the esophagus. **Diffuse esophageal spasm** causes intermittent dysphagia to solids and liquids. It is most commonly described seconds after initiating a swallow. Retrosternal pain is common. Esophageal manometry is diagnostic, showing increased or premature contractions in the distal esophagus in at least 20% of swallows. Barium esophagram may show corkscrew esophagus but has poor sensitivity and specificity. Upper endoscopy with biopsy should be done to evaluate for structural disease.

CASE 3 | Zenker's Diverticulum

A 70-year-old man presents with dysphagia for the past 4 weeks with associated foul-smelling breath. He regurgitates food into his mouth hours after eating, and now has a new fever, cough, and shortness of breath for the past 2 days. The patient's temperature is 38.5°C, heart rate is 88/min, respiratory rate is 20/min, blood pressure is 130/80 mmHg, and oxygen saturation is 94%. He has normal dentition and no cervical lymphadenopathy. Audible crackles are noted in the right lower lung. He has no abdominal tenderness or masses, and his neurological exam is normal.

Evaluation/Tests	Barium swallow (esophogram) shows a sac or pharyngoesophageal false diverticulum (Zenker). CXR shows right lower lobe infiltrate.
Treatment	Surgery is the definitive treatment of the diverticulum. Treat aspiration pneumonia with antibiotics.
Discussion	This presentation is consistent with **aspiration pneumonia** due to **Zenker's diverticulum**. Herniation of mucosal tissue at Killian triangle (between thyropharyngeal and cricopharyngeal parts of the inferior pharyngeal constrictor) results in Zenker's diverticulum. It commonly presents with dysphagia, regurgitation of undigested food, aspiration, foul breath (halitosis), noisy swallowing, cough, and weight loss. **Strictures**, **esophageal cancers**, or **strokes** can cause aspiration. Dysphagia affects 50% of stroke patients, and most recover function within 1 week. Initial presentation would typically have additional stroke-like findings (e.g., right-sided weakness, facial droop, etc.). Swallowing physiology includes oral preparatory stage, oral propulsive stage, pharyngeal phase, and esophageal phase. Any of these can be affected, and diagnosis is made by videofluorographic swallow study. Affected individuals may require enteral feeding or a modified diet to decrease risk of aspiration.
Additional Considerations	Newborns presenting with aspiration pneumonia may have a **tracheoesophageal fistula**, which is an abnormal connection between the trachea and esophagus. It typically occurs in association with **esophageal atresia** but may present without it. Polyhydramnios may be found on prenatal ultrasound, and it can be associated with **CHARGE syndrome** (coloboma, heart defects, atresia choanae, growth retardation, genital abnormalities, and ear abnormalities) or **VACTERL association** (vertebral defects, anal atresia, cardiac defects, TEF, renal anomalies, and limb abnormalities).

CASE 4 | Esophageal Squamous Cell Carcinoma

A 75-year-old man with a history of chronic alcohol and tobacco abuse presents with progressive dysphagia to solids for the past 3 months, and he has had difficulty swallowing liquids for the past 2 weeks. He has noticed a 15-pound weight loss over the past 3 months. On exam, he has temporal wasting, conjunctival pallor, and poor dentition. He has no abdominal tenderness or masses.

Evaluation/Tests	Endoscopy with biopsy shows squamous cell carcinoma.
Treatment	Squamous cell carcinoma is treated with a combination of surgical resection, neoadjuvant chemoradiation, and adjuvant chemoradiation depending on staging.
Discussion	Esophageal cancer has two common histologies: squamous cell and adenocarcinoma. Patients with esophageal cancer frequently describe difficulty swallowing (dysphagia) and weight loss. Dysphagia usually starts with solid foods and progresses to liquids over time. This stands in contrast to neuromuscular causes of dysphagia, such as achalasia and diffuse esophageal spasm, which present with simultaneous solid and liquid dysphagia. By the time symptoms develop, esophageal cancer is usually advanced. Esophageal cancer spreads to adjacent and supraclavicular lymph nodes, liver, lungs, and bone. Advanced disease is best treated with a multidisciplinary approach that can include chemotherapy, radiation, and surgery. **Squamous cell cancers** are found in the upper 2/3 of the esophagus, and adenocarcinoma is found in the lower 1/3. Esophageal squamous cell carcinoma is often due to specific exposures such as alcohol abuse, nitrate consumption, smoking and opiate use. Other risk factors include male sex, ingestion of hot liquids, and caustic strictures. Staging workup includes endoscopic ultrasound and CT neck/chest/abdomen with contrast. Brain imaging is only needed if patients have symptoms of brain metastases. **Esophageal adenocarcinoma** risk factors include male sex, chronic GERD, history of Barrett esophagus, obesity, smoking, and achalasia. Adenocarcinoma typically occurs in the lower 1/3 of esophagus. Barrett's esophagus is a premalignant finding often seen as a result of chronic gastroesophageal reflux (GERD). In Barrett's esophagus, stratified squamous epithelium that normally lines the esophagus is replaced by intestinal columnar epithelium due to chronic inflammation caused by GERD. As metaplasia advances, it can eventually lead to esophageal adenocarcinoma. Given the poor prognosis, surveillance is recommended in patients at risk for Barrett's.

ABDOMINAL AND RECTAL PAIN

The most common sources for abdominal pain are the gastrointestinal tract and genitourinary system. Description of the severity and quality of abdominal pain may be misleading, and the diagnosis should rely on a thorough evaluation of history and careful assessment of physical examination and laboratory findings. The perception of abdominal pain has three sensory components: visceral, somatic, and referred.

Visceral pain originates from the organs in the abdomen that are typically covered with visceral peritoneum and are innervated by visceral nerves. Visceral pain is usually poorly localized and may be perceived in a separate area from the affected organ. However, *foregut organs* (stomach, duodenum, liver, gallbladder, and pancreas) are generally associated with *upper abdominal pain*; midgut organs (small bowel, proximal colon, and appendix) are associated with periumbilical pain; and hindgut organs (distal colon and genitourinary tract) are associated with lower abdominal pain. Visceral pain is caused by distension, stretching, inflammation, ischemia, and peristalsis in a hollow organ. The sensations are conveyed to the spinal cord via sympathetic and parasympathetic nerves. Severe pain can be associated with autonomic responses (vomiting, nausea, and sweating).

Somatic pain originates from the parietal peritoneum and is precisely localized. Somatic pain is caused by infection, injury, inflammation, chemical irritation, and hemorrhage. Somatic pain could also originate from the body wall due to exertion of abdominal muscles, injury, and inflammation of the skin or peripheral nerves (herpes zoster). The sensations are conveyed to the spinal cord by somatic nerves. The pain is aggravated by coughing or movement.

Some cases are associated with both visceral and parietal pain. In early appendicitis, the pain is visceral and perceived in the periumbilical region. When the peritoneum covering the appendix is irritated, the pain becomes localized to the lower right quadrant (McBurney's point).

Referred pain originates from a certain region in the abdomen but is perceived in an area away from its origin. The differential could be broad, but it should include possible involvement of organs in the area where the pain is perceived. Irritation of the diaphragm (from ruptured spleen, perforated duodenal ulcer, or intra-abdominal abscess) may cause pain in the shoulder. Biliary colic can cause back pain in the right lower area of the thorax. Pain radiating to the back is a classic finding of acute pancreatitis. Renal colic can cause back and flank pain that radiates to the lower abdomen and groin. Pain originating from the uterus or the rectum can cause lower back pain. Referred pain occurs because afferent fibers carrying sensations from different locations enter the spinal cord via the same nerve root and can be interpreted as originating from a different area of the same spinal segment.

Pelvic pain is generally more difficult to characterize than pain from abdominal structures. Rectal pain is often described as low in the pelvis and may radiate to the back or sacrum, while bladder and prostate pain are described more often in the lower abdomen. Bowel movements may relieve the pain of rectal distension in constipation but increase with inflammation or spasm of the pelvic floor muscles. **Tenesmus**, the sensation of persistent feeling of rectal fullness despite rectal evacuation, often suggests rectal inflammation commonly from ulcerative proctitis. It can also arise from radiation injury (complicating treatment of cervical or prostate cancer) or from rectal infection (often from a sexually transmitted pathogen). Painless bleeding post bowel movement suggests the presence of internal hemorrhoids, while pain and bleeding with defecation suggests anal fissures that can present with anal carcinoma.

The location, onset, duration, and character of pain should be considered when making the diagnosis.

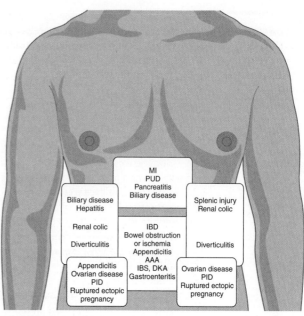

AAA, abdominal aortic aneurysm; DKA, diabetic ketoacidosis; IBD, inflammatory bowel disease; IBS, irritable bowel syndrome; MI, myocardial infarction; PID, pelvic inflammatory disease; PUD, peptic ulcer disease.

The differential diagnosis of abdominal pain by location. Reproduced with permission from Stern S, Cifu AS, Altkorn D: Symptom to Diagnosis: An Evidence-Based Guide, 4th ed. New York, NY: McGraw Hill; 2020.

Differential Diagnosis of Abdominal Pain Based on Location

RUQ	Epigastric	LUQ	Diffuse	GI Chest Pain
Biliary colic	GERD	Splenic pathology	Peritonitis	GERD
Choledocholithiasis	Gastritis	Referred from cardiac	Bowel perforation	Esophageal
Cholecystitis	Gastric cancer	source (ACS, pericarditis,	Gastroenteritis	Spasm
Ascending cholangitis	PUD	myocarditis)	Sickle cell crisis	Boerhaave
Hepatitis	Pancreatitis	Referred from lung source	Superior mesenteric	syndrome
Hepatic abscess	Referred from	(pneumonia, pleural effusion)	artery syndrome	
Hepatic adenoma	cardiac source		Dissection or	
Hepatic vein or portal vein	(ACS, pericarditis,		ruptured aneurysm	
thrombosis	myocarditis)		Diabetes ketoacidosis	
Referred from lung source			(DKA)	
(pneumonia, pleural effusion)			IBD	
			IBS	
			Intestinal obstruction	
			Volvulus	
			Intussusception	

RLQ	Periumbilical	LLQ	Suprapubic	Rectal
Appendicitis	Early appendicitis	Sigmoid diverticulitis	Bladder (UTI)	Hemorrhoids
Meckel's diverticulitis	Aortic aneurysm	Psoas abscess	Uterine etiology	Fissure
Cecal diverticulitis		Ureteral calculi	(PID, fibroids,	Abscess
Psoas abscess		Ovarian etiology	endometriosis,	Cancer
Ureteral calculi		(Mittelschmerz, ectopic	pregnancy)	Proctitis
Ovarian etiology (Mittelschmerz,		pregnancy, ovarian cyst,	Referred from	
ectopic pregnancy, ovarian cyst,		torsion, or abscess)	prostate	
torsion, or abscess)		Incarcerated/strangled hernia	Referred from rectum	
Incarcerated/strangled hernia				

General Characteristics and Abdominal Pain Differential Diagnoses

General Characteristics		Abdominal Pain Differential
Onset		
Sudden	- →	Perforation, rupture, torsion, bleeding into peritoneum
Gradual	- →	Distension of a hollow organ (obstruction causing backup), vascular insufficiency, peritoneal irritation
Duration		
Seconds to minutes	- - - - - - - - - - - - - - - - - - - →	Distension or spasm in a hollow organ
15–45 minutes	- →	Peptic ulcer (relieved by food or antacids)
Hours to days	- →	Biliary colic, pancreatitis
Weeks	- →	Pancreatic cancer, lymphoma
Months to years	- →	Opioid-induced constipation, emotional disturbances, functional disorders
Pain character		
Burning, aching	- →	Peptic ulcer
Cramping, stabbing	- - - - - - - - - - - - - - - - - →	Spasm, distension, or obstruction of a hollow organ
Squeezing, steady	- - - - - - - - - - - - - - - - - - →	Biliary colic

Key History Findings and Abdominal Pain Differential Diagnosis

Abdominal Pain with Key Associated History Findings	Diagnoses
Burning epigastric pain, worse with lying down and aggravated by spicy foods and caffeinated beverages and improved with TUMS, PPI. Associated globus sensation, sore throat, hoarse voice, asthma, regurgitation	GERD
NSAID use, epigastric pain, history of *H. pylori*	Peptic ulcer disease (PUD), gastritis
Improved with PPI/H2-blockers or antacids	GERD, PUD, gastritis
Chest pain, dyspnea after violent vomiting or post EGD	Boerhaave syndrome
Female, 40s, parous, RUQ colicky pain aggravated by fatty foods; referred right shoulder/scapular pain	Biliary colic, cholecystitis
RUQ pain, fevers/chills, jaundice (Charcot triad) The preceding plus mental status changes, hypotension (Reynold's pentad)	Ascending cholangitis
RUQ pain associated with jaundice	Hepatitis, choledocolithiasis
Upper abdominal pain, radiating to the back, vomiting and history of ETOH abuse	Pancreatitis, PUD, gastritis, alcoholic hepatitis
Cardiac risk factors and abdominal pain after eating causing food fear	Superior mesenteric artery syndrome (acute or chronic mesenteric ischemia)
Sickle cell patient (SC disease) with LUQ pain	Splenic infarct
Initial periumbilical pain, then localized RLQ	Appendicitis
History of diverticulosis with LLQ pain	Sigmoid diverticulitis
Severe intermittent crampy abdominal pain, vomiting, currant jelly stools, RUQ mass in kids	Intussusception
Alternating constipation, diarrhea, associated bloating	IBS
Abdominal pain associated with diarrhea, which may be bloody, weight loss, rash, arthralgias, eye irritation/redness	IBD
Pelvic pain with vaginal discharge, fever	PID, abscess
Young sexually active female, missed menses, and now with pelvic pain	Ectopic pregnancy
Weight loss, abdominal pain, older age, family history of colon cancer or not up-to-date on screening, change in stool caliber, iron deficiency anemia, ulcerative colitis	Colorectal cancer
Dysuria, frequency, hematuria, fever, and suprapubic pain	UTI (consider pyelonephritis if back pain)
Flank pain radiating down groin with associated hematuria and history of kidney stones	Nephrolithiasis

Key Physical Exam Findings and Abdominal Pain Differential Diagnoses

Abdominal Pain with Key Associated Exam Findings	Diagnoses
Jaundice, scleral icterus, hepatosplenomegaly	Liver, gallbladder, or pancreatic causes
RUQ tenderness, inspiratory arrest (positive *Murphy's sign*)	Cholecystitis
Diffuse pain out of proportion to exam	Superior mesenteric artery syndrome
Rebound tenderness	Peritonitis
McBurney's sign (RLQ tenderness: 1/3 distance from anterior superior iliac spine and umbilicus). (Rovsing's sign (pain in RLQ with palpation of LLQ), psoas sign (pain RLQ right lower quadrant with passive extension of the right hip), and obturators sign (pain RLQ with flexion and internal rotation of the right hip))	Appendicitis
LLQ tenderness, fever, elevated WBC	Diverticulitis, ovarian abscess
Cervical motion tenderness, vaginal discharge	PID
Suprapubic tenderness	UTI, uterine source (e.g., PID, endometriosis)
Prostate tenderness	Prostatitis
Periumbilical (Cullen's sign) and flank (Turner's sign) ecchymosis	Hemoperitoneum (pancreatitis, dissection)

Gastric Cancers and Associated Findings

Key Feature	Diagnosis
Signet ring cells Reproduced with permission from Reisner H. Pathology: A Modern Case Study, 2nd ed. New York, NY: McGraw Hill; 2020.	Diffuse-type gastric adenocarcinoma
Linitis plastica	Diffuse-type gastric adenocarcinoma
H. pylori infection	Intestinal-type gastric adenocarcinoma or MALT lymphoma
HER-2 mutation Ingestion of nitrates	Intestinal-type gastric adenocarcinoma
c-kit mutation	Gastrointestinal stromal tumor (GIST)
Virchow node	Gastric cancer metastasis to the left supraclavicular lymph node
Krukenberg tumor	Gastric cancer metastasis to the ovaries, often mucin secreting
Sister Mary Joseph nodule	Gastric cancer metastasis to subcutaneous periumbilical region

Initial tests and evaluation to confirm or refute diagnoses for patients presenting with abdominal pain include upper endoscopy to assess the esophagus and stomach and lower endoscopy (colonoscopy) to evaluate the colon. If indicated, biopsies can be done at the time of the procedures. Plain radiographs can be useful to assess for intestinal obstruction (dilation proximal to obstruction) or perforation (air under the diaphragm). RUQ ultrasound is useful for assessing gallbladder pathology, and CT scans are useful to assess other intra-abdominal pathology such as appendicitis and nephrolithiasis. Initial useful blood tests include CBC, BMP, LFTs, amylase, and lipase (pancreatitis), urinalysis, and pregnancy tests in female patients. Lactic acid levels and blood cultures may also be useful in the appropriate setting.

CASE 5 | Cholecystitis

A 43-year-old obese woman presents with right upper quadrant pain radiating to her right shoulder for 10 hours. She is also having nausea, vomiting, and loss of appetite. She has had similar intermittent pain in the past after eating fatty meals, but this episode is more severe and constant. On exam, she is in moderate distress, and her vital signs are notable for tachycardia. She has anicteric conjunctiva, hypoactive bowel sounds, tenderness in the RUQ, inspiratory arrest with deep palpation of the RUQ (Murphy's sign), guarding, and rebound tenderness.

Evaluations/Tests	CBC shows elevated WBC count. AST/ALT, alkaline phosphatase, and direct bilirubin were slightly elevated. Amylase and lipase are within normal limits. RUQ ultrasound shows gallstones and a thickened gallbladder wall with pericholecystic fluid. Gallbladder is not visualized on HIDA scan (suggestive of obstruction).
Treatment	The patient should be made NPO (nothing by mouth) and given IV fluids and medication for pain control. Treat the infection with IV antibiotics and urgent cholecystectomy.
Discussion	**Acute cholecystitis** refers to the presence of acute inflammation in the gall bladder. Ninety to 95% of the cases are due to **cholelithiasis**, which refers to the presence of biliary stones. Composition of stones vary and may include cholesterol, pigment (bilirubin), or mixed/brown (cholesterol and salts). After a fatty meal, cholecystokinin (CCK) is released, and the gallbladder contracts. Stone impaction in the cystic duct (**calculous cholecystitis**) causes obstruction and stasis, which leads to thickening and inflammation of the gallbladder wall and allows infection to set in proximal to the obstruction. Risk factors include drugs that promote stone formation (fibrate, progesterone, estrogen) and obesity. Cholecystitis is the second most common cause for acute abdominal pain in pregnant women, following appendicitis. Patients with cholecystitis have strong associations with the 5 Fs: fair, fat, female, fertile, and forty. High levels of estrogen and progesterone are common in all individuals with the 5 Fs.
Additional Considerations	**Ascending (acute) cholangitis** is due to an infection in the biliary tract, usually as a result of stasis caused by obstruction (typically a gallstone obstructing the common bile duct). Classical presentation is known as Charcot's triad: fever, RUQ abdominal pain, jaundice. As the infection progresses and becomes more severe, patients may also develop hypotension and alterations in mental status (Reynold's pentad). Patients with cholangitis frequently present with abnormal liver tests, typically in a cholestatic pattern (elevated serum total bilirubin and alkaline phosphatase), as well as a direct hyperbilirubinemia due to the inability of the bile to effectively drain from the liver. Abdominal ultrasounds can show signs of bile duct dilation or bile duct stones. CT scans may also detect bile duct dilatation, but they are less adept at identifying bile duct stones. If both of these scans are normal in a patient suspected of having acute cholangitis, magnetic resonance cholangiopancreatography (MRCP) is performed. Treatment includes intravenous hydration, correction of electrolyte disorders, and empiric antibiotics with activity against streptococci, *Escherichia coli*, and anaerobes. In addition to antibiotics, most patients will require biliary drainage, the timing of which depends on the severity of the presentation. The treatment of choice is endoscopic sphincterotomy via ERCP with stone extraction and possible stent placement. Cholecystitis could lead to the formation of a fistula between the gallbladder and the duodenum. The fistula may lead to drainage of the gallbladder and resolution of symptoms. **Acalculous cholecystitis** is a form of cholecystitis caused by dysfunction or hypokinesis of the gallbladder. It can result from CMV infection, stasis, or hypoperfusion of the gallbladder, as seen in critically ill patients. Long fasting, total parenteral nutrition (TPN), and weight loss may also predispose to acalculous cholecystitis. **Choledocholithiasis** is the presence of stones in the common bile duct, which can obstruct both the biliary system and the pancreatic duct. Labs will typically show elevated ALP and direct bilirubin. Jaundice suggests common bile duct obstruction or cholangitis. **Biliary colic** occurs when a stone temporarily blocks the cystic duct. Pain is typically <8 hours, and RUQ US will show gallstones (cholelithiasis) but no inflammation. Labs will be normal. **Chronic cholecystitis** is a condition associated with ongoing inflammation of the gallbladder. It is mostly associated with cholelithiasis and may occur because of recurrent episodes of acute cholecystitis or chronic irritation of the gallbladder by stones, leading to inflammatory response. **Porcelain gallbladder** refers to calcification of the gallbladders that could be a consequence of chronic inflammatory processes. Porcelain gallbladder is considered a risk for carcinoma of the gallbladder. Cholecystectomy should be performed when this condition is suspected.

CASE 6 | Acute Pancreatitis

A 44-year-old obese woman with a history of alcohol abuse presents with severe abdominal pain. The pain presents in her upper abdomen and radiates to her back and is associated with nausea, vomiting, and abdominal bloating. She has had similar but less severe symptoms in the past related to eating fatty foods. She is in acute distress secondary to pain. Her temperature is 38°C, respiratory rate is 24/min, pulse is 100/min, and blood pressure is 100/60 mmHg. She has epigastric tenderness, periumbilical (Cullen's sign) and flank ecchymosis (Turner's sign), decreased breath sounds, and dullness to percussion at both lung bases.

Evaluation/Tests	Amylase/lipase are >3× the upper limits of normal. Calcium is low. CBC shows elevated WBC and Hgb 10. Abdominal US shows gallstones that appear nonobstructive. CT abdomen shows the pancreas surrounded by edema.
Treatment	The patient should be NPO and receive supportive care including IV fluids and pain management.
Discussion	This patient is presenting with symptoms classic for acute pancreatitis: epigastric pain radiating to the back along with nausea and vomiting. The most common causes include gallstones, alcohol use, and hypertriglyceridemia. Other important etiologies include post-ERCP, trauma, autoimmune, steroid-related, mumps, hypercalcemia, scorpion sting, and drugs (protease inhibitors, sulfa, nucleoside reverse transcriptase inhibitors (NRTIs)). To make the diagnosis of acute pancreatitis, two of three criteria need to be positive: classic presentation (epigastric pain radiating to the back with associated nausea/vomiting), serum lipase >3× upper limit of normal, or radiological evidence (typically CT scan) of pancreatitis. Additional lab tests, including a CBC, BMP, and liver functional tests (LFTs) should be obtained to assess for alternative/additional diagnoses. Patients with pancreatitis may present with pleural effusion (dullness to percussion) and **signs of hypocalcemia**: facial muscles twitch with tapping over facial nerve (Chvostek's sign) and carpopedal twitching/spasm with inflated BP cuff (Trousseau's sign). Complications include hypocalcemia (precipitation of calcium soaps), hemorrhage, abscess, necrosis, organ failure (ARS, shock, renal failure), and pseudocyst. Patients with acute pancreatitis may require varying levels of supportive care based on the severity of presentation, but the initial management consists of aggressive fluid resuscitation and symptomatic pain and nausea control. The timing of restarting oral feedings is controversial, but early feeding as soon as the patient can tolerate is the favored approach.

CASE 7 | Gastric Cancer

A 62-year-old man with a history of tobacco use, alcohol use, and prior treatment of *H. pylori* infection presents with abdominal pain and weight loss. He has some nausea and occasional vomiting. He denies hematemesis, melena, or blood in stool. His diet consists of salty, fatty, fried foods. On exam, he has a palpable left supraclavicular lymph node, mild epigastric tenderness, a palpable abdominal mass, and a hard lymph node around the umbilicus.

Evaluation/Tests	Upper gastrointestinal endoscopy shows suspicious-appearing ulcers with raised margins. Biopsy reveals cells with peripheral nuclei or adenocarcinoma consistent with gastric malignancy.
Treatment	Surgery/chemotherapy.
Discussion	Clinically, gastric cancer usually presents late. Patients will report weight loss with early satiety and can present with an upper GI bleed. You should suspect gastric cancer in patients with alarm symptoms (new dyspepsia in patients >55 years, weight loss, bleeding, iron deficiency anemia, progressive dysphagia/odynophagia, jaundice, vomiting, palpable mass/lymph nodes). Risk factors include tobacco use, alcohol use, prior *H. pylori* infection, and consumption of nitrosamines and salty, fatty, processed foods. The most common type of gastric cancer is adenocarcinoma. Subtypes include intestinal and diffuse adenocarcinoma. Intestinal-type is often associated with *H. pylori* infections, occur on lesser curvature and look like ulcers with raised margins. Diffuse carcinomas are not typically associated with *H. pylori*, occur on the stomach wall, and have a grossly thickened/leathery (linitis plastica) appearance and characteristic signet ring cells (mucin-filled cells with peripheral nuclei) under microscopy. Other gastric cancers include lymphoma, gastrointestinal stromal tumors (GISTs), and carcinoid. Once a primary tumor is identified on endoscopy and a tissue diagnosis is made, pursue further staging with imaging studies. Metastasis can occur locally to the liver and lymph nodes or distally. The left supraclavicular node (Virchow node), subcutaneous periumbilical area (Sister Mary Joseph nodule), and, in females, bilateral ovaries (Krukenberg tumor) are common areas for metastasis. Treatments vary based on clinical stage. Early disease is treated with resection and may benefit from chemotherapy perioperatively. Advanced and metastatic disease is treated with systemic chemotherapy or palliative therapy. Patients with advanced HER2-positive adenocarcinoma of the stomach or gastroesophageal junction might benefit from the addition of trastuzumab, a monoclonal antibody that targets the HER2 receptor.

CASE 7 | Gastric Cancer (continued)

Discussion	Consider **malignancy** in patients presenting abdominal pain, weight loss, and supraclavicular lymphadenopathy. If EGD is not diagnostic, CT scan should be obtained to look for pancreatic and other cancers.
Additional Considerations	In **chronic gastritis**, mucosal inflammation leads to atrophy and intestinal metaplasia and is associated with increased risk of gastric cancers. *H. pylori* affects the antrum first and is associated with **MALT lymphoma**.

CASE 8 | Appendicitis

A 24-year-old woman presents with progressively worsening abdominal pain for the past 24 hours. The pain started in the periumbilical area but is now primarily in the right lower quadrant. She is unable to tolerate any foods or liquids due to nausea and vomiting. On physical exam, she is in moderate distress secondary to pain. Her temperature is 37.8°C, blood pressure is 120/80 mmHg, and pulse is 90/min. She has RLQ tenderness 1/3 of the distance from the anterior superior iliac spine to the umbilicus (McBurney's point), as well as guarding and rebound tenderness. She has pain in the RLQ with palpation of LLQ (Rovsing's sign) and pain in the RLQ with passive extension of the right hip (psoas sign).

Evaluation/Tests	CBC shows elevated WBC, and beta-hcg is negative. CT scan with contrast shows an enlarged appendix with wall thickening, fat stranding (signs of appendiceal inflammation).
Treatment	Appendectomy.
Discussion	Appendicitis symptoms may be subtle at first but progressively worsen with increasing inflammation. Inflammation and infection are proximal to an obstruction of the appendix by either a fecalith or lymphoid hyperplasia (children). The typical history is abdominal pain that starts periumbilically then migrates to the right lower quadrant; however, this migratory pain occurs in only about half of patients. Nausea and vomiting are frequently associated symptoms, and fever may develop later in the course. Guarding and rebound tenderness may present if the appendicitis is complicated by perforation and subsequent peritonitis. Rovsing's, psoas, obturator (pain in the RLQ with flexion and internal rotation of the right hip), and rebound are signs of peritonitis. **Pseudoappendicitis** presents similarly and is associated with *Yersinia enterocolitica* infections. Patients with **IBD** typically have diarrhea. In woman of childbearing age, consider **ovarian pathologies** such as ectopic pregnancy, ovarian torsion, ovarian cysts or abscess, or even normal pregnancy as they may present in a similar fashion. If the patient is pregnant, then an ultrasound may be obtained in lieu of CT scan. Ovarian torsion is a gynecologic emergency. It typically presents with acute moderate to severe pain on the affected side, along with nausea or vomiting. An adnexal mass is often present. Ectopic pregnancy can be ruled out with a negative pregnancy test. PID and tubo-ovarian abscess can be ruled out with STI testing and pelvic exam.

CASE 9 | Diverticulitis

A 78-year-old obese man with a history of diverticulosis presents with left lower quadrant abdominal pain. He also reports chronic constipation, mild nausea, and a subjective low-grade fever. His temperature is 38.5°C, blood pressure is 110/80 mmHg, and pulse is 88/min. He has LLQ tenderness to palpation, rebound tenderness, and guarding.

Evaluation/Tests	CBC shows elevated WBC. BMP and urinalysis are within normal limits. Abdominal CT scan with oral and intravenous contrast shows numerous small out-pouches in the colon filled with contrast (diverticulosis). The sigmoid shows thickening and pericolic fat stranding (inflammation) and a possible abscess.
Treatment	Treat with bowel rest: NPO, IV fluids, and pain management. IV antibiotics that cover gram negatives and anaerobes (e.g., pipercillin-tazobactum) should be given.
Discussion	**Diverticulosis** is commonly seen in older patients and is associated with low-fiber and high-fat/red meat diet and obesity. These outpouches of the colon or false diverticula involving the mucosa and muscularis mucosa only are caused by focal weakness in the wall and increased intraluminal pressure. They can occur anywhere but are typically seen in the sigmoid colon. Patients may be asymptomatic or present with bleeding from the diverticulum (painless hematochezia) or with **diverticulitis** (inflammation of diverticulae). Typical symptoms of diverticulitis include LLQ pain, fever, and leukocytosis. Patients may have abdominal tenderness to palpation, typically in the LLQ due to involvement of the sigmoid colon, as well as guarding or rebound depending on the level of inflammation. If severe, such as from

CASE 9 | Diverticulitis *(continued)*

Discussion	perforation, patients may present with fever, tachycardia, and/or hypotension. A CT scan can localize the area of inflammation/infection and may aid in identifying if perforation is present. Mild presentations can be managed in the outpatient setting while more serious presentations are managed in the hospital. Additional complications seen in diverticulitis that may require hospitalization include complex presentations (abscess, perforation/peritonitis, obstruction from inflammation causing stenosis), or fistulas. Patients with **acute appendicitis** typically present with RLQ pain. And, given recent negative colonoscopy, **colorectal cancer** is not likely. Patients with **colitis** typically have diarrhea.

CASE 10 | Chronic Mesenteric Ischemia

A 75-year-old woman with a history of tobacco use and coronary artery disease presents with generalized dull, cramping abdominal pain for the past several months. The pain occurs about 15–20 minutes after meals and is associated with nausea and vomiting. The pain lasts about 30 minutes before going away on its own. She has limited her food intake and has lost weight because of the pain. On physical exam, she has a documented 10-pound weight loss and appears to be in moderate distress secondary to pain. Her vital signs are normal, and the abdomen is soft and nontender.

Evaluation/Tests	Angiography shows partial occlusion of the superior mesenteric artery.
Treatment	Advise smoking cessation. Treat with antiplatelet medication and statins, and consider mesenteric angioplasty and stenting of the atherosclerotic vessel(s).
Discussion	This is a classic presentation of chronic mesenteric ischemia due to atherosclerosis. Patients are typically elderly and have numerous comorbid conditions including smoking, hypertension, diabetes mellitus, and hypercholesterolemia. Symptoms include postprandial dull abdominal pain associated with weight loss, food aversion, nausea, vomiting, or diarrhea. Atherosclerosis of the vasculature of the GI tract (celiac artery, superior mesenteric artery, and/or inferior mesenteric artery) over time results in a gradual decrease in blood flow to the intestines. The diseased blood vessels cannot meet the increased demand for blood flow to the intestines after meals, which results in temporary ischemia to the intestines. Therefore, the pathophysiology of mesenteric ischemia is similar to that of angina pectoris or claudication. After eating, the patient is essentially "exerting" the gut, and, due to atherosclerosis, the O_2 demand cannot be met. A key finding is pain "out of proportion" to physical exam, where the patient voices severe pain and appears uncomfortable, but the exam is benign with a soft, nontender abdomen. CT with contrast or MR angiogram can identify atherosclerosis and partial or complete occlusion of vessels of the intestines: *Celiac artery*: Supplies blood to the foregut—liver (common hepatic artery), stomach (left gastric artery), abdominal esophagus, spleen (splenic artery), and portions of the duodenum and pancreas. *Superior mesenteric artery (SMA)*: Supplies blood to the midgut—distal duodenum through much of the transverse colon and pancreas. *Inferior mesenteric artery (IMA)*: Supplies blood to the hindgut—colon from splenic flexure to upper rectum. **Acute mesenteric ischemia** refers to inadequate blood flow to the small intestine (arterial or venous) and is often caused by an acute thrombosis, embolism, or low blood-flow state. It can result in severe, "pain out of proportion to exam" abdominal pain, peritonitis, and bowel necrosis and possibly "currant jelly" stools. In **colonic ischemia or ischemic colitis**, patients may present with hematochezia and crampy abdominal pain. The splenic flexure and the rectosigmoid junction are areas of high risk and are referred to as watershed areas (receive dual blood supply from the most *distal* branches of two large *arteries* (i.e., SMA and IMA). In the case of severe hypoperfusion, blood supply through these end arteries becomes insufficient). Mucosal edema/hemorrhage may show thumbprint sign on imaging. **Abdominal aortic aneurysm (AAA)** are often asymptomatic unless they become very large or rupture. Pain with AAA typically radiates to the back, and a pulsating abdominal mass may be palpated. A bedside ultrasound can be used to quickly assess for an aneurysm.

CASE 11 | Intussusception

A 2-year-old boy is brought to the emergency department for evaluation of acute lower abdominal pain. The mother says the patient has been crying inconsolably with legs drawn up to his abdomen for the past 4 hours. The child is recovering from a cold. The mother noted stool with mixed mucous and blood in the toddler's diaper. On exam, his abdomen is rigid with diffuse abdominal tenderness. A sausage-shaped abdominal mass is palpated in the RUQ.

CASE 11 | Intussusception *(continued)*

Evaluation/Tests	Ultrasound of the abdomen shows "target sign."
Treatment	Air enema or reduce telescoping bowel via hydrostatic (contrast/saline) with or without ultrasound/fluoroscopic guidance.
Discussion	Intussusception is the result of telescoping of a part of the intestine into itself. The classic triad is crampy abdominal pain, vomiting, and currant jelly stools. Most cases occur in infants/toddlers. A lead point can be from Meckel diverticulum (children), Peyer's patch, mass/tumor (adults), or idiopathic. Typical location is at the ileocecal junction and can be associated with Henoch-Schönlein purpura (HSP), rotavirus vaccine, or recent viral infection. Peyer patch hypertrophy creates the lead point. Ultrasound is the diagnostic method of choice and can show "target sign," which is a cross section of the telescoping bowel. Initial treatment is reduction with enemas; surgery is indicated if enemas fail or if symptoms are worrisome for perforation or peritonitis. **Meckel diverticulum** results from incomplete closure of the vitelline (omphalo-mesenteric) duct; it is the most common congenital abnormality of the small intestine. Meckel diverticulum is a true diverticulum because it contains all layers of the GI wall. Remember the rule of 2s: presentation before the age of 2, 2% of the population, 2 inches in length, within 2 feet of the ileocecal valve, and 2 types of heterotopic mucosa. Although Meckel diverticulum can be a lead point causing intussusception, the typical presentation is painless hematochezia in a child. This congenital anomaly of the GI tract typically contains gastric and pancreatic mucosa. Meckel's scan would show uptake of 99m technetium pertechnetate by gastric mucosa. Treatment is surgical resection of the diverticulum. **Midgut volvulus** is the result of malrotation of a segment of the small intestine around the superior mesenteric artery, which can lead to obstruction, ischemia, and infarction. This condition commonly presents during the first year of life, and infants may present with vomiting, abdominal distension, shock, abdominal pain, peritonitis, or hematochezia. Stable patients can be evaluated by upper GI series, which will show a corkscrew appearance of the duodenum or jejunum and displacement of the duodenum with the ligament of Treitz to the right. Abdominal xray (XR) will show "double bubble" sign in cases of duodenal obstruction.
Additional Considerations	**Sigmoid volvulus** is more commonly seen in the elderly. The disorder is multifactorial and could be congenital in rare cases. Factors that may lead to this condition include redundancy of the sigmoid colon (too long to fit in the body), dolichomesentery (mesentery that is wider than long), and narrowing of the base of the sigmoid mesentery. XR may show coffee bean sign.

GI BLEED

A helpful approach in finding the cause of GI bleeding is by distinguishing between an upper GI (UGI) tract source (proximal to the ligament of Treitz) and a lower GI (LGI) tract source (distal to the ligament of Treitz). An upper GI bleed typically presents as hematemesis or melena (dark, tarry stool). Although a brisk upper GI bleed may present with hematochezia (bright red blood in stool), this is usually from a lower GI bleed (colon).

Hematemesis and Melena

Hematemesis can look like frank blood, or it may look like coffee grounds in the case of smaller volume or slower bleeding. When it is unclear whether a patient truly has hematemesis, nasogastric lavage may be helpful. Generally, the longer the blood stays in the GI tract, the darker the stool will appear. The black, tarry appearance of stool is thought to be from oxidation of heme products and from blood acting as a cathartic. Keep in mind that it is possible for melena to be from a naso-/oropharyngeal source if the patient has been swallowing blood or has significant epistaxis. Bismuth or iron supplements can also make stools dark.

Hematochezia

Maroon-colored stool is suggestive of a more proximal source of bleed in the lower GI tract than bright red blood. The presence or absence of associated pain may also provide clues to the source of the bleed.

Being attuned to clues for the potential location of the source of the bleed will help narrow down the DDx and determine what diagnostic workup is most appropriate.

Differential Diagnoses GI Bleed

UGI Source	LGI Source

Esophageal varices (gastric varices)
 Boerhaave syndrome
 Mallory-Weiss tear
 Esophagitis, gastritis, duodenitis
 Peptic ulcer disease (gastric, duodenal)
 (NSAID induced or *H. pylori* associated)
 Dieulafoy's vascular malformation
 Gastric cancer
	Arteriovenous malformations (AVM) or angiodysplasia
	 Meckel diverticulum
	 Inflammatory bowel disease (IBD)
	 Ischemic colitis
	 Infectious colitis
	   E coli O157:H7
	   Salmonella
	   Shigella
	   Campylobacter
	   Entamoeba histolytica
	 Colorectal cancer
	 Diverticulosis
	 Hemorrhoids/fissures

Key Associated Findings and GI Bleed Differential Diagnosis

GI Bleed with Key Associated Findings	Diagnoses
Coffee grounds emesis, melena	UGI bleed
NSAID use, epigastric pain, history of *H. pylori*	Peptic ulcer disease (PUD), gastritis
Improved with PPI/H2-blockers or antacids	GERD, PUD, gastritis
Hematemesis or large Hgb drop in a patient with stigmata of liver disease: ascites, scleral icterus, splenomegaly, spider angioma, telangiectasias, palmar erythema, gynecomastia, testicular atrophy, fluid wave, and shifting dullness	Esophageal varices
Hematemesis, chest pain in setting of recurrent vomiting—2:1 AST:ALT elevation (alcoholic) or finger calluses and eroded tooth enamel (bulimic)	Mallory-Weiss tear
Weight loss, early satiety, history of tobacco, EtOH	Gastric cancer
Fever, diarrhea, recent travel or restaurant/picnic food, sick contacts	Bacterial gastroenteritis
Weight loss, diarrhea, rash, arthralgias, eye irritation/redness	Inflammatory bowel disease (IBD)
Cobblestone mucosa and transmural inflammation with skip lesions and rectal sparing, noncaseating granulomas on colonoscopy; string sign on barium swallow X-ray, fistulas	Crohn disease
Continuous colonic inflammation with rectal involvement, crypt abscesses on colonoscopy	Ulcerative colitis
Lateral abdominal pain	Ischemic colitis
Abdominal pain, currant jelly stools	Intussusception (child), acute mesenteric ischemia (adult)
Abdominal pain after eating, food fear	Chronic mesenteric ischemia
Tenesmus, rectal pain after bowel movement	Anal fissure
Painless bright red blood per rectum (BRBPR), constipation	Diverticulosis, internal hemorrhoid
Weight loss, conjunctival pallor (iron deficiency anemia), abdominal pain, older age, strong family history of colon cancer, or not up-to-date on screening, change in stool caliber, ulcerative colitis, apple core lesion on barium enema; *Streptococcus bovis* bacteremia (rare)	Colorectal cancer
Iron deficiency anemia, weight loss, bleed	Ascending (right) colorectal cancer
Colicky pain, partial obstruction, apple core lesion on barium enema; *S. bovis* bacteremia (rare)	Descending (left) colorectal cancer
Immunocompromised, fever, abdominal pain, diarrhea with hematochezia	CMV colitis

Colorectal Cancers and Associated Features

Key Features	Diagnosis
"Apple core" lesion Reproduced with permission from Jameson JL, Fauci AS, Kasper DL, et al: Harrison's Principles of Internal Medicine, 20th ed. New York, NY: McGraw Hill; 2018.	Colon adenocarcinoma
S. bovis bacteremia	Colon adenocarcinoma
Iron deficiency anemia and positive FOBT or FIT test	Colon adenocarcinoma
Autosomal dominant mutation of *APC* tumor suppressor gene with nearly 100% risk of colorectal cancer	Familial adenomatous polyposis (FAP)
Germline mutation in the *APC* gene and supernumerary teeth	Gardner syndrome
Numerous hamartomas throughout the GI tract and increased risk of breast and GI cancers	Peutz-Jeghers syndrome
Hamartomatous polyps in GI tract in children <5 years old and increased risk of colorectal cancer	Juvenile polyposis syndrome
Autosomal dominant mutation of DNA mismatch repair (MMR) genes, leading to microsatellite instability (MSI) with increased risk of colorectal, endometrial, ovarian, and skin cancer	Lynch syndrome

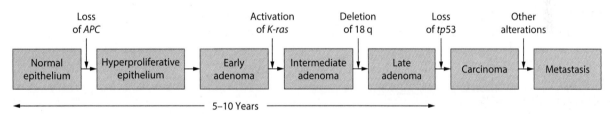

Modified with permission from Fearon ER, Vogelstein B. A genetic model for colorectal tumorigenesis, Cell 1990 Jun 1;61(5):759–767.

The evaluation of active GI bleeding should start with assessing for hemodynamic instability or significant blood loss. If the patient is unstable with active bleeding, immediately obtain reliable IV access (preferably two large-bore IVs) for resuscitation with IV fluids and blood transfusions as necessary. Look for findings of hypotension and tachycardia, conjunctival or general skin pallor, and blood or melena on rectal exam. Physical exam should also focus on assessing for abdominal tenderness, organomegaly, and stigmata of cirrhosis (jaundice, ascites, spider angiomas, palmar erythema, gynecomastia, caput medusae).

Along with checking the CBC and obtaining a type and screen/cross for possible transfusion, laboratory workup should include coagulation studies. Abnormalities may necessitate further assessment for bleeding disorders. Liver studies are especially relevant if the patient has known or suspected liver disease (e.g., cirrhosis).

Esophagogastroduodenoscopy (EGD) is used to visualize the upper GI tract, and flexible sigmoidoscopy or colonoscopy for the lower GI tract. Other procedures, such as push enteroscopy and video capsule endoscopy, can help visualize the part of the small bowel that EGD and colonoscopy are unable to reach. In some situations, a tagged RBC scan or angiography may be considered to localize the source of a bleed.

When treating a patient, remember the ABCs (airway, breathing, circulation), IV access for blood transfusion or fluids, stop bleeding, and correct any possible coagulopathies. Some of the preceding diagnostic procedures can also be useful therapeutic tools. For instance, bleeding ulcers can be cauterized or clipped during an EGD, or the blood vessel supplying the bleeding source can be embolized during angiography. For uncontrollable bleeding, surgical intervention may be necessary. In addition to endoscopy, acute medical management of upper GI bleeds often includes starting a proton pump inhibitor (PPI), and other medications may be added depending on the suspected bleeding source and patient's other medical problems.

CASE 12	Mallory-Weiss Tear
A 40-year-old man with a history of alcohol abuse presents with 1 day of severe epigastric pain and hematemesis. He has been drinking vodka heavily throughout the day, and he started vomiting a few hours ago. The pain started shortly after a particularly violent episode of vomiting. Initially, the vomitus was yellow, but now he is vomiting up bright red blood. On exam, he is tachycardic, mildly hypotensive, and in moderate distress. Patient is retching violently; he vomits again, and emesis appears to resemble coffee grounds. On exam, he has epigastric tenderness to palpation.	
Evaluation/Tests	CBC and PT/PTT and INR are within normal limits. Upper endoscopy showed a red longitudinal tear at the esophagogastric junction.
Treatment	Proton pump inhibitor and antiemetic if vomiting is persistent.
Discussion	Mallory-Weiss tears are partial thickness, longitudinal mucosal lacerations in the submucosa of the distal esophagus and proximal stomach thought to result from increased intra-abdominal pressure related to actions such as retching, coughing, or straining/lifting. The classic presentation is of an alcoholic or bulimic patient who has been retching/vomiting. It can also occur in other patients who are experiencing multiple episodes of emesis (e.g., hyperemesis gravidarum). The severe epigastric pain is secondary to the tear in the esophagus/proximal stomach. Hematemesis or coffee ground emesis occurs when submucosal vasculature is exposed from under the tear. Depending on the size of the tear and the blood vessel, the bleeding can be brisk and result in significant hemodynamic changes. Rebound and/or voluntary guarding can be signs of perforation and peritonitis. Presence of **esophageal varices** should be suspected in patients with portal hypertension. It would be difficult to definitively rule out variceal bleeding in this patient with a risk factor for cirrhosis until an upper endoscopy is done. As opposed to Mallory-Weiss tears, the presentation of **gastric ulcer** is typically more chronic, with patients experiencing prolonged symptoms such as abdominal pain, nausea/vomiting, or weight loss. **Boerhaave syndrome**, or distal esophageal transmural rupture, classically presents with chest pain and dyspnea after violent vomiting and is a surgical emergency. Pneumomediastinum, or air in the mediastinum, occurs due to leakage through the rupture. Crepitus in the neck and/or chest is a sign of subcutaneous emphysema, meaning that air has migrated into subcutaneous tissue.

CASE 13	Esophageal Varices
A 55-year-old man with alcoholic cirrhosis presents with 2 days of dark, tarry stools and an episode of hematemesis. His face and clothes are covered in bright red blood, and he has a waxing level of consciousness. On exam, he is tachycardic, hypotensive, and has cold/clammy extremities. Epigastric tenderness is present with rebound and guarding, and the patient has a distended abdomen with fluid wave. On skin exam, spider angiomata, telangiectasias, and palmar erythema are seen.	
Evaluation/Tests	ABCs—stabilize the patient first! Order type and screen/cross (in case transfusion is needed). CBC shows low hemoglobin and platelets. Coagulation studies show elevated PT/INR. EGD reveals dilated submucosal veins in lower esophagus.
Treatment	Give IV fluids and transfuse to stabilize the patient. Treat with octreotide and endoscopy to stop bleeding. Give prophylactic antibiotics.
Discussion	Esophageal varices are dilated veins in the distal esophagus that result from high pressures in the portal system. A stiff and fibrotic liver, as found in cirrhosis, causes portal hypertension and blocks normal blood flow through the portal system. Blood then gets shunted to the systemic circulation (by draining into the azygous vein) via small collateral vessels, which are fragile, get dilated, and are at risk for rupture. Acute variceal bleeding is life-threatening and results in approximately 1/3 of all deaths related to cirrhosis. All patients should receive octreotide infusion and antibiotic prophylaxis. Octreotide is a somatostatin analog thought to temporarily lower portal pressures. Antibiotic prophylaxis has been linked to decreased infectious complications, including spontaneous bacterial peritonitis and mortality. Though **PUD** and **Mallory-Weiss tear** are in the differential, urgent endoscopy is indicated for diagnosis and treatment.

CASE 14 | Peptic Ulcer Disease

A 45-year-old man with a history of chronic low back pain presents with epigastric pain for the past 2 weeks. The pain is gnawing and localized to the upper abdomen. It sometimes wakes him up at night, is associated with some nausea, and is better with eating or over-the-counter antacids. He is concerned because he noticed a small amount of blood in his vomit earlier today. He is taking ibuprofen a few times a week for his chronic low back pain. He appears comfortable and nontoxic but has mild to moderate epigastric tenderness to palpation.

Evaluation/Tests	*Helicobacter pylori* stool antigen is positive. EGD shows duodenal mucosal break >5 mm covered with fibrin (ulcer). Biopsy is positive for *H. pylori* and negative for malignancy.
Treatment	Treat *H. pylori* with triple therapy: clarithromycin, amoxicillin or metronidazole, and a PPI, or with quadruple therapy: bismuth subsalicylate, metronidazole, tetracycline, and a PPI or H-2 blocker. Advise patient to stop NSAIDS.
Discussion	Peptic ulcers can occur within the stomach or within the duodenum and are associated with two major factors: ***Helicobacter pylori* infection** and use of nonsteroidal anti-inflammatory drugs (**NSAIDs**). The ulcerations can expose submucosal vasculature resulting in hematemesis and/or melena. Duodenal ulcers are more common and are typically due to *H. pylori* infection and acid hypersecretion. Symptoms of PUD generally include epigastric pain, weight loss, nausea, and vomiting. Anterior duodenal ulcers may perforate, causing pneumoperitoneum, whereas posterior duodenal ulcers may penetrate the gastroduodenal artery, leading to major bleeding. **Gastric ulcers** tend to present with pain exacerbated by meals, while duodenal ulcer pain is classically improved with meals and may awaken patients from sleep. Gastric ulcers can be caused by NSAIDs or *H. pylori* infection and are associated with an increased risk of gastric cancer. In **acute gastritis**, EGD would show erosions in the gastric mucosa but no ulcers. Erosions can be caused by NSAIDS, burns (causing hypovolemia and leading to mucosal ischemia (Curling ulcer)), or brain injury (causing increased vagal stimulation and increased Ach, which increases acid production (Cushing ulcer)).
Additional Considerations	**Zollinger-Ellison syndrome** can also cause duodenal ulcers and is associated with hypertrophy of Brunner glands. Although it can present with a single ulcer, suspicion should be raised when there are multiple or refractory ulcers or when the patient has MEN1.

CASE 15 | Crohn's Disease

A 21-year-old woman presents to clinic for diarrhea and intermittent abdominal cramping for the past 6 months. She reports up to 5 watery stools per day with occasional mucus and blood, which sometimes wakes her up at night. Her past medical history includes recurrent urinary tract infections and a recent bout of tender, reddish lumps on the front of her legs. Her abdominal pain is intermittent, and she has lost weight. Exam reveals pallor, generalized abdominal tenderness to palpation, erythematous nodules on her anterior shins bilaterally (erythema nodosum), perianal skin tags, and aphthous oral ulcers.

Evaluation/Tests	CBC reveals low hemoglobin. ESR and CRP are both elevated. Stool testing is negative for ova and parasites, *Clostridium difficile* toxin is negative. Fecal markers of inflammation (calprotectin and lactoferrin) were elevated. Colonoscopy shows cobblestone appearance of bowel mucosa, areas of normal appearing mucosa, and fistula near bladder; pathology report of biopsies later showed noncaseating granulomas and lymphoid aggregates. Upper GI barium XR series with small bowel follow through showed "string sign" (*see* image). 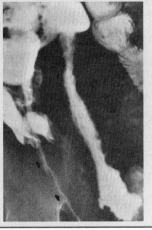 Reproduced with permission from Chen MYM, Pope TL, Ott DJ: Basic Radiology, 2nd ed. New York, NY: McGraw Hill; 2011.
Treatment	Corticosteroids should be given in the acute setting, and immunomodulators such as azathioprine or anti-TNF inhibitors (infliximab, adalimumab) are given as maintenance therapy. Advanced disease involving strictures and/or fistula formation may require surgical resection.

CASE 15 | Crohn's Disease *(continued)*

Discussion	This patient has Crohn's disease, an inflammatory bowel disease that results in chronic symptoms such as abdominal pain and diarrhea. Crohn's disease can involve any portion of the GI tract but most often involves the distal ileum and colon; unlike **ulcerative colitis (UC)**, it spares the rectum. As opposed to UC, which exhibits continuous colonic involvement, Crohn's disease is characterized by "skip lesions" involving various noncontinuous portions throughout the GI tract. The transmural inflammation specific to Crohn's disease results in fistula formation, which can create tracts between bowel and the genitourinary tract. This can result in recurrent UTIs, as seen in this patient. Ulcerative colitis involves only the mucosa and submucosa in the colon, so fistulas are not typically formed. Chronic transmural inflammation in Crohn's disease can also lead to the development of strictures sometimes seen on imaging as a "string sign," which can result in abdominal pain and symptoms similar to bowel obstruction. On biopsy, noncaseating granulomas and lymphoid aggregates are present, whereas biopsy of ulcerative colitis typically shows crypt abscesses without granulomas. Extraintestinal manifestations of Crohn's disease commonly include rashes such as pyoderma gangrenosum, erythema nodosum (reddish lumps on the front of the patient's legs), ocular involvement including episcleritis and uveitis, oral ulcerations, kidney/gallstones, and spondyloarthropathy. The classic extraintestinal manifestation of ulcerative colitis is primary sclerosing cholangitis, which ultimately may lead to liver failure and is associated with p-ANCA antibodies. The signs and symptoms of **chronic ischemic colitis**, such as weight loss, malnutrition, abdominal pain, and bloody diarrhea, may be similar to IBD. However, chronic ischemic colitis is most commonly due to atherosclerosis and is typically seen in the elderly with risk factors for cardiac disease. **Diverticular bleed** due to diverticulosis is typically seen in older, obese patients with lower-fiber/high-fat diets and physical inactivity. Imaging or colonoscopy would show small sac-like outpouchings in the colon, which are thought to be caused by increased intraluminal pressure in focal areas of weakness in the colonic wall.

CASE 16 | Angiodysplasia

A 52-year-old woman with a history of end-stage renal disease on hemodialysis presents for evaluation of iron deficiency anemia. Overall, she feels well and denies any issues with abdominal pain or nausea/vomiting. She does occasionally note a small amount of "maroon" colored blood in her stools, which she attributed to her hemorrhoids. She recently had an EGD and colonoscopy to evaluate for a source of possible GI bleeding, both of which were negative. Her physical exam revealed no abnormalities.

Evaluation/Tests	She was referred for a video capsule endoscopy (VCE), which identified several small cherry-red vascular lesions in the jejunum.
Treatment	Treat lesions with electrocautery.
Discussion	Angiodysplasias, or arteriovenous malformations (AVM), are small vascular malformations that can occur anywhere in the GI tract. They are composed of small, tortuous, dilated, thin-walled vessels that are susceptible to rupture and bleeding. Patients may present with hematochezia but are often asymptomatic. The classic presentation is iron deficiency anemia with unrevealing upper and lower endoscopies. A video capsule endoscopy (VCE) should be completed if both upper and lower endoscopies are negative for a source of bleeding. Alternatively, a special endoscopy called small bowel enteroscopy can be used. CT or MRI angiography can be done for colonic angiodysplasia evaluation. Patients at highest risk of angiodysplasias include older patients, those with end-stage renal disease, aortic stenosis, and von Willebrand disease. Incidentally found angiodysplasias does not require treatment. Actively bleeding lesions or lesions suspected of causing clinically significant anemia/bleeding can be treated endoscopically or during angiography. Lower GI bleeding is also often caused by **hemorrhoids**, which are large dilated veins in the rectum most commonly resulting from straining with defecation due to constipation. Classically, **internal hemorrhoids** (dilated veins above the dentate line) are painless but can bleed. Treatment includes a bowel regimen such as a stool softener or ligation of the hemorrhoids.

CASE 17 | Colorectal Cancer

A 64-year-old woman with a history of heavy tobacco use presents with several days of hematochezia. She denies any past medical history but has not seen a doctor in decades. She has noticed abdominal cramping, generalized malaise, and weight loss despite a normal appetite. Her father had colon cancer. Her physical exam is pertinent for conjunctival pallor, mild abdominal tenderness, but no guarding. There is no palpable mass on digital rectal exam (DRE), but dark stool is found, which is positive for occult blood.

CASE 17 | Colorectal Cancer (continued)

Evaluation/Tests	Colonoscopy shows an exophytic mass in the ascending (right) colon, and biopsy showed adenocarcinoma. On CBC and iron studies, there are low levels of Hgb, MCV, and ferritin, consistent with iron deficiency anemia. Baseline CEA is elevated.
Treatment	Resection of the primary colon tumor followed by chemotherapy.
Discussion	This patient has unexplained weight loss along with changes in stool, which are concerning for GI malignancy. Iron deficiency anemia in male patients and postmenopausal female patients should raise concern for colorectal cancer. Colorectal cancer is the third most common cancer in men and woman worldwide. Pathology is typically adenocarcinoma, but squamous cell, carcinoid, and stromal tumors can be found. Given the high risk of malignancy in older adults and that treatment can be curative in early stages, screening is recommended. Recently, the American Cancer Society (ACS) decreased their recommended age for screening from 50 to 45 years old due to the increasing prevalence of rectal cancer in younger patients. Patients with IBD or with familial syndromes associated with colon cancer such as Lynch syndrome or familial adenomatous polyposis (FAP) have earlier and more frequent screening recommendations. As this patient also has a first-degree relative with a history of colon cancer, she should have started screening 10 years prior to her father's age at presentation. Typically, colon cancer involving the ascending (right) colon presents insidiously with iron deficiency anemia, weight loss, and anemia. Cancer affecting the descending (left) colon often results in intermittent obstruction (causing constipation and thin caliber stools), abdominal pain, and frank hematochezia. CEA is a tumor marker that is used for monitoring for recurrence. Treatment is primarily resection and, depending on stage, may be followed by adjuvant chemotherapy. If there are a few sites of metastases (oligometastatic), colon cancer may still be treated with curative intent. Unresectable metastatic disease is treated with palliative chemotherapy, possibly in combination with a biologic agent. Although hematochezia can be due to **diverticulosis** or **hemorrhoids**, these conditions should not cause weight loss. **Ulcerative colitis** can cause hematochezia as an initial presenting symptom; it also carries higher risk of colorectal cancer that increases with duration and severity of the disease.

CASE 18 | Lynch Syndrome

A 29-year-old man with no past medical history presents to clinic with intermittent abdominal pain and nonbloody diarrhea over the past year. Both his grandfather and father died from colon cancer. His 48-year-old cousin was recently diagnosed with colon cancer, and this prompted him to seek medical attention. The patient's physical exam is notable for mild, diffuse abdominal tenderness but is otherwise unremarkable. Digital rectal exam is negative for hematochezia or hemorrhoids.

Evaluation/Tests	Colonoscopy shows several proximal large flattened adenomas. Biopsy is consistent with adenocarcinoma. Genetic testing reveals an MSH2 germline mutation.
Treatment	Total colectomy.
Discussion	Lynch syndrome (also known as hereditary nonpolyposis colorectal cancer or HNPCC) is an autosomal dominant disorder of DNA mismatch repair genes. Consider Lynch syndrome if the family history is notable for 3 or more cases of colorectal cancer (CRC), one or more cases diagnosed before age 50, one is a first-degree relative of the other two, and at least two generations are affected. In addition to colorectal cancer, patients are at an increased risk for endometrial, gastric, ovarian, and skin cancers among others. A total colectomy would be the only way to prevent disease recurrence. Other important familial cancer syndromes are as follows.
Additional Considerations	**Familial adenomatous polyposis** is an autosomal dominant mutation of the APC tumor suppressor gene, and prophylactic total colectomy is recommended for these patients. It is also associated with other cancers. **Juvenile polyposis syndrome** typically affects children (<5 years of age) but may also affect adults. The term "juvenile" refers to the polyps, and this autosomal dominant syndrome is characterized by numerous hamartomatous polyps in the colon, stomach, and small bowel. They are initially benign but may become malignant in the future. **Peutz-Jeghers syndrome** is autosomal dominant, and patients present with numerous hamartomas in the GI tract and hyperpigmented mouth, lips, and hands. It is associated with increased risk of breast and other GI cancers.

CASE 19 | Anal Cancer

A 57-year-old man with a history of genital warts and HIV presents with rectal pressure and itching. He also has intermittent rectal bleeding. Physical exam shows inguinal adenopathy, and digital rectal exam reveals a small palpable lesion.

Evaluation/Tests	Anoscopy and rigid proctoscopy with biopsy helps to further visualize a nodular, ulcerated lesion. Biopsy reveals keratinized squamous cell hyperplasia with central necrosis, indicative of anal squamous cell carcinoma.
Treatment	Combined fluorouracil or capecitabine plus mitomycin and radiation therapy.
Discussion	Rectal bleeding is the most common initial symptom, followed by anorectal pain, in anal cancer. Human papillomavirus (HPV) is closely linked to malignancies of the genital tract, anus, and rectum. The majority of anal squamous cell carcinomas (SCC) are associated with HPV 16. Other risk factors include high-risk sexual behavior, HIV, IV drug use, history of genital warts, and cigarette smoking. Among women, additional risk factors include a history of cervical cancer, vulvar cancer, cervical or vulvar intraepithelial neoplasia, and immunosuppression. **Internal hemorrhoids** and adenocarcinoma are above the pectinate line and typically are not painful.
	External hemorrhoids, fissures, and squamous cell cancer are below the pectinate line and can be painful.
	Anal fissures are tears that typically occur posteriorly where there is less perfusion. They are associated with constipation and low-fiber diets and can occur secondary to IBD, infections, or cancer. If a patient presents with associated rectal bleeding, endoscopy should be performed to evaluate for underlying malignancy.

NAUSEA AND VOMITING

Nausea and vomiting are controlled by pathways and neurotransmitters involving the brainstem chemoreceptor trigger zone, gut neurons, and smooth muscle cells. Medications, toxins, mechanical blockages, and even behavioral disorders can initiate this reflex. The list of causes is extensive, but initial focus should be on associated gastrointestinal symptoms, neurologic/vestibular symptoms, and medications to help narrow the differential. This section will focus on causes related to the GI system and associated symptoms and signs of abdominal pain, diarrhea, fever, or an abnormal abdominal examination.

Regardless of the varying causes of nausea and vomiting, the medications that treat these symptoms focus on blocking receptors in the chemoreceptor trigger zone (e.g., 5HT3 (ondansetron), dopamine (metoclopramide), or act as prokinetic agents (erythromycin).

Differential Diagnoses for Nausea and Vomiting

GI/Biliary/Liver	Neuro	Other
Small bowel obstruction	Intracranial mass versus bleed	MI
Large bowel obstruction	Posterior circulation stroke	Pregnancy
Gastric outlet obstruction	Hydrocephalus	Post-tussive emesis
Gastroparesis	Idiopathic intracranial hypertension	Motion sickness
Dyspepsia, GERD, PUD	Migraine	Vestibular neuritis
Crohn disease	**Infectious**	Alcohol intoxication
Acute cholecystitis, ascending cholangitis	Viral versus bacterial gastroenteritis	Uremia
Acute pancreatitis	Pyelonephritis	DKA
Acute hepatitis	Meningitis	Adrenal crisis
Appendicitis	Otitis media	Bulimia
Intussusception	**Drugs**	Psychogenic
Malrotation, midgut volvulus	Chemotherapy	Cyclic vomiting syndrome secondary to marijuana use
Incarcerated hernia	Metformin, GLP1 antagonists	
Pyloric stenosis	Alzheimer medications	Acute intermittent porphyria
Intestinal atresia	Antibiotics	Inborn errors of metabolism
Hirschsprung's disease	Opioids	Toxic ingestion (e.g., iron, vitamin A, vitamin C, lithium)
Food protein–induced enteropathy (e.g., milk protein)	Opiate withdrawal	
	Inhaled anesthetics	

Key History Findings and Nausea/Vomiting Differential Diagnoses

Nausea/Vomiting with Key Associated Findings	Diagnoses
Associated diarrhea, recent travel or unusual/picnic food	Gastroenteritis
Cruise ship, associated diarrhea	Gastroenteritis—specifically norovirus
Uncontrolled diabetes mellitus, postprandial fullness	Gastroparesis, DKA
Chemotherapy, new prescriptions	Medication induced
Accompanying vertigo, worse with movement	Benign paroxysmal positional vertigo
Abdominal distension, high pitched, tinkling bowel sounds	Small bowel obstruction
Hypoactive bowel sounds	Ileus, opioids
Calluses on fingers, dental caries/enamel erosion	Bulimia
Recent aspirin use, hepatomegaly, hypoglycemia	Reye syndrome
Infancy, projectile vomiting, palpable "olive-like mass"	Pyloric stenosis
Failure to pass meconium within the first 48 hours after birth	Hirschsprung's disease, cystic fibrosis
Within first 2 days of life, "double bubble" sign on X-ray	Duodenal atresia
Poor feeding, smells like maple syrup	Maple syrup urine disease

CASE 20 | Hypertrophic Pyloric Stenosis

A 4-week-old boy is brought for evaluation of nonbloody, nonbilious, projectile vomiting after each feed for the past 24 hours. Parents deny fever or diarrhea. After vomiting, the infant appears hungry and wants to feed, only to vomit again. On exam, a small abdominal mass is palpated in the epigastric area.

Evaluation/Tests	BMP reveals hypochloremic hypokalemic metabolic alkalosis from the vomiting. Abdominal ultrasound shows increased pyloric muscle thickness length and diameter.
Treatment	Treat with surgical pyloromyotomy.
Discussion	Pyloric stenosis is caused by hypertrophy of the pyloris, effectively causing gastric outlet obstruction. The classic triad for pyloric stenosis includes projectile vomiting immediately after feeds, palpable olive-like mass, and visible peristalsis. Typical age at presentation is 2–12 weeks old. **Annular pancreas** and **intestinal atresia** can present similarly with vomiting, abdominal distension, and feeding intolerance in this age group; however, physical exam findings and ultrasound results help confirm the diagnosis in this case. Annular pancreas occurs when the ventral pancreatic bud fails to rotate during development, causing encirclement of the second part of the duodenum. Intestinal atresia can occur due to failure of the intestine to recanalize during development and would present with *bilious* vomiting. **Hirschpung's** or **tracheoesophageal fistula** causes vomiting within the first few *days* of birth.

CASE 21 | Small Bowel Obstruction Secondary to Incarcerated Hernia

A 25-year-old man presents with acute abdominal pain, nausea, and bilious emesis. His only medical history is of a reported "lump" in his groin area that has been present since birth. The abdominal pain is crampy, severe, initially intermittent, and now persistent. He is passing less gas and has not had a bowel movement in a few days. On exam he is tachycardic and mildly hypotensive. Abdominal auscultation reveals "tinkling" high-pitched bowel sounds. His abdomen is distended, tympanic to percussion, and tender to palpation. There is a nonreducible and extremely tender inguinal mass with overlying normal appearing skin.

Evaluation/Tests	Upright chest/abdominal X-ray shows dilated loops of small bowel with multiple horizontal lines that are radiolucent above and radiopaque below.
Treatment	General surgery consultation for resection of incarcerated bowel.
Discussion	The classic high-pitched, "tinkling" bowel sound pattern of **small bowel obstruction (SBO)** results from the bowel contracting against the obstruction; this differs from what is classically observed in intestinal **ileus**, which is defined as intestinal hypomobility (and thus hypoactive bowel sounds) without obstruction. Common causes of SBO include hernias, adhesions, or strictures from prior surgeries, tumors. Therefore, it is important to ask about prior surgeries and check for surgical scars on examination. Along

CASE 21 | Small Bowel Obstruction Secondary to Incarcerated Hernia (continued)

Discussion	with looking for the presence of air–fluid levels on an upright X-ray, assessing for free air under the diaphragm from possible perforation is important because presence of this is an indication for emergent surgery. Abdominal CT with PO contrast can identify a transition point at the site of the obstruction, assess for causes of mechanical obstruction, and evaluate whether the obstruction is partial or complete. Patients with gastroenteritis, pancreatitis, or cholecystitis would not present with signs and symptoms of bowel obstruction.

DIARRHEA, CONSTIPATION, AND STEATORRHEA

The goal of the digestive tract is to move ingested food down a path from the mouth to anus, whereby nutrients are extracted and absorbed for use by the body and wastes are excreted. This requires coordination among multiple organs such as mechanical breakdown by the stomach, enzyme/hormonal release by the pancreas, bile from the liver, and finally absorption via villi throughout the intestines. When this process is disrupted because of inflammation, infection, dysmotility, or alteration in the usual interplay of necessary enzymes/hormones, the result is diarrhea, constipation, or steatorrhea. History should focus on travel and exposures, the presence or absence of fever or hematochezia, potential for immunosuppression, and the chronicity of symptoms to help guide relevant laboratory testing. Direct visualization by endoscopy/colonoscopy and tissue sampling may be required.

Differential Diagnosis for Diarrhea, Constipation, and Steatorrhea

Diarrhea	Constipation	Steatorrhea

Infectious (viral, bacterial, parasitic)
Inflammatory/IBD (UC, Crohn)
Malabsorptive (celiac, tropical sprue, short gut syndrome, lactose intolerance)
Functional (IBS)
Malignancy—VIPoma, neuroendocrine tumor, carcinoid tumor
Drugs:
  Antibiotic (adverse effect vs. *C. difficile* infection)
  Metformin (other diabetic medications)
  Magnesium, laxatives
	Functional (IBS)
	Malignancy (obstructive colorectal tumor)
	Hirschsprung's disease
	Toxic megacolon (secondary to UC)
	Drugs:
	  Iron
	  Loperamide
	  Bismuth
	  Opiates/opioids
	  Anticholinergics (tricyclics)
		Pancreatic insufficiency
		Bile salt disorder

Diarrhea

Acute symptoms (<14 days) are usually caused by infections; conversely, chronic diarrhea (>30 days) is not usually due to an infectious cause with the exception of immunocompromised hosts. Most acute diarrhea can be traced to viral or bacterial causes. Patients usually present with watery diarrhea, and most episodes will be self-limited and resolve with supportive care. Special consideration should be given to patients presenting with systemic symptoms of fever or with bloody diarrhea (dysentery). These are usually caused by invasive bacteria or toxins such as *Salmonella, Shigella, Campylobacter,* EHEC *E. coli* O157:H7, or the protozoa *Entamoeba histolytica,* and these patients can have a more severe clinical course. Depending on the clinical scenario, antibiotics may play a role in treatment except for EHEC *E. coli* O157:H7 because they can precipitate hemolytic uremic syndrome (HUS). As diarrhea becomes more chronic, the likelihood of underlying organic pathology increases. Focus should first be on evaluating the nature of the stool, an assessment of alarm symptoms, presence or absence of blood, triggers such as certain foods/stress, and an evaluation of the host (other medical illnesses, immunocompromised states). Alarm symptoms include age >50 with change in symptoms, weight loss, fever, bloody stools, nocturnal diarrhea, family history of colon cancer/IBD/MEN/celiac sprue, or an immunocompromised host.

If exam and history are not suggestive of an identifiable cause, then further testing can be performed. Stool can be tested for blood, WBCs, osmotic gap, electrolytes, and fat. Any possible culprit medications should be evaluated and eliminated because these are very common causes. In addition, hormonal testing can be helpful in the setting where secretory diarrhea is suggested. Colonoscopy is diagnostic for causes such as IBD and ruling out pathology when diagnosing IBS. Upper endoscopy with small bowel biopsies showing blunted villi can be diagnostic for celiac sprue.

Differential Diagnosis for Diarrhea

Infection	Inflammatory	Malabsorption
Infection	**Inflammatory**	**Malabsorption**
Gastroenteritis	IBD: UC, Crohn's	Lactose intolerance
Viral: _Norovirus, Rotavirus_		Chronic pancreatitis
Bacterial: _E. coli, Shigella, Salmonella, Yersinia, Campylobacter, Vibrio_	**Endocrine**	Bile salt disorder
	Hyperthyroid	Celiac disease
Toxin producing: _B. cereus, C. perfringens, Staphylococcus aureus, C. difficile_	Diabetes	Tropical sprue
	Gastrinoma	Short gut syndrome
	VIPoma	
Colitis	Carcinoid	**Other**
C. difficile, Klebsiella, E. coli, Shigella, Salmonella, Yersinia, Campylobacter		IBS
		Colon cancer
	Medication/substances	
Other:	Metformin	
Parasites: _Giardia, Cryptosporidium, Entamoeba histolytica_; small bowel bacterial overgrowth	Antibiotics	
	Laxatives	
	Sorbitol, fructose	

Key Associated Findings and Diarrhea Differential Diagnosis

Diarrhea with Key Associated Findings	Diagnoses
Watery stool, nausea/vomiting, abdominal cramps, fever	Gastroenteritis
Children, adolescents, and young adults with nonbloody diarrhea	_Rotavirus_
Diarrhea within 6 hours of ingestion	_Staphylococcus aureus_ or _Bacillus cereus_ (preformed toxins)
Diarrhea and recent camping	_Giardia_
Diarrhea with fever, travel	Gastroenteritis including travelers (ETEC) and _Norovirus_ (cruise ship)
Diarrhea with recent antibiotic use, health care exposure	_C. difficile_ diarrhea
Hemolytic uremic syndrome (microangiopathic hemolytic anemia with acute kidney injury)	_E Coli_ O157:H7
CD4 < 100	_Cryptosporidium, Isospora, Cyclospora,_ CMV
Bloody diarrhea, fever, tenesmus	Colitis
Diarrhea worse with dairy products, bloating/cramping	Lactose intolerance
Diarrhea worse with wheat products (breads/pasta) Dermatitis herpetiformis Blunted villi on endoscopy	Celiac disease
Alternating constipation and diarrhea, no weight loss, associated with stress	Irritable bowel syndrome
Chronic diarrhea, weight loss, hematochezia	Inflammatory bowel disease (UC, Crohn's)
Crypt abscesses Lead pipe on barium X-ray	Ulcerative colitis
Skip lesions, cobblestoning, fistulae, transmural inflammation, granuloma String sign on barium X-ray	Crohn's disease
Weight loss, decreased stool caliber, iron deficiency anemia Apple core lesion	Colorectal cancer
Nighttime diarrhea/awakening from sleep	Secretory diarrhea (VIPoma, gastrinoma, carcinoid)
Steatorrhea, chronic alcoholism, pancreatic calcifications on CT	Chronic pancreatitis
Constipation, black hard stools	Iron supplement, bismuth

CASE 22 | Irritable Bowel Syndrome (IBS)

A 27-year-old woman with a history of generalized anxiety presents with intermittent crampy abdominal pain for the past 6 months. The pain comes and goes 2–3 times per week and is associated with alternating diarrhea and constipation and flatulence. She denies any blood in her stools, nighttime stools, or weight loss. Symptoms are aggravated at times of stress, and abdominal discomfort is better after a bowel movement. She is mildly tender to palpation diffusely, without rebound or guarding.

Evaluation/Tests	Clinical diagnosis with suggestive history and exclusionary evaluation (as listed), CBC, CRP, TSH, BMP are all within normal limits. Celiac testing and fecal calprotectin negative. Endoscopic studies may be performed for recalcitrant symptoms.
Treatment	Lifestyle changes and antispasmodics.
Discussion	IBS is clinically diagnosed and is a diagnosis of exclusion. Age-appropriate colon cancer screening should be completed, and any red flag symptoms should be investigated. Rome IV criteria for diagnosis: presence of intermittent abdominal pain at least once a week for 3 months with 2 of the following:
	1. Related to defecation
	2. Associated with change in stool frequency
	3. Associated with change in stool appearance
	Initial management is nonpharmacologic, including lifestyle management (avoid gas-producing foods) and dietary changes (low FODMAP diet) +/− trial of psyllium. FODMAP stands for fermentable oligo-, di-, monosaccharides, and polyols, which are short-chain carbohydrates that are poorly absorbed and can aggravate gut symptoms. Antispasmodics such as dicyclomine or hyoscyamine can decrease cramps, and TCAs may help slow transit time and improve diarrhea.
	Negative fecal calprotectin and celiac testing make IBD and celiac disease unlikely.

CASE 23 | Celiac Disease

A 12-year-old girl is brought to clinic for evaluation of abdominal discomfort and chronic diarrhea with foul smelling stools. She also reports weight loss, fatigue, and an intensely pruritic rash on her elbows. Her symptoms are aggravated after eating bread and other grain-based foods. On physical exam, she has pale conjunctivae, abdominal distension, and a papulovesicular rash on her elbows (dermatitis herpetiformis).

Evaluation/Tests	IgA antitissue transglutaminase (IgA tTG) is positive. EGD with small bowel biopsy shows villous atrophy, crypt hyperplasia, and intraepithelial lymphocytosis. CBC reveals low Hg and low MCV. Ferritin is low.
Treatment	Treatment is a lifelong gluten-free diet.
Discussion	Celiac disease is an autoimmune-mediated gluten-sensitive enteropathy that is associated with the DQ2/DQ8 HLA subtype. Exposure to gluten protein (gliadin) found in wheat causes destruction of the villi via an immune-mediated process, leading to malabsorption in distal duodenum/proximal jejunum. Patients may present with signs and symptoms of malabsorption such as diarrhea, abdominal discomfort, iron deficiency anemia, fat-soluble vitamin deficiencies, and dermatitis herpetiformis. Villous atrophy can be seen on biopsy with resolution of mucosal lesions within weeks to months after eliminating gluten-containing foods. There is an increased risk of lymphoma in patients with celiac disease. Diagnosis is made by tissue biopsy, but the following antibodies are useful confirmatory tests: IgA antitissue transglutaminase (IgA tTG), IgA antiendomysial, IgA, and IgG deamidated gliadin peptide.
	Tropical sprue also affects the small bowel, but it is typically seen in patients who visit or reside in the tropics and responds to antibiotics.
	Lactose intolerance is due to lactase deficiency. Symptoms occur after dairy consumption and include flatulence/bloating. On endoscopy and biopsy, villi will appear normal.
	Carcinoid is a neuroendocrine tumor of the gastrointestinal tract that secrete a variety of molecules into the blood, the most common is serotonin (5-HT). Typical symptoms of carcinoid syndrome include diarrhea and facial flushing.
Additional Considerations	**Whipple disease** is more common in older men and is an infection due to *T. whipplei*. It is also associated with cardiac symptoms, arthralgia, and neurologic symptoms. Foamy macrophages are seen in the lamina propria on biopsy.

CASE 24	Chronic Pancreatitis
A 40-year-old man with a history of alcohol abuse presents with abdominal pain radiating to the back, vomiting, and frequent bowel movements with fatty, bulky stools that are difficult to flush (steatorrhea). He also reports weight loss as well as polyuria and polydipsia. He has a history of recurrent abdominal pain but came in now because he is feeling worse. Review of systems is notable for impaired night vision and muscle spasms. His BMI is 18, and his abdomen is mildly distended with epigastric tenderness to palpation.	
Evaluation/Tests	Random glucose is 240, and HgbA1c is 8. Amylase/lipase are both slightly elevated. BMP reveals elevated BUN/Cr ratio, and low K and Mg. Imaging shows pancreatic calcifications, pseudocysts, beading of the main pancreatic duct or ectatic side branches.
Treatment	Treat with analgesics, IV fluids, bowel rest with low-fat meals, pancreatic enzyme supplements, and avoid alcohol.
Discussion	The classic triad of chronic pancreatitis includes pancreatic calcifications, steatorrhea, and diabetes mellitus. Chronic pancreatitis typically occurs secondary to alcoholism in adults and cystic fibrosis in children. Other causes of chronic pancreatitis include hyperparathyroidism and pancreatic divisum, and it can also be idiopathic. Pancreatic insufficiency and malabsorption of fat and fat-soluble vitamins can occur. Deficiency in A (impaired night vision), D (osteoporosis/fragility fractures), E (neuropathy neuromuscular weakness and hemolysis), and K (coagulopathy/elevated INR due to inability to make coagulation factors) are common. In the setting of steatorrhea and/or abnormal pancreatic imaging, stool studies are obtained. Sudan stain of stool will be consistent with fecal fat. Fecal elastase-1 (FE-1) being low is also suggestive of pancreatic exocrine insufficiency. If qualitative fecal fat is positive, a secretin stimulation test is performed. Imaging findings can confirm if calcifications are within the pancreas on abdominal computed tomography (CT) scan, US, or MRI. During and ERCP a pancreatogram will reveal beading of the main pancreatic duct or ectatic side branches. **Celiac disease** can also cause malabsorption. Consider **bile salt deficiency** for patients who have had ileal resection for any reason. **Whipple's disease** would present with abdominal pain, weight loss, and diarrhea but would also present with arthralgias.

CASE 25	Hirschsprung's Disease
A 3-day-old boy with Down syndrome presents with bilious emesis and failure to pass meconium. He has abdominal distension, a tight anal sphincter, and a positive squirt sign on digital rectal exam (an empty rectum with stool higher up in the colon and an explosive passage of stool upon withdrawal of the examining finger).	
Evaluation/Tests	Abdominal radiograph shows dilation of proximal bowel with absence of air in the rectum. Anorectal manometry with suction rectal biopsy shows absence of ganglion cells in Auerbach and Meissner plexuses in the distal colon. Contrast enema shows a funnel-shaped transition zone.
Treatment	Treat with IV fluids, decompression, and surgical resection of the aganglionic segment of bowel.
Discussion	Hirschsprung's disease is due to a RET mutation and should be highly suspected in the following: • Failure to pass meconium in the first 48 hours of life • Symptoms of obstruction due to failure of neural crest cells to migrate to the colon leading to disinhibited smooth muscle contracture • Constipation in a neonate with trisomy 21 **Meconium plug** would be diagnosed by contrast enema, which would reveal the meconium plug and lack of a transition point. **Meconium ileus** occurs when thickened meconium obstructs the ileum; this can be seen in cystic fibrosis, and genetic testing can confirm the diagnosis.

Approach to Liver Disease

The liver plays an important role in digestion, metabolism, storage of glycogen, vitamins and minerals, synthesizing plasma proteins, enzyme activation, and detoxification. When the liver is damaged for any reason, these essential functions may be compromised.

In evaluating a patient with liver disease, the key historical features include assessing possible exposure history such as alcohol, drug, medication usage, exposures to contaminated foods, or blood transfusions. It is important to elicit a sexual history, relevant family history, and history of diabetes or obesity. On review of systems (ROS), inquire about jaundice, pruritus, abdominal pain, swelling, changes in bowels, nausea/vomiting, fevers, joint aches, pains or rashes, urine color, and stool color. Finally, perform a thorough physical exam looking for stigmata of liver disease such as ascites, conjunctival icterus, splenomegaly, spider angioma, telangiectasias, palmar erythema, gynecomastia, testicular atrophy, fluid wave, and shifting dullness.

On physical exam, pay attention to the following findings and signs and symptoms.

System	PE Findings	Signs and Symptoms
Skin	Jaundice, palmar erythema, spider angiomas, caput medusa, purpura, petechiae	Pruritis
HEENT	Icteric conjunctiva, fetor hepaticus	Yellow eyes and skin
Lungs	Decreased breath sounds or dullness to percussion from ascites	Dyspnea
CV	Peripheral edema	Swelling
GI	Ascites, hepatosplenomegaly	Nausea/vomiting, anorexia, abdominal distension/pain, hematemesis, melena, cirrhotic liver, esophageal, gastric and anorectal varices
GU/renal	Gynecomastia, testicular atrophy	Amenorrhea, erectile dysfunction, hepatorenal syndrome
Neuro	Altered mental status, asterixis	Hepatic encephalopathy
Hematologic	Pale conjunctiva, skin bruising	Anemia, thrombocytopenia, coagulation disorders
Metabolic	Jaundice	Hyperbilirubinemia, hyponatremia

The following are common and important initial labs to obtain: liver function tests (including AST, ALT, ALP, and albumin), coagulation studies (PT/PTT/INR), CBC, and hepatitis serologies. Aspartate aminotransferase (AST) and alanine aminotransferase (ALT) are typically elevated with hepatocellular injury while alkaline phosphatase (ALP) and bilirubin elevations typically occur due to cholestasis and biliary tract disease. For example, direct hyperbilirubinemia associated with an isolated increase in the transaminases (AST/ALT) is suggestive of disorders affecting the hepatocytes (e.g., viral hepatitis, drug-induced liver injury). Predominantly elevated ALP +/− AST/ALT is suggestive of cholestasis and of a disease process that is blocking/damaging the bile ducts (e.g., primary sclerosing cholangitis, pancreatic tumor, choledocholithiasis). Of note, ALP can also be elevated due to bone disease; in this case, an elevated GGT level not found in the liver will help confirm that liver injury is the most likely source. Indirect hyperbilirubinemia with associated abnormalities with CBC (low hemoglobin (Hgb) and platelets), elevated lactate dehydrogenase (LDH) and low haptoglobin, is suggestive of hemolysis.

Common Radiologic Tests	Indications
Ultrasound (US)	Visualize biliary tree/liver (assess liver morphology and rule out bile duct dilation)
CT scan with contrast of the abdomen	Can characterize any liver lesions and visualize the pancreas
Magnetic resonance cholangiopancreatography (MRCP)	Noninvasive test, can delineate biliary and pancreatic anatomy
Endoscopic retrograde cholangiopancreatography (ERCP)	Invasive test, can delineate biliary and pancreatic anatomy. Can be used to diagnose a biliary obstruction and pancreatic mass with the ability to obtain tissue diagnosis and intervene with stent placement to restore biliary drainage
Endoscopic ultrasound (EUS)	Can be used to better visualize the extent of diseases such as cancer affecting the intestinal walls as well as to see structures surrounding the digestive tract (lymph nodes, pancreatic masses, liver). This also allows for fine-needle aspiration (FNA) and can be a therapeutic tool.

JAUNDICE

Jaundice occurs when there is buildup of bilirubin (hyperbilirubinemia is usually defined as total bilirubin >2.5 mg/dL). Clinically, patients present with yellowing of the skin and/or eyes (conjunctival icterus). Normally, when red cells break down, heme is converted to bilirubin and sent to the liver to be conjugated prior to its excretion. Therefore, hyperbilirubinemia can consist of either unconjugated (indirect) or conjugated (direct) bilirubin. Direct hyperbilirubinemia occurs when there is damage to the hepatocytes or bile ducts after conjugation has taken place. Indirect hyperbilirubinemia occurs when there is overproduction of bilirubin (e.g., hemolysis) or problems with uptake and conjugation of indirect bilirubin (e.g., Gilbert, Crigler-Najjar).

Differential Diagnosis of Jaundice

Prehepatic Unconjugated	Intrahepatic/Hepatocellular	Post-/Extrahepatic/Obstruction
Decreased uptake or conjugation (Gilbert, Crigler-Najjar, drugs, breast milk jaundice) Hemolysis (hemoglobinopathy, enzyme deficiency, drugs, autoimmune, infectious, DIC (disseminated intravascular coagulation), TTP (thrombotic thrombocytopenic purpura), HUS (hemolytic-uremic syndrome), vasculitis, or malignancy) Hematoma reabsorption	Viral hepatitis (A (HAV), B (HBV), C (HCV), D (HDV), E (HEV)) Nonalcoholic fatty liver disease/nonalcoholic steatohepatitis (NAFLD/NASH) Autoimmune hepatitis Wilson's disease Hemochromatosis/iron overload Drugs/toxins Ischemia/sepsis HELLP (hemolysis, elevated liver enzymes, low platelets) Intrahepatic cholestasis of pregnancy (IHCP) Hereditary dysfunction (Dubin-Johnson)	Biliary obstruction (stones, tumors, cysts, congenital, pancreatitis, strictures, surgical ligation) Primary sclerosing cholangitis (PSC) Primary biliary cholangitis (PBC) Cholangiocarcinoma Pancreatic cancer Budd-Chiari syndrome Portal HTN

Key Associated Findings and Jaundice Differential Diagnoses

Jaundice with Key Associated Findings	Diagnoses
Travel to endemic country, contaminated water, fever	Hepatitis A or E
Obese, T2DM	Nonalcoholic fatty liver disease/nonalcoholic steatohepatitis (NAFLD/NASH)
IVDA, multiple tattoos or remote blood transfusions (pre-1992)	Hepatitis C
Hypercoagulable state (OCPs, protein C/S deficiency, JAK2 disorders)	Budd-Chiari
Painless jaundice, weight loss	Pancreatic cancer, cholangiocarcinoma
Female, history of autoimmune disorders, ALP elevation	PBC
PSC with worsening jaundice, weight loss	Cholangiocarcinoma
Skin hyperpigmentation, diabetes, cardiomyopathy, joint pains, elevated ferritin	Hemochromatosis
Conjunctival pallor, anemia, low haptoglobin, elevated indirect bilirubin	Hemolysis
Keyser-Fleischer rings on slit lamp exam, low ceruloplasmin, neuropsychiatric symptoms	Wilson's disease
"Beads on a string" on cholangiogram; ulcerative colitis, ALP elevation	Primary sclerosing cholangitis (PSC)
Children, adolescents, and young adults	Congenital causes of hyperbilirubinemia: Gilbert, Crigler-Najjar, Dubin-Johnson, Rotor syndromes Breast-feeding jaundice and breast milk jaundice are causes of neonatal jaundice.
Adolescents and young adults	Consider drug or toxin ingestions or viral hepatitis.
Women	Fulminant hepatic failure in pregnant female—hepatitis E PBC is much more common in female patients.
Pregnancy	HELLP, acute fatty liver of pregnancy, intrahepatic cholestasis of pregnancy (IHCP) are all causes of abnormal liver tests and jaundice in pregnancy.

Diagnostic Labs

Condition	Useful Labs
Wilson disease	Low ceruloplasmin
Hemochromatosis	High ferritin and transferrin saturation (high iron, low TIBC)
PSC	+pANCA; IgM: high
PBC	+antimitochondrial Ab (AMA); IgM: high
HAV	Anti-HAV IgM Ab+ (acute); anti-HAV IgG Ab+ (chronic)
HBV	HBsAg+ (infection/carrier); HBsAb+ (immunity due to vaccine or previous infection); anti-HBcAg Ab+ (IgM: current infection/IgG: prior exposure or chronic infection)
HCV	HCV Ab+ (prior or current infection)
Autoimmune hepatitis	ANA+; antismooth muscle Ab (ASMA)+; IgG: high

CASE 26 | Acute Hepatitis A

A 28-year-old man presents to clinic with new onset jaundice. He recently came back from a trip to South America. He initially had abdominal pain with nausea, vomiting, and generalized malaise and fatigue, followed by his eyes turning yellow and his urine turning tea colored. He denies taking any medications or supplements and denies drinking alcohol. He is hemodynamically stable with a temperature of 38°C. He has conjunctival icterus and jaundice, mild right upper quadrant tenderness to palpation and hepatomegaly. No asterix is present.

Evaluation/Tests	Labs show AST 1300, ALT 2700, alkaline phosphatase 377, direct bilirubin 8.4, and normal PT/PTT. Hepatitis A antibody IgM is positive. Hepatitis B surface antigen and hepatitis B core antibody IgM: negative. Ceruloplasmin is normal. ANA, ASMA, and IgG are negative. Abdominal US shows no evidence of biliary obstruction.
Treatment	The treatment is supportive.
Discussion	Hepatitis A is confirmed by a positive hepatitis A antibody IgM. It is endemic in developing countries and transmitted by the fecal-oral route from contaminated food or water. Acute hepatitis A is usually self-limited, and only 1% of patients will develop fulminant liver failure that would require liver transplantation.
	Hepatitis E is also fecal-oral transmission with a similar presentation to hepatitis A. In pregnant patients, hepatitis E can lead to fulminant liver failure.
	Acute or reactivation of **hepatitis B** can have a similar presentation. Two common ways hepatitis B is acquired are through unprotected sex or from mother to child at birth.
	Wilson's disease is a genetic liver disease related to abnormal copper metabolism. A low plasma ceruloplasmin level with a high urine 24-hour urine copper excretion and Kaiser-Fleischer rings on slit lamp examination can confirm the diagnosis.
	Autoimmune hepatitis (AIH) is more common in female patients, associated with other autoimmune disorders, with a positive ANA, smooth muscle antibody, and an elevated IgG level. AIH is very responsive to treatment with steroids.
	Drug-induced liver injury related to prescription or OTC medications—acetaminophen being the most common—or supplements can present with acute hepatitis of variable severity; the key to the diagnosis is the history and timing of exposure.

CASE 27 | Pancreatic Cancer

A 64-year-old man with recently diagnosed type 2 diabetes mellitus presents with anorexia, malaise, nausea, fatigue, and midepigastric pain for several weeks. He notes the epigastric pain is dull, constant, and worsened by eating. He also notes an unintentional 15-pound weight loss over the last month and has noticed dark brown urine, pale stools, and generalized pruritus. He denies fevers, chills, vomiting, or dysphagia but was diagnosed with superficial thrombophlebitis 4 weeks ago. Exam reveals yellowing of the skin and conjunctiva, with mild abdominal tenderness to deep palpation in the epigastrium.

Evaluation/Tests	Liver chemistries show AST 47, ALT 59, alkaline phosphatase 983, total bilirubin 10.7, PT/PTT normal. CA 19-9 tumor marker is elevated.
	CT of the abdomen shows a mass in the uncinate process of the pancreas. Fine-needle aspiration reveals an infiltrating epithelial neoplasm with glandular (ductal) differentiation and intracellular mucin (adenocarcinoma).

CASE 27 | Pancreatic Cancer *(continued)*

Treatment	The only curative treatment for pancreatic cancer is surgical resection, typically with a Whipple procedure.
Discussion	A presentation with painless jaundice and weight loss in a middle-aged patient is highly suspicious for pancreatic adenocarcinoma. Pancreatic adenocarcinoma, is a very aggressive tumor arising from the pancreatic ducts. Patients often are not diagnosed until the cancer is advanced or has metastasized. Clinical presentation may be vague with fatigue and weight loss, but patients can also present with backache, new-onset diabetes, or acute pancreatitis. Pancreatic head lesions can block the common bile duct, resulting in the classic "painless jaundice" presentation. Pancreatic cancer can be associated with superficial migratory thrombophlebitis (Trousseau's syndrome) as seen in this case. Diagnosis can be associated with elevated CA 19-9 tumor marker. If CA 19-9 is elevated, it can be followed to monitor treatment response. Surgical resection is the only curative treatment for pancreatic cancer; however, there is a high rate of recurrence even with early stage disease. Chemotherapy is often used prior to surgery to shrink the tumor, or after surgery to reduce the risk of recurrence. For patients with advanced disease (unresectable or metastatic), palliative chemotherapy is the only treatment option. Patients with **cholangiocarcinoma** may present similarly, however, abdominal ultrasound would show dilated biliary ducts, and diagnosis would be confirmed with tissue biopsy.
Additional Considerations	**Cholangiocarcinomas** are bile duct cancers arising from the epithelial cells of the bile ducts (commonly the extrahepatic ducts). They are grouped based on their anatomic site of origin: intrahepatic, perihilar, or extrahepatic. Intrahepatic cholangiocarcinoma is the second most common primary liver tumor. Symptoms occur once the tumor obstructs the biliary system. Patients may present with jaundice, pruritus, clay colored stools, and dark urine. Primary sclerosing cholangitis increases the risk of cholangiocarcinoma. In Asia (particularly Thailand), infection with Clonorchis sinensis (liver flukes) is associated with cholangiocarcinoma of the intrahepatic bile ducts. This parasitic infection is transmitted via undercooked fish. Adult liver flukes lay eggs in the biliary system, causing chronic inflammation and increasing the risk of malignancy. The only curative treatment is surgical resection. Advanced cancers are treated with palliative chemotherapy.

CASE 28 | Primary Sclerosing Cholangitis (PSC)

A 42-year-old man with a history of ulcerative colitis (UC) presents with pruritis and new onset jaundice. He denies any weight loss or bloody diarrhea. His ulcerative colitis has been in remission on treatment. He does not drink alcohol and has not started any new medications or supplements. On exam, he is hemodynamically stable, well nourished, with icteric conjunctiva and jaundice. The liver edge is soft and palpable 2 cm below the right lower rib at the level of the midclavicular line.

Evaluation/Tests	His laboratory studies are as follows: AST 57, ALT 64, Alk Phos 583, total bilirubin 2.8, and PT/PTT normal. MRCP or ERCP shows intra- and extrahepatic bile duct stricturing and dilation (beaded appearance). Liver biopsy reveals bile duct fibrosis (onion skinning).
Treatment	Liver transplantation.
Discussion	Primary sclerosing cholangitis is an inflammatory disease involving the biliary tree. It is mostly seen in middle-aged men and has a strong association with IBD (ulcerative colitis). The progression of PSC is independent of the activity of UC. Diagnosis is confirmed by cholangiography revealing bile duct structuring and dilatation. Laboratory testing may reveal p-ANCA positive antibodies. Management of PSC includes treatment of manifestations of cirrhosis and portal hypertension (ascites, edema, gastroesophageal varices). Liver transplant can be considered for advanced disease. Cholangiocarcinoma is one of the complications of PSC. **Primary biliary cholangitis (PBC)** mostly affects middle-aged female patients, and characteristic US findings make **alcoholic hepatitis** and **drug-induced liver injury** unlikely.

CASE 29 | Primary Biliary Cholangitis (PBC)

A 43-year-old woman with a history of Sjögren syndrome presents with new onset jaundice, fatigue, and itching. She denies drinking alcohol or taking any new medications or supplements. On exam, she is hemodynamically stable, afebrile, with conjunctival icterus. She is jaundiced, and her abdomen is soft and nontender to palpation. The liver edge is soft and palpable 2 cm below the right lower rib at the level of the midclavicular line.

CASE 29 | Primary Biliary Cholangitis (PBC) (continued)

Evaluation/Tests	Her laboratory tests are as follows: AST 43, ALT 52, Alk Phos 489, T bili 4.8, serum antimitochondrial antibody (AMA) >1:40 (strongly positive). US abdomen is negative for biliary obstruction and PSC. Liver biopsy shows noncaseating granulomas with bile duct injury.
Treatment	Treat with ursodeoxycolic acid (UDCA) and cholestyramine for pruritis. Liver transplantation is the only curative treatment.
Discussion	PBC is an autoimmune disease of the liver with the injury centered on the biliary canaliculi leading to progressive cholestasis. PBC mostly affects middle-aged females. Diagnosis is made with a combination of serologic testing (AMA) and liver biopsy. IgM antibody levels are also elevated. The disease has a course that may extend over many decades with progression to cirrhosis and portal hypertension. Ursodeoxycolic acid (UDCA) is proven to delay the progression of the disease and improve survival, especially if started at an early stage of the disease. It can be associated with other autoimmune diseases such as Sjögren's, scleroderma, rheumatoid arthritis, and celiac disease. Liver transplantation is a curative treatment in advanced PBC with decompensated cirrhosis. Other treatment is aimed at the management of manifestations of cirrhosis and portal hypertension, including ascites, lower extremity edema, and esophageal varices. Hyperlipidemia and xanthomas/xanthalesmas are treated with lipid-lowering medications. In contrast to the elevated IgM level and positive AMA seen in PBC, in **autoimmune hepatitis**, ANA and antismooth muscle antibodies are positive with an elevated IgG level.

CASE 30 | Hemochromatosis

A 52-year-old man with a history of uncontrolled type 2 diabetes mellitus, hypertension, and congestive heart failure presents for evaluation of abnormal liver chemistries. The patient denies drinking alcohol, using illicit drugs, or taking supplements or herbal preparations. He was diagnosed with diabetes 3 years ago and was recently started on insulin. Review of symptoms is notable for erectile dysfunction and bilateral knee and shoulder pains. On exam, he is afebrile with normal vital signs. He has icteric conjunctiva, jugular venous distension, an S3, an enlarged liver, and bilateral lower extremity pitting edema. He has decreased range of motion of both knees with mild effusion, and there is diffuse hyperpigmentation of the skin with a bronze discoloration.

Evaluation/Tests	His laboratory studies are as follows: AST 97, ALT 74, ALP 273, T bili 2.5, albumin 2.8, and PT/PTT are normal. CBC and iron studies show hemoglobin 14.0 g/dL, ferritin 1100 ng/mL, transferrin saturation 82%. *HFE* gene mutation is positive for C282Y mutation.
Treatment	Treat iron overload with repeated phlebotomy. Chelation therapy with deferoxamine, deferasirox, or deferiprone will bind excess iron.
Discussion	Hereditary hemochromatosis is an autosomal recessive disease related to *C282Y* mutation defect in the *HFE* gene on chromosome 6. Iron accumulates in the liver and can lead to cirrhosis. Extrahepatic manifestations include "bronze diabetes," or new onset diabetes mellitus with associated skin discoloration. Other manifestations are cardiomyopathy, arthropathy, hypogonadism, and erectile dysfunction. Extrahepatic manifestations are the result of iron deposited elsewhere in the body. Hemochromatosis is a risk factor for HCC. Phlebotomies and iron chelation can prevent the progression to cirrhosis and other manifestations of HH. The overall goal of treatment is to reduce iron body stores. This can be achieved by scheduled phlebotomies and maintenance with iron chelators. It is also important to manage the manifestations of cirrhosis and extrahepatic manifestations of hemochromatosis such as cardiomyopathy and diabetes. The constellation of symptoms and bronze skin make other diagnoses such as **chronic viral hepatitis**, **alcoholic liver disease**, and **nonalcoholic steatohepatitis** (NASH) unlikely.

CASE 31 | Hepatocellular Carcinoma (HCC)

A 67-year-old woman with a 40-year history of alcohol abuse presents with poor appetite, abdominal distension, and jaundice. Her physical exam is notable for conjunctival icterus, abdominal distension, anasarca, and a palpable right upper quadrant mass.

Evaluation/Tests	Triple-phase CT of the abdomen and pelvis reveals a 6-cm mass in the right lobe of the liver demonstrating arterial phase enhancement and delayed phase washout. AFP is elevated.
Treatment	Surgical resection or liver transplant.

CASE 31 | Hepatocellular Carcinoma (HCC) *(continued)*

Discussion	Hepatocellular carcinoma (HCC) is the most common malignant tumor of the liver. Risk factors include all causes of cirrhosis such as hepatitis B and C, alcohol abuse, and nonalcoholic steatosis (NASH). It is recommended to screen patients with cirrhosis for developing HCC with imaging and serum alpha-fetoprotein (AFP). HCC is one of the few malignancies that can be diagnosed without biopsy in the appropriate setting with radiographic findings and elevated AFP. Triple-phase abdominal CT findings will reveal a mass with arterial phase enhancement and venous phase washout. In the setting of localized disease and for those ineligible to receive resection or transplant, treatment options include radioembolization, transarterial chemoembolization (TACE), and systemic chemotherapy. **Hepatic adenomas** are rare, benign liver tumors that are most frequently associated with oral contraceptive or androgen use. They are typically diagnosed incidentally in patients undergoing imaging studies for other reasons. Diagnosis can be made with ultrasound or CT scan, demonstrating features of adenomas, such as well demarcated margins and hyperechogenicity. Laboratory abnormalities are not typically seen. Biopsies for the evaluation of suspected hepatic adenomas are not routinely performed due to the high risk of bleeding and lack of diagnostic benefit. Surgical resection is the definitive treatment of hepatic adenomas and is recommended for patients with large, symptomatic adenomas or those that have ruptured.

ASCITES

Ascites is the accumulation of fluid within the abdominal cavity and manifests as abdominal distension, shifting dullness, or fluid wave on physical examination. Ascites occurs because of various factors such as portal hypertension, loss of oncotic pressure related to hypoalbuminemia, or peritoneal diseases secondary to infection, inflammation, or malignancy.

Key Findings and Ascites Differential Diagnosis

Ascites with Key Associated Findings	Diagnoses
Chronic liver disease of any type	Cirrhosis
Severe congestive heart failure or pulmonary hypertension	Cardiac ascites
Foamy urine, chronic kidney disease	Nephrotic syndrome; hypoalbuminemia causing ascites secondary to low oncotic pressure
Cachexia, severely low BMI, malnourished	Hypoalbuminemia causing ascites secondary to low oncotic pressure
Intra-abdominal/gynecologic malignancy	Malignant ascites
Abdominal pain, fever	Spontaneous bacterial peritonitis (SBP)
Person from endemic area of TB (e.g., Mexico, South East Asia)	TB ascites

Ultrasound can easily confirm the presence of fluid within the abdomen. It can also assess for liver disease; cirrhosis is the most common cause of ascites. A diagnosis of the underlying cause is necessary for treatment. Ascites should be assessed by paracentesis with lab testing (total protein, albumin, serum-ascites albumin gradient (SAAG), gram stain and culture, cell count with differential, and cytology). The most useful initial tests on ascitic fluid are the total protein and SAAG. Total protein >2.5 g/dL suggests appropriate synthetic function of protein by the liver. Therefore, cardiac causes such as right-sided heart failure should be considered in the DDx. If total protein is <2.5 g/dL, it suggests either poor synthetic function by the liver or loss by another means (nephropathy, enteropathy, malnutrition). SAAG, serum-ascites albumin gradient = serum albumin minus ascitic fluid albumin. SAAG >1.1 g/dL is indicative of portal hypertension, while a SAAG <1.1 g/dL indicates lack of portal hypertension as the primary cause of ascites. A diagnostic paracentesis should always be performed for a patient with new-onset ascites or in a patient with known ascites presenting with acute abdominal pain and fever (to rule out spontaneous bacterial peritonitis (SBP)). If the neutrophil count is greater than 250 cells/μL, then the diagnosis of SBP is confirmed, and antibiotics should be started. In addition, a therapeutic paracentesis removing large volumes of fluid can be performed electively when the volume of fluid in the abdomen causes physical discomfort or pushes on the diaphragm, causing dyspnea.

Paracentesis Findings and Differential Diagnosis

Protein	SAAG >1.1	SAAG <1.1
Low (<2.5)	Cirrhosis: (ETOH, hep C, etc.) Budd Chiari (late, with cirrhosis)	Nephrotic syndrome Protein losing enteropathy Severe malnutrition
High (>2.5)	Constrictive pericarditis Right heart failure Portal or splenic vein thrombosis Budd-Chiari syndrome (early) Schistosomiasis	Pancreatitis Peritoneal carcinomatosis (e.g., ovarian) TB

CASE 32 | Alcoholic Cirrhosis

A 54-year-old man with a history of alcohol abuse presents with worsening abdominal distension and lower extremity edema for the past 4 weeks. He has been drinking about 10 beers daily for the past 18 years. He denies any illicit drug use. He has had problems with alcohol withdrawal symptoms, including tremors and seizures in the past. Two months ago, he had esophageal variceal bleeding that was treated with banding. On exam, he is cachectic. He has slow speech, icteric conjunctiva, and asterixis. Vital signs are BP 105/70 mmHg, heart rate 88/min, and respirations 18/min. He has decreased breath sounds and dullness to percussion at bilateral lung bases. Abdomen is distended with caput medusae and a positive fluid wave. Bilateral lower extremity pitting edema is present up to the knees. Skin is notable for jaundice with multiple spider angiomas on the chest.

Evaluation/Tests	LFTs show AST 68, ALT 32, ALP 269, T bili 3.8, albumin 2.5, INR 2.3, and CBC shows a platelet count of 59,000/μL. US abdomen with Doppler shows ascites and cirrhotic liver morphology with severe liver steatosis, patent hepatic vessels, and no evidence of liver lesions. Viral hepatitis serologies are negative for HBV and HCV. Ascitic fluid analysis shows protein 1.8, albumin 1.2, cell count 389 with 28% neutrophils. SAAG >1.1.
Treatment	Diagnostic and therapeutic paracentesis. Advise alcohol cessation, low-salt diet, and diuretics (furosemide or spironolactone). Upper endoscopy should be done to evaluate esophageal varices and repeat banding to prevent recurrent bleeding. Nonselective beta blockers (propranolol or nadolol) can be used for prophylaxis of variceal bleeding. Lactulose is used for management of hepatic encephalopathy.
Discussion	A prolonged history of daily alcohol use is highly suggestive of alcoholic cirrhosis. Other causes of chronic liver disease, mainly chronic viral hepatitis B and C, should always be ruled out because their presence may potentiate the toxicity of alcohol and accelerate the development of cirrhosis. Patients presenting with ascites should have abdominal US with Doppler performed to assess for cirrhotic liver morphology, to rule out hepatic or portal vein thrombosis, and to evaluate for liver lesions. Diagnostic and therapeutic paracentesis should be done for symptomatic relief and to check ascitic fluid albumin, protein, cell count, and differential to confirm portal hypertension and rule out spontaneous bacterial peritonitis. AST and ALT mildly elevated with AST/ALT ratio >2 is suggestive of alcohol abuse. Ascitic fluid analysis showed that the serum-ascites albumin gradient (SAAG, serum albumin minus ascitic albumin) is >1.1, confirming that ascitic fluid is due to portal hypertension, and neutrophil <250 cells/mm³, ruling out spontaneous bacterial peritonitis. Alpha fetoprotein is indicated every 6 months for screening for hepatocellular carcinoma in the setting of cirrhosis. Without a known exposure to significant alcohol, one must continue assessing risk factors to determine the likely cause. Workup should include assessing risk factors for hepatitis B or C and testing for those etiologies. **Nonalcoholic steatohepatitis (NASH)** is a cause of chronic liver disease and cirrhosis related to obesity. Risk factors include obesity, diabetes, hyperlipidemia, and hypertension.

CASE 33 | Chronic Hepatitis C

A 64-year-old man with a history of intravenous drug abuse presents with worsening abdominal distension and lower extremity edema for the past 4 weeks. He denies drinking alcohol but admits to using intravenous heroin 20 years ago. On exam, he appears cachectic with poor muscle mass. Vital signs show blood pressure of 105/70 mmHg, pulse 88/min, and respirations 18/min. He has conjunctival icterus, decreased breath sounds, and dullness to percussion at lung bases. Abdomen is large and distended with a positive fluid wave. Bilateral lower extremity edema is present.

CASE 33 | Chronic Hepatitis C *(continued)*

Evaluation/Tests	LFTs are significant for AST 57, ALT 28, T bili 3.4, albumin 2.8, INR 1.9, platelet count 79,000/uL. US abdomen with Doppler shows large-volume ascites and cirrhotic liver morphology with severe liver steatosis, patent hepatic vessels, and no evidence of liver lesions. HCV antibody is positive with HCV RNA PCR positive. Serologies are negative for HBV and HIV.
Treatment	Treat with diagnostic and therapeutic paracentesis. Treat hepatitis C with direct acting antiviral therapy. Manage cirrhosis complications and monitor for HCC.
Discussion	Hepatitis C remains one of the major causes of cirrhosis in the United States. This is slowly changing with the advent of the new highly effective antiviral therapies. Modes of transmission of HCV involve contact with contaminated blood either through sharing needles in IV drug users or blood transfusions received prior to 1990. HCV is very rarely sexually transmitted. It is recommended that all adults between 18 and 79 years of age be screened for HCV. If hepatitis C infection is confirmed with hep C antibody followed by HCV RNA PCR tests, then an HCV genotype should be performed. Diagnostic and therapeutic paracentesis should be done for symptomatic relief and to rule out spontaneous bacterial peritonitis. Note that thrombocytopenia indicates portal hypertension and hypersplenism; hypoalbuminemia indicates advanced cirrhosis. **Hepatitis B** is more prevalent in Asia and Eastern Europe. HBV is transmitted through unprotected sexual contact, at birth from mother to child, and by contact with contaminated blood, mainly when sharing needles. An HBV vaccine is available and highly effective in preventing HBV infections. Chronic HBV infection is defined by a persistently positive HBV surface antigen for more than 6 months after initial exposure. About 80% of patients who acquire the infection at birth will develop chronic HBV. When acquired as an adult, the risk of chronic HBV is 20–30% after an acute infection. Antiviral therapy for HBV aims at suppressing viral replication that will reduce liver inflammation and prevent liver cirrhosis.

CASE 34 | Budd-Chiari Syndrome

A 43-year-old woman with no known medical problems presents with progressive ascites and lower extremity edema. She reports that for the past 2–3 weeks, she has had right upper quadrant discomfort followed by progressive abdominal distension and lower extremity edema and significant weight gain. She denies drinking alcohol. She has been taking oral contraceptives for the past 5 years. On exam, she is jaundiced, afebrile, and her vital signs are normal. She has a distended tense abdomen, with bilateral flank dullness to percussion suggestive of large ascites, right upper quadrant tenderness, and bilateral lower extremity edema.

Evaluation/Tests	Her laboratory test show ALT 157, AST 213, ALP 352, T bili 2.8, albumin 2.3, INR 1.6, hemoglobin 16.8 g/dL. Abdominal US with Doppler shows the absence of normal flow in the hepatic veins.
Treatment	Stop oral contraceptives and start anticoagulation. Manage cirrhosis and its complications.
Discussion	Budd-Chiari syndrome is defined as the presence of hepatic outflow obstruction, either acute or progressive, from a thrombus or tumor invasion. The diagnosis is made with abdominal US with Doppler showing the absence of normal flow in the hepatic veins. Contrast imaging with CT scan or MRI can confirm the diagnosis and rule out compression of the hepatic veins by benign lesions or invasion by malignancy. The etiologic workup for Budd-Chiari syndrome should include an evaluation for hypercoagulable states (i.e., factor V Leiden mutation, protein C and S deficiency, or JAK2 mutation), myeloproliferative disorders, vasculitis, and inflammatory diseases, and benign or malignant lesions. Oral contraceptives and a recent pregnancy are important risk factors for Budd-Chiari syndrome as well. Paracentesis can be performed for diagnostic and therapeutic purposes. In this case, anticoagulation can be used, and a transjugular intrahepatic portosystemic shunt (TIPS) can be placed, when technically possible, to restore patency of the hepatic veins and bypass the liver. Any diagnosis that can cause ascites can be considered in this situation. However, the acuity of the development of ascites leads away from more chronic processes such as congestive heart failure, cirrhosis related to viral hepatitis, or NASH. In addition, the US imaging with Doppler is key for proving obstruction within the hepatic veins that would not be present in other scenarios.

CASE 35 | Spontaneous Bacterial Peritonitis (SBP)

A 62-year-old woman with a history of hepatitis C cirrhosis complicated by ascites and esophageal varices is brought for evaluation of diffuse abdominal pain and confusion. Her vitals are notable for a fever of 38.2°C, heart rate 102/min, and blood pressure of 95/60 mmHg. On physical exam, she is jaundiced and has a tense, protuberant abdomen with a fluid wave and rebound tenderness.

Evaluation/Tests	Fluid collected through abdominal tap of ascitic fluid (paracentesis) shows >250 cells/μL polymorphonuclear cells (PMNs). Fluid cultures are pending.
Treatment	Treat with IV antibiotics to cover gram negatives (third-generation cephalosporins).
Discussion	Spontaneous bacterial peritonitis (SBP) is a common but potentially fatal infection in patients with advanced cirrhosis and ascites. The infection develops due to the translocation of gut enteric bacteria into the ascitic fluid. SBP frequently presents with fever, diffuse abdominal pain, or worsening encephalopathy, but it can also be asymptomatic. Jaundice, ascites, and rebound tenderness (a sign of peritonitis) are frequently present. Systemic signs of infection, such as fever, tachycardia, and hypotension, may also be present. Since early detection and treatment are key, patients with ascites of any cause who display the preceding symptoms should undergo diagnostic paracentesis. The diagnosis of SBP is established if the ascitic fluid polymorphonuclear cell (i.e., neutrophil) count is ≥250 cells/mm³. It is important to perform the abdominal paracentesis prior to administering any antibiotics. Ascitic fluid cultures may aid in identifying the causative organism. While SBP is most commonly caused by infection from gut enteric bacteria, such as *Escherichia coli* or *Klebsiella*, streptococcal and, less frequently, staphylococcal infections may also occur. As a result, empiric broad-spectrum antibiotics, as with a third-generation cephalosporin, are recommended with subsequent de-escalation pending ascitic fluid culture results and susceptibility testing. In addition, patients with cirrhosis presenting with upper gastrointestinal bleeding should have SBP prophylaxis initiated, usually with trimethoprim-sulfamethoxazole therapy or fluoroquinolone therapy.

10

Hematology and Oncology

Rozina Chowdhery, MD
Ardaman Shergill, MD
John Galvin, MD

ANEMIA

Anemia is defined as a hemoglobin or hematocrit below the lower limit of normal. It varies by lab assay, though in general it is a hemoglobin <13 g/dL or hematocrit <42% in male patients and hemoglobin <12 g/dL or hematocrit <37% in female patients. It is important to remember that anemia is not a primary disease process itself but rather a manifestation of another condition or disease process that causes anemia. The easiest way to understand anemia is to divide it into smaller categories. One of the most common methods to categorize anemia is by red blood cell (RBC) size. Normal red blood cell size (**MCV**, mean corpuscular volume) is approximately **80–100 fL**, with smaller cells being referred to as "microcytic" and larger cells being referred to as "macrocytic."

Microcytic anemia is usually the result of the disordered production of hemoglobin, and the most common cause is iron deficiency; other causes include thalassemias and lead poisoning.

Macrocytic anemias refer to anemias in which the MCV is >100 fL. This can be either **megaloblastic**, meaning accompanied by hypersegmented neutrophils, or **nonmegaloblastic**, in which case neutrophils appear normal. Macrocytic anemias become megaloblastic if DNA synthesis is impaired. This usually occurs in the context of deficiencies of vitamins important for DNA synthesis, such as **folate** or **B12** (see "Biochemistry" chapter). In nonmegaloblastic anemias, DNA synthesis is unimpaired; the causes include liver disease, alcohol use, and certain medications.

Microcytic	Normocytic	Macrocytic
Iron deficiency	Aplastic anemia	Folate deficiency
Anemia of chronic disease	Chronic kidney disease	B12 deficiency
Thalassemias	Spherocytosis	Liver disease
Sideroblastic anemia	Glucose-6-phosphate dehydrogenase (G6PD) deficiency	Alcoholism
Lead Poisoning	Paroxysmal nocturnal hemoglobinuria (PNH)	
	Sickle cell anemia	
	Autoimmune hemolytic anemia (AIHA)	
	Microangiopathic hemolytic anemia	
	Malaria	

Anemia of chronic disease can have a mildly low MCV or may be normocytic. The total body iron is normal but sequestered and unable to be used by RBC precursors.

Hemolytic anemias occur with increased destruction of RBCs. They can be **intrinsic** (a problem with the erythrocyte itself leading to hemolysis) or **extrinsic** (erythrocytes are normal but another process causes hemolysis). Hemolysis may also be differentiated as **intravascular** (within blood vessels) or **extravascular** (usually within the spleen). Intravascular hemolytic anemias are often accompanied by an *increase in indirect and total bilirubin, LDH,* and *reticulocyte count* if the bone marrow is functioning normally and a *decrease in haptoglobin.* **Sickle cell anemia** is a normocytic anemia associated with intravascular and extravascular hemolysis. Extravascular hemolysis occurs in **hereditary spherocytosis** as the spleen tries to destroy the abnormally shaped red blood cells. In **glucose-6-phosphate dehydrogenase (G6PD) deficiency**, both intravascular and extravascular hemolysis can occur after oxidative stress.

Decreased production of erythrocytes resulting in anemia is due to primary or secondary bone marrow failure. **Aplastic anemia** is caused by either the failure or the destruction of myeloid stem cells. It has a multitude of potential causes, including radiation, medications, viruses, and genetic disorders. It also can be idiopathic. Typical findings include a decrease in reticulocyte count, increase in erythropoietin, and pancytopenia. In **chronic kidney disease (CKD)**, the failing kidney will produce decreased levels of erythropoietin (a hormone that stimulates RBC production), resulting in anemia. This generally does not occur until later stages of CKD. Erythropoietin analogs such as epoetin alfa can be given as treatment as long as the other mineral and vitamin levels are within normal limits.

Differential Diagnosis of Anemia

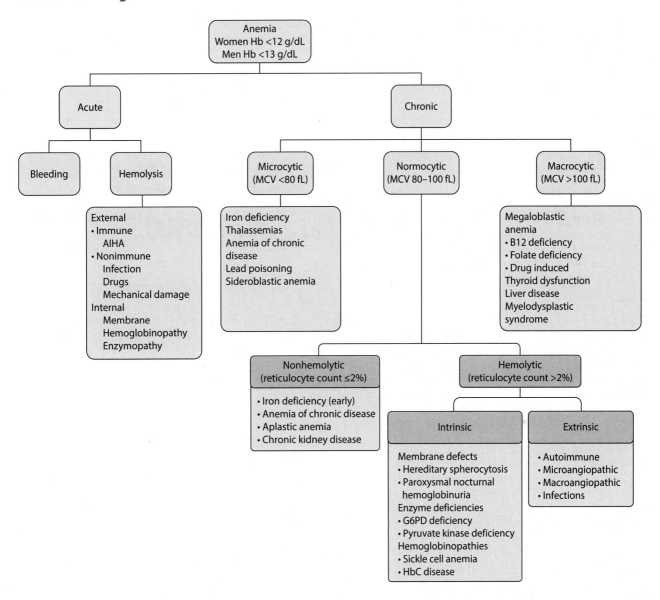

Key Associated Findings and Anemia Differential Diagnoses

Anemia with Key Associated Findings	Diagnoses
History of heavy menses, GI bleed, pica, or esophageal webs (Plummer-Vinson syndrome) Spoon nails (koilonychia), or cheilosis Lab findings: low ferritin, low iron, high TIBC	Iron deficiency anemia (IDA)
Chipped paint exposure, encephalopathy, or abdominal colic Foot/wrist drop, or gingival lines Lab findings: erythrocyte basophilic stippling, sideroblastic anemia	Lead poisoning
Family history of anemia Asian, African, or Mediterranean descent	Thalassemia
History of autoimmune or inflammatory disease Lab findings: high ferritin and low TIBC, mildly low or normal MCV	Anemia of chronic disease
Travel to endemic regions	Malaria
Family history sickle cell Priapism, dactylitis Asplenia, avascular necrosis (AVN), or pulmonary HTN	Sickle cell disease

(continued)

Key Associated Findings and Anemia Differential Diagnoses (*continued*)

Anemia with Key Associated Findings	Diagnoses
Drug exposure (classically sulfas) African or Middle Eastern decent Lab findings: Heinz bodies, bite cells	G6PD
Lab findings: increased indirect/total bilirubin, LDH, retic count; decreased haptoglobin	Hemolytic anemia (intravascular)
Lab findings: pancytopenia, decrease reticulocyte count, increase erythropoietin	Aplastic anemia

CASE 1 | Iron Deficiency Anemia

A 43-year-old woman with a history of uterine fibroids and heavy menses presents with several months of progressive fatigue. Vital signs are normal. Physical exam reveals a pale, fatigued individual with conjunctival pallor and spoon-shaped nails (koilonychia).

Evaluations/Tests	Hemoglobin 9.5 g/dL; MCV 75 fL; RDW 17%. Iron and ferritin are low and TIBC is high. Examination of the peripheral blood reveals small red blood cells with marked central pallor but no other morphologic abnormalities. Microcytosis and hypochromasia (central pallor) Reproduced with permission from Reisner H. Pathology: A Modern Case Study, 2nd ed. New York, NY: McGraw Hill; 2020.
Treatment	Iron replacement therapy and evaluation of underlying blood loss.
Discussion	Iron deficiency anemia (IDA) is a microcytic, hypochromic anemia that can be caused by nutritional deficiency, poor absorption (malabsorption syndromes), or chronic blood loss (e.g., colon cancer). Patient presentation can vary depending on age, comorbid conditions, and chronicity of the deficiency. Symptoms may include fatigue, weakness, shortness of breath, dizziness, conjunctival pallor, pica symptoms (consumption of ice, dirt, clay, or other nonfood substances), or headaches. Physical exam findings may include conjunctival pallor, cheilosis, tachycardia, and koilonychia (spoon nails). Typical lab findings include *a low ferritin, low iron, and high TIBC*. Treatment includes replacing iron with either oral (preferred) or IV therapy and determining and treating the underlying cause. A common cause in young women is blood loss from menorrhagia. However, in men or postmenopausal women, a complete GI evaluation is warranted to rule out underlying GI malignancies.
Additional Considerations	**Lead poisoning** can also cause microcytic anemia. Consider this in children due to ingestion/exposures (lead-based paint) and in adults through occupational hazards. Classic signs and symptoms of lead poisoning include sideroblastic anemia, erythrocyte basophilic stippling, lead lines on gingivae and on metaphyses of long bones on X-ray, abdominal pain, encephalopathy, and wrist and foot drop (neuropathy). Bone marrow biopsy would reveal ringed sideroblasts. Treat advanced cases of lead poisoning with Dimercaprol or EDTA. Erythrocyte basophilic stippling Used with permission from Herbert L. Fred, MD and Hendrik A. van Dijk - Images of Memorable Cases: Case 81. Dec 8, 2008 http://cnx.org/content/m15003/latest/

CASE 1 | Iron Deficiency Anemia *(continued)*

Additional Considerations	**Sideroblastic anemias** occur when the patient is not iron deficient but is unable to use available iron to create red blood cells. The result is the formation of sideroblasts in the bone marrow, which are Prussian blue staining of iron-laden mitochondria.

CASE 2 | β-Thalassemia

A 16-year-old boy of Greek descent presents for evaluation of incidentally discovered anemia on routine lab work. He denies bleeding or bruising and otherwise feels well. He denies fevers, chills, weight loss, irregular bowel movements, chest pain, dyspnea, or palpitations. On exam, he looks healthy, and his vital signs and oxygen saturation are normal. On exam, his spleen is easily palpated, and the rest of the exam is unremarkable.

Evaluations/Tests	CBC: hemoglobin 11.4 g/dL, MCV 64 fL, WBC 8600/mm^3, platelets 284,000/mm^3. Ferritin is 150 ng/mL. Hemoglobin electrophoresis demonstrates an increased amount of HbA$_2$.
Treatment	Supportive care and RBC transfusion when symptomatic.
Discussion	This patient with asymptomatic, microcytic anemia likely has β-thalassemia trait (thalassemia minor). Electrophoresis showing increased HbA$_2$ yields the diagnosis. β-thalassemia major, on the other hand, can have a variety of manifestations. **Hemoglobinopathies**, such as **thalassemias**, are a frequent cause of microcytic anemias. **α-Thalassemia** is caused by a mutation coding α-globin chain. α-Thalassemia is more common in African and Asian populations. **β-Thalassemia** is a mutation of the gene encoding β-globin and is more common in Mediterranean populations. Heterozygotes are usually asymptomatic but mildly anemic with underproduced β-chains. Homozygotes have a severe microcytic hypochromic anemia with target cells, and they generally require frequent blood transfusions. They can develop hepatosplenomegaly as well as multiple other systemic manifestations (e.g., iron overload, skeletal deformities, cholelithiasis, jaundice, and pulmonary hypertension). β-Thalassemia presents with HbA$_2$ ($\alpha_2\delta_2$), while the electrophoresis of a patient with **α-thalassemia** would be predominantly HbA, which is the normal hemoglobin molecule. In severe disease, HbH (four β-chains) or HbF may be present. In general, the microcytosis of thalassemia is greater in magnitude than the microcytosis of **iron deficiency**. **Lead poisoning** will often present with other symptoms such as lead lines on gingivae and metaphyses of long bones, encephalopathy, abdominal pain, and neuropathies. **Sickle cell** and **hemoglobin C disease** usually cause normocytic anemias. Electrophoresis would show evidence of HbS or HbC, as well as relatively increased amounts of HbF (fetal hemoglobin), especially if the patient is on hydroxyurea.

CASE 3 | Anemia of Chronic Disease

A 54-year-old woman with a history of systemic lupus erythematosus (SLE) presents with generalized fatigue. She denies any recent illnesses or changes in medications. Her last menses was 2 years ago, and she denies any melena or blood in her stools. Her SLE has been well controlled on hydroxychloroquine for the past year. On exam, her vital signs are normal and she is in no acute distress. Her conjunctivae are normal and there are no rashes, joint tenderness, or swelling. One week ago, her hemoglobin was 11 g/dL with a normal MCV, which is unchanged over the past 2 years.

Evaluations/Tests	CBC: hemoglobin 11 g/dL, MCV 89 fL, WBC 4200/mm^3, platelets 190,000/mm^3. Reticulocyte count is low. Iron and TIBC are low, and ferritin is high. Peripheral smear shows normocytic RBCs. BMP and LFTS are normal. TSH, B12, and folate levels are normal. Hemoccult stool test is negative for blood and she is up to date on screening colonoscopy.
Treatment	Continue to treat underlying cause of anemia, in this case SLE.
Discussion	Anemia of chronic disease is generally seen in conditions causing chronic inflammation such as autoimmune diseases, chronic liver or kidney disease, infections, or cancers. Systemic, chronic inflammation causes elevated acute phase reactants such as interleukin-6 (IL-6) and ferritin. IL-6 can promote increased synthesis and the release of hepcidin from the liver. Hepcidin affects iron transport by decreasing iron absorption from the gut and preventing release of intracellular iron from macrophages. This results in low serum iron levels. Elevated ferritin promotes increased intracellular storage of iron, further contributing to low serum iron levels. Peripheral smear typically shows a normocytic or microcytic anemia with a low reticulocyte count. Underlying causes should be treated appropriately. Typical findings may include a *high ferritin* and *low TIBC* in the setting of chronic conditions causing inflammation such as cancers or autoimmune diseases.

CASE 3 | Anemia of Chronic Disease *(continued)*

| Discussion | **Anemia of chronic kidney disease** can be normocytic, and treating significant anemia in this setting with erythropoiesis-stimulating agents such as epoetin alfa (EPO) can be helpful.
Nutritional deficiencies, such as folate and B12, are common, and **alcohol** can be directly toxic to the bone marrow. However, these disorders usually cause macrocytosis.
End-stage liver disease–associated anemia can be multifactorial as well. Anemia can be due to portal hypertension (resulting from acute blood loss from ruptured esophageal varices or chronic loss from portal hypertensive gastropathy) and/or from splenic sequestration. Peripheral smear may show spur cells, burr cells, or target cells. |

CASE 4 | Sickle Cell Disease

A 22-year-old woman with family history of sickle cell diseases is brought via ambulance for shortness of breath. When paramedics initially arrived, her vitals were temperature 38°C, pulse 128/min, respirations 32/min, blood pressure 92/53 mmHg, and O_2 saturation 72%. She is urgently intubated with an improvement in her O_2 saturation to 92%. On exam, she is tachycardic, has conjunctival icterus, and diffuse crackles on lung exam. Abdomen is soft and there is no rash or lower extremity edema. STAT CBC shows hemoglobin 5.7 g/dL.

Evaluations/Tests	CBC: WBC 16,500/mm³, hemoglobin 5.7 g/dL, platelets 268,000/mm³. LDH is 1273 U/L. Absolute reticulocyte count is 253×10^3/uL. Hemoglobin electrophoresis reveals HbS and HbF. Peripheral blood smear shows sickle and target cells. Peripheral blood smear with sickle cells. Reproduced with permission from Laposata M. Laposata's Laboratory Medicine Diagnosis of Disease in Clinical Laboratory, 3rd ed. New York, NY: McGraw Hill; 2019.	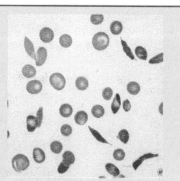
Treatment	Supportive care (aggressive hydration, oxygenation) as well as treatment of the underlying cause (pneumonia) of acute chest syndrome. Patients with sickle cell disease who have acute pain require aggressive pain control, often with opioid pain medications. Exchange transfusion may be needed in severe cases with end-organ complications.
Discussion	Severe anemia with elevated LDH and reticulocyte count is suggestive of hemolysis and peripheral smear showing sickle-appearing cells is consistent with the diagnosis of sickle cell disease. Sickle cell anemia causes a normocytic anemia, and it results from a single amino acid replacement in the β-globin molecule (glutamic acid → valine), leading to cytoplasmic polymerization of hemoglobin molecules and the classic sickling shape, resulting in intravascular and extravascular hemolysis. Additionally, these abnormal cells do not flow through the vasculature as well and can occlude capillaries, triggering very painful vaso-occlusive crises. **Acute chest syndrome** is a serious complication, which can be precipitated by pneumonia, asthma, pulmonary embolus, or other infections. It is defined as the presence of new pulmonary infiltrates with respiratory complaints and hypoxia, with or without fever. Increased adhesion of sickled red cells to pulmonary vasculature is the cause of hypoxia. It has a high mortality and potential for developing into chronic lung disease. This is a medical emergency, and treatment for severe cases is exchange transfusion. Other indications for exchange transfusion include acute stroke, multiorgan failure, and severe priapism. Chronic complications of sickle cell anemia include asplenia, aplastic crisis (often precipitated by Parvovirus B19 infection), avascular necrosis (AVN), pulmonary HTN, and renal papillary necrosis resulting in chronic kidney disease. **Hemoglobin C disease** is related to sickle cell disease, but glutamic acid is substituted for lysine, and patients may still undergo hemolysis. However, cells in hemoglobin C disease do not sickle; instead, hemoglobin crystals form within the RBCs. **Pyruvate kinase deficiency** is another genetic disorder predisposing cells to hemolyze because the RBCs are no longer able to complete anaerobic respiration. These cells do not appear to sickle in the periphery.

CASE 5 | Glucose-6-Phosphate Dehydrogenase Deficiency (G6PD Deficiency)

A 28-year-old woman presents with fatigue and yellowing of her eyes after starting a course of sulfamethoxazole/trimethoprim for a urinary tract infection (UTI). Her UTI symptoms have significantly improved, but her urine is significantly darker. On exam, her pulse is 96/min, respirations are 18/min, blood pressure is 106/76 mmHg, O_2 saturation is 98% on room air, and she has conjunctival icterus. The rest of her exam is normal.

Evaluations/Tests	Repeat urinalysis shows hemoglobinuria and is negative for RBCs, WBCs, leukocyte esterase, or nitrites. CBC: WBC 9200/mm³, hemoglobin 7.3 g/dL, platelets 172,000/mm³. LDH is 1362 U/L, total bilirubin is 8.6 mg/dL (direct bilirubin 2.4 mg/dL), and haptoglobin is undetectable. Her MCV is normal, reticulocyte count is increased, and Heinz bodies and bite cells are noted on the blood smear. 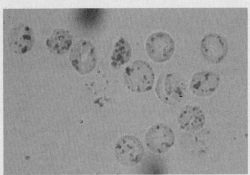 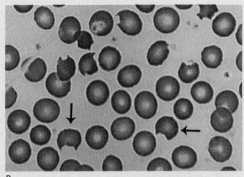 A B **A.** Heinz bodies. Blood mixed with hypotonic solution of crystal violet. The stained material is precipitates of denatured hemoglobin within cells. **B.** Degmacytes ("bite cells") on peripheral smear, classically seen with G6PD Deficiency. Part A Reproduced with permission from Jameson JL, Fauci AS, Kasper DL, et al: Harrison's Principles of Internal Medicine, 20th ed. New York, NY: McGraw Hill; 2018; part B Reproduced with permission from Kaushansky K, Lichtman MA, Prhal JT, et al: Williams Hematology, 9th ed. New York, NY: McGraw Hill; 2016.
Treatment	Supportive care (hydration) and avoid drugs and chemicals that can cause oxidant stress. Consider transfusion in severe, symptomatic cases.
Discussion	This patient has significant normocytic anemia due to hemolysis, as evidenced by elevated indirect bilirubin and LDH, as well as undetectable haptoglobin. Her history of taking a sulfa-containing medication, as well as the peripheral smear showing bite cells, also supports the diagnosis of G6PD deficiency, which is an X-linked recessive disorder most common in African and Middle Eastern populations. A defect in G6PD enzyme results in decreased levels of the antioxidant molecule glutathione, which in turn renders the RBC more susceptible to oxidative stress. G6PD normally catalyzes the rate-limiting step in the pentose phosphate pathway (hexose monophosphate shunt). In this pathway, a series of enzymatic reactions converts glucose-6-phosphate to form NADPH, which is an important reducing agent used in antioxidant defenses in RBCs. Decreased NADPH results in decreased levels of glutathione and leads to increased RBC susceptibility to oxidant stress. Common oxidizing agents include sulfonamides, primaquine, chloroquine, antituberculosis drugs, nitrofurantoin, and fava beans. Exposure to these agents or infections (because the RBCs can no longer detoxify free radicals) can trigger both intravascular and extravascular hemolysis and formation of Heinz bodies (denatured hemoglobin that has precipitated in RBCs). Bite cells result from the phagocytic removal of Heinz bodies by splenic macrophages. Therefore, bite cells will not be seen in patients with a splenectomy. In **microangiopathic hemolytic anemias** (e.g., TTP, HUS, HELLP syndrome, DIC) schistocytes would be seen on the peripheral smear. Additionally, DIC would be accompanied by derangements in coagulation factors (i.e., elevated PT/INR, PTT, and D-dimer, and low fibrinogen). **Autoimmune hemolytic anemia** would not be accompanied by bite cells.

CASE 6 | Hereditary Spherocytosis

A 32-year-old woman presents with fatigue, dyspnea on exertion, and yellow eyes. She notes that her urine has been darker lately. She recently started training for a marathon but had to stop when these symptoms developed. She denies chest pain, fevers, or chills. Her last menstrual period was 2 weeks ago and her menses are normal; she denies any bruising or bleeding. Her mother had anemia and had to have her spleen removed in her twenties. On exam, her vital signs are respirations 14/ min, pulse 112/min, blood pressure 128/86 mmHg, and SpO₂ 99% on RA. She is not in any distress, but her conjunctiva are yellow and she has splenomegaly. Stat hemoglobin is 8.2. Last year, it was normal.

CASE 6 | Hereditary Spherocytosis *(continued)*

Evaluations/Tests	WBC 5.2/mm³, hemoglobin 8.2 g/fL, MCV 87, platelets 180,000/mm³, LDH 400 U/L, haptoglobin <10 mg/dL, total bilirubin 8.2 mg/dL with direct component 2.6 mg/dL, reticulocyte count >6%, LFTs otherwise unremarkable. Urinalysis shows increased urobilinogen. A direct Coombs test is negative. Peripheral smear shows small spherical cells without central pallor (spherocytes). 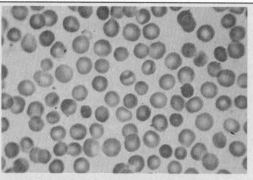 Spherocytosis. Note small hyperchromatic cells without the usual clear area in the center. Reproduced with permission from Jameson JL, Fauci AS, Kasper DL, et al: Harrison's Principles of Internal Medicine, 20th ed. New York, NY: McGraw Hill; 2018.
Treatment	Splenectomy; severe, symptomatic anemia may require blood transfusion.
Discussion	Hereditary spherocytosis is a genetic red blood cell membrane disorder. Patients present with anemia secondary to hemolysis and spherocytes are seen on peripheral blood smear. Patients may be asymptomatic or in severe cases present in a hemolytic crisis. Mild cases may present with jaundice, fatigue, and dyspnea after hemolytic exacerbation secondary to pregnancy, exercise, or illnesses. Hemolytic workup includes CBC with differential, reticulocyte count, haptoglobin, LDH, bilirubin, BMP, LFTS, as well as Coombs testing. Hereditary spherocytosis occurs when a defect in erythrocyte membrane skeleton proteins (e.g., ankyrin, band 3, protein 4.2, or spectrin proteins) causes the erythrocyte to be unable to hold its normal discoid shape. These cells are less resilient against osmotic changes and thus will show increased fragility in an osmotic fragility test. Extravascular hemolysis occurs in hereditary spherocytosis as the spleen tries to destroy the abnormally shaped RBCs. Thus, a splenectomy helps reduce the hemolysis. Patients with **autoimmune hemolytic anemia** may present very similarly but would not have spherocytes and may have a positive direct Coombs test. Autoimmune hemolytic anemia occurs as either IgG or IgM antibodies are created against erythrocyte antigens. It can present in the context of autoimmune disease, some malignancies (e.g., CLL), drugs (α-methyldopa), and infections (*Mycoplasma pneumoniae*, infectious mononucleosis). **Microangiopathic hemolytic anemias** (TTP, HUS, DIC, HELLP) can cause hemolysis; however, **schistocytes** ("helmet cells") would be seen in the peripheral smear.

PORPHYRIA

The porphyrias are a group of hereditary or acquired conditions resulting in defective heme synthesis that lead to the accumulation of heme precursors. Affected individuals may present with a constellation of symptoms. The two most common types are acute intermittent porphyria and porphyria cutanea tarda.

CASE 7 | Acute Intermittent Porphyria (AIP)

	A 50-year-old woman is brought to the emergency department for evaluation of severe abdominal pain, nausea, and vomiting for the past 24 hours. While on the way to the hospital, she had a witnessed seizure by her sister. The patient has had similar episodes that last a few days that had completely resolved. Per her sister, the patient had been on a "crash diet" for the last week. On exam, the patient is disoriented and tachycardic with a heart rate of 110/min. Neurologic exam shows 2/5 reflexes in her lower extremities, and she has diffuse abdominal tenderness. Urine collected for analysis is noted to be dark and wine colored.
Evaluations/Tests	Urine has an increased porphobilinogen level. She is mildly hyponatremic. Urine toxicology screen and blood alcohol level are negative. Head CT and EEG are normal.

CASE 7 | Acute Intermittent Porphyria (AIP) *(continued)*

Treatment	Treat with glucose as it will inhibit aminolevulinic acid (ALA) synthase or heme infusion for severe attacks.
Discussion	The constellation of symptoms and the chronic, intermittent nature of her condition are consistent with **acute intermittent porphyria (AIP)**. AIP is an autosomal dominant disorder caused by a mutation of porphobilinogen deaminase, leading to an accumulation of porphobilinogen. Symptoms include the 5 Ps: painful abdomen, port wine–colored urine, peripheral neuropathy, psychological disturbances (anxiety, confusion, psychosis, dementia), and precipitation by starvation and drugs (sulfa drugs, barbiturates, cytochrome P-450 inducers antipsychotics, alcohol). Goals of treatment are to avoid precipitants and treat with carbohydrates/glucose or heme infusion for severe attacks that will inhibit ALA synthase, thereby inhibiting the mechanism for hemolysis. A normal head CT and EEG rules out other neurologic causes such as an ischemic stroke, while normal toxicology screen rules out drug overdose or alcohol withdrawal.

CASE 8 | Porphyria Cutanea Tarda (PCT)

A 40-year-old man presents with painful blisters on his hands and forearms after he spent the morning gardening. This happens every time he gardens or landscapes. One day prior, he was at a winery sampling different wines and spirits. He feels tired but has no fevers or chills. Physical exam reveals raised and open blisters on his fingers extending to the wrists bilaterally. The lesions are blanching, purple, and erythematous.

Evaluation/Tests	CBC and chemistry panel are normal. Urine porphyrins are elevated.
Treatment	Avoidance of sun exposure and alcohol consumption.
Discussion	This patient has the classic findings of **porphyria cutanea tarda (PCT)**, the most common type of porphyria. PCT is an autosomal dominant disorder caused by deficiency of uroporphyrinogen decarboxylase. The deficiency results in the accumulation of uroporphyrin. As a result, blistering cutaneous lesions and hyperpigmentation can occur in sun-exposed areas. Attacks are often exacerbated by alcohol consumption. The blisters will resolve over time. Though other causes such as contact dermatitis should be high on the differential, the elevated porphyrins are consistent with the diagnosis of PCT.

THROMBOCYTOPENIA

Thrombocytopenia is defined as a platelet count less than $150,000/mm^3$, but it is most clinically significant when the count is below $100,000/mm^3$. There are many etiologies for a low platelet count. Some require urgent intervention, while others can be safely monitored. Common presentations include epistaxis, easy bruising, menorrhagia, hematuria, or gastrointestinal bleeding. The clinical context of each presentation can greatly aid in determining the underlying cause. Infections, medications, chronic liver disease, and bone marrow disorders can all cause decreased platelets. Platelets, which are an integral part of the primary coagulation cascade, are derived from megakaryocytes in the bone marrow. Thrombocytopenia can result from decreased production (seen in bone marrow failure syndromes such as aplastic anemia or myelodysplastic syndromes (MDS)) or increased destruction (such as disseminated intravascular coagulation (DIC) or thrombotic microangiopathies). Though less common, platelet sequestration can be seen with congestive splenomegaly, during which platelets exit the circulation and enter the splenic pool.

Key Associated Findings and Thrombocytopenia Differential Diagnoses

Thrombocytopenia with Key Associated Findings	Diagnoses
Classic pentad: neurologic changes, renal dysfunction, fever, thrombocytopenia, and microangiopathic hemolytic anemia (schistocytes) Lab findings: ADAMTS13 decreased	Thrombotic Thrombocytopenic purpura (TTP)
Classic triad: renal dysfunction, thrombocytopenia and microangiopathic hemolytic anemia (schistocytes) GI infection (EHEC)	Hemolytic uremic syndrome (HUS)
Heparin use 4 Ts: **t**hrombocytopenia, **t**iming, **t**hrombosis, likelihood of other causes	Heparin induced Thrombocytopenia (HIT)

(continued)

Key Associated Findings and Thrombocytopenia Differential Diagnoses (*continued*)

Thrombocytopenia with Key Associated Findings	Diagnoses
HIV Autoimmune diseases Lab findings: anti-GPIIb/IIIa antibodies	Idiopathic thrombocytopenic purpura (ITP)
Sepsis Lab findings: elevated PT/PTT and D-dimer; decreased fibrinogen, factor V, and factor VIII	Disseminated intravascular coagulation (DIC)

CASE 9 | Idiopathic Thrombocytopenic Purpura (ITP)

A 65-year-old woman is found to have thrombocytopenia on a routine blood test. She otherwise feels well. She has no personal or family history of a bleeding disorder and takes no medications. Physical exam is normal, without lymphadenopathy or hepatosplenomegaly.

Evaluation/Tests	CBC: hemoglobin 14.8 g/dL, WBC 7000/mm³, platelets 67,000/mm³. Peripheral blood smear shows thrombocytopenia with mildly enlarged platelets but no other abnormalities. Coags (PT/INR and PTT) are normal.
Treatment	Steroids, intravenous immunoglobulin (IVIG), possibly splenectomy.
Discussion	Idiopathic thrombocytopenic purpura (ITP) is usually an incidental finding in patients and is a diagnosis of exclusion after more serious etiologies have been ruled out. With no evidence of hemolysis or coagulopathy, TTP and DIC are ruled out. In ITP, antiplatelet antibodies, often against the GPIIb/IIIa fibrinogen receptor on platelets, lead to splenic macrophage destruction of the platelet-antibody complex. ITP can be idiopathic (primary) or due to autoimmune disease, viral infection, malignancy, or drug reaction (secondary). Severe bleeding can occur depending on the degree of thrombocytopenia (primarily when <10,000/mm³. Treatment includes steroids, IVIG, or splenectomy in refractory disease.

CASE 10 | Thrombotic Thrombocytopenic Purpura (TTP)

A 45-year-old woman presents with 2 weeks of fatigue and malaise. Her symptoms have progressed with worsening confusion and lethargy. On examination, she has a temperature of 101°F, mild scleral icterus, and purpuric lesions are noted on her upper and lower extremities and back.

Evaluation/Tests	Notable labs include hemoglobin 10 g/dL, hematocrit 23%, and platelets 12,000/mm³. LDH is elevated. Serum creatinine is 1.6 mg/dL. Haptoglobin is decreased, and indirect bilirubin and reticulocyte count are elevated. PTT, PT/INR, and fibrinogen are normal, and Coombs test is negative. Peripheral blood smear shows fragmented RBCs (schistocytes). ADAMTS13 activity is decreased.
Treatment	Plasmapheresis, steroids, rituximab.
Discussion	The classic pentad of symptoms in thrombotic thrombocytopenic purpura (TTP) includes fever, anemia with fragmented RBCs (schistocytes), thrombocytopenia, kidney injury, and neurologic symptoms. TTP is due to inhibition or deficiency of the von Willebrand factor (vWF) metalloproteinase ADAMTS13, which helps breakdown vWF multimers. Defects in ADAMTS13 result in large vWF multimers, which promote platelet adhesion, aggregation, and formation of microthrombi. LDH will be elevated and coagulation studies will be normal. It is important to rule out infectious causes in this type of presentation. **Hemolytic uremic syndrome (HUS)** presents similarly, but there is usually a history of bloody diarrhea, most classically due to *E. coli* (EHEC, e.g., O157:H7 strain). Children tend to be affected by HUS more often than adults. **ITP** would also present with thrombocytopenia but would not typically present with anemia, renal failure, or neurologic signs. Normal PT/INR and PTT also helps distinguish TTP from **disseminated intravascular coagulation (DIC)**, in which the coagulation pathway would be activated.

CASE 11 | Hemolytic Uremic Syndrome (HUS)

A 9-year-old boy is brought in for evaluation of abdominal pain and bloody diarrhea for the past 3 days. He has no nausea or vomiting. Prior to the onset of symptoms, he had visited the carnival with his family and ate an undercooked cheeseburger. Examination is normal except for mild confusion and scattered petechiae on the extremities.

Evaluation/Tests	CBC: hemoglobin 9.7 g/dL, platelets 74,000/mm^3. Serum LDH is elevated. Schistocytes are observed on peripheral blood smear. Serum creatinine is elevated to 2.3 mg/dL.
Treatment	Supportive care including IV hydration.
Discussion	**Hemolytic uremic syndrome (HUS)** has a characteristic triad of thrombocytopenia, microangiopathic hemolytic anemia, and acute renal failure, usually accompanied by bloody diarrhea. It is typically seen in children and often associated with enterohemorrhagic *E. coli* (EHEC) infection, specifically the serotype O157:H7. This serotype releases Shiga-like toxin, which enhances release of pro-inflammatory cytokines. *E. coli* O157:H7 is often transmitted in food such as raw or undercooked meat and leafy green vegetables. **TTP** is also a thrombotic microangiopathy; however, patients usually do not have diarrhea and instead would present with fever and neurologic symptoms.

CASE 12 | Disseminated Intravascular Coagulation (DIC)

A 55-year-old woman is admitted to the intensive care unit for management of pyelonephritis and bacteremia. She has been in septic shock since her admission 24 hours ago and now has developed purpuric lesions on her arms and bleeding at her IV sites. Blood cultures are growing gram negative rods and she has new thrombocytopenia.

Evaluation/Tests	CBC: hemoglobin 15.5 g/dL, WBC 17,000/mm^3, platelets 73,000/mm^3. Coagulation panel shows increased PT/PTT, thrombin, D-dimer, and decreased fibrinogen level.
Treatment	Treat the sepsis and provide supportive care. Cryoprecipitate and vitamin K can be given depending on the degree of coagulopathy and severity of disease.
Discussion	Thrombocytopenia with these accompanying lab abnormalities in the setting of sepsis is consistent with **disseminated intravascular coagulation (DIC)**. There is large-scale activation of the clotting cascade, resulting in depletion of clotting factors and increased propensity to bleed. Causes include sepsis (gram negative bacteria), trauma, obstetric complications, acute pancreatitis, malignancy such as acute promyelocytic leukemia (APL), nephrotic syndrome, and transfusions. Abnormal labs classically include low platelet count, increased bleeding time, prolonged PT/INR and PTT, increased fibrin degradation products (D-dimers), decreased fibrinogen, and decreased factors V and VIII. In the setting of sepsis, DIC is far more likely than other causes. **TTP** would present with neurologic symptoms and other signs of end-organ damage due to microangiopathy, such as renal failure. **ITP** is typically found incidentally in an asymptomatic patient.

CASE 13 | Heparin-Induced Thrombocytopenia (HIT)

A 55-year-old man develops right calf pain and swelling in the hospital despite treatment with heparin to prevent deep vein thromboses. He was initially admitted several days ago with acute coronary syndrome and aspiration pneumonia. His physical exam is unremarkable except for newly developed right-leg edema and tenderness.

Evaluation/Tests	His platelet count has declined from 240,000/mm^3 at the start of his hospitalization to 60,000/mm^3. Lower extremity doppler ultrasound of the right leg shows a deep vein thrombosis. Autoantibodies to platelet factor 4 (PF4) are detected.
Treatment	Heparin products should be stopped immediately, and anticoagulation with nonheparin products should be initiated such as direct thrombin inhibitors (argatroban, bivalirudin) or direct oral anticoagulants (apixaban, rivaroxaban).
Discussion	Heparin treatment or exposure leading to thrombosis and a decreased platelet count with no other explanation is consistent with **heparin-induced thrombocytopenia (HIT)**. This occurs in a small percentage of patients receiving unfractionated heparin. Platelets clump excessively and cause vessel obstruction and paradoxical arterial and venous thrombosis. Bleeding is rare. Heparin should be stopped in patients who become thrombocytopenic and develop a new clot or who have a 50% decrease in their

CASE 13 | Heparin-Induced Thrombocytopenia (HIT) *(continued)*

Discussion	platelet count. Tests should be performed to detect IgG autoantibodies that recognize heparin bound to platelet factor 4 (PF4), particularly in patients with an intermediate to high pretest probability based on the 4 Ts: thrombocytopenia, timing relative to heparin exposure, thrombosis, and the likelihood of other causes of thrombocytopenia. The complex of antibody, heparin, and PF4 that forms results in platelet activation, causing thrombosis and reducing platelet count. Anticoagulation with nonheparin products is necessary until platelets recover.

COAGULOPATHIES

Disorders of coagulation can cause venous thromboembolism or bleeding disorders. The risk of developing a thrombus can increase due to a temporary disruption of Virchow's triad (blood stasis, endothelial injury, and hypercoagulable state), such as long airplane flights or immobility due to hospitalization. For thrombi without clear disruptions of Virchow's triad, hypercoagulable disorders must be explored. Bleeding disorders typically present with varying degrees of bleeding in friable tissues such as gums or easy bruising or bleeding with mild injury.

Hypercoagulable States

Antithrombin III deficiency	Antithrombin inhibits the action of factor IIa and factor Xa; deficiency of this protein results in hypercoagulation. Antithrombin III may be decreased as an inherited deficiency or it can be lost in the urine of patients with nephrotic syndrome or renal failure.
Factor V Leiden	Factor V Leiden is the most common cause of hypercoagulability in Caucasians. It is caused by an autosomal dominant point mutation (Arg506Gln) with incomplete penetrance that results in factor V being resistant to cleavage by protein C, causing a hypercoagulable state.
Prothrombin gene mutation	A DNA mutation results in increased production of prothrombin, a procoagulant, resulting in a hypercoagulable state.
Protein C and S deficiency	Proteins C and S are involved in inhibiting the actions of factor Va and factor VIIIa; deficiency of these proteins results in less cleavage of these factors, leading to thrombosis.
Antiphospholipid syndrome (APS)	APS is an autoimmune condition involving the development of antiphospholipid antibodies that cause activation of the complement system and coagulation cascade. This process also inhibits the action of proteins C and S.

CASE 14 | Von Willebrand Disease, Type 1

A 14-year-old girl presents with prolonged and heavy menstrual cycles since undergoing menarche last year. She also notices bleeding gums and easy bruising. Her father and brother have a history of recurrent nosebleeds. Her platelets are normal, but the bleeding time is prolonged.

Evaluation/Tests	Mild elevation in PTT, ristocetin cofactor assay reveals poor platelet aggregation, bleeding time is prolonged, and vWF and factor VIII levels are decreased.
Treatment	Desmopressin; vWF/factor VIII complex.
Discussion	This patient likely has **von Willebrand disease** (vWD), given her clinical history and lab values showing low vWF antigen, low factor VIII, and elevated PTT. vWD is the most common heritable bleeding disorder that is present in all ethnicities. Women are more frequently diagnosed than men due to mild disease becoming apparent during menstruation. It is characterized by an abnormal quantity or quality of von Willebrand factor (vWF), which is a glycoprotein produced by endothelial cells and is involved in hemostasis. This factor forms high-molecular-weight multimers, which are significantly more effective at mediating hemostasis than the individual units. vWF acts by binding to the glycoprotein Ib (GpIb) receptor on platelets, which allows adhesion to sites of endothelial injury. It also stabilizes the half-life of factor VIII in circulation. Ristocetin promotes the binding of vWF with platelet GpIb; patients with vWF will have poor platelet aggregation with the ristocetin cofactor assay. Patients can be treated with desmopressin for mild bleeding and vWF/factor VIII complex for severe bleeding or for surgery preparation. Desmopressin works by binding to the V2 receptor on endothelial cells, causing them to release vWF into the blood.

CASE 14 | Von Willebrand Disease, Type 1 *(continued)*

Discussion	**Hemophilia A** or **B** is much more likely to present in men as their inheritance is X-linked recessive. In addition, a prolonged bleeding time is more suggestive of a platelet disorder than a coagulation factor disorder. **Bernard-Soulier syndrome** is a disorder of platelet adhesion caused by low GpIb on platelets. It presents with thrombocytopenia and normal levels of vWF and factor VIII. **Glanzmann thrombasthenia** is a disorder of platelet aggregation due to low glycoprotein IIb/IIIa. Platelet count, vWF and factor VIII levels, and the ristocetin cofactor assay will all be normal.

CASE 15 | Hemophilia A

A 12-year-old boy presents with painful swelling of his right knee after a soccer injury. There is overlying bruising and developing hematoma in the joint. He has a history of easy bruising with minor trauma. He has two maternal uncles with a similar history of easy bleeding and bruising, but his sisters have no problems.

Evaluation/Tests	Factor VIII level is low and PTT is prolonged. Factor IX, factor XI, vWF antigen, and ristocetin cofactor assay are all unremarkable.
Treatment	Recombinant factor VIII.
Discussion	This patient likely has hemophilia A given the presentation of hemarthrosis and easy bruising. In addition, his family history is suggestive of an X-linked recessive disorder. Hemophilia is a bleeding disorder characterized by spontaneous bleeding and/or bruising occurring internally or externally. There are three types of hemophilia: types A, B, and C. A is the most common, followed by B. Hemophilia A and B show X-linked recessive inheritance. Daughters of affected males are carriers. It is extremely rare for females to have symptomatic disease, but it is possible if born to an affected male and a carrier female. Hemophilia C is inherited in an autosomal recessive pattern. Common sites for bleeding include the joints (hemarthrosis) or muscles after trauma. Repeated episodes of hemarthrosis may lead to permanent joint damage. Hemophilia A involves deficiency in factor VIII, **hemophilia B** is deficiency in factor IX, **hemophilia C** is deficiency in factor XI. **Von Willebrand's disease** would also present with low factor VIII. However, vWF antigen would be low, and ristocetin cofactor assay would be abnormal.

MYELOPROLIFERATIVE DISORDERS

Myeloproliferative disorders are diseases of the bone marrow that cause abnormalities in WBCs, RBCs, or platelet production. Patients can present with a constellation of symptoms including fatigue, weakness, dyspnea, anorexia, weight loss, pallor, easy bruising, bleeding, or infections.

CASE 16 | Polycythemia Vera (PV)

A 60-year-old woman with a past history of splenic vein thrombosis presents with burning of the extremities and generalized pruritis, which is worse after hot showers. She notes that her feet intermittently turn red, warm, and puffy and intensely burn (erythromelalgia). Review of systems is notable for intermittent headaches. She does not smoke. On exam, she has a blood pressure of 150/90 mmHg, enlarged liver, erythematous and swollen extremities with excoriations, areas of bluish discoloration, and hypersensitivity to touch.

Evaluation/Tests	CBC: hemoglobin 17.5 g/dL, hematocrit 50%, WBC 8000/mm³, platelets 300,000/mm³. BMP and LFTs are normal. Bone marrow biopsy reveals hypercellularity and erythroid hyperplasia without dysplasia or blasts. Erythropoietin level is low. JAK2 V617F mutation detected.
Treatment	Aspirin, phlebotomy, hydroxyurea, or ruxolitinib (JAK1/2 inhibitor) and anticoagulation for thrombosis.
Discussion	Polycythemia vera (PV) patients can be asymptomatic or present with pruritis, neuropathy, hypertension, and symptoms of hyperviscosity (headaches, thrombosis, and Raynaud phenomena). PV is a myeloproliferative disorder marked by a high red blood cell mass and occasional leukocytosis and thrombocytosis. Bone marrow biopsy will be positive for hypercellularity of all cell lines. Erythropoietin (EPO) levels will be low, as the elevated RBC levels due to PV will cause the kidneys to secrete less

CASE 16 | Polycythemia Vera (PV) (continued)

Discussion	erythropoietin. PV is due to JAK2 V617F tyrosine kinase or exon 12 mutation, resulting in proliferation of myeloid cell lines. Symptoms of PV are thought to be related to the release of inflammatory markers or from microthrombi. Patients may have a history of thrombosis as well as splenomegaly. Treatment is targeted at reducing the risk of thrombosis in these patients with phlebotomy (hematocrit goal of <45%) and cytoreductive therapy like hydroxyurea. It is important to rule out **secondary causes of polycythemia** such as chronic hypoxic states (e.g., chronic lung diseases, tobacco use, high altitude, hypoventilation (sleep apnea)), and those related to high EPO levels (e.g., renal or liver cancers).
Additional Considerations	**Essential Thrombocytosis** (ET) is another myeloproliferative disorder that can be associated with a JAK2 mutation. Other common mutations include CALR and MPL. It is a primary disorder of platelets with clonal excessive production. It is associated with thrombosis, hemorrhage and vasomotor symptoms. Bone marrow biopsy would reveal increased number and size of megakaryocytes (platelet precursors) without dysplasia. Treatment is based on risk (age, history of thrombosis) and includes aspirin and cytoreductive therapy (hydroxyurea). Both ET and PV need to be monitored for progression to myelofibrosis, myelodysplastic syndrome or acute leukemia.

CASE 17 | Myelofibrosis

A 65-year-old man presents with fatigue, low-grade fevers, sweats, weight loss, early satiety, and abdominal fullness. On physical exam, conjunctival pallor and hepatosplenomegaly are noted.

Evaluation/Tests	CBC reveals pancytopenia, and peripheral smear shows leukoerythoblastosis (nucleated red cells, immature granulocytes, and teardrop-shaped erythrocytes). Abdominal ultrasound shows hepatosplenomegaly. Bone marrow aspirate results in dry tap. Bone marrow biopsy shows extensive fibrosis with diffusely positive collagen stain.
Treatment	Ruxolitinib (JAK1/2 inhibitor), stem cell transplant, hydroxyurea.
Discussion	Myelofibrosis is a chronic myeloproliferative disorder that is marked by the presence of reticulin or collagen fibrosis in the bone marrow due to increased fibroblast activity. Myelofibrosis can sometimes be the end-stage manifestation of other myeloproliferative conditions like polycythemia vera or essential thrombocytosis. At other times, it is diagnosed de novo (primary myelofibrosis). About 8–23% of patients with primary myelofibrosis will progress to acute leukemia within 10 years of diagnosis. Patients present with nonspecific symptoms such as fatigue, weight loss, and abdominal pain and are noted to be anemic and sometimes pancytopenic. Imaging often reveals splenomegaly. Peripheral smear shows "teardrop" cells, nucleated RBCs, and immature forms of WBCs (leukoerythroblastosis), which are signs of the replacement of normal bone marrow with fibrosis. Bone marrow biopsy is required for diagnosis, and aspiration of marrow contents is often difficult due to fibrosis, yielding a "dry tap." Specific molecular mutations are associated with primary myelofibrosis, including the JAK1/2 mutations seen in other myeloproliferative disorders such as essential thrombocythemia and polycythemia vera. Stem cell transplant is the treatment of choice for high-risk disease in patients with a good functional status, while hydroxyurea or JAK1/2 inhibitors can be used for those with low-risk disease and significant comorbidities. Observation with serial clinical evaluation is an option for those with low-risk disease. Myelofibrosis could present similarly to **CML** with features of splenomegaly, thrombocytosis, and leukocytosis. However, the dry tap, fibrotic bone marrow, and tear drop cells are all more indicative of myelofibrosis. **Granulomatous diseases**, such as **TB** or **histoplasmosis**, may have similar constitutional symptoms but would have risk factors or exposures.

LEUKEMIA

Leukemia is a malignancy of white blood cells resulting from unregulated growth and differentiation in the bone marrow. This leads to marrow failure, decrease in other cell lines, and nonfunctional circulating WBCs. The presentation of leukemia can vary widely. Acute leukemia can present with signs and symptoms related to cytopenias. Patients may have fatigue and flu-like symptoms. Thrombocytopenia can cause mucocutaneous bleeding and petechiae, while patients with severe leukopenia (ANC <500 cells/µL) may present with neutropenic fever and sepsis. Initial diagnostic workup includes CBC with manual differential, comprehensive metabolic panel, and coagulation studies. Bone marrow aspirate and biopsy are essential for confirmation of diagnosis.

Key Associated Findings and Abnormal WBC Differential Diagnoses

Abnormal WBC with Key Associated Findings	Diagnoses
Lab findings: myeloblasts, Auer rods, myeloperoxidase+	Acute myelogenous leukemia (AML)
Lab findings: myeloblasts, Auer rods, myeloperoxidase+, coagulopathy (DIC), t(15;17)	Acute promyelocytic leukemia (APL) (RX: all-*trans* retinoic acid)
Down syndrome	AML, ALL
CNS or testes involvement Lab findings: lymphoblasts, TdT+ SVC syndrome	ALL
Splenomegaly Lab findings: t(9;22), BCR-ABL (Philadelphia chromosome)	Chronic myelogenous leukemia (CML) (RX: tyrosine kinase inhibitors)
Lab findings: smudge cells, autoimmune hemolytic anemia Richter transformation into diffuse large B-cell lymphoma (DLBCL)	Chronic lymphocytic leukemia/small lymphocytic lymphoma (CLL/SLL)

CASE 18 | Acute Myelogenous Leukemia (AML)

A 67-year-old woman with no significant past medical history presents with fatigue, bleeding gums, and shortness of breath for 2 weeks. Physical examination is notable for low-grade fever, tachycardia, tachypnea, sternal tenderness, erythematous papules and nodules on her chest and back, and scattered ecchymosis on the extremities.

Evaluation/Tests	CBC: hemoglobin 8.0 g/dL, WBC 90,000/mm³, platelets 25,000/mm³. Bone marrow biopsy reveals hypercellular marrow with 70% myeloblasts. Peripheral blood smear shows Auer rods inside blasts. Acute myeloid leukemia. Leukemic myeloblast with an Auer rod. Note two to four large, prominent nucleoli in each cell. Reproduced with permission from Jameson JL, Fauci AS, Kasper DL, et al: Harrison's Principles of Internal Medicine, 20th ed. New York, NY: McGraw Hill; 2018.
Treatment	Hydration and allopurinol to help prevent tumor lysis, chemotherapy with cytarabine and an anthracycline, stem cell transplant.
Discussion	AML is most often a disease of older adults and can arise as primary de novo disease or secondary disease following myeloproliferative disorders or previous exposure to alkylating chemotherapy or radiation. There is also an association with Down syndrome. Myeloblasts with Auer rods are characteristically seen in the peripheral smear, and myeloperoxidase (MPO) staining is positive in myeloid leukemias. Common chromosomal abnormalities include t(8;21), inv(16), t(16;16), t(9;11), t(6;9), inv(3). Treatment is usually 7 + 3 (cytarabine + daunorubicin) and allogeneic stem cell transplant in fit patients. Patients typically present with pancytopenia, but some may present with markedly elevated WBC and are at risk for tumor lysis syndrome, which is an oncologic emergency. **Tumor lysis syndrome** is seen in patients with leukemias and lymphomas in which massive tumor destruction causes elevations in potassium, phosphorus, and uric acid levels and decreases in calcium (due to sequestration by phosphate). This can result in acute kidney injury, arrhythmias, and death. Prevention and treatment involve aggressive hydration, allopurinol, rasburicase, and/or dialysis. To distinguish the different types of AML, analysis of the nucleated cells in the blood and marrow, cytogenetic markers, and immunophenotyping is needed. Peripheral smear with a large promyelocyte population and labs indicative of DIC should raise strong suspicion for **acute promyelocytic leukemia (APL)**. APL is a subtype of AML with t(15;17) translocation, creating a PML-RARA fusion gene that blocks the maturation of promyelocytes (blasts). Promyelocytes contain cytoplasmic granules, which can lead to DIC. Peripheral blood smear shows a characteristic population of promyelocytes with reddish-blue or dark purple cytoplasmic granules and dumbbell-shaped nuclei. Treat with all-*trans* retinoic acid (ATRA), which promotes the maturation of promyelocytes.

CASE 19 | Acute Lymphoblastic Leukemia (ALL)

A 2.5-year-old child with Down syndrome is brought to the emergency department for evaluation of fever, lethargy, and bleeding gums. On exam, he is febrile, tachycardic, pale, and has petechiae on his extremities. Additionally, there is notable cervical lymphadenopathy and hepatosplenomegaly.

CASE 19 | Acute Lymphoblastic Leukemia (ALL) *(continued)*

Evaluation/Tests	CBC: hemoglobin 9.0 g/dL, hematocrit 26%, MCV 97 fL, WBC 59,000/mm³, platelets 15,000/mm³, absolute neutrophil count 700/mm³. Bone marrow aspirate and biopsy shows 90% lymphoid blasts positive for CD19, CD20, CD22, CD10, CD34, TdT, and HLA-DR. Reproduced with permission from Jameson JL, Fauci AS, Kasper DL, et al: Harrison's Principles of Internal Medicine, 20th ed. New York, NY: McGraw Hill; 2018.
Treatment	Chemotherapy including vincristine, prednisone, anthracycline, and asparaginase. Stem cell transplant.
Discussion	ALL is diagnosed by finding 20% or more lymphoblasts in the peripheral circulation and bone marrow. Nuclear staining is positive for terminal deoxynucleotidyltransferase (TdT), a marker of pre-T- and pre-B-cells. ALL is the most common malignancy in children, and it can be associated with Down syndrome. The presence of the t(9;22) Philadelphia (Ph) chromosome translocation confers a poor prognosis, while t(12;21) translocation confers a better prognosis. **B-cell ALL** is positive for CD10, CD19, and CD20. Classic presentation includes lymphadenopathy, hepatosplenomegaly, bone pain, and leukemia cutis. **T-cell ALL** is positive for CD2, CD3, CD4, CD5, and CD7. Presentation includes lymphadenopathy and/or a mediastinal mass, which can cause SVC syndrome. **Lymphoma** can present with similar bulky lymphadenopathy, but the presence of hyperleukocytosis and blasts makes ALL more likely.
Additional Considerations	**Hairy cell leukemia (HCL)** is most often diagnosed in adult men. It classically presents with massive splenomegaly and pancytopenia; lymphadenopathy is uncommon. HCL may cause marrow fibrosis leading to a dry bone marrow aspiration. Stain for tartrate-resistant acid phosphatase (TRAP) is positive in HCL, although this has largely been replaced by flow cytometry for diagnostic testing, and treatment is with cladribine.

CASE 20 | Chronic Myelogenous Leukemia (CML)

A 66-year-old man presents to his primary care doctor for a routine exam. Review of systems is positive for mild fatigue, night sweats, and some weight loss. Physical exam is unremarkable except for splenomegaly.

Evaluation/Tests	CBC: hemoglobin 10.9 g/dL, WBC 50,000/mm³, platelets 100,000/mm³. Peripheral blood smear reveals predominantly mature neutrophils. Leukocyte alkaline phosphatase (LAP) activity is low. Bone marrow biopsy reveals granulocyte hyperplasia. Cytogenetic testing shows the presence of a *BCR-ABL1* fusion protein resulting from a t(19;22), Philadelphia chromosome.
Treatment	Tyrosine kinase inhibitors (imatinib, dasatinib, nilotinib).
Discussion	CML is a neoplastic proliferation of mature granulocytes. It has a characteristic cytogenetic abnormality of t(9;22), resulting in the chimeric *BCR-ABL* gene. CML can be chronic phase (about 90% of cases), accelerated phase, or blast phase. It is diagnosed incidentally in about 50% of cases, and it may present with fatigue, night sweats, splenomegaly, and bone pain. Tyrosine kinase inhibitors (TKIs) that bind to the BCR-ABL tyrosine kinase such as imatinib or dasatinib prevent autophosphorylation, thereby preventing downstream signaling pathways that promote proliferation of leukemia. Though this patient has hyperleukocytosis that may be seen with **AML**, the chronic nature and lack of acuity is more suggestive of a chronic leukemia. Cytogenetic testing demonstrating BCR-ABL fusion confirms the diagnosis. **Leukemoid reaction** refers to hyperleukocytosis >50,000/mm³, most often due to infection. Leukocyte alkaline phosphatase (LAP) activity will be high in leukemoid reaction, but it will be low in CML due to the low activity of malignant neutrophils. **Chronic lymphocytic leukemia (CLL)** is mostly seen in older adults as well. Patients may be asymptomatic or present with fatigue, lymphadenopathy, and hepatosplenomegaly. Smudge cells, which are fragile leukemia cells, can be seen in the peripheral smear. Complications include hemolytic anemia, infections, and transformation into more aggressive disease such as diffuse large B-cell lymphoma (DLBCL), known as Richter's transformation.

LYMPHOMA

A lymphoma is a solid tumor arising from lymph nodes. In advanced stages, it can involve extranodal sites as well as the bone marrow. Presentation is classically associated with B Symptoms, including fevers, night sweats, and weight loss. It is primarily categorized as Hodgkin's lymphoma (HL) or non-Hodgkin's lymphoma.

Key Findings and Lymphoma Differential Diagnosis

Lymphoma with Key Associated Findings	Diagnosis
Contiguous spread of lymphadenopathy Pathologic findings: Reed-Sternberg cells (CD15+ and CD30+) Reproduced with permission from Kaushansky K, Prhal JT, Burns LJ, et al: Williams Hematology, 10th ed. New York, NY: McGraw Hill; 2021.	Hodgkin's lymphoma (HL)
Jaw lesion in a patient from Africa Pathologic findings: starry sky appearance Viral association (EBV and HIV)	Burkitt lymphoma
Lymphadenopathy Organomegaly Indolent course	Small lymphocytic lymphoma (SLL)/chronic lymphocytic leukemia (CLL)
Lymphadenopathy Rapidly progressive Lab findings: cytopenias	Diffuse large B-cell lymphoma (DLBCL)
Association with chronic inflammation	Marginal zone lymphoma

Non-Hodgkin's Lymphoma Cytogenetics

Cytogenetics	NHL Type
t(8;14)	Burkitt lymphoma
t(14;18)	Follicular Lymphoma
t(11;14)	Mantle cell lymphoma
t(11;18)	Marginal zone lymphoma
Bcl-2, Bcl-6 alterations	DLBCL

CASE 21 | Hodgkin's Lymphoma (HL)

A 20-year-old man presents with a 2-month history of a 20-pound weight loss, low-grade fevers, and night sweats. Physical exam reveals a chronically ill appearing man with two 3-cm palpable nontender, immobile, firm right axillary lymph nodes.

Evaluation/Tests	Excisional lymph node biopsy shows giant tumor cells with bilobed "owl eyes" nuclei (Reed-Sternberg cells), which are CD15+ and CD30+. CBC does not show atypical lymphocytes. HIV test is negative.
Treatment	Chemotherapy—ABVD (adriamycin, bleomycin, vinblastine, and dacarbazine).
Discussion	A young patient with lymphadenopathy and constitutional (B) symptoms (fever, night sweats, weight loss) warrants workup for Hodgkin's lymphoma (HL). HL is a malignancy affecting B lymphocytes and is broadly classified as classical or nonclassical HL. It presents in a bimodal age distribution, affecting young adults approximately 20 years of age and older adults with average age of 65 years. HL classically presents with painless lymphadenopathy, mediastinal mass, weight loss, night sweats, and chills. Risk factors include a history of infectious mononucleosis caused by EBV, immunosuppression, or autoimmune disease such as rheumatoid arthritis, SLE, or sarcoidosis. Survival is excellent, >75% of patients are cured of their disease, though some may require stem cell transplant to achieve remission. **Infectious mononucleosis** is due to EBV infection, which may also play a role in the pathogenesis of Hodgkin's lymphoma. However, biopsy results showing Reed-Sternberg cells confirm the diagnosis of HL.

CASE 22 | Burkitt Lymphoma

A 10-year-old African boy who recently immigrated to the United States presents with a rapidly growing mass on his right jaw for the past 6 weeks. He also reports pain with eating, weight loss and night sweats. On exam, he has difficulty speaking and opening the right side of his mouth. A firm 3-cm mass arising from the right mandible with central necrosis and purulent drainage is noted.

Evaluation/Tests	Biopsy reveals a "starry-sky" pattern. Cytogenetics are positive for t(8;14) mutation. EBV is positive. Tumor lysis labs reveal elevated LDH, hyperkalemia, hyperuricemia, hyperphosphatemia, and hypocalcemia.
Treatment	Initiate chemotherapy and start aggressive hydration, and allopurinol to treat tumor lysis syndrome (TLS).
Discussion	This is a classic presentation of Burkitt lymphoma (a child from Africa presenting with jaw lesion). **Non-Hodgkin's lymphomas (NHL)** are malignant neoplasms that may arise from multiple cell lines including B-cells, T-cells, and NK-cells; they may be indolent or aggressive. Indolent lymphomas such as chronic lymphocytic leukemia/small lymphocytic lymphoma (CLL/SLL) may present with slow growing lymphadenopathy, cytopenias, or organomegaly, whereas aggressive NHL, like Burkitt lymphoma or diffuse large B-cell lymphoma (DLBCL), present with rapidly growing lymphadenopathy, night sweats, weight loss, chills, elevated LDH, and tumor lysis syndrome. **Burkitt lymphoma** is an aggressive NHL also affecting B-cells, and it is strongly associated with both EBV and HIV. The endemic form may present as a jaw lesion in patients from Africa, and the sporadic form may present as a pelvic or abdominal mass. Burkitt lymphoma is diagnosed by biopsy of the involved tissue, which reveals a "starry-sky" morphology, and cytogenetics will reveal a t(8;14) mutation. **Diffuse large B-cell lymphoma (DLBCL)** is the most common type of NHL, and it affects mature B-cells. DLBCL is more commonly seen in elderly patients and may present with Bcl-2 and Bcl-6 rearrangements. A **jaw abscess** or **osteosarcoma** may present in similar fashion, but the biopsy and cytogenetics results confirm the diagnosis of NHL.
Additional Considerations	**Mucosa-associated lymphoid tissue (MALT) lymphoma** is a marginal zone lymphoma commonly associated with chronic inflammation (secondary to *H. pylori*, hepatitis C or B, or autoimmune disease). In gastric MALT lymphoma, the most likely source of inflammation is *H. pylori* gastritis. Therefore, *H. pylori* eradication with triple therapy is an essential part of treatment. Biopsy of suspicious lesions would show lymphocytes with t(11;18) mutation.

PLASMA CELL DYSCRASIAS

Plasma cell dyscrasias (PCDs) are disorders that cause excessive proliferation of a single clone of plasma cells resulting in excess immunoglobulins and immunoglobulin fragments (heavy chains and/or light chains). They produce monoclonal antibodies called the M protein. The two most common conditions are multiple myeloma and monoclonal gammopathy of undetermined significance.

CASE 23 | Multiple Myeloma (MM)

A 66-year-old man presents with lower back pain, progressive fatigue, and a 15-pound weight loss over the last 6 months. He attributes the weight loss to two separate episodes of pneumonia in the last year. He denies incontinence of bowel or bladder or lower extremity weakness. He has paresthesias in his upper and lower extremities. Physical exam reveals focal spinal tenderness over his lower lumbar spine.

Evaluation/Tests	Hemoglobin 8.4 g/dL, MCV 87 fL, creatinine 2.4 mg/dL, calcium 12.3 mg/dL. Peripheral blood smear reveals stacks of RBCs in Rouleaux formation. Serum protein electrophoresis (SPEP) reveals an M spike >3 g/dL. Skull and spine X-ray reveals multiple "punched-out" lesions in the skull and other bones, along with compression fracture of L3 vertebra. Bone marrow biopsy shows monoclonal plasma cell population of 43%. Urinalysis reveals presence of Ig light chains (Bence Jones protein).

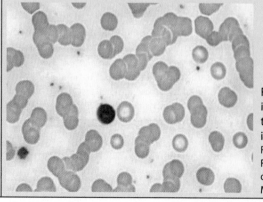

Rouleaux formation. Small lymphocyte in center of field. These red cells align themselves in stacks and are related to increased serum protein levels.
Reproduced with permission from Jameson JL, Fauci AS, Kasper DL, et al: Harrison's Principles of Internal Medicine, 20th ed. New York, NY: McGraw Hill; 2018.

CASE 23 | Multiple Myeloma (MM) *(continued)*

Treatment	Targeted therapy, which may include: chemotherapy, bisphosphonates or radiation to lytic vertebral lesion.
Discussion	Multiple myeloma (MM) is a plasma cell malignancy that arises from the bone marrow. In MM, constitutional symptoms like fatigue and weight loss are common, but symptoms that should raise high suspicion for MM include CRAB (hyperCalcemia, Renal involvement, Anemia, and lytic Bone lesions). Patients may present with a history of recurrent infections (due to abnormal clonal plasma cell line–producing abnormal/defective antibodies), paresthesias/neuropathy, and renal disease due to cast nephropathy. Hypercalcemia (due to osteolysis), abnormal renal function, and anemia can be detected on routine laboratory evaluation. Elevated serum protein levels are also commonly seen, usually due to large amounts of IgG or IgA produced by monoclonal plasma cells. Peripheral smear of MM patients may show numerous plasma cells (clock-face nuclei with a "fried-egg" appearance) and Rouleaux formation (RBCs stacked like poker chips). Urine studies often reveal Bence Jones protein (Ig light chains in urine). Particular attention should be given to complaints of low back pain (as in this patient) because it may indicate risk of spinal cord compression. **Metastatic cancer** to the spine could also cause a compression of the L3 vertebra, and a chronic infection such as tuberculosis could spread to the spine (Pott's disease); however, the other constellation of findings on blood tests and bone marrow biopsy are consistent with multiple myeloma. **Monoclonal gammopathy of undetermined significance (MGUS)** is another example of a plasma cell dyscrasia. MGUS is an asymptomatic disorder due to monoclonal expansion of plasma cells without classic symptoms of myeloma such as hypercalcemia, renal disease, and lytic bone lesions. Many patients with MGUS are diagnosed incidentally as part of an evaluation for other problems. Clonal M proteins are identified consistent with plasma cell dyscrasias, but evaluation reveals no evidence of end-organ damage from the proteins. The hallmark of diagnosis for MGUS is via bone marrow biopsy, which reveals a plasma cell population <10%, whereas it is >10% in MM. Likewise, an M protein may be detected in serum studies in patients with MGUS but will generally be at concentrations <3 g/dL (>3 g/dL in MM). While the disorder is asymptomatic, timely diagnosis remains relevant as patients with MGUS may progress to multiple myeloma (rate of 1–2% per year).
Additional Considerations	**Waldenstrom macroglobulinemia** is a clonal B-cell disorder that causes monoclonal immunoglobulin M (IgM) gammopathy. Elderly patients may present with fatigue, B symptoms, GI symptoms, unsteady gait, and symptoms related to hyperviscosity from high levels of IgM and abnormal plasma cells infiltrating tissue. Exam may be notable for lymphadenopathy, rash, hepatosplenomegaly, and neuropathy.

11

Musculoskeletal, Dermatology, and Connective Tissue

Michael Charles, MD
Anne Polick, MD
Suzanne Falck, MD

Musculoskeletal Concerns

Wrist/Hand Symptoms
1. Rheumatoid Arthritis
2. Psoriatic Arthritis
3. Scaphoid Fracture
4. Carpal Tunnel Syndrome
5. Wrist Drop (Radial Nerve Damage)

Elbow Symptoms
6. Lateral Epicondylitis (Tennis Elbow)

Shoulder/Neck Symptoms
7. Rotator Cuff Tear
8. Cervical Radiculopathy

Distortions of the Upper Extremity
9. Klumpke's Palsy
10. Winged Scapula (Long Thoracic Nerve (C5–C7) Injury)

Ankle/Foot Symptoms
11. Ankle Sprain (Anterior Talofibular Ligament Injury)
12. Tarsal Tunnel Syndrome (Tibial Nerve Injury)

Knee Symptoms
13. Anterior Cruciate Ligament (ACL) Tear

Hip Symptoms
14. Paget's Disease
15. Avascular Necrosis (AVN) of the Hip

Miscellaneous Presentations
16. Gout
17. Leg Compartment Syndrome
18. Common Peroneal Nerve Injury

Musculoskeletal Presentations in Children
19. Slipped Capital Femoral Epiphysis (SCFE)
20. Osteomalacia (Rickets)
21. Greenstick Fracture

MUSCULOSKELETAL CONCERNS

Joint, bone, and muscle symptoms can result from a myriad of causes. The history and physical exam will help determine the etiology in most cases. Initially, it is important to establish if the pain or concern is related to trauma or associated with other illnesses, if there are systemic signs (fever, rash, or weight loss), weakness, or paresthesias. It is also important to determine if a given symptom is confined to the bones, muscles, soft tissues, or joints (single vs. multiple). The affected area(s) should be assessed for evidence of trauma, deformity, swelling, erythema, warmth, tenderness, range of motion, weakness, and sensation. Other areas such as the neck, chest, back, and abdomen may need to be evaluated to distinguish if the symptom is intrinsic to the joint or referred from another site. Common initial tests and evaluations to confirm or refute diagnoses for patients presenting with musculoskeletal (MSK) concerns include X-rays, aspiration and analysis of fluid, and basic blood tests including muscle enzymes (e.g., CK) and inflammatory markers such as erythroid sedimentation rate (ESR), C-reactive protein (CRP), and autoantibodies such as antinuclear antibody (ANA), rheumatoid factor (RF), and anticitrullinated protein antibodies (ACPAs).

Differential Diagnosis for Musculoskeletal Concerns

Wrist/Hand	Elbow	Shoulder	Spine
Trauma/infection Arthritis Carpal tunnel Guyon's canal syndrome De Quervain's Tenosynovitis Scaphoid fracture Metacarpal neck fracture (boxer's)	Trauma/infection Arthritis Lateral epicondylitis Medial epicondylitis Cubital tunnel syndrome Olecranon bursitis Radial head subluxation	Trauma/infection Arthritis Rotator cuff Tendinopathy/tear Adhesive capsulitis	Trauma/infection Arthritis Cervical radiculopathy Lumbar strain/sprain Herniated disk Ankylosing spondylitis Compression fracture Spinal stenosis Cauda equina Tumors Referred pain (e.g., pyelonephritis, kidney stones)
Ankle/Foot (MSK)	**Knee**	**Hip**	**Miscellaneous**
Trauma/infection Arthritis Ankle sprain (Anterior talofibular ligament injury) Plantar fasciitis Foot drop (common peroneal nerve injury)	Trauma/infection Arthritis Ligament/cartilage tears (ACL, PCL, MCL, LCL, Medial meniscus tear) Prepatellar bursitis Patellofemoral syndrome Osgood-Schlatter disease (Traction apophysitis) Iliotibial band syndrome Baker's cyst	Trauma/infection Arthritis Avascular necrosis Greater trochanteric bursitis Slipped capital femoral epiphysis (SCFE) Legg-Calve-Perthes disease	Trauma Fractures (green stick) Torus (buckle), spiral, compression Arthritis (rheumatoid arthritis, osteoarthritis, psoriatic, infectious, reactive, postinfectious) Crystalline disease (gout, CPPD) Infections (osteomyelitis, septic arthritis) Nerve injuries/entrapment Compartment syndrome Tumors (benign vs. malignant) Fibromyalgia Autoimmune-systemic (polymyalgia rheumatic, SLE, Sjögren's, scleroderma, polymyositis, dermatomyositis, myasthenia gravis, Lambert-Eaton, sarcoidosis)

Some conditions may present in one or multiple joints and may be associated with inflammation. Signs of inflammation include warmth, swelling, and tenderness. The following table shows more common presentations.

	Monoarticular	Polyarticular
Noninflammatory	Trauma, OA, avascular necrosis	Osteoarthritis (OA)
Inflammatory: infectious	Gonococcal (GC) arthritis, septic arthritis, Lyme disease	HIV, Hep B, Parvovirus, Rubella, post-infectious (secondary to GI, GU infection or rheumatic fever)
Inflammatory: crystalline	Monosodium urate (gout) Calcium pyrophosphate dihydrate deposition disease (pseudogout or CPPD)	Polyarticular gout
Inflammatory: noninfectious, noncrystalline		Rheumatoid arthritis (RA), systemic lupus erythematous (SLE), psoriatic arthritis, other rheumatologic diseases

Joint Concern Definitions

Sprain: injury to ligaments

Strain: injury to muscles

Bursa: fluid-filled sac around joints prone to friction

Bursitis: inflammation of bursa usually due to repetitive movements

Enthesis: site where tendons or ligaments insert into the bone

Enthesitis: inflammation of the entheses

Tenosynovitis: infectious or noninfectious inflammation of the fluid-filled sheath (synovium) that surrounds a tendon resulting in joint pain, swelling, and/or stiffness

Dactylitis: inflammation of a digit (finger or toe) resulting in pain and swelling (sausage shaped)

Spondyloarthropathies: chronic diseases of joints include ankylosing spondylitis, reactive arthritis, psoriatic arthritis, and joint problems linked to inflammatory bowel disease (enteropathic arthritis)

Raynaud phenomenon: main cause of color changes in the hands. During an attack, digits may be white (indicating ischemia), blue (indicating hypoxia), or red (which is seen in reperfusion).

WRIST/HAND SYMPTOMS

Pain: A common presentation is wrist/hand pain, swelling, or deformity. In assessing patients, consider trauma, fracture, infection, nerve entrapment/injury, and arthritis in the differential diagnoses.

If multiple joints are involved, it is helpful to consider the following when trying to determine if a presentation is consistent with rheumatoid arthritis vs. osteoarthritis.

	Rheumatoid Arthritis	Osteoarthritis
Age/speed onset	20–40 years old; rapid	>50 years old; slow
Pain	Better throughout the day	Worse throughout the day
Stiffness	>30 minutes–1 hour	<30 minutes
Joint characteristics	Symmetric; boggy, warm, tender Swan neck (C), Boutonniere (D) and Ulnar deviation deformities	Asymmetric; hard and bony Heberden (A), Bouchard (B) nodes
Joints involved	Spares the DIP May also have extra-articular joint manifestations	PIP, DIP
Radiographic findings	Erosions, osteopenia	Osteophytes, joint space narrowing
Lab findings	RF, ACPA, ESR, CRP	None

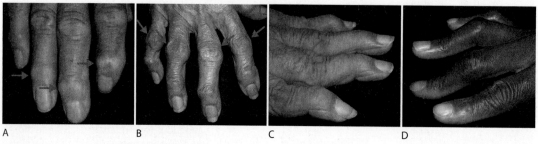

A   B   C   D

Used with permission from Richard Usatine, MD.

Key Associated Findings and Wrist/Hand Pain Differential Diagnosis

Wrist/Hand Pain with Key Associated Findings	Diagnosis
Bony, hard enlargement of the DIP (Heberden nodes) and PIP (Bouchard nodes) joints of the hand.	Osteoarthritis (OA)
Symmetric erythema, swelling, and tenderness of MCP/MTP and PIP joints of the hands and feet (sparing DIP), ulnar deviation of fingers, swan neck deformities, boutonniere deformities, and nodules in skin	Rheumatoid arthritis (RA)
Asymmetric erythema, swelling and tenderness of MCP/PIP/DIP, sausage digits (dactylitis), red patches with silvery scale on extensor surfaces (psoriasis), and nail pits	Psoriatic arthritis
Tenderness in the anatomic snuffbox and volarly over the scaphoid tubercle	Scaphoid fracture

Weakness and paresthesias: Hand weakness, along with tingling, numbness, and pain, can result from pathology anywhere from the head/neck, shoulder, elbow, and wrist down to the fingertips. In assessing patients, consider nerve entrapment/injury from trauma, fracture, or infection. Patients with median nerve pathology at the wrist may present with pain, paresthesias, and weakness along the median nerve distribution (first 3 digits). Decreased grip strength, along with sensory loss in the 4th–5th digits, indicates damage or entrapment of the ulnar nerve as seen in **cubital tunnel syndrome**. "Wrist drop," along with sensory loss on the dorsal aspect of the forearm and hand, indicate damage to the radial nerve. In a posterior interosseous nerve injury, patients present with painless inability to extend finger and thumb, but wrist drop does not occur because the extensor carpi radialis is spared.

Key Associated Findings and Wrist/Hand Pain and/or Weakness/Paresthesia Differential Diagnosis

Wrist/Hand Pain and/or Weakness/Paresthesia with Key Associated Findings	Diagnosis
Wasting thenar eminence and/or pain and/or paresthesia in the median nerve distribution (first 3 digits) elicited via Phalen, Tinel, or Durkan test Tinel's sign: tapping median nerve at carpal tunnel elicits symptoms Phalen's sign: symptoms elicited when patient presses dorsal surface of wrists together while maintaining wrist in flexion for 60 seconds Durkan's test: examiner applies pressure over carpal tunnel with both thumbs for 30 seconds	Carpal tunnel syndrome
Finkelstein's test: pain is elicited when patient grasps their thumb in their fist and ulnar deviates the wrist	De Quervain's tenosynovitis
Pain and/or paresthesia in ulnar nerve distribution (4th and 5th digits) may be aggravated by the pressure from handlebars in cyclists.	Guyon's canal syndrome (ulnar nerve entrapment at wrist)
Pain in elbow and/or paresthesia in ulnar nerve distribution (4th and 5th digits)	Cubital tunnel syndrome (ulnar nerve entrapment at elbow)

CASE 1 | Rheumatoid Arthritis

A 33-year-old woman presents with worsening joint pain in her bilateral hands, wrists, ankles, and knees for over 4 months. She has morning joint stiffness that lasts approximately 90 minutes. The pain gets better throughout the day. She has swelling, erythema, and tenderness of the MCP and PIP joints of the hands, as well as the metatarsophalangeal (MTP) and PIP of the feet. She has ulnar deviation of the fingers and swan neck deformities, as well as nodules on her arms.

Evaluation/Tests	Rheumatoid factor (RF) and ACPA are positive. Bilateral hand X-rays show periarticular osteopenia, marginal erosions, and joint space narrowing.
Treatment	NSAIDs and disease-modifying antirheumatic drugs (DMARDs).
Discussion	This is a classic case of rheumatoid arthritis, which is an autoimmune inflammatory arthritis that causes symmetric erosion of cartilage, bone, and tendons, as well as proliferation (synovial hypertrophy and pannus formation). In addition to typical erythema, swelling, and tenderness of MCP/MTP and PIP joints of the hands and feet, findings may include rheumatoid nodules in skin, ulnar deviation of fingers, swan neck deformities, and boutonniere deformities. Common risk factors for RA include age (35–50), gender

CASE 1 | Rheumatoid Arthritis *(continued)*

Discussion	(with women more at risk), HLA-DR4, and smoking. There is usually symmetric, polyarticular involvement (>3 joints), and morning stiffness (>60 minutes) and systemic symptoms such as fatigue, weight loss, and fevers. Laboratory tests include rheumatoid factor (RF) and anticitrullinated protein antibodies (ACPAs) (more specific); however, 10–20% of patients are seronegative. Patients may have normocytic, normochromic anemia and elevated ESR and CRP. Synovial fluid is inflammatory (WBC 3000–50,000). Treatment generally consists of disease-modifying antirheumatic drugs (DMARDs) such as methotrexate, sulfasalazine, or hydroxychloroquine. NSAIDs can be used for minor cases. For severe cases, the addition of TNF-alpha inhibitors (rituximab, leflunomide) and other biologic agents can be used. Steroids can be used for short-term relief. **Osteoarthritis (OA)** typically has DIP and PIP involvement. It is characterized by progressive degradation of the synovial joints or articular cartilage (degenerative joint disorder (DJD)) mediated by abnormal chondrocyte activity. Common risk factors for OA include age, obesity, previous joint trauma, and family history. There can be polyarticular involvement, particularly in the hands, with characteristic deterioration of articular cartilage and osteophyte bone formation at the joint surfaces resulting in crepitus, bony hypertrophy, and decreased range of motion. No specific laboratory tests are diagnostic. Inflammatory markers are usually normal, and synovial fluid is noninflammatory (WBC <2000). **Psoriatic arthritis** typically has DIP and spinal involvement, as well as skin and nail abnormalities. **Gout** and **pseudogout** are typically monoarticular, and they rarely cause joint destruction.
Additional Considerations	Rheumatoid arthritis may present with extra-articular manifestations such as **Caplan syndrome** (pulmonary fibrosis or pneumoconiosis), **Felty syndrome** (splenomegaly and neutropenia), pleuritis, pericarditis, interstitial lung disease, amyloidosis, Sjögren's syndrome, or scleritis.

CASE 2 | Psoriatic Arthritis

A 45-year-old woman is evaluated for worsening joint pain in her left thumb, left index finger, and right foot over the past 4 months. She has had chronic lower back pain for the past 3 years. She has morning joint stiffness that lasts approximately 2 hours. On exam, she has swelling and tenderness of the DIP joint on the left hand with several sausage-shaped digits. She has patches of erythema and silvery scaling on the skin, as well as nail pitting.

Evaluation/Tests	Clinical diagnosis.
Treatment	NSAIDs and disease-modifying antirheumatic drugs (DMARDs). Exercise is important to preserve joint strength and range of motion.
Discussion	Psoriatic arthritis is an inflammatory seronegative spondyloarthropathy, which involves inflammation of the axial skeleton, asymmetric peripheral arthritis, enthesopathy, eye inflammation (uveitis), and a strong association with the genetic expression of HLA-B27. The other three subtypes of **spondyloarthritis** are ankylosing spondylitis, inflammatory bowel disease, and reactive arthritis. In psoriatic arthritis, patients may present with tenderness and swelling of involved joints, tendons, and ligaments. Psoriasis precedes arthritis in most cases. Characteristic exam findings include psoriasis (red patches with silvery scale on extensor surfaces such as elbows), nail pits, scaly sausage digits (dactylitis) caused by tenosynovitis and arthritis, multiple asymmetric joint involvement (including wrists, MCP, PIP, DIP), and arthritis of the spine. Laboratory tests such as rheumatoid factor (RF) and ACPA are usually negative. There is a strong association with HLA-B27, but this test alone cannot independently support or exclude a diagnosis. Radiographs may show "pencil-in-cup" deformity of the DIP due to bony destruction around joints. Skin, nail findings, and dactylitis are commonly seen in psoriasis. **OA** does not classically present with skin changes and nail involvement. DIP and spine abnormalities are not common in **RA**. **Gout** and **pseudogout** are typically monoarticular, and they do not cause joint destruction. **Reactive arthritis** also presents as an additive, asymmetric arthritis often involving the knees, ankles, or feet. It may involve the fingers and wrists with dactylitis being a distinctive feature similar to psoriatic arthritis. However, it occurs 1–4 weeks after an infection (e.g., *Shigella*, *Yersinia*, and *Chlamydia*), and patients often have other symptoms such as urethritis, conjunctivitis, or uveitis, nonpainful mucocutaneous ulcers, or keratoderma blennorrhagica.

CASE 3 | Scaphoid Fracture

A 20-year-old man presents with 3-day history of right wrist pain after falling onto outstretched hands while snowboarding. The pain did not improve with acetaminophen and ibuprofen. Patient has tenderness in the anatomic snuffbox, as well as tenderness volarly over the scaphoid tubercle. Resisted pronation also elicits pain.

Evaluation/Tests	X-ray (XR) confirms fracture.
Treatment	Immobilization with cast.
Discussion	Pain in the anatomic snuffbox following a fall on the outstretched hands is indicative of a potential scaphoid fracture. This injury has a high risk of nonunion or avascular necrosis (AVN), which can lead to early-onset arthritis in the wrist. Risk of AVN increases with the more proximal the location of the fracture due to the retrograde blood supply of the scaphoid. For acute onset of pain after trauma, it's important to rule out fractures. Surgical treatment is reserved for unstable or displaced fractures and involves open reduction and internal fixation with a screw.
Additional Considerations	**Metacarpal neck fracture** or **boxer's fracture** is more commonly seen in the 4th and 5th metacarpals, and they usually occur due to a direct blow with a closed fist. Most boxer's fractures can be treated nonoperatively with immobilization.

CASE 4 | Carpal Tunnel Syndrome

A 55-year-old woman with a history of hypothyroidism presents with a 6-month history of numbness and tingling in the right thumb, index, and middle fingers. She reports pain in her forearm and her hand that wakes her up at night. She is a typist and is right-handed. On exam, there is wasting of her thenar muscles. Tapping over the carpal tunnel elicits pins-and-needles sensation in the thumb and index fingers. She experiences increased numbness and tingling in the median nerve distribution with carpal tunnel compression, as well as after holding the wrist in a flexed position for 1 minute.

Evaluation/Tests	Clinical diagnosis. Her hemoglobin A1C is normal.
Treatment	Wrist splint and NSAIDs.
Discussion	Carpal tunnel syndrome is often diagnosed clinically. When the median nerve gets compressed or entrapped under the carpal tunnel, patients may present with pain over the proximal forearm and thenar area and with paresthesias in the median nerve distribution. Symptoms can be worse with repetitive movements and flexion and is also worse at night. Potential comorbidities include diabetes, hypothyroidism, amyloidosis, hemochromatosis, rheumatoid arthritis, acromegaly, and pregnancy. The diagnosis is often made by history and physical exam alone (positive Phalen and/or Tinel tests). Electromyography (EMG) and nerve conduction velocity (NCV) are largely confirmatory tests. Failure to treat carpal tunnel syndrome may lead to irreversible sensory loss in the median nerve distribution, as well as significant wasting of the thenar muscles which, in turn, can cause weak grasp and thumb opposition. Surgery is reserved for refractory cases. The patient has no neck pain, is not diabetic, and has no symptoms in the ulnar distribution; therefore, cervical pathology, diabetes, cubital tunnel syndrome, and Guyon's canal syndrome are less likely etiologies.
Additional Considerations	Ulnar nerve entrapment can occur at the elbow **(cubital tunnel syndrome)** or the wrist **(Guyon's canal syndrome)**; symptoms occur in the 4th and 5th digits and may be aggravated by the pressure from handlebars in cyclists. **De Quervain's tenosynovitis** often presents in golfers and racket-sport athletes. It may also present postpartum or post-traumatically. The first dorsal extensor compartment contains the abductor pollicis longus and the extensor pollicis brevis. Pain is elicited due to swelling and thickening of the first dorsal compartment, which may present as a painful bump over the wrist.

CASE 5 | Wrist Drop (Radial Nerve Damage)

A 24-year-old man presents with right wrist weakness for one day. He was drinking the previous night and passed out with his right arm draped over a chair. When he woke up, he was unable to bend his right wrist backwards. On exam, he is afebrile and has wrist drop. He has difficulty in extending his hand and fingers and has decreased sensation of posterior forearm.

Evaluation/Tests	Clinical diagnosis.
Treatment	Conservative treatment as spontaneous recovery is likely. This can include NSAIDs for pain and physical therapy to maintain range of motion.

CASE 5 | Wrist Drop (Radial Nerve Damage) *(continued)*

Discussion	Wrist drop can occur secondary to compression of the radial nerve at the axilla secondary to prolonged use of crutches or falling asleep with the arm draped over a chair (Saturday night palsy).
Additional Considerations	**C7 radiculopathy** will typically have pain in the neck with radiation into the middle finger. There is also usually weakness of the triceps muscle, wrist flexion, and extension fingers. Sensory loss involves the middle finger, and loss of the triceps reflex is also seen. See chart for other DDx.

Nerve damage	Axillary (C5–C6)	Radial (C5–T1) Wrist drop	Median (C5–T1) Pope's blessing (median nerve damage) Ape hand (recurrent branch of median nerve damage)	Ulnar (C8–T1) Ulnar claw
Causes	Humeral neck fracture Anterior dislocation humerus	Humeral midshaft fractures Tumors compressing nerve Compression of the radial nerve at the spiral groove ("Saturday night palsy"/ prolonged use of crutches)	Supracondylar humeral fracture Carpal tunnel syndrome	Compression of ulnar nerve due to prolonged elbow resting on desk, osteophytes, or other mass lesions. Ulnar nerve injury at the wrist due to constant use of hand tools, bicycling, or hook of hamate fracture
Symptoms and signs	Decreased sensation over deltoid Flattened deltoid Decrease abduction	Decreased sensation of posterior forearm and dorsum of hand (radial) Weakness in hand and finger extension: wrist drop	Decreased sensation in first 3 half digits and thenar area Inability to make a fist Loss of thumb opposition	Decreased sensation in 4th and 5th digits Medial elbow pain if injury is at the elbow Weak grip Clawing of 4th and 5th fingers

ELBOW SYMPTOMS

Key Associated Findings and Elbow Pain and/or Weakness/Paresthesia Differential Diagnoses

Elbow Pain and/or Weakness/Paresthesia with Key Associated Findings	Diagnosis
Tennis or racquetball player with tenderness to palpation over lateral epicondyle	Lateral epicondylitis (tennis elbow)
Golfer with tenderness to palpation over medial epicondyle	Medial epicondylitis (golfer's elbow)
Pain and swelling over olecranon process, often from someone resting the elbows on a hard surface for long periods of time "student's elbow"	Olecranon bursitis
Pain in elbow and/or paresthesia in ulnar nerve distribution (4th and 5th digits)	Cubital tunnel syndrome (ulnar nerve entrapment at elbow)
Child with elbow pain and refusing to move forearm after being suddenly pulled/grabbed. Exam: tenderness at radial head; arm is pronated, partially flexed elbow, held close to the body	Radial head subluxation (Nursemaid's elbow)

CASE 6 | Lateral Epicondylitis (Tennis Elbow)

A 40-year-old man presents with right elbow pain for the past month. He started playing tennis a few months ago and now can no longer play due to worsening pain, especially when performing backhand shots. The pain is localized to the lateral elbow and forearm and is exacerbated with gripping and resisted wrist extension. The pain improves with ibuprofen and rest. On exam, there is tenderness at the lateral epicondyle at the insertion of extensor carpi radialis brevis, and this is exacerbated by wrist and third digit extension.

Evaluation/Tests	Clinical diagnosis.
Treatment	Conservative treatment with rest, NSAIDs, avoidance of aggravating activity.
Discussion	Pain at the level of the elbow either medially or laterally can indicate epicondylitis. Lateral epicondylitis (tennis elbow) is due to overuse of the common extensor tendon by repetitive wrist extension, which often occurs in racket ball players or laborers. The repetitive motions (i.e., backhand shots) may lead to vascular hyperplasia, fibroblast hypertrophy, and disorganized collagen resulting in tendinopathy or tendonitis. This is similar to findings in patellar or Achilles tendonitis. The lateral epicondyle is the origin for several muscles that extend the wrist, which comprise the common extensor tendon. The extensor carpi radialis brevis (ECRB) is stressed during wrist extension and forearm pronation, like when hitting a backhand shot. The ECRB inserts at the base of the third metacarpal distally. As a result, resisted extension of the third digit may reproduce the pain. **Medial epicondylitis (golfer's elbow)** results from repetitive flexion as seen in forehand shots. Pain is characteristically near the medial epicondyle and is elicited with forearm pronation or wrist flexion. Pain associated with swelling over the olecranon process may be indicative of **olecranon bursitis**. Patients with **cervical radiculopathy** typically have associated neck pain.
Additional Considerations	The classic mechanism of injury for **radial head subluxation** or **Nursemaid's elbow** is sudden pulling or grabbing a child's arm in order to prevent an injury or incident. The annular ligament slips into the radiohumeral joint and becomes trapped between the two joint surfaces, where it remains stuck. Exam will reveal a pronated arm and partially flexed elbow that is held close to the body, as well as tenderness of the radial head.

SHOULDER/NECK SYMPTOMS

Presenting shoulder symptoms include pain, swelling, decreased range of motion, weakness, and paresthesias. Consider trauma, fracture, infection, nerve entrapment/injury, and arthritis in the differential diagnosis. Damage to the rotator cuff often causes shoulder pain, but it is important to rule out cervical pathology causing referred pain. Associated decreased range of motion and stiffness in a patient with diabetes or hypothyroidism may point toward adhesive capsulitis.

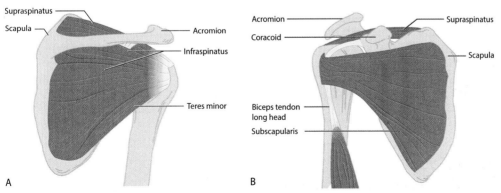

A, Posterior view of the shoulder illustrating rotator cuff muscles. B, Anterior view of the shoulder illustrating the supraspinatus muscle and the long head of the biceps.
Reproduced with permission from Tintinalli J, Ma O, Yealy DM, et al: Tintinalli's Emergency Medicine: A Comprehensive Study Guide. 9th ed. New York, NY: McGraw Hill; 2020.

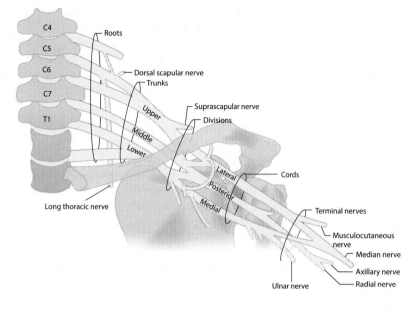

Brachial plexus.
Reproduced with permission from Tintinalli J, Ma O, Yealy DM, et al: Tintinalli's Emergency Medicine: A Comprehensive Study Guide. 9th ed. New York, NY: McGraw Hill; 2020.

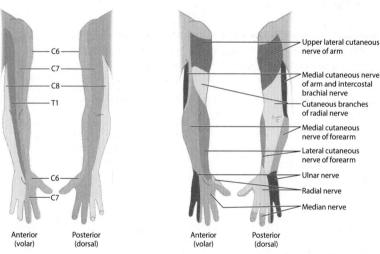

Sensory distribution of the brachial plexus.
Reproduced with permission from Tintinalli J, Ma O, Yealy DM, et al: Tintinalli's Emergency Medicine: A Comprehensive Study Guide. 9th ed. New York, NY: McGraw Hill; 2020.

Specific tests can be helpful in identifying which of the four components of the rotator cuff (supraspinatus, infraspinatus, subscapularis, or teres minor) are affected. Pain with a positive empty can test/Jobe's test without arm drop may indicate tendinopathy, whereas arm drop during the test is more likely due to a rotator cuff tear. Other physical exam maneuvers such as the Hawkins and Neer's tests are useful in diagnosing impingement of the supraspinatus tendon. Speed's test is helpful in diagnosing biceps tendon pathology, while O'Brien's test is useful in detecting a superior labral tear from anterior to posterior (SLAP tear).

Key Physical Exam Maneuvers and Findings and Shoulder and/or Neck Pain Differential Diagnosis

Shoulder and/or Neck Pain with/without Weakness/Paresthesia and Key Associated Exam Findings	Diagnoses
Hawkins-Kennedy test: Patient flexes elbow and shoulder forward 90 degrees while examiner internally rotates arm, bringing forearm downward reproducing pain. **Painful arc test:** Patient abducts arms (pain with abduction between 60 and 120 degrees is positive). **Neer's test:** Raising internally rotated (thumb pointing down) and extended arm forward in scapular plane elicits pain.	Subacromial impingement rotator, cuff tendonitis or tendonosis

(continued)

Key Physical Exam Maneuvers and Findings and Shoulder and/or Neck Pain Differential Diagnosis (*continued*)

Shoulder and/or Neck Pain with/without Weakness/Paresthesia and Key Associated Exam Findings	Diagnoses
Jobe's test/empty can test: Internally rotate fully extended arms with thumb pointing down, and elevate while the examiner applies resistance reproducing weakness. **Drop arm sign:** Examiner fully abducts patient's arm and then asks patient to slowly lower and attempt to hold at 90 degrees (inability to hold is positive for weakness or tear).	Rotator cuff injury, supraspinatus pathology
Elbow flexed to 90 degrees and rotated externally while the examiner applies resistance (pain and/or weakness with external rotation is positive).	Rotator cuff injury, infraspinatus or teres minor pathology
Lift-off test: Patient places hand behind (midlumbar and slightly off back) and attempts to push away from the body while the examiner applies resistance (inability to hold extremity in position is positive). **Belly press test:** Patient presses hand against their abdomen with elbow abducted away from the body while the examiner tries to pull hand away from belly (inability to hold extremity in position is positive).	Rotator cuff injury, subscapularis pathology
Apprehension test: Patient lies supine, and examiner flexes elbow to 90 degrees, abducts shoulder to 90 degrees, and then maximally externally rotates (apprehension to this position can be positive for anterior shoulder dislocation). **Relocation test:** As with the apprehension test, but the examiner simultaneously applies pressure to the shoulder posteriorly (less apprehension or pain with posterior glide of humerus is positive).	Shoulder dislocation, subluxation or glenohumeral instability
O'Brien test: Shoulder is flexed 90 degrees and slightly adducted and internally rotated (with thumb pointing down), and patient raises arm while the examiner applies resistance. Repeat with palm facing upward. Test is positive if pain or crepitus in internally rotated position and better with palm facing up.	Glenohumeral joint labral tears (superior labral tear from anterior to posterior (SLAP tear)) or impingement
Speed's test: Patient extends elbow, supinates arm, and attempts to flex elbow while examiner resists. Test is positive if pain is reproduced in anterior shoulder/bicipital groove.	Biceps tendinopathy
Axial loading or compression: Pressing downward on the seated patient's head reproduces radicular symptoms (pain and/or paresthesia into upper extremity). **Spurling's test:** Pressing downward on the patient's head (axial loading or axial compression) while the neck is extended and flexed to the affected side reproduces radicular symptoms.	Cervical radiculopathy (cervical nerve root impingement)
Atrophy of intrinsic hand muscles (claw hand), diminished pulses and edema of hand.	Thoracic outlet syndrome
Atrophy of intrinsic hand muscles (claw hand).	Klumpke's palsy
Arm hangs by side medially rotated; wrist is flexed and pronated (waiter's tip).	Erb palsy
Protrusion of scapula when patient leans with arms against the wall (winged scapula).	Winged scapula (C5–C7 injury)

CASE 7 | Rotator Cuff Tear

A 55-year-old carpenter presents with right shoulder pain for the past 2 weeks. He reports that he tripped and fell 2 weeks ago. He had immediate pain in his shoulder, which has failed to improve with NSAIDs. He reports difficulty reaching into the overhead cabinets. He denies any neck pain or tingling/numbness in his right arm. On exam, there is tenderness over the lateral aspect of the right shoulder, and with abduction, there is pain and limited range of motion. There is no weakness with external rotation with the elbow at the patient's side (infraspinatus test) or with patient holding his hand behind his back and trying to push away from his body against resistance (subscapularis test/liftoff test). There is weakness and pain with resisted elevation in the plane of the scapula (supraspinatus test/empty can test). When the patient's arm is passively abducted and then let go, patient is unable to hold the position in the horizontal plane, reports pain, and "drops" the arm (positive drop arm test). Shoulder X-rays were negative for fracture.

Evaluation/Tests	Clinical diagnosis. MRI can confirm rotator cuff tear.
Treatment	Treatment includes NSAIDs, physical therapy, or surgical repair.
Discussion	This is a common presentation for a rotator cuff injury, specifically a **supraspinatus tear**. The rotator cuff consists of four muscle groups: supraspinatus, infraspinatus, teres minor, and subscapularis, and it is innervated mostly by C5–C6. The primary function of the rotator cuff is to provide dynamic stability by keeping the humeral head against the glenoid. Supraspinatus pathology (tendinosis or tendonitis) is the most common cause of shoulder pain and can result from trauma, impingement, or degeneration. It is

CASE 7 | Rotator Cuff Tear *(continued)*

Discussion	innervated by the suprascapular nerve, abducts the arm initially (before deltoid), and can be assessed by the empty can test. Patients often complain of shoulder pain in the lateral deltoid region, exacerbated by overhead activities and weakness with active range of motion of the shoulder.
	The **infraspinatus** externally rotates the arm (pitching injury) and is supplied by the suprascapular nerve. The **teres minor** adducts and externally rotates arm and is innervated by the axillary nerve. The **subscapularis** internally rotates and adducts arm and is supplied by lower subscapular nerves. X-rays are usually obtained to rule out fractures, dislocations, and osteoarthritis. Findings consistent with rotator cuff pathology may include cystic changes in the greater tuberosity at the location of the tendon insertion, calcific tendonitis of the rotator cuff, or a hooked morphology of the acromion. Chronic rotator cuff injuries may exhibit proximal migration of the humeral head. MRI is the study of choice and will show the size and shape of the rotator cuff tear, as well as degree of retraction. The first line of treatment is physical therapy and NSAIDs. Rotator cuff repair is offered to patients who have failed conservative treatment or who have a full tear.
	Common differential diagnosis for shoulder pain includes fracture and/or dislocation, but these would have been detected on X-ray.
	Patients with **adhesive capsulitis** or frozen shoulder typically present with insidious pain and decreased range of motion. Adhesive capsulitis is caused by adhesions and scar tissue and classically affects women over 40 years with diabetes. Histology shows fibroblastic proliferation of the joint capsule.

CASE 8 | Cervical Radiculopathy

A 50-year-old man presents with neck and right upper extremity pain after a motor vehicle accident 1 week ago. He describes pain as an electric shock that is aggravated with certain movements of his neck. On physical exam, he has decreased sensation in his thumb and lateral forearm. He has weakness with wrist extension and a diminished brachioradialis deep tendon reflex compared to the contralateral arm. Symptoms are reproduced with simultaneous neck extension, rotation to the affected side, lateral bend, and vertical compression of his head (Spurling's test). Passive shoulder abduction of more than 90 degrees relieves symptoms. His right hand has no gross deformity, and his pulses are intact. Tinel, Phalen, and rotator cuff testing is unremarkable.

Evaluation/Tests	X-rays of cervical spine show no fractures or dislocations. MRI of cervical spine reveals a right-sided C5–C6 disc herniation.
Treatment	NSAIDs and physical therapy. Surgery if there is no improvement or if any upper motor neuron signs or symptoms are present.
Discussion	Cervical radiculopathy is an important cause of neck pain that can radiate to the upper extremities. Other symptoms may include numbness, tingling, and weakness in the affected arms. Cervical radiculopathy can result from degenerative cervical spondylosis resulting from age-related loss of disc height and formation of spurs at the uncovertebral joints and facets, decreasing the space available for the exiting nerve root in the neuroforamen. Disc herniation may be another cause of cervical radiculopathy. Disc herniations are most commonly posterolateral between the posterior edge of the uncinate and the lateral edge of the posterior longitudinal ligament (PLL). This similarly causes impingement on the nerve root. The level of disc herniation may be elucidated based on clinical findings. See image showing cervical nerve distribution. C5 radiculopathy presents with decreased sensation over the lateral shoulder, deltoid and biceps weakness, and diminished biceps reflex. C6 radiculopathy presents with paresthesias in the thumb and radial side of the hand, weakness with brachioradialis and wrist extension, and diminished brachioradialis reflex. C7 radiculopathy presents with paresthesias of the index/middle/ring finger, weakness of wrist flexion and elbow extension, and diminished triceps reflex. C8 radiculopathy presents with decreased sensation in the small finger, diminished finger flexion, and diminished grip strength. T1 radiculopathy presents with medial forearm and elbow paresthesias and weak finger abduction.
	MRI can help localize the nerve root compression spinal level. EMG/NCV is performed to help distinguish peripheral (carpal tunnel) from central processes (cervical radiculopathy). In this scenario, the patient likely suffered a cervical disc herniation as a result of the motor vehicle accident.
	Thoracic outlet syndrome can result from cervical rib or Pancoast tumor, and patients typically present with symptoms of compression of the lower trunk and subclavian vessels (atrophy of intrinsic hand muscles and/or pain, edema, and ischemia).
	Cervical ribs predispose to thoracic outlet syndrome by causing compression of the scalene muscular triangle, which in turn may lead to neurologic or vascular compromise (causing ischemia, pain, and edema).

DISTORTIONS OF THE UPPER EXTREMITY

Though rare, upper extremity distortions often stem from brachial plexopathy due to trauma in adults and due to neonatal birth injuries in infants. The brachial plexus is an intricate network of cervical and thoracic nerves that are conventionally divided into roots, trunks, divisions, cords, and branches. Familiarity with the most common syndromic presentations helps localize nerve injuries and arrive at a diagnosis.

CASE 9	Klumpke's Palsy
	An 18-year-old man slipped while climbing a tree. On his way down, he stretched out his right arm and grabbed a tree branch in an attempt to catch himself. Since then, he has been experiencing hand weakness, difficulty grasping objects, and closing his fingers into a fist. *Or:* After a difficult delivery, a newborn boy is found to have left arm weakness, forearm supination, and wrist and finger hyperextension with DIP and PIP flexion. Exam is notable for decreased grasp strength and claw hand. Pulses are equal bilaterally.
Evaluation/Tests	Clinical diagnosis.
Treatment	Observation, physical therapy.
Discussion	Hand paralysis in adults or arm weakness at birth with ptosis and miosis are classic features suggestive of Klumpke's palsy, which is described as "total claw hand" due to the appearance of the flexed fingers on physical exam. This uncommon brachial plexus injury involves the lower trunk nerves C8–T1 and is often accompanied by ptosis and miosis (Horner's syndrome) secondary to damage to the sympathetic fibers of T1. In neonates, Klumpke's palsy often results from upward arm traction during delivery. In adults, this injury stems from trauma associated with a similar mechanism or tumor of shoulder or lung.
Additional Considerations	**Pancoast tumors** are a type of lung cancer (usually nonsmall cell) that occur at the pulmonary apex. Patients may present with shoulder pain, weakness, or paresthesias of the hand and upper arm swelling. **Erb's palsy**, also known as Erb-Duchenne palsy or "waiter's tip," is the most common neonatal brachial plexus palsy. Resulting from traction or tear of the upper trunk nerve roots of C5–C7, it is often associated with the following risk factors: difficult deliveries, instrumentation, macrosomia, and shoulder dystocia. Injury to C5–C6 results in forearm extension and arm adduction and internal rotation. C7 injury results in wrist and finger flexion. It is important to note that respiratory distress may also present in brachial plexus injuries that involve the phrenic nerve. **Thoracic outlet syndrome** may also present with a claw hand, but this is usually due to compression of the lower trunk and subclavian vessels from a cervical rib or Pancoast tumor. Vascular compression features may present in thoracic outlet syndrome, while Klumpke's palsy is due to traction or tear of the lower trunk at C8–T1 root from trauma.

CASE 10	Winged Scapula (Long Thoracic Nerve (C5–C7) Injury)
	A 47-year-old woman with breast cancer, status post left-sided mastectomy and axillary node dissection, presents with left arm swelling and difficulty combing her hair. Exam reveals mild edema of the left forearm and inability to abduct the left arm above 90 degrees. When the patient leans against the wall using her arms, there is protrusion of her scapula (winged scapula).
Evaluation/Tests	Clinical diagnosis.
Treatment	Physical therapy.
Discussion	**Long thoracic nerve (C5–C7) injury** typically results from thoracic surgeries or procedures but may also result from a stab wound. Injury to the nerve leads to serratus anterior deficit and the pathognomonic "winged scapula" on exam. **Thoracodorsal nerve injury** may present similarly but with the additional findings of shoulder abduction and internal rotation deficit.

ANKLE/FOOT SYMPTOMS

Presenting ankle/foot symptoms include pain, swelling, decreased range of motion, weakness, and paresthesias. Consider trauma, sprains/strains, fracture, infection, nerve entrapment/injury, arthritis, and crystalline diseases in the differential diagnosis.

Key Findings and Ankle/Foot Pain Differential Diagnosis

Ankle/Foot Pain and Key Associated Findings	Diagnosis
Anterior drawer test: Distal tibia is stabilized with one hand, while the heel is pulled forward with the other hand. The test is positive if the talus moves more anteriorly compared to the contralateral side.	Anterior talofibular ligament laxity/injury
Talar tilt or inversion stress test: When the ankle is inverted or adducted, the test is positive if there is instability or inversion greater than the contralateral side.	Calcanofibular ligament laxity/injury
Pain in the plantar region of the midfoot near the heel, which is worse with the first steps in the morning. Tenderness over the medial tuberosity of the calcaneus. Dorsiflexion of the foot and extension of the toes increase patient's pain.	Plantar fasciitis
Painful, swollen big toe in an alcoholic	Podagra (gout)

CASE 11 | Ankle Sprain (Anterior Talofibular Ligament Injury)

A 33-year-old woman presents with right ankle pain after "rolling it" while running. She is able to walk, but she has a limp. On exam, the patient has swelling over the lateral aspect of the ankle and tenderness just distal and anterior to the distal tip of the fibula. With the ankle in slight plantar flexion, the talus translates significantly more anteriorly with anterior pull on the foot when compared to the contralateral side (anterior drawer test). There is no instability or pain when varus stress is applied with the ankle in dorsiflexion (talar tilt test).

Evaluation/Tests	Clinical diagnosis. X-rays are negative for fracture.
Treatment	Conservative treatment with rest, ice, compression, and elevation (RICE).
Discussion	This patient has a low ankle sprain. The most commonly injured ligament in a low ankle sprain is the anterior talofibular ligament (ATFL). The mechanism of injury is plantar flexion and inversion, which stresses the ATFL. The calcaneofibular ligament (CFL) is the second most sprained ligament in the ankle. The injury takes place during dorsiflexion and inversion. Patients with ATFL injury typically show pain with weight bearing but are still able to walk. They often have focal tenderness and swelling over the ATFL or CFL. The anterior drawer test may show anterior translation of the talus. Additionally, increased foot inversion compared to the noninjured ankle may be seen with the tilt test. X-rays are usually negative. Diagnosis is typically made by history and exam, and imaging can rule out other causes such as fracture or osteochrondal lesions of the talus.

CASE 12 | Tarsal Tunnel Syndrome (Tibial Nerve Injury)

A 55-year-old woman with diabetes presents with pain at her right medial foot over the ankle, radiating to the sole of the foot for the past month. She describes it as a sharp, shooting pain and indicates that the sole of her foot feels numb. She reports that her symptoms get worse with standing, walking, as well as at nighttime. She also reports spraining her right ankle shortly before her symptoms started. On physical exam, she is afebrile, and tapping over the tarsal tunnel reproduces her pain (positive Tinel's sign). She also has sensory loss of the right plantar foot.

Evaluation/Tests	Clinical diagnosis. Comparison with the contralateral, unaffected body part is usually helpful. Imaging, such as foot and ankle X-ray, can be used to ensure there are no bony abnormalities such as bone spurs or changes due to previous trauma. Ultrasound can be used to evaluate for soft tissue structures such as ganglion cysts. EMG/NCS would reveal decreased amplitude in the sensory/motor components of the medial and lateral plantar nerves.
Treatment	Nonsteroidal anti-inflammatory drugs (NSAIDs), physical therapy (PT), and orthotic shoes. If there is a source of compression of the tibial nerve such as a ganglion cyst, operative decompression can be helpful.
Discussion	This presentation is consistent with tarsal tunnel syndrome. The tibial nerve gets compressed/injured in the ankle area as it passes through the tarsal tunnel. This usually occurs due to trauma (ankle sprain/fracture). Other causes and risk factors include diabetes, hypothyroidism, space-occupying lesions such as lipomas, or ganglion cysts. The tarsal tunnel also contains the medial and lateral plantar nerves. **Plantar fasciitis** is usually described as heel pain that is worse in the morning with taking a few steps. On physical exam, with dorsiflexion of the toes/foot, palpation of the fascia from the heel to the forefoot will elicit tenderness. It is caused by inflammation of the plantar aponeurosis near its origin on the calcaneus

CASE 12 | Tarsal Tunnel Syndrome (Tibial Nerve Injury) *(continued)*

Discussion	(heel bone). Plantar fasciitis can be caused by chronic overuse or stress on the plantar fascia, leading to microtears and recurrent inflammation. Dancing and running are common causes. Diagnosis is made clinically. X-rays are usually normal, but they may show a bone spur off the calcaneus.
	L5–S1 radiculopathy will usually have back pain with radiation of pain down the leg into the foot. With **L5 radiculopathy**, patients may have decreased strength foot eversion, inversion, dorsiflexion, and toe extension. With **S1 radiculopathy**, patients may have weakness with plantar flexion with sensation loss along the posterior leg and lateral foot, with decreased ankle reflex. The straight leg raise test involves having the patient lie supine, raising the leg while dorsiflexing the foot; this may reproduce the patient's pain, making it a positive test.
	Femoral nerve injury can occur secondary to hip or pelvic fractures, abdominal/pelvic operations, or hematoma. Patients typically present with numbness/tingling in the thigh/medial leg and knee buckling. Exam findings include decreased strength of the quadriceps, sensory loss in the medial thigh, absent knee jerk, and sparing of adduction.

KNEE SYMPTOMS

A common presentation is knee pain or swelling. Consider trauma, sprains/strains, fracture, infection, nerve entrapment/injury, arthritis, and crystalline diseases when assessing patients. Pain resulting from injury is often due to a cruciate ligament, collateral ligament, or meniscus problem.

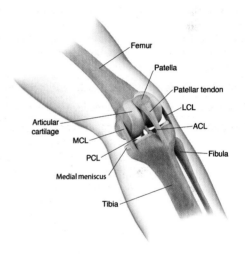

Internal anatomy of the knee and major stabilizers.
Reproduced with permission from Elsayes KM, Oldham SA: Introduction to Diagnostic Radiology. New York, NY: McGraw Hill; 2014.

Key Findings and Knee Pain Differential Diagnosis

Knee Pain and Key Associated Exam Findings	Diagnosis
Increased anterior translation of the tibia relative to femur compared with the unaffected side with the following tests: **Anterior drawer test:** Patient lies with feet flat on table, hips flexed, and knee bent at 90 degrees while examiner pulls the tibia forward with both hands. *Or:* **Lachman's test** (more sensitive): Patient lies with knee bent 30 degrees, and examiner places one hand on thigh and pulls the tibia forward with the other hand.	Anterior cruciate ligament (ACL) tear 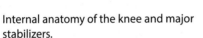 **ACL tear** **Anterior drawer sign**
Increased posterior translation of tibia relative to femur compared with unaffected side with the following test: **Posterior drawer sign:** Patient lies with feet flat on table, hips flexed, and knee bent at 90 degrees while examiner pushes the tibia posteriorly with both hands. *Or:* **Posterior sag test:** Place patient's feet on elevated surface so knees and hips are bent to 90 degrees, and observe for excessive posterior positioning of tibia.	Posterior cruciate ligament (PCL) tear **PCL tear** **Posterior drawer sign**

(continued)

Key Findings and Knee Pain Differential Diagnosis (*continued*)

Knee Pain and Key Associated Exam Findings	Diagnosis
Increased laxity along medial joint compared to unaffected side with: **Valgus** (lateral force) **stress test** (abnormal passive abduction): Examiner places one hand laterally against knee and pushes inward and with the other hand pushes ankle away from the body.	Medial collateral ligament (MCL) tear Abduction (valgus) forve — MCL tear
Increased laxity along lateral joint compared to unaffected side with: **Varus** (medial force) **stress test** (abnormal passive adduction): Examiner places one hand medially against knee and pushes out and with the other hand pulls ankle toward the body.	Lateral collateral ligament (LCL) tear Abduction (valgus) forve — LCL tear
Pain and/or clicking or popping reproduced in knee with: **Thessaly's test:** Patient stands on affected leg with knee bent 20 degrees and rotates knee internally and externally. **McMurray's test:** Examiner places one hand along medial and lateral joint line and with other hand grasps heel and flexes and extends knee while providing internal and external rotation to the tibia.	Meniscal injury External rotation — Medial tear Internal rotation — Lateral tear

CASE 13 | Anterior Cruciate Ligament (ACL) Tear

A 20-year-old woman presents with acute left knee pain and swelling. She was playing soccer when she made a cutting move and felt a sudden "pop" in her left knee. She developed significant swelling and pain with range of motion. On physical exam, the left knee is swollen, but there is no point tenderness. With the knee bent at 30 degrees, the tibia translates anteriorly approximately 1 cm without a firm endpoint (positive Lachman's test). With the knee at 90 degrees, the tibia similarly translates anteriorly with stress, compared to the contralateral side (positive anterior drawer test); however, the tibia does not translate posteriorly (negative posterior drawer test) or medially.

Evaluation/Tests	X-rays of knee are negative for fracture or dislocation.
Treatment	Conservative treatment or surgical correction in younger, active patients.
Discussion	This patient suffered an ACL tear. This injury is common in sports requiring sudden twisting and pivot motions. Patients often note a "pop" or snapping sensation in their knee at the time of injury and a bloody effusion quickly builds within the knee. They may report a feeling of instability while walking or when pivoting. With chronic ACL tears, patients may report their knee unexpectedly "giving out." MRI of the knee is the study of choice to confirm the diagnosis and identify any associated injuries, such as a meniscus tear. The "unhappy triad" of ACL, MCL, and medial meniscus tears is seen in contact sports when lateral force is applied to a planted leg. Patients with the "unhappy triad" present with acute knee pain, knee instability, and signs of joint injury. **Medial meniscus tear** injuries often happen as a result of a twisting injury to the knee. Medial meniscus tears are more common than lateral tears. Diagnosis is often made clinically with a positive McMurray's or Thessaly's test. Treatment of meniscal tears depends on the location and size of the tear. Most patients are treated nonoperatively with physical therapy, and others may require partial meniscectomy or meniscal repair. **Lateral tears** often occur in the setting of an acute ACL injury. **PCL injuries** can be caused by several mechanisms, one of which is a direct blow to the tibia with a posteriorly directed force as seen when a dashboard slams into the proximal tibia of a flexed knee. Hyperextension of the knee can also cause PCL damage. PCL injuries are commonly associated with injuries to other structures that support the knee, including collateral ligaments and occasionally the popliteal tendon (during posterolateral corner knee injuries). The majority of isolated PCL injuries may be treated nonoperatively because its blood supply is often maintained after the injury due to its extrasynovial location and close association with the well-vascularized posterior capsule.

CASE 13 | Anterior Cruciate Ligament (ACL) Tear *(continued)*

Additional Considerations	**Patellofemoral pain syndrome** presents with dull aching pain under or around patella. **Prepatellar bursitis** presents with pain and swelling of the patella with overlying erythema, warmth, and swelling that worsens with knee flexion. Patients with **iliotibial band syndrome** present with lateral knee pain due to friction of the IT band against the lateral femoral epicondyle secondary to overuse of the lateral knee (e.g., in runners).

HIP SYMPTOMS

Hip problems often present as hip pain. In assessing patients, consider arthritis, bursitis, trauma, fracture, infection, nerve entrapment/injury, avascular necrosis, and crystalline diseases.

Key Associated Findings and Hip Pain Differential Diagnosis

Hip Pain with Key Associated Findings	Diagnoses
Log roll test (specific test to confirm hip pathology): While patient is supine, extended leg is internally and externally rotated. If pain, clicking, or increased or decreased range of motion is detected, it helps confirm hip pathology vs. pain from outside the hip joint (i.e., referred from back).	Hip pathology (e.g., arthritis (OA), osteonecrosis, slipped capital femoral epiphysis (SCFE), piriformis syndrome)
FADIR test (flexion, adduction, internal rotation): Pain is reproduced with flexing the hip of a supine patient to 90 degrees and internally rotating and adducting the hip by placing one hand on bent knee and ankle.	Anterior pain: intra-articular pathology (e.g., OA)
FABER test (flexion, abduction, external rotation): Examiner lexes, externally rotates and abducts the hip of a supine patient so the ankle is lying just above the opposite knee. Then gentle pressure is applied to the bent knee while the opposite pelvic bone is stabilized. Test is positive if pain is elicited.	Posterior pain: SI joint, lumbar spine, or posterior hip pathology Groin pain: intra-articular pathology
Asymmetric thigh skin folds, leg length discrepancy, abnormal gait, and limited hip abduction in an infant/toddler **Ortolani maneuver:** Infant is supine with hip flexed at 90 degrees. While the thumb is placed at the inner thigh and the index and middle finger held firmly at the greater trochanter, the examiner gently abducts the hip by lifting the trochanter anteriorly; a "clunk" appreciated while reducing the abducted hip constitutes a positive test. **Barlow maneuver:** Infant is supine with hip flexed at 90 degrees. While the thumb is at the inner thigh and the index and middle fingers held firmly at the greater trochanter, the examiner gently adducts the thigh while palpating the head of the femur; a "clunk" appreciated while the femur dislocates or subluxates from the acetabulum constitutes a positive test.	Developmental dysplasia of the hip

CASE 14 | Paget's Disease

A 75-year-old man presents with right hip pain. He describes 6 months of progressive achy right hip pain worse at night. He also notes headache and hearing loss and thinks his head has gotten bigger because his hat size has increased. Exam reveals decreased range of motion for the right hip, which is moderately warm to the touch on the lateral aspect of the proximal thigh. Reduced hearing is noted bilaterally to finger rub.

Evaluation/Tests	Alkaline phosphatase levels are elevated. X-ray of the affected area: mixed lytic/sclerotic lesions with candle flame sign (area of lucency with a V-shaped area of bone destruction extending out of it).
Treatment	Bisphosphonates.
Discussion	Paget's disease is a disorder of bone metabolism isolated to one (mono-ostotic) or several (polyostotic) bones in the skeleton. It is marked by accelerated bone turnover resulting in thickened/enlarged bone but with weakened bone strength. Any bone can be involved, including the skull where overgrowth can cause headaches and narrowing of cranial nerve canals can lead to deafness. Symptoms depend on the site and extent of disease involvement but include pain, warmth, and fracture at sites of pagetic change.

CASE 14 | Paget's Disease *(continued)*

Discussion	Some lesions are found incidentally on imaging and are asymptomatic. Patients are at higher risk of primary bone tumors, specifically osteosarcoma. Elevated levels of alkaline phosphatase (bone specific) indicate increased bone formation, help support the diagnosis, and are useful as follow-up for recurrence. Plain X-ray imaging is often diagnostic but depends on the age of the lesion. Treatment is given for all symptomatic patients and asymptomatic patients when involving weight-bearing sites and the skull. Intravenous bisphosphonate therapy is the treatment of choice with preference for zoledronic acid. **Osteoarthritis** is a degenerative disease characterized by joint pain with loss of articular cartilage, and it is typically seen in elderly patients. Patients typically note pain in their groin that eventually impairs their day-to-day activities. Night pain and hip stiffness are often seen as well. However, alkaline phosphatase levels are not elevated as seen in this patient. **Greater trochanteric pain syndrome (bursitis)** is caused by inflammation of the gluteal tendon and trochanteric bursa of the femur. It is common in female runners. The trochanteric bursa is deep to the iliotibial band and superficial to the hip abductor muscles. During running, the iliotibial band repeatedly rubs over the bursa, which can lead to irritation and inflammation. On exam, the patient would have tenderness over the greater trochanter. Diagnosis is clinical, and X-rays are typically done to rule out other pathologies, but they are usually unremarkable in bursitis.
Additional Considerations	**Osteopetrosis** is increased bone density. In infants, it is associated with renal tubular acidosis and increased risk for fractures. There are different forms, but most would be apparent much earlier than with this patient.

CASE 15 | Avascular Necrosis (AVN) of the Hip

A 35-year-old man with sickle cell disease presents with 2 months of worsening right hip pain. He reports that the pain is localized to his groin. Pain is made worse with walking, climbing stairs, and prolonged standing. Recently, his left hip has started to hurt as well. Patient denies any falls or trauma. Physical exam reveals normal range of motion of the hip. However, hip movement elicits pain in the groin region.

Evaluation/Tests	X-rays of the pelvis and hips are negative for fractures or dislocations but do show sclerosis at the superior aspect of the right femoral head. MRI of the hips shows increased signal at the anterior-superior aspect of the femoral head.
Treatment	Hip surgery.
Discussion	Risk factors for AVN (osteonecrosis) of the hip include chronic steroid use, alcoholism (most common cause), sickle cell disease, trauma, "the bends" (caisson/decompression disease), Legg-Calve-Perthes disease (idiopathic), Gaucher disease, slipped capital femoral epiphysis (SCFE), and hypercoagulable states. Painful infarction of bone typically occurs at the watershed zone of the femoral head due to insufficiency of the medial circumflex femoral artery. AP and frog leg lateral X-rays of the hip are used as an initial evaluation. Earlier stages of AVN may show either a normal radiograph or sclerotic changes in the superior-anterior portion of the femoral head. A "crescent sign," a sign of subchondral collapse, may be seen in more advanced stages. MRI is the study of choice when X-rays are negative but AVN is suspected. Bilateral hips are involved 80% of the time; therefore, both hips should be imaged. Early stages of AVN may be treated with bisphosphonates to help prevent femoral head collapse. Once femoral head collapse has occurred, a total hip arthroplasty (reconstruction or replacement) is the treatment of choice. Patients with **septic arthritis** typically present with fever, erythema, and swelling of the joint. Osteoarthritis may present similarly but is typically seen in older patients, and fractures typically present acutely after trauma.

MISCELLANEOUS PRESENTATIONS

Crystalline Diseases

	Gout	Calcium Pyrophosphate Deposition Disease (CPPD)
Joint involvement	Smaller joints (classically MTP of big toe)	Larger joint (knee most common)
Synovial fluid	Needle-shaped crystals, negatively birefringent (yellow under parallel light)	Rhomboid-shaped crystals, positively birefringent (blue under parallel light)

(continued)

	Gout	Calcium Pyrophosphate Deposition Disease (CPPD)
Acute treatment	NSAIDs, colchicine, glucocorticoids	NSAIDs, colchicine, glucocorticoids
Chronic/preventative treatment	Xanthine oxidase inhibitors	Colchicine
Age	Generally middle-aged men or postmenopausal women	Typically >50-year-old men or women

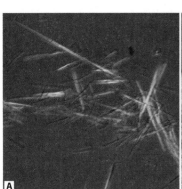
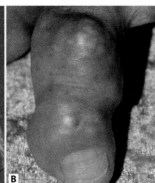

A: Gout crystals are needle shaped and negative birefringent under polarized light (yellow under parallel light, blue under perpendicular light). B: Tophus formation seen in gout.

Part A used with permission from Bobjgalindo/Wikimedia Commons. Part B reproduced with permission from Roddy E. Revisiting the pathogenesis of podagra: why does gout target the foot? J Foot Ankle Res 2011 May 13;4(1):13.

CASE 16 | Gout

A 60-year-old man with a history of diet-controlled diabetes, obesity, and HTN presents with severe right big toe pain and swelling. He is on a thiazide diuretic and drank 10 beers the night before. On exam, his right first MTP joint is erythematous, swollen, warm, and very tender to touch (podagra).

Evaluation/Tests	Clinical diagnosis. Aspiration of the joint shows needle-shaped, negatively birefringent crystals under polarized light.
Treatment	Acute: high-dose NSAIDs (indomethacin), colchicine, or glucocorticoids. Preventive: xanthine oxidase inhibitors (allopurinol, febuxostat).
Discussion	Gout typically occurs in middle-aged men and postmenopausal women. Patients present with recurrent attacks of monoarthritis due to deposition of monosodium urate crystals. Potential triggers are purine-rich meals (shellfish, red meats), trauma, surgery, ethanol, or serious medical illnesses. Hyperuricemia can occur either due to undersecretion of uric acid (most cases), which is worsened by renal failure or certain medications (thiazides), or due to overproduction (Lesch-Nyhan syndrome, tumor lysis syndrome). The MTP joint of the first toe is classically affected, but any joint can be involved. Tophi (soft tissue deposition of urate crystals) can be seen on the joints, external ear, olecranon bursa, or Achilles tendon. Joint aspiration will show needle-shaped monosodium urate crystals that are negatively birefringent. The synovial fluid white count will often elevate to between 2000 and 60,000/µL. Radiographs may show soft tissue masses (in tophaceous gout), cystic changes, and erosions with sclerotic margins. A serum uric acid level may be normal during an acute attack but is helpful later if starting hypouricemic medications. Long-term treatment with hypouricemic therapy may be necessary after repeat acute attacks with uric acid stones or those with tophi or chronic gout. Options to lower uric acid include probenecid, allopurinol, and febuxostat. Therapy should be delayed until resolution of the acute flare. Aspiration and analysis of fluid will help distinguish between an infection and crystalline disease. **Pseudogout** or calcium pyrophosphate deposition disease (CPPD) tends to affect larger joints (knee, hip, wrist). It can be idiopathic, associated with joint trauma, or associated with other diseases such as hemochromatosis or hyperparathyroidism. Joint aspiration analysis will show rhomboid, weakly positive birefringent crystals. Radiographs may show cartilage calcification (chondrocalcinosis). Patients with **septic arthritis** may also present with an erythematous, swollen joint; however, they typically have a fever, and arthrocentesis findings include markedly elevated WBC with predominant neutrophils and positive gram stain and cultures.

CASE 17 | Leg Compartment Syndrome

A 21-year-old man presents with a comminuted, midshaft tibia fracture after a car accident. He is splinted and admitted for preoperative clearance. Overnight, nursing staff notes more frequent requests for pain medication. The patient reports excruciating pain as well as new-onset numbness and tingling in his foot. On physical exam, the patient has hard, noncompressible compartments of the leg. His pain seems to be out of proportion to exam. The foot is pale, and he has decreased sensation in the peroneal and tibial nerve distributions and diminished dorsalis pedis and posterior tibial arterial pulses.

Evaluation/Tests	Diagnosis is confirmed if compartment pressures are >30 mmHg in all leg compartments or the diastolic blood pressure (DBP) minus compartment pressure is <30 mmHg.
Treatment	Emergent fasciotomy and debridement of devitalized tissue.
Discussion	This patient is presenting with compartment syndrome. The lower leg (calf) has four compartments: anterior, lateral, superficial posterior, and deep posterior. These compartments are surrounded by tough layers of fascia that restrict the amount of distension that can take place. When compartment pressures rise significantly after injury, and fascial compartment pressure exceeds perfusion pressure, blood perfusion is cut off via the tamponade effect, leading to tissue ischemia/necrosis. Any number of compartments can be involved. Later signs may include paresthesias in the peroneal and/or tibial nerve distributions and diminished dorsalis pedis and posterior tibial arterial pulses. The most sensitive findings are pain out of proportion to the injury and pain with passive movement of the foot and ankle. While compartment syndrome is a clinical diagnosis, it may be confirmed by measuring compartment pressures if a device is readily available. CPK levels may be elevated, indicating muscle damage/ischemia. Compartment syndrome is treated with emergent fasciotomy and debridement of devitalized tissue. Treatment should not be delayed for compartment pressure checks if a measurement device is not readily available. Compartment pressures are not typically elevated in arterial thrombus, deep vein thrombosis (DVT), or nerve injury.

CASE 18 | Common Peroneal Nerve Injury

A 47-year-old man undergoes a 3-hour-long surgery in the left lateral decubitus position. When the patient attempts to walk later in the day, he walks with a high stepping gait and is not able to dorsiflex his left foot. On exam, there is no lower extremity edema, erythema, or warmth. Lower extremity pulses are intact. He has numbness on the dorsal aspect of his left foot and cannot extend his left big toe or dorsiflex his ankle and has limited foot eversion.

Evaluation/Tests	Clinical diagnosis.
Treatment	Ankle-foot-orthosis (AFO) brace.
Discussion	This is a classic case of common peroneal/fibular nerve injury. The patient is not able to activate the tibialis anterior, extensor digitorum longus, or extensor hallucis longus. The patient also exhibits decreased foot eversion due to weakness of the peroneal longus and peroneal brevis. When the common peroneal nerve is involved, patients will have decreased sensation on the dorsum of the foot and the area between all toes. When the deep peroneal nerve alone is involved, the patient will present with drop foot only and decreased sensation in the first web space between the great and second toes. The injury often occurs when a patient is placed on their side during surgery without adequate padding to the lateral side of the knee. The common peroneal nerve runs laterally around the fibular neck and can be damaged with prolonged pressure. Over 50% of cases resolve with expectant management. Patients are given an ankle-foot-orthosis (AFO) brace to help with ambulation and to help prevent plantar contracture of the ankle.
Additional Considerations	The **lateral femoral cutaneous nerve** is a purely sensory nerve that can be compressed on its way from the lumbosacral plexus through the abdominal cavity and under the inguinal ligament into the subcutaneous tissue of the thigh. Patients present with intermittent numbness and tingling sensation on the lateral aspect of the thigh (**meralgia paresthetica**). Risk factors are diabetes, obesity, and surgery.

MUSCULOSKELETAL PRESENTATIONS IN CHILDREN

Immature bone in children is more elastic than mature bone, so children can fracture differently than in adults. For example, a pediatric patient with a recent fall or trauma may have a greenstick or torus fracture. Be suspicious of child abuse in a pediatric patient with a spiral fracture.

A new soft tissue mass, swelling, and pain are the most common presentations of a primary bony tumor in children. Systemic signs of illness such as fever, malaise, and weight changes are usually indicative of infection or malignancy. The location of the tumor and its radiographic and/or histologic characteristics are very helpful in differentiating the various benign and malignant bone tumors.

CASE 19 | Slipped Capital Femoral Epiphysis (SCFE)

A 13-year-old obese boy with hypothyroidism presents with a limp and left groin pain for several months. He denies any recent illnesses or trauma. Exam is notable for antalgic gait, difficulty with weight bearing, and limited range of motion of the hip (abduction, flexion, and internal rotation).

Evaluation/Tests	X-ray of the hip and femur shows anterior translation and external rotation of metaphysis relative to epiphysis ("scoop of ice cream slipping off a cone") but no fracture.
Treatment	Surgery.
Discussion	SCFE occurs more frequently in overweight adolescents. Endocrinopathies (e.g., hypothyroidism or growth hormone deficiency) can be another important risk factor. A common presentation is hip/knee pain and limp/altered gait due to posterior and inferior translation of femoral epiphysis relative to metaphysis secondary to mechanical axial overload on the femoral head. The goal of treatment is hip stabilization, non-weight-bearing crutches, and urgent referral to orthopedics for surgical correction. **Hip fracture** is unlikely as there is no history of trauma and X-ray is negative for fracture. **Septic arthritis** of the hip joint may also present with antalgic gait and limited range of motion, but it is also accompanied by signs of systemic illness (e.g., fever). **Legg-Calve-Perthes disease** leads to ischemic necrosis of the femoral head, and X-ray findings are initially normal. It occurs mostly in males ages 5–7 who tend to present with insidious pain with a limp. MRI may be more sensitive to detect early changes suggestive of infarction of the femoral head.
Additional Considerations	**Development dysplasia of the hip (DDH)** (abnormal formation of the femoral head and acetabulum) causes hip joint instability. Risk factors include female sex, family history of DDH, and oligohydramnios. Exam findings may vary by age. In early infancy, the Ortolani and Barlow maneuvers help identify any joint instability due to abnormal femoral head development. Other helpful findings are asymmetric thigh skin folds, limb length discrepancy, abnormal gait, and limited hip abduction. Ultrasound can help confirm diagnosis and is the main imaging modality as the femoral head may not be well appreciated on plain films before 4 months of age because cartilage is not ossified.

CASE 20 | Osteomalacia (Rickets)

A 15-month-old boy is brought for evaluation of bowlegs and difficulty walking. His parents are concerned that he is short for his age. He has been exclusively breast-fed and does not take any vitamins. On exam, the child appears to have short stature, an open anterior fontanelle, bossing of the forehead, tooth abnormalities, swelling of the wrists, and bowing of the knees.

Evaluation/Tests	Low vitamin D, increased PTH, increased alkaline phosphatase, and low calcium on lab studies. X-ray of the knees shows widened growth plates, metaphyseal cupping or fraying, and lateral bowing (genu varum).
Treatment	Vitamin D supplementation.
Discussion	

A: Genu varum. B: Bead-like costochondral junctions (rachitic rosary).
Part A reproduced with permission from Linglart A, Biosse-Duplan M, Briot K, et al: Therapeutic management of hypophosphatemic rickets from infancy to adulthood, Endocr Connect 2014 Mar 14;3(1):R13-R30. Part B reproduced with permission from Essabar L, Meskini T, Ettair S, et al: Malignant infantile osteopetrosis: case report with review of literature, Pan Afr Med J 2014 Jan 27;17:63.

CASE 20 | Osteomalacia (Rickets) *(continued)*

Discussion	While osteomalacia describes a defect in bone mineralization, **rickets** implies resultant growth plate changes. These conditions occur due to **vitamin D deficiency**. Vitamin D is responsible for increasing intestinal absorption of calcium, magnesium, and phosphate. It is obtained both through a chemical reaction that occurs in the skin that converts cholesterol to cholecalciferol, as well as through the diet. It is further converted to an active form by enzymes in the liver and kidney. Prolonged, severe vitamin D deficiency causes reduced intestinal absorption of calcium and phosphorus, causing hypocalcemia which in turn causes secondary hyperparathyroidism. This leads to phosphaturia and demineralization of bones, ultimately causing rickets in children and osteomalacia in children and adults.
	Bowed legs are commonly seen in skeletal dysplasia. Classic X-ray features include osteopenia, cupping or fraying of the metaphyses of the knees/wrists, widening of the wrists or ankles, bowing of the long bones (radius/ulna), and lateral bowing of the weight-bearing extremities (genu varum). Bead-like enlargement of the costochondral joints, also known as "rachitic rosary," is another classic radiologic finding. Usually, a metabolic profile suggestive of rickets includes decreased serum 25-hydroxyvitamin D, elevated PTH and serum alkaline phosphatase, decreased phosphate, and a normal or decreased calcium level. Treatment includes correction of vitamin D and electrolyte deficiencies.
	In **hypophosphatemic rickets**, PTH is typically normal.
	Hypoparathyroidism is typically caused by parathyroid excision or autoimmune destruction, and vitamin D levels may be normal.

CASE 21 | Greenstick Fracture

A 3-year-old is brought for evaluation of left distal forearm pain after tripping over his toy. The father reports the child fell forward on his outstretched hand. Physical exam does not reveal any gross deformity, breaks in the skin, or bruising. However, there is focal point tenderness to palpation and swelling at the radial side of the distal forearm.

Evaluation/Tests	X-ray of the distal radius demonstrates mild bending (or bowing) of the bone on one side, with complete fracture on the opposite cortex (side of tension) that does not completely cross the bone.
Treatment	Immobilization with splint or cast.
Discussion	In a fracture, bone failure depends on the mechanism of injury, loading forces, and compressive stress. Greenstick fracture, plastic deformity, and buckle (torus) fracture all refer to unique patterns commonly seen in pediatric patients. The typical mechanisms of injury include a fall on an outstretched hand and extended wrist, direct blow, or motor vehicle accidents. Greenstick fracture occurs when there is a fracture on the side where there was tension, but the fracture does not extend all the way through the bone.
	Plastic deformity implies bending of the bone without necessarily breaking.
	A **buckle (torus) fracture** results from cortical fracture of the compression side, while the tension side remains intact.
	Spiral fracture of long bones is usually caused by a twisting force that produces the injury. Fractures of the long bones (femur, humerus, and tibia) are commonly found in cases of child abuse. A focal area of tenderness, swelling, and overlying ecchymosis of a long bone of a child who is nonambulatory is suggestive of abuse. Additional findings in cases of physical abuse include shaped bruises (e.g., belt), shaped burns (e.g., cigarette), and fractures in various stages of healing. Children with complex medical needs or children with conditions that may promote parental anxiety are at a higher risk for child abuse.

MUSCULOSKELETAL TUMORS

Primary bone cancers are exceedingly rare. Compared to most other solid tumors, bone cancers disproportionately affect children and young adults. The initial diagnostic workup typically starts with an X-ray, which may be followed by more advanced imaging. Outside of osteochondroma, a benign tumor with characteristic features on X-ray, definitive diagnosis is made by a bone biopsy. The clinical spectrum of bone cancers ranges from benign tumors to aggressive and fatal malignancies.

Key Findings and Musculoskeletal Tumor Differential Diagnosis

Musculoskeletal Tumor with Key Associated Findings	Diagnosis
Li-Fraumeni syndrome Codman triangle "Sunburst" subperiosteal tumor	Osteosarcoma
t(11;22) Malignant bone tumor in young boy (<15 years old)	Ewing sarcoma
Painless benign bony growth in metaphysis of distal femur or humerus	Osteochondroma
"Soap bubble" pattern on X-ray RANK-L expression on osteoclasts	Giant cell tumor

CASE 22 | Osteochondroma

A 13-year-old boy presents for evaluation of a painless but firm swelling that has been slowly growing below his right knee for 1 month. He denies any fever, malaise, weight changes, or trauma. The patient has a palpable, painless mass at the medial aspect of his proximal tibia. There is no bony deformity, redness, or impairment in range of motion.

Evaluation/Tests	X-ray of the lower extremities shows a cartilage-capped mass, which is continuous with the marrow space. It arises from the cortex and projects away from the knee joint.
Treatment	Observation; surgical excision in some cases.
Discussion	Benign bone tumors (e.g., osteoid osteoma, osteochondroma) are not associated with systemic signs of illness, and they can typically be diagnosed radiographically. Osteochondroma is the most common benign bone tumor. It is classified as a cartilage-producing tumor that often occurs at the metaphysis of growth plate of long bones. They may be diagnosed incidentally in younger men and usually do not require any medical intervention. Lesions typically grow throughout childhood, then remain static in adulthood after the growth plates close. New symptoms or tumor growth after adulthood may signal a need for additional workup. **Osgood-Schlatter disease**, or traction apophysitis, results from joint overuse or repetitive strain and chronic avulsion of the secondary ossification center of the proximal tibial tubercle. It often presents in preadolescents/adolescents. Patients present with pain below the anterior knee that worsens with activity and with soft tissue swelling and tenderness at the tibial tuberosity. **Osteoid osteoma** classically presents as bone pain that is worse at night and relieved by NSAIDs. It is most common in adults under the age of 25, and it disproportionately impacts men. X-ray shows a bony mass <2 cm with radiolucent osteoid core. **Osteoblastoma** is an uncommon benign bone tumor that can present at any age. It is histologically similar to osteoid osteoma, but it more typically presents in the vertebrae. Osteoblastoma is also larger in size >2 cm, and pain is unresponsive to NSAIDs.
Additional Considerations	**Lipomas** are benign tumors, typically occurring on the trunk and upper extremities of adults. On exam, they are skin-colored, typically 1–10 cm, nontender, mobile tumors made of adipocytes. They very rarely transform into liposarcomas. **Ganglion cysts** are also benign tumors found in adults, typically on the dorsum of the hand at the wrist.

CASE 23 | Ewing Sarcoma

A 12-year-old boy has had intermittent aching over his right thigh for 1 month. He has experienced fever, malaise, and weight loss over the past few days, and he began noticing swelling near the middle of his right thigh yesterday. He denies any trauma to his leg. On exam, the patient has localized pain and swelling of the middle of the right thigh.

Evaluation/Tests	X-ray of his femur demonstrates destruction of the femoral diaphysis with "onion skin" periosteal reaction. Further testing reveals anaplastic small blue cells and t(11;22) chromosomal translocation.
Treatment	Chemotherapy, local treatment with surgery and/or radiation therapy.
Discussion	This is a classic presentation for Ewing sarcoma, a malignant bone tumor that occurs most often in Caucasian males at the diaphysis of a long bone. It is the most aggressive bone cancer and has the worst prognosis, with long-term survival only recently approaching 50% despite treatment with chemotherapy, surgery, and radiation. Roughly 30% of patients already have overt metastases at the time of diagnosis—most

CASE 23 | Ewing Sarcoma *(continued)*

Discussion	often in the lungs, bones, or bone marrow. It is more common in younger boys, usually younger than age 15, and it is associated with a (11;22) translocation resulting in the EWS-FLI1 fusion protein. Given that the differential diagnoses include both malignant (osteosarcoma) and nonmalignant (osteomyelitis) conditions on presentation, further imaging studies and bone aspiration help in establishing a definitive diagnosis and treatment plan. **Growing pain** is common in this age group, but it should not be associated with any physical signs of inflammation. **Osteosarcoma** is a common primary malignant bone tumor associated with loss of tumor suppressor genes, such as RB1 in familial retinoblastoma or p53 in Li-Fraumeni syndrome. Other risk factors include personal history of Paget's disease of bone, radiation treatment, or bone infarcts. X-rays reveal destruction of the bony cortex at the metaphysis with periosteal new bone formation in a so-called Codman triangle and associated soft tissue mass ossifying in a "sunburst" pattern. Bone aspiration yields pleomorphic osteoid-producing cells.

CASE 24 | Giant Cell Tumor

A 32-year-old woman presents to clinic with worsening pain with flexion/extension and stiffness in her left wrist over the past several weeks. Physical exam shows no distinguishing exam features besides decreased range of motion in the left wrist.

Evaluation/Tests	X-ray shows a "soap bubble" appearance with multiple lytic lesions in the epiphyseal region. Biopsy results demonstrate histology significant for >50% multinucleated giant osteoclast cells expressing RANK-L. Chest X-ray subsequently reveals numerous pulmonary nodules.
Treatment	Surgery is the first-line treatment in appropriate patients. Other considerations include denosumab (a RANK-L inhibitor) and radiation therapy.
Discussion	Although technically classified as benign, giant cell tumors are often locally aggressive and typically require surgical treatment. They tend to present at the epiphysis of long bones. Tumors present in young adults (ages 20–40) with a slight predominance in women. Giant cell tumors make up 15–20% of benign tumors. Most cases are solitary, though a small percentage may present with benign pulmonary lesions that resemble metastases and have identical histology to the primary tumor. However, they do not carry the same clinical and prognostic implications as typical metastatic solid tumors. The bones are a common site for **lytic metastases**, particularly from lung, thyroid, and kidney cancer. However, this patient would likely present with other features demonstrating a different primary cancer. **Brown tumors** occur in the setting of hyperparathyroidism and patients typically have other symptoms associated with hypercalcemia.

BACK SYMPTOMS

When presented with a patient with low back pain (LBP), in addition to the usual history, it is important to inquire about alarm or "red flag" symptoms such as trauma history, extremes of age (<16 or >50) with new-onset pain, severe nighttime pain or rest pain, duration >1 month, history of cancer or osteoporosis, fevers/chills or history of significant infection or injection drug use, unexplained weight loss, malaise, or other systemic symptoms. It is also important to ask about pain in the chest, abdomen, pelvis, or other joints; chronic steroid use or immunosuppression; saddle anesthesia; bowel/bladder incontinence or urinary retention; or new neurological deficit (weakness, tingling, numbness). If a history of trauma is present, imaging studies such as X-rays, MRI, and/ or CT scans are warranted, in addition to possibly urgent/emergent surgical evaluation.

It is important to determine if the source of the patient's pain is *intrinsic* to the back or *extrinsic* to the back (referred from another part of the body). Intrinsic back pain may emanate from skeletal, neurologic, muscular, and other soft-tissue structures of the back. Pain referred to the lower back may originate within abdominal, pelvic, and retroperitoneal structures. Systemic symptoms such as fever, night sweats, or weight loss may suggest etiologies such as cancer, infection, or inflammatory arthritis. If abdominal or pelvic symptoms are elicited, focused questioning can further narrow the differential.

Differential Diagnosis for Back Pain

Back Trauma	Mechanical (Musculoskeletal) Back Pain	Referred from Intra-Abdominal/Pelvic/Retroperitoneal Sources	Tumors
Fracture Muscular sprain/strain/tear Joint disruption	Lumbar strain/sprain Degenerative disease Spondylolisthesis Spondylolysis Scoliosis Kyphosis Lordosis Spinal stenosis Disk herniation Vertebral compression fracture Cauda equina syndrome	Pancreatitis or pancreatic cancer Cholecystitis Penetrating peptic ulcer Nephrolithiasis Pyelonephritis Perinephric abscess Retroperitoneal lymphadenopathy or mass Abdominal aortic aneurysm/rupture Endometriosis Pelvic inflammatory disease Prostatitis	Multiple myeloma Metastatic cancer Lymphoma Leukemia Primary spinal cord tumors Retroperitoneal tumors
Infection	**Inflammatory Arthritis**	**Skin**	**Other**
Osteomyelitis Diskitis Paraspinal or epidural abscess	Ankylosing spondylitis Inflammatory bowel disease (IBD)–associated arthritis Reactive arthritis Psoriatic arthritis	Zoster	Cauda equina syndrome Malingering

Key Associated Findings and Back Pain Differential Diagnoses

Back Pain with Key Associated Findings	Diagnosis
Sideways curvature of the spine	Scoliosis
Exaggerated rounding of the upper back	Kyphosis
Inward curvature of lower back	Lordosis
Forward displacement of a vertebra on the vertebra immediately below it	Spondylolisthesis
Fracture or defect of the vertebral pars interarticularis	Spondylolysis
Focal point spinal tenderness	Infection, tumor, or compression fracture
Costovertebral angle (CVA) tenderness	Pyelonephritis
Sacroiliac (SI) joint tenderness and/or other joint inflammation/tenderness	Inflammatory arthritis
Weak hip flexion, weak knee extension, diminished patellar reflex, diminished sensation behind medial malleolus	L4 spinal nerve pathology (L3–L4 disc)
Abnormal heel walking (weak dorsiflexion and great toe extension), diminished sensation of dorsum of foot and 1st/2nd web space	L5 spinal nerve pathology (L4–L5 disc)
Abnormal toe walking (weak plantar flexion), diminished Achilles tendon reflex, diminished sensation of the lateral aspect of foot and/or posterior calf	S1 spinal nerve pathology (L5–S1 disc)
Straight leg raise test (SLR): Reproduction of shooting pain down affected leg (posterior calf) when affected straight leg is passively raised between 30 and 70 degrees: this is a positive SLR test (more sensitive). **Crossed straight leg raise (cSLR):** Reproduction of shooting pain down affected leg (posterior calf) when unaffected straight leg is passively raised between 30 and 70 degrees: this is a positive (cSLR) test (more specific).	Herniated disk L5–S1
Diminished anal sphincter tone or perianal sensation	Cauda equina syndrome
Hyperreflexia, presence of Babinski, positive Romberg test	Myelopathy

CASE 25 | Herniated Disk

A 45-year-old obese man presents with a 2-day history of acute low back pain after picking up a heavy box. The pain was sudden, gripping, and localized to the left lower back with radiation down the posterior aspect of the left leg. He denies any weakness or bladder/bowel incontinence. His exam is notable for tenderness over left paraspinal muscles and shooting pain to his left calf when his left leg is raised to 60 degrees off the table. There is no focal spinal tenderness. His left Achilles reflex is absent, and he has diminished sensation in the lateral aspect of his left foot and mildly impaired left toe walking.

Evaluation/Tests	Clinical diagnosis.
Treatment	Conservative treatment with NSAIDs and early mobilization.
Discussion	Diagnosis of a **herniated L5–S1 disk** with nerve root impingement (L5–S1 radiculopathy or sciatica) is made clinically, and imaging is not indicated as there are no red flag symptoms. If there is no improvement after conservative treatment or if there is any worsening of neurological deficits or symptoms, then consider ordering MRI, referring the patient to a spine specialist, and/or referring for physical therapy. Intervertebral disks typically herniate posteriorly because the posterior ligament is thinner than the anterior ligament. Symptoms depend upon which disk herniates. L3–L4 can lead to weakness of knee extension and a decreased patellar reflex. L4–L5 can cause weakness with dorsiflexion and difficulty with heel walking. **Mechanical low back pain (lumbar strain)** is in the differential, but the characteristics of the shooting pain and physical exam findings of a positive SLR test and neurological deficits are more consistent with nerve root impingement secondary to herniated disk. **Vertebral fracture** and **spinal infection** would present with focal spinal tenderness.
Additional Considerations	**Cauda equina syndrome** is a polyradiculopathy resulting from injury to the bundle of nerves situated below the end of the spinal cord. Symptom onset can be gradual or sudden with variable degrees of neurologic dysfunctions depending on the involved nerve roots. Any patient with symptoms of saddle anesthesia and/or bilateral lower extremity weakness or loss of bowel or bladder control should undergo immediate surgical consultation for decompression and intervention to minimize chances of permanent neurologic injury. Emergent MRI is indicated for anyone presenting with cauda equina symptoms due to the MRI's ability to detect soft tissue detail.

CASE 26 | Compression Fracture (Osteoporosis)

A 75-year-old woman presents with acute back pain after slipping in her bathtub. She slipped and fell, hitting her back against the edge of the tub. The pain started immediately after the fall. It is constant, sharp, most intense in the midline at the mid-lower back, and wraps around her abdomen. It worsens with any kind of movement. The patient denies any lower extremity weakness/numbness or any incontinence/retention of bowel or bladder. Her exam is notable for focal spinal tenderness around the T10 level. She has full range of motion of both hips, her SLR test is negative bilaterally, and her rectal tone is normal. Her lower extremity strength, sensation, and reflexes are normal.

Evaluation/Tests	Thoraco-lumbar films reveal diffuse vertebral lucency, decreased cortical thickness (suggestive of osteopenia/osteoporosis), loss of anterior vertebral height, and a wedge-shaped deformity consistent with T10 vertebral compression fracture.
Treatment	Pain control and physical therapy for mobility and strength rehabilitation. Treat osteoporosis.
Discussion	**Traumatic vertebral compression fractures** (with predisposition from osteoporosis) is the most likely diagnosis given the patient's age, characteristic of the pain with midline tenderness, and no known diagnosis of cancer. The cause of thoraco-lumbar compression fractures is usually osteoporosis. **Osteoporosis** is trabecular and cortical bone loss due to or exacerbated by menopause (increase bone resorption secondary to decrease estrogen levels), use of prednisone and other medications (anticonvulsants, anticoagulants), poor nutrition, alcohol, malabsorption syndromes, vitamin D deficiency, hyperthyroidism, hyperparathyroidism, multiple myeloma, and renal or liver failure. In osteoporosis, there is a decrease in generalized bone density as osteoclastic activity exceeds osteoblastic activity. The weakened bone is prone to fracturing even with minor injuries or falls. Low back pain is the hallmark symptom for compression fractures. A patient's posture may change to compensate for vertebral deformities resulting from height loss (kyphosis). This in turn can result in secondary pain in hips, sacroiliac joints, and spinal joints. Additionally, these patients are at risk for falls and accidents, increasing the risk of secondary fractures in the femoral neck, spine, and distal radius (Colles fracture). X-rays are the standard imaging study for spine fractures, and they usually show osteopenia with a wedge-shaped compression fracture with loss of

CASE 26 | Compression Fracture (Osteoporosis) *(continued)*

Discussion	vertebral height on lateral views. Dual-energy X-ray absorptiometry (DEXA) scanning measures bone mineral density, and it is used for diagnosis of osteopenia and osteoporosis. Osteoporosis is treated with adequate calcium, vitamin D, and weight-bearing exercises in addition to medications such as bisphosphonates, teriparatide, SERMs (selective estrogen receptor modulators), or denosumab.

CASE 27 | Ankylosing Spondylitis

A 25-year-old man presents with low back pain and stiffness for five months. Pain and stiffness are worse in the morning (lasting >30 minutes) and improve through the day and with physical activity. He denies lower extremity weakness, numbness, or tingling. He has no other joint pains. He is well appearing and in no acute distress. Spinal exam shows no deformities; however, he has limited lumbar flexion, tenderness over bilateral sacroiliac joints, and pain upon external rotation of the hip joints. His straight leg test is normal.

Evaluation/Tests	ESR and CRP are elevated. X-ray of the hip shows bilateral sacroiliitis, and anteroposterior (AP) radiograph of the spine shows early ossification of annulus fibrosus at multiple levels and squaring of vertebral bodies (bamboo spine).
Treatment	NSAIDs, physical therapy.
Discussion	Ankylosing spondylitis (AS), a spondyloarthropathy, is a chronic, multisystem inflammatory disorder involving the spine and sacroiliac (SI) joints and is associated with the *HLA-B27* gene. Clinical criteria to diagnose AS include: pain/stiffness >3 months, onset <45 years, sacroiliitis on X-ray, or *HLA-B27* plus at least two spondyloarthritis features (e.g., inflammatory back pain, arthritis, enthesitis, uveitis, dactylitis, IBD, psoriasis, elevated CRP). Initially, symptoms are generally unilateral and intermittent. However, with disease progression, pain and stiffness become more severe and constant. Characteristic features include bamboo spine (outer fibers of the intervertebral discs undergo ossification to form syndesmophytes). A stooped posture is characteristic of advanced-stage AS. Early diagnosis is important because early medical and physical therapy may improve symptoms and functional outcomes. Peripheral enthesitis, arthritis, and extra-articular involvement such as anterior uveitis, aortitis with aortic regurgitation, restrictive lung disease, pulmonary fibrosis, neurologic sequelae (cauda equina), or amyloidosis can occur. Elevation in ESR/CRP is not seen in **lumbar strain**, and patients with **inflammatory bowel disease** typically have gastrointestinal symptoms (e.g., diarrhea), while patients with **rheumatoid arthritis** have other joint involvement.

OTHER RHEUMATIC AND AUTOIMMUNE DISEASES

Rheumatic diseases can affect the bones, joints, muscles, skin, blood vessels, tendons, ligaments, and other connective tissues. They are inflammatory conditions that are often autoimmune. Patients can present with a constellation of symptoms including aches, pains, swelling, fatigue, malaise, stiffness, fever, and weight loss.

Key Findings and Rheumatologic/Autoimmune Condition Differential Diagnoses

Rheumatologic or Autoimmune Conditions with Key Associated Findings	Diagnosis
White, blue, or red color changes in digits precipitated by cold or stress	Raynaud's
Elderly woman with progressively worsening bilateral shoulder/hip pain and stiffness and elevated ESR	Polymyalgia rheumatica (PMR)
Elderly woman with PMR, temporal headache with visual changes, jaw claudication, tender temporal artery and elevated ESR	Temporal arteritis
Proximal muscle weakness, heliotrope and malar rash (involving nasolabial folds), shawl, and/or V sign rash on torso, Gottron's papules, "mechanic" hands	Dermatomyositis
Proximal muscle weakness, worsened with repetitive muscle use	Myasthenia gravis

(continued)

Key Findings and Rheumatologic/Autoimmune Condition Differential Diagnoses (*continued*)

Rheumatologic or Autoimmune Conditions with Key Associated Findings	Diagnosis
History of small cell lung cancer with proximal muscle weakness, diminished or absent reflexes and autonomic symptoms (orthostatic hypotension, dry mouth, erectile dysfunction). Weakness improves with repetitive muscle use.	Lambert-Eaton syndrome
Sicca (dry eyes and mouth)	Sjögren's syndrome
Calcinosis cutis, Raynaud's phenomenon, Esophageal dysmotility, sclerodactyly, and telangiectasias	Scleroderma (systemic sclerosis, CREST syndrome)
Female of childbearing age with malar rash (sparing the nasolabial fold), oral ulcers, arthritis, multiple affected organs, cytopenias and +ANA	Systemic lupus erythematosus (SLE)
SOB/cough and systemic symptoms, uveitis, erythema nodosum, and hilar adenopathy	Sarcoidosis

Useful Diagnostic Labs

Sjögren's syndrome	Positive anti-SSA (anti-Ro) and anti-SSB (anti-La)
Scleroderma	Diffuse systemic sclerosis: anti-scl-70 (anti-topoisomerase 1) CREST: anti-centromere antibody
PMR	ESR, CRP
RA	RF, ACPA
SLE	ANA, anti-dsDNA; anti-Smith (anti-Sm), low complements C3, C4 Drug-induced SLE: anti-histone
Mixed connective tissue disease	U1RNP
Autoimmune hepatitis	Anti-smooth muscle
Primary biliary cirrhosis	Anti-mitochondrial
Vasculitis	Granulomatosis with polyangiitis (GPA): c-ANCA Microscopic polyangiitis: p-ANCA
Polymyositis/dermatomyositis	Anti-Jo-1; anti-SRP, anti-Mi2
Lambert-Eaton myasthenic syndrome (LEMS)	Antibodies to presynaptic Ca++ channel (decreased Ach release)
Myasthenia gravis	Antibodies to postsynaptic Ach receptor

CASE 28 | Sjögren's Syndrome

A 50-year-old woman presents with an ongoing gritty/dry sensation in both of her eyes, dry mouth, generalized fatigue, and generalized joint pain for months. She has no known medical problems, and she is not on any medications. On exam, there is fullness of her parotid and submandibular glands and conjunctival injection. Her oral mucosa is dry, she has multiple dental caries, and her tongue appears lobulated, depapillated, and red.

Evaluation/Tests	Positive anti-SSA (anti-Ro) and anti-SSB (anti-La).
Treatment	Symptomatic relief with eye and mouth lubricants. Nonpharmacologic treatments are the mainstay and include exercise, physical therapy, sleep hygiene, cognitive behavior therapy, and antidepressants such as SNRIs and tricyclic antidepressants, as well as neuropathic pain agents such as gabapentin.
Discussion	Sjögren's syndrome is an autoimmune disease primarily affecting exocrine glands (lymphocytic infiltrates in the lacrimal and salivary glands) of middle-aged women characterized by sicca symptoms (dry eyes and mouth). It can be a primary disorder, or it can present with other autoimmune disorders (e.g., SLE, RA, hypothyroidism, scleroderma). Patients can have joint tenderness/swelling, scattered palpable purpura, conjunctival injection from dry eyes (keratoconjunctivitis: corneal damage from decreased tear production), and dry mouth (xerostomia). Complications include dental caries and non-Hodgkin's

CASE 28 | Sjögren's Syndrome (continued)

Discussion	lymphoma (primarily MALT lymphoma), which may present as parotid gland enlargement. Positive anti-SSA (anti-Ro) and anti-SSB (anti-La) support the diagnosis. ANA and RF antibodies may also be positive. ESR may be elevated, and cytopenias may be present. Schirmer test is useful to measure tear production. Biopsy of salivary glands can be helpful if the diagnosis is uncertain. Symptomatic treatment includes eye and mouth lubricants. Pilocarpine is a direct cholinergic agonist at muscarinic receptors, which results in increased secretion of exocrine glands. This increases salivation and ocular lubrication, which is useful in relieving the symptoms of Sjögren syndrome, but it may also increase sweating and increase muscle tone in GI and urinary tracts. **Anticholinergic medications** can also cause dry mouth and eyes but not the other symptoms in the vignette. **Fibromyalgia** is characterized by widespread noninflammatory skin and muscle pain, fatigue, and exercise intolerance; exam is normal except for widespread soft tissue/muscle tender points and sensitivity to light touch/palpation (allodynia).

CASE 29 | Scleroderma (Systemic Sclerosis)

A 44-year-old woman presents for evaluation of progressive skin tightness in her hands and face for several months. She also notes generalized aches, constipation, heartburn, mild difficulty swallowing and that her fingers change colors when exposed to the cold. On exam, her skin is shiny and tight distal to her MCP joints as well as on her face. She has difficulty opening her mouth fully and has scattered telangiectasias on her face. She has sclerodactyly, pits on her fingertips, and cutaneous calcium deposits on the hands (calcinosis cutis). Fine crackles are noted on lung exam.

Evaluation/ Tests	Anti-scl-70 and anticentromere antibody positive. Barium esophagram shows absent peristalsis with dilation of distal 2/3 of the esophagus.
Treatment	Treatment is largely focused on symptomatic relief, but immunosuppressive therapy may be used to decrease the progression of disease. ACE inhibitors are used for renal crisis, PPIs for GERD, and vasodilators for Raynaud's.
Discussion	Scleroderma is an autoimmune disease characterized by collagen deposition with fibrosis that affects the skin and other organs (lungs, kidneys, heart, and GI tract). Patients typically present with tight skin, but they may also have digital ulceration, calcinosis cutis, and telangiectasias. Microstomia (decreased ability to open mouth) also may be seen. Crackles and edema may be present if there is cardiac/pulmonary involvement. Almost all patients with systemic sclerosis experience **Raynaud's phenomenon**, which is described as color changes in the digits precipitated by cold or stress. If a patient is actively experiencing a vasospasm, then there may be a notable color change. Depending on the phase of the attack, digits may be white (ischemia), blue (hypoxia), or red (reperfusion). Digital ulceration and gangrene may be present. If idiopathic (primary), it is labeled as Raynaud disease. If secondary, it is called Raynaud syndrome. Subtypes of scleroderma include limited cutaneous (fingers and face) and diffuse cutaneous (widespread skin involvement). **CREST** (Calcinosis cutis, Raynaud's phenomenon, Esophageal dysmotility, Sclerodactyly, and Telangiectasias) syndrome is a limited cutaneous form of systemic sclerosis that this patient has. Labs may be positive for ANA, anti-scl-70 (generally associated with diffuse systemic sclerosis), and anticentromere antibody (generally associated with CREST syndrome).

CASE 30 | Systemic Lupus Erythematosus (SLE)

A 34-year-old woman presents with fatigue, headache, weight loss, intermittent fevers, and pain in her bilateral hands and knees for a few months. She has also noticed a rash on her cheeks and nose and discoloration of her hands when she goes out in the cold. On exam, temperature is 38°C, pulse is 90/min, and blood pressure is 146/82 mmHg. An erythematous rash on her cheeks and nose that spares the nasolabial fold, patchy erythema, and oral ulcers are noted. She has fine crackles in her posterior lung fields and mild hepatomegaly. There is mild swelling and tenderness of the knees and of the MCP and PIP joints of the hands bilaterally.

Evaluation/Tests	ANA, anti-dsDNA, and anti-Smith antibodies are present. ACPA, RF, and anti-smooth muscle antibodies are negative.

CASE 30 | Systemic Lupus Erythematosus (SLE) (continued)

Treatment	Antimalarials (hydroxychloroquine or chloroquine) are the first-line treatments. If the patient is unresponsive or has severe disease, steroids and other immunomodulating/immunosuppressive agents can be used.
Discussion	Systemic lupus erythematosus (SLE) is a relapsing, intermittent autoimmune disease seen predominantly in women of childbearing age. Patients will often come in with flares of the disease and then may have periods of quiescence. Virtually any organ can be involved in SLE, and diagnosis is based on clinical findings and autoantibody testing. Damage is mostly due to a type III hypersensitivity reaction which causes activation of complement (i.e., complements proteins get "used up," forming activated complexes that are harder for the body to clear). Therefore, the measured labs will show a decrease in complement protein (C1Q, C4, C2) levels. SLE should be suspected if more than two organs are involved, and it is diagnosed when >4 of 17 criteria from Systemic Lupus International Collaborating Clinics (SLICC) are met. These criteria include acute cutaneous lupus (malar rash); chronic cutaneous lupus (discoid rash with raised erythematous patches with scale); nonscarring alopecia; oral or nasal ulcers; joint disease; serositis (pericardial or pleural effusions, pericardial rub, or pericarditis on ECG); renal involvement; neurological involvement (seizures or psychosis); hemolytic anemia; lymphopenia or leukopenia; thrombocytopenia; ANA; anti-dsDNA antibodies; anti-Sm antibodies; antiphospholipid antibodies; low complement; and direct coombs. ANA is sensitive but not specific, while anti-dsDNA and anti-Sm antibodies are specific but not sensitive. **Dermatomyositis** is characterized by diffuse muscle weakness and a malar rash that extends beyond nasolabial folds. In **autoimmune hepatitis**, ANA and anti-smooth muscle antibodies are positive with an elevated IgG level.
Additional Considerations	Important complications of SLE include **Libman-Sacks endocarditis** (noninfectious thrombi on the mitral or aortic valve), nephritis, infections, and accelerated CAD. Most patients will be treated with antimalarials, and some will also receive steroids for acute exacerbations. Several B-cell-directed antibodies (e.g., belimumab) have also been approved for treatment. Specific treatments are often used for certain complications such as renal disease (e.g., cyclophosphamide or mycophenolate mofetil). **Antiphospholipid antibody (APLA) syndrome** is also associated with SLE, but APLA syndrome can occur independently. It should be considered in any young patient with unprovoked venous thromboembolism, anyone with an arterial thrombus, or any young person with renal disease and renal vein thrombosis. The classic presentation is a young woman with clots and multiple fetal losses. Antiphospholipid antibody, anticardiolipin and B2 glycoprotein titers, and aPT, PTT, and INR are typically elevated. Treatment with lifelong anticoagulation is indicated.

CASE 31 | Polymyalgia Rheumatica (PMR)

A 75-year-old woman is evaluated for progressively worsening shoulder and hip pain and stiffness bilaterally for several months. Stiffness is worse in the morning and lasts greater than 30 minutes. She has difficulty rising from a chair and combing her hair. She denies any weakness but reports some occasional fevers, malaise, and a recent 10-pound weight loss. Exam is notable for mild proximal joint swelling and reduced range of motion in the shoulders bilaterally. Upper and lower extremity strength and sensation are intact.

Evaluation/Tests	ESR and CRP are elevated. TSH and CK are normal. Anti-cyclic citrullinated peptide (APCA) and ANCA are negative.
Treatment	Low-dose corticosteroids.
Discussion	Polymyalgia rheumatica is an inflammatory condition characterized by pain and stiffness in the proximal muscles (neck, shoulders, and hips). Strength is preserved, but other systemic symptoms such as fever, fatigue, and weight loss may be present. It is more common in women >50 and has an association with **giant cell arteritis**. Diagnosis is made clinically and is supported by elevated ESR/CRP, TSH, CPK, RA, and APCA; other tests are helpful in ruling out other etiologies. Low-dose oral steroids are used initially for treatment. If **temporal arteritis** is suspected, urgent temporal biopsy and higher-dose steroids are indicated.

CASE 32 | Dermatomyositis

A 40-year-old woman reports generalized muscle weakness for months. She has difficulty rising from a chair, combing her hair, and climbing stairs. She denies any joint pain, but she has noticed a rash along her knuckles, eyes, upper neck, and back. On exam, she has symmetric proximal muscle weakness that is most prominent in the shoulders, hip, and neck. On skin exam, there is an erythematous/violaceous periorbital (heliotrope) rash, a malar rash involving the nasolabial folds, an upper back/shoulders/chest (shawl and "V" sign) rash, and an erythematous, scaly, papular rash (Gottron's papules) over bony areas on hands, elbows, and just below the knees, as well as "dirty" appearing marks on hands/fingertips (mechanic hands).

Evaluation/Tests	CK is elevated and anti-Jo-1, anti-SRP, and anti-Mi-2 Ab are present. Muscle biopsy shows perimysial inflammation with CD4+ T-cells.
Treatment	High-dose steroids followed by steroid-sparing agents (methotrexate, azathioprine, or mycophenolate mofetil).
Discussion	**Dermatomyositis** and **polymyositis** are examples of idiopathic, progressive, inflammatory myopathies. Both disorders are clinically similar with symmetrical proximal muscle weakness, but dermatomyositis has skin findings. Both are also associated with elevated muscle enzyme (CK, aldolase, LDH) levels and elevation in the following antibodies: ANA, anti-Jo-1, anti-SRP, and anti-Mi-2 Ab. In polymyositis, T-cell-mediated muscle fiber necrosis occurs while dermatomyositis is complement-mediated microangiopathy; complement activation damages muscle capillaries, resulting in necrosis and muscle fiber atrophy. Biopsy shows endomysial inflammation in polymyositis (CD8+ T-cells) and perimysial inflammation and atrophy in dermatomyositis (CD4). Both are associated with interstitial lung disease, and there is an increased risk for occult malignancy in dermatomyositis. It is important to consider other diagnoses, especially **muscular dystrophies**, when a patient presents with weakness. However, the characteristic skin finding makes other diagnoses less likely. Symptoms of **statin-induced myopathy** are similar to the other inflammatory myopathies, but patients will have a history of statin medication usage.

CASE 33 | Lambert-Eaton Myasthenic Syndrome (LEMS)

A 62-year-old man with a history of significant tobacco use presents with increasing weakness over several weeks. He initially noticed difficulty rising from a chair and climbing stairs, and now he notes shoulder weakness and lightheadedness with standing. He also reports chronic cough and unintentional weight loss. Exam is notable for orthostatic hypotension and proximal lower extremity weakness. His grip strength improves with repeated testing (Lambert sign). His deep tendon reflexes are diffusely diminished and absent in the ankles.

Evaluation/Tests	Clinical diagnosis with positive antibodies to voltage-gated calcium channels and confirmatory features on EMG. CT scan shows lung nodule that is concerning for cancer. CK level is normal.
Treatment	Treat underlying malignancy if found; otherwise: 3,4-diaminopyridine (3,4 DAP). Acetylcholinesterase inhibitors (pyridostigmine) can be added. If there is severe weakness, IVIG, in addition to immunosuppressive agents (steroids, azathioprine), can be tried.
Discussion	Lambert-Eaton syndrome is a paraneoplastic (associated with small cell lung cancer) autoimmune disorder characterized by autoantibodies to the presynaptic calcium ion channels. Patients present with proximal muscle weakness (typically in the legs, followed by arms), diminished or absent reflexes, and autonomic symptoms (orthostatic hypotension, dry mouth, and erectile dysfunction). Weakness often improves with repetitive muscle use. Antibodies to voltage-gated calcium channels may be present. CT scan should be done to diagnose occult malignancy (i.e., small cell lung cancer). The results of an edrophonium test will be negative. (Edrophonium allows for more acetylcholine in the neuromuscular junction, which makes acetylcholine more available to the receptors.) This test will be positive in myasthenia gravis. The underlying malignancy should be treated if found; otherwise: 3,4-diaminopyridine (3,4 DAP) is first line. **Myasthenia gravis** is characterized by the formation of autoantibodies to the postsynaptic AChR. Hallmarks of myasthenia gravis include ptosis, diplopia, and weakness that worsens with increased muscle use. The goal of treatment is to increase available ACh in the neuromuscular junction cleft, which can overcome the autoantibodies. Thus, use of the acetylcholinesterase inhibitor pyridostigmine is first line.

DERMATOLOGY

Common skin concerns include rashes, moles and growths, blisters, infections, and pigment changes (hyperpigmentation or depigmentation). When evaluating a patient with skin concerns, the following information should be elicited:

When, where, and how did it start?
Was it present since birth (congenital)?
Did individual lesions evolve/change or spread?
Is there itching, burning, bleeding, or pain?
Any associated fevers, rash, illness, or joint pains?
Are there any identifiable provoking or exacerbating factors?
Any previous episodes or treatment?
Any exposures to new products, medications, sun exposure, environmental, travel history?
Any significant personal history: systemic illnesses, atopic triad (asthma, allergies, atopic dermatitis), sunburns, radiation, or family history of skin conditions?

A physical examination of the entire body and joints should be performed and any findings—especially any suspicious characteristics—should be noted.

ABCDE's of a Suspicious Mole

A – Asymmetry
B – Borders irregular
C – Colors changing, or multiple colors in one lesion
D – Diameter >6 mm
E – Evolution of mole/change in mole as per patient

The following table describes basic morphologic descriptions of skin lesions.

Primary Skin Lesions—Terminology	Secondary Skin Lesions—Terminology
Macule: flat area of discoloration, <1 cm	**Scale:** dead, exfoliating (flaking) epidermal cells
Patch: flat area of discoloration, >1 cm	**Crust:** dried serum, blood, or purulent exudates that accumulates on the skin, e.g., scab
Papule: elevated solid area, <1 cm	**Erosion:** superficial loss of epidermis
Plaque: elevated solid area, >1 cm	**Excoriation:** linear erosion produced by scratching
Vesicle: elevated fluid-filled lesion, <1 cm	**Fissure:** linear split or crack of the skin from tension or lack of elasticity
Bullae: elevated fluid-filled lesion, >1 cm	**Ulcer:** loss of epidermis extending into the dermis
Pustule: elevated pus-filled lesion, <1 cm	**Lichenification:** thickening of epidermis with accentuation of normal skin markings
Nodule: elevated, hard, solid lesion, >1 cm	**Scar:** replacement of normal skin with fibrous tissue
Wheal: transient papule or plaque	**Atrophy:** thinning of skin

Additional Terminology	Characteristics
Cyst	Fluid-filled papule or nodule (Sac) with epithelial lining
Abscess	A localized pocket of pus, >1 cm
Purpura	red/purple, nonblanching lesion due to hemorrhage into the skin
Ecchymoses	Larger bruises
Petechiae	Small red, purple or brown macules, <2 mm, usually round
Telangiectasia	Blanchable dilated blood vessel

Differential Diagnoses for Skin Conditions

Bumps/Lesions			Rash			Pigmentation
Cancers	Not Cancer	Vascular	With Fever	Blister/ Bullae	No Fever	
Basal cell carcinoma Squamous cell carcinoma Melanoma Kaposi sarcoma Angiosarcoma **Premalignant:** Actinic keratosis Keratoacanthoma Sunburns	Acne rosacea Seborrheic keratosis Pseudofolliculitis barbae Herpes Molluscum contagiosum Verrucae/warts Dermatofibroma Erythema nodosum Hairy leukoplakia Epidermoid cysts Ganglion cysts Lipomas Xanthomas Melanocytic nevi Ephelis/ephelides (freckle(s))	Kaposi sarcoma Bacillary angiomatosis Cherry hemangioma Strawberry hemangioma Cystic hygroma Glomus tumor Pyogenic granuloma Angiosarcoma	Drug reaction Cellulitis Impetigo Erysipelas Abscess Necrotizing fasciitis Measles Mumps Rubella Rubeola Secondary syphilis Rocky mountain spotted fever Meningococcal meningitis	Bullous pemphigoid Pemphigus vulgaris Dermatitis herpetiformis Stevens-Johnson syndrome Erythema multiforme DRESS Staph-scalded skin syndrome Herpes Varicella zoster	Atopic dermatitis (eczema) Allergic contact dermatitis Seborrheic dermatitis Psoriasis Pityriasis rosea Lichen planus Dermatitis herpetiformis Tinea corporis/ capitis Scabies Urticaria Scleroderma Malar rash (SLE)	Albinism Melasma Vitiligo Acanthosis nigricans Tinea versicolor

Key Associated Findings and Skin Lesion(s) Differential Diagnoses

Skin Lesion(s) with Key Associated Findings	Diagnoses
Gritty/rough, scaly patch or plaque, usually pink/red (atypical keratinocytes)	Actinic keratosis (premalignant)
Persistent patch or plaque, usually pink/red, can bleed or ulcerate (keratin pearls)	Squamous cell carcinoma
Pink pearly papule with telangiectasia and a rolled border (palisading nuclei)	Basal cell carcinoma
Dark macule or patch, often with irregular borders, various colors, and history of the mole changing; can itch or bleed	Melanoma
Sharply demarcated, well circumscribed, hyperpigmented lesion with a waxy texture and appears to be "stuck on"	Seborrheic keratosis
Untreated HIV/AIDS patient with multiple red-violaceous macules and papules on back and legs	Kaposi sarcoma Bacillary angiomatosis (bitten by a cat)

(continued)

Key Associated Findings and Skin Lesion(s) Differential Diagnoses (continued)

Skin Lesion(s) with Key Associated Findings	Diagnoses
Teenager with open and closed comedones and erythematous papules and pustules scattered in the T-zone (on the face), upper back, and chest	Acne
Fair-skinned adult with flushing aggravated by alcohol, with erythematous papular/pustular lesions with telangiectasias without comedones extending beyond nasolabial folds	Rosacea
Erythematous patches on both cheeks and bridge of the nose, sparing the nasolabial folds in a butterfly pattern	Malar rash (SLE)
Hyperpigmented tan patches on cheeks in a pregnant woman	Melasma
Razor bumps	Pseudofolliculitis barbae
Recurrent blisters on lip associated with tingling	Herpes simplex
Multiple flesh-colored papules with central umbilication (dimple in the center) in clusters	Molluscum contagiosum
Cauliflower-like lesions	Verruca (warts)
Diabetic or obese patient with dark velvety discoloration noted in the folds of the neck and axilla	Acanthosis nigricans
Large, tense blisters and bullae over bilateral legs, thighs, groin, and abdomen. When the skin surrounding the lesion is pulled laterally, there is no separation of the epidermis or creation of an erosion (negative Nikolsky sign)	Bullous pemphigoid
Tugging skin with lateral traction induces exfoliation of outer layer or necrosis/blister formation (positive Nikolsky sign)	SJS-TENS Pemphigus vulgaris Staphylococcal-scalded skin syndrome
Multiple types of lesions (macules, papules, target lesions) associated with drugs (sulfa, B-lactams, phenytoin), infections (HSV, mycoplasma pneumoniae), autoimmune disease or cancer	Erythema multiforme
Intensely pruritic vesicles in groups (usually on elbows) seen in patients with celiac disease	Dermatitis herpetiformis
Infection of the skin that involves the deeper dermis and subcutaneous fat	Cellulitis
Infection usually confined to superficial layers of skin with more distinct demarcation	Erysipelas
Kids with maculopapular, erythematous lesions with overlying honey-colored crust and pustules	Impetigo
Swollen erythematous fluctuant area with purulent drainage	Abscess
Dandruff and scaly, erythematous patches on eyebrows and nasolabial folds	Seborrheic dermatitis
Atopic individual with recurring pruritic rash on neck, arms, and legs	Atopic dermatitis (eczema)
Erythematous "silvery-scaled" plaques on extensor surfaces and may be associated with arthritis	Psoriasis
3-cm well demarcated salmon-colored lesion (Herald's patch) precedes multiple small erythematous plaques with collarette scales, in a "Christmas tree" distribution on the trunk	Pityriasis rosea
Lacy (reticular) whitish lines on buccal mucosa (Wickham's striae) and rash on flexor surface of wrists, forearms, and legs with grouped pink-purplish, polygonal, flat-topped (planar), pruritic papules and plaques	Lichen planus

RAISED SKIN LESIONS

CASE 34 | Acne Vulgaris

A 14-year-old girl presents with concerns about bumps all over the face, especially over the forehead, nose, and cheeks. Exam is notable for open and closed comedones and erythematous papules and pustules scattered on the central face, forehead, upper back, and chest.

Evaluation/Tests	Clinical diagnosis.
Treatment	Treatment for mild disease includes topical medications: benzoyl peroxide, salicylic acid, azelaic acid, or topical antibacterials (clindamycin, erythromycin or dapsone) and retinoic acid. For more moderate disease with inflammation, oral antibiotics such as the tetracyclines are used, and for severe cases, oral retinoids may be used.
Discussion	Acne vulgaris affects the majority of young people, particularly after they reach puberty and can continue into adulthood. The etiology is multifactorial. Excess sebum from hormonal stimulation can block pilosebaceous follicles, causing the formation of closed (whiteheads) or open (blackheads) comedones. *Cutibacterium acnes* (formerly *Propionibacterium acnes*) can cause inflammation resulting in pustules/papules. Some may develop large inflammatory cysts

A, Acne vulgaris showing papulonodular lesions along with areas of scarring on the face. B, Acne. Papules, pustules, and open comedones.
Part A reproduced with permission from Kelly AP, Taylor SC, Lom HW, et al: Taylor and Kelly's Dermatologyfor Skin of Color, 2nd ed. New York, NY: McGraw Hill; 2016. Part B reproduced with permission from Soutor C, Hordinsky MK: Clinical Dermatology. New York, NY: McGraw Hill; 2013.

and nodules, which may lead to significant scarring. Endocrine diseases and medications such as steroids, oral contraceptives, phenytoin, and phenobarbital can also cause acne.

Rosacea might occur similarly but typically occurs on the face of middle-aged, fair-skinned adults and is associated with flushing, which can be aggravated by alcohol or other stimuli. Lesions are erythematous papules/pustules, with telangiectasias but without comedones; they respond to treatment with topical metronidazole or oral tetracyclines for severe disease. Connective tissue overgrowth, especially of the nose (rhinophyma), can occur.

A, Erythematotelangiectatic rosacea. Erythema on nose, cheeks, and chin with telangiectasia and a few small papules. B, Malar rash of systemic lupus erythematosus. C, Pseudofolliculitis barbae. Multiple perifollicular papules in beard of an African-American patient due to curved hair fibers reentering the skin.
Part A and C reproduced with permission from Soutor C, Hordinsky MK: Clinical Dermatology. New York, NY: McGraw Hill; 2013. Part B reproduced with permission from Imboden JB, Hellmann DB, Stone JH: Current Diagnosis & Treatment: Rheumatology, 3rd ed. New York, NY: McGraw Hill; 2013.

CASE 34 | Acne Vulgaris *(continued)*

Additional Considerations	**Malar rash** is seen in patients with SLE and is characterized by erythematous patches on both cheeks and the bridge of the nose, sparing the nasolabial folds in a butterfly pattern. **Pseudofolliculitis barbae** typically happens in areas that are shaved and is related to curving of the hair follicles beneath the skin, causing a foreign-body reaction and inflammation. Secondary infection with *Staphylococcus aureus* is common. The treatment is allowing the hair to get long enough to prevent it from curling back into the skin.

CASE 35 | *Herpes Simplex* Virus Skin Infection

A 19-year-old woman comes in with painful bumps along the side of her lip. She has been feeling poorly with fevers and malaise and has had some tingling and burning sensation prior to the development of the rash. On exam, temperature is 37.7°C. There are multiple papular and vesicular lesions on an erythematous base on her upper lip and face. She also has painful anterior cervical and submandibular lymphadenopathy.

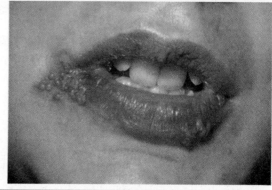

Herpes simplex on lips and oral commissure. Grouped vesicles.
Reproduced with permission from Soutor C, Hordinsky MK: Clinical Dermatology. New York, NY: McGraw Hill; 2013.

Evaluation/Tests	Clinical diagnosis, with viral culture, PCR testing for HSV DNA, or Tzanck smear showing multinucleated giant cells, can be confirmatory tests.
Treatment	Treat with antivirals such as acyclovir, famciclovir, and valacyclovir that help reduce severity and shedding. For recurrent disease, patients can receive chronic suppressive treatment as well.
Discussion	HSV skin infections can occur anywhere but are often seen on mucosal surfaces. Oral-labial lesions typically occur due to HSV-1 and genital lesions due to HSV-2. Herpetic whitlow is a lesion on the finger. Primary infection occurs from direct contact and tends to be more severe. Patients may present with a prodrome (fevers, malaise, lymphadenopathy and tingling, numbness, burning, and pain in the affected area). Recurrent episodes tend to be milder than initial infection. **Impetigo** is a bacterial infection due to *Staph.* or *Strep.* species. Thelesions typically have an overlying honey-colored crust. **Varicella** zoster can also present with vesicles, but HSV-1 typically causes cold sores.
Additional Considerations	**Verruca (warts)** are cauliflower-like lesions caused by HPV. **Molluscum contagiosum** is caused by a *Poxvirus*. It is common in children but can be sexually transmitted in adults and is more severe in immunosuppressed patients (HIV). It is characterized by multiple 2- to 5-mm flesh-colored papules with central umbilication (dimple in the center) in clusters. It's diagnosed clinically, but if a biopsy is taken, histology shows cytoplasmic inclusion bodies (molluscum bodies). Lesions will eventually resolve or can be treated with cryotherapy and curettage or topical agents. 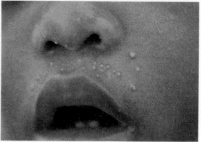 Molluscum contagiosum on face. 1 to 2 mm dome-shaped papules. Reproduced with permission from Soutor C, Hordinsky MK: Clinical Dermatology. New York, NY: McGraw Hill; 2013.

CASE 36 | Seborrheic Keratosis

A 56-year-old man presents for evaluation of a long-standing skin lesion on his back. It is not itchy or painful. Exam shows a sharply demarcated, well-circumscribed, hyperpigmented lesion with a waxy texture and appears to be "stuck on."

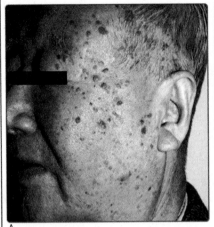

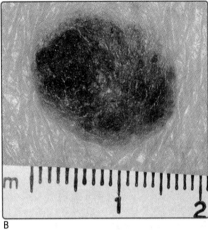

A, Multiple small seborrheic keratoses. B, Seborrheic keratosis showing a rough surface and stuck-on appearance.
Reproduced with permission from Kang S, Amagai M, Bruckner AL, et al: Fitzpatrick's Dermatology, 9th ed. New York, NY: McGraw Hill; 2019.

Evaluation/Tests	Clinical diagnosis.
Treatment	No treatment needed. Can be excised if it bothers the patient.
Discussion	Seborrheic keratoses are common, benign, pigmented neoplasms that give a well-demarcated, stuck-on appearing lesion. They are caused by proliferation of epidermal keratinocytes with hyperkeratosis, papillomatosis, and pseudohorn cysts. No biopsy or further testing is indicated as the diagnosis is made by history and exam. Biopsy may be done to rule out other causes. No treatment is needed, but it can be excised if it bothers the patient. **Leser-Trelat sign** is the sudden appearance of numerous lesions, which can indicate underlying neoplasm. **Melanocytic nevi (common mole)** are benign, usually less than 6 mm, uniformly pigmented, and well-defined with rounded borders. They are subcategorized and clinically differ based on location of cells: epidermal flat macules (junctional); raised papules in the dermis (intradermal) or both areas (compound).

CASE 37 | Kaposi Sarcoma (KS)

A 29-year-old man presents for evaluation of multiple enlarging, purplish lesions. They are not itchy or painful. He is sexually active with men and uses inconsistent protection. He also has unintentional weight loss, fatigue, and fevers. On exam, he has a temperature of 38°C, a few scattered purplish macules on his palate, and generalized lymphadenopathy of cervical and inguinal chains. On skin exam, there are multiple red-violaceous macules and papules on his back and legs with patches and plaques.

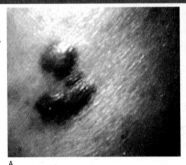

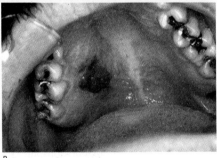

A, Kaposi sarcoma in an AIDS patient. B, Involvement of oral cavity in AIDS patient with Kaposi sarcoma.
Reproduced with permission from Stern S, Cifu AS, Altkorn D: Symptom to Diagnosis: An Evidence-Based Guide, 4th ed. New York, NY: McGraw Hill; 2020.

Evaluation/Tests	Biopsy shows predominantly spindle cells and dilated capillaries, usually HIV positive, can confirm exposure to human herpesvirus 8 (HHV-8) by antibody testing.
Treatment	HAART and local treatment (surgery, radiation, cryotherapy, intralesional, or topical treatment) or systemic chemotherapy for more widespread disease.

CASE 37 | Kaposi Sarcoma (KS) (continued)

Discussion	Kaposi sarcoma is a human herpesvirus 8 (HHV-8)–associated malignancy typically involving the skin, GI, or respiratory tracts. Risk factors include immunosuppression. The lesions typically start as macules and patches. They can progress to papules, plaques, and ultimately to nodules or tumors. They tend to be purplish, reddish, or dark brown/black depending upon the patient's skin tone. **Bacillary angiomatosis** is caused by Bartonella infections (cat-scratch disease) and typically occurs in advanced HIV disease. The papules and nodules look like angiomas: bright red, violaceous, or skin-colored. They can grow up to 3 cm, and they can have thinning, erosions, and ulcerations. Biopsy and/or culture help with diagnosis. Treatment includes antibiotics (macrolide or doxycycline) and HAART if HIV positive.
Additional Considerations	**Cherry hemangiomas** are benign, occur in the elderly, and may increase with age. **Strawberry hemangioma** are benign, are seen in infants, but regress over time.

CASE 38 | Hairy Leukoplakia

A 54-year-old male with HIV, not on HAART, presents with 2 weeks of white painless patches on his tongue. Oropharyngeal exam reveals bilateral white patches on the lateral tongue, which cannot be scraped off.

Evaluation/Tests	Clinical diagnosis; can be confirmed with biopsy.
Treatment	Not required, but HAART and acyclovir may help.
Discussion	Hairy leukoplakia is due to Epstein-Barr virus (EBV) infection, which is also the cause of infectious mononucleosis and Burkitt lymphoma. It typically occurs in immunocompromised patients. **Oral leukoplakia** can also present as white patches/plaques that cannot be scraped off. Risk factors include tobacco or alcohol use. It can develop into squamous cell carcinoma over time, in contrast to hairy leukoplakia which does not lead to malignancy.
Additional Considerations	**Oropharyngeal candidiasis** can also present with white patches/plaques on the tongue in a patient who is immunocompromised or using certain medications, such as inhaled steroids. These lesions can be scraped off, and diagnosis can be confirmed with potassium hydroxide prep.

CASE 39 | Actinic Keratosis

A 67-year-old man with significant sun exposure presents for evaluation of a skin lesion. Exam is notable for a 4.5-mm gritty/rough papule with an erythematous base that is covered with white-yellow scale on the dorsum of his left hand. On palpation, it has a rough, sandpaper-like consistency.

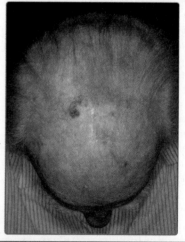

Field cancerization. There are several ill-defined erythematous and scaly plaques, crusts, and ulcerations affecting a large area ("field") of the balding scalp. Further alterations, such as mottled hypopigmentation and hyperpigmentation, are present and indicate actinic damage.
Reproduced with permission from Kang S, Amagai M, Bruckner AL, et al: Fitzpatrick's Dermatology, 9th ed. New York, NY: McGraw Hill; 2019.

Evaluation/ Tests	Clinical diagnosis. Biopsy would show atypical keratinocytes that do not invade the dermis.
Treatment	Cryotherapy, topical agents (5-FU, imiquimod), phototherapy, or dermabrasion.
Discussion	Actinic keratoses are precursor lesions tosquamous cell carcinoma. Cumulative UV exposure is the most common risk factor in lesion development, but fair skin, age, and immunosuppression also contribute. **SCC** is typically a persistent patch or plaque, is usually pink/red, can bleed or ulcerate, and typically grows rapidly (>1 cm). **BCC** is typically a pink, waxy, pearly nodule with rolled borders and telangiectasias on sun-exposed areas.

CASE 39 | Actinic Keratosis *(continued)*

Additional Considerations	**Psoriasis** is characterized by plaques with silvery scales on extensor surfaces (knees, elbows) and may be associated with nail pitting and arthritis. 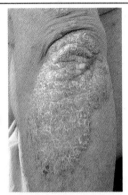 Psoriasis. Pink, well-demarcated plaque with silvery scale on elbow is a characteristic finding. Reproduced with permission from Soutor C, Hordinsky MK: Clinical Dermatology. New York, NY: McGraw Hill; 2013.

CASE 40 | Squamous Cell Carcinoma (SCC) of the Skin

A 65-year-old man with a history of a renal transplant presents for evaluation of a rapidly growing, firm bump on his lower lip. He was an archeologist until he retired a year ago. Exam is notable for an ulcerated erythematous nodule that is 3 cm in diameter.

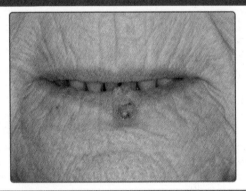

Hyperkeratotic squamous cell carcinoma located centrally on the lower lip.
Reproduced with permission from Kang S, Amagai M, Bruckner AL, et al: Fitzpatrick's Dermatology, 9th ed. New York, NY: McGraw Hill; 2019.

Evaluation/Tests	Excisional biopsies will show keratin pearls.
Treatment	Treatment depends upon tumor site, size, depth, and histological features, as well as the patient's comorbidities and ability to tolerate treatment. Surgical excision or Mohs surgery (thin slices taken and examined under microscope) are treatment options.
Discussion	Squamous cell carcinoma occurs most commonly in sun-exposed areas, particularly on the head and neck. Lesions are often irregular, with scaling and ulcerations. Despite its increased propensity for local invasion and spread to regional lymph nodes, SCC rarely progresses to distant metastases, and typically can be managed surgically. Cumulative sun exposure is a higher risk than the early sunburns associated with basal cell carcinoma (BCC) and melanoma. Risk factors also include immunosuppression and chronically draining sinuses. Lesions are a persistent patch or plaque, usually pink/red, which can bleed or ulcerate. They grow rapidly, are >1 cm, and are usually locally invasive but may spread to LN. They rarely metastasize. SCCs more often affect the lower lip, and **BCCs** more often affect the upper lip. Telangiectasias are uncommon (unlike in BCC), and there is often keratosis on the lesion. **Keratoacanthoma** is a rapidly growing variant of SCC that may spontaneously regress.

CASE 41 | Basal Cell Carcinoma (BCC)

A 75-year-old man comes in for a bump on his face. He recalls multiple severe sunburns as a child. On exam, there is a pink, waxy, pearly, ulcerated nodule with rolled borders and telangiectasias.

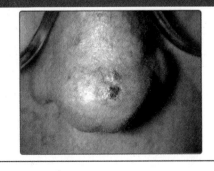

Basal cell carcinoma, nodular type.
Reproduced with permission from Kang S, Amagai M, Bruckner AL, et al: Fitzpatrick's Dermatology, 9th ed. New York, NY: McGraw Hill; 2019.

CASE 41 | Basal Cell Carcinoma (BCC) *(continued)*

Evaluation/Tests	Skin biopsy showing palisading nuclei.
Treatment	Surgical excision, Mohs micrographic surgery, topical or intralesional therapy, radiation, or electrodissection and curettage.
Discussion	There are five histological types of BCC tumors. The two most common are nodular and superficial. Nodular are the pink- or flesh-colored nodules that often have telangiectasias, may have ulceration, and have a "rolled" border where they are higher on the sides than in the middle. They are most typically found on the face and head. The superficial type is more commonly on the trunk, may have a scale, and tends to be flatter. BCCs are more commonly seen in Caucasian elderly men with significant sun exposure.

CASE 42 | Melanoma

A 44-year-old woman comes in for evaluation of a "mole" on her leg. She noticed it a few months ago while shaving. It occasionally bleeds, itches, and has grown in size. She recalls multiple severe sunburns as a child. On exam, she is a red-headed woman with fair complexion and multiple nevi on the skin. On her leg, there is a dark patch with irregular borders and various colors that measures 1.2 cm in diameter.

Evaluation/Tests	Full-thickness excisional biopsy shows atypical melanocytes and architectural disorder.
Treatment	Excision, chemotherapy, radiation; immunotherapy (nivolumab) for metastasis or recurrence.
Discussion	

A
B

A, Dermatoscopic image of a malignant melanoma showing an atypical pigment network, structural asymmetry, a white veil, and regression changes. B, Advanced acral melanoma. Irregular patch with central verrucous nodule on the heel of a foot.
Part A reproduced with permission from Soutor C, Hordinsky MK: Clinical Dermatology. New York, NY: McGraw Hill; 2013.
Part B reproduced with permission from Kelly AP, Taylor SC, Lom HW, et al: Taylor and Kelly's Dermatology for Skin of Color, 2nd ed. New York, NY: McGraw Hill; 2016.

Malignant melanoma is the most aggressive and deadly form of skin cancer.
Those restricted to the epidermis are in the radial growth phase, the subtypes of which are lentigo maligna, superficial spreading and acral/mucosal lentiginous (more common in darker skinned patients). Those with only a vertical growth phase have invaded downward into the dermis and are termed nodular melanomas. Risk factors include: fair complexion, red/blond hair, light eye color, many common nevi, or atypical melanocytic nevi. Visual exam with ABCDE criteria assists in identifying high-risk lesions requiring biopsy. Common/melanocytic nevi can be difficult to differentiate without biopsy. In some cases, other additional considerations include pigmented BCC and seborrheic keratosis. Wide excision down to the deep fascia with a margin of normal tissue surrounding the lesion is indicated to decrease local recurrence. Immunotherapy is the backbone of treatment in stage 3 and 4 disease because it offers the most potential for long-term durable responses. The presence of a BRAF mutation allows for treatment with targeted BRAF inhibitors such as dabrafenib, trametinib, and vemurafenib.

SKIN PIGMENT CHANGES

Complete lack of pigment is albinism. When the loss of pigment is patchy and progressive, it is called vitiligo. Hyperpigmentation of the face in pregnant women is called melasma. Acanthosis nigricans is hyperpigmentation usually seen in the axillae and neck, and it is associated with insulin resistance. Hyperpigmentation can also be postinflammatory.

CASE 43 | Vitiligo

A 25-year-old woman with Graves's disease presents with diffuse, white patches on multiple parts of her body for several months. Exam shows discrete white macules/patches on the skin exhibiting depigmentation. There are no associated signs of inflammation.

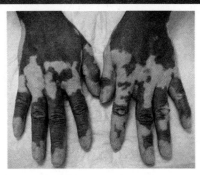

Vitiligo on dorsum of hands.
Reproduced with permission from Soutor C, Hordinsky MK: Clinical Dermatology. New York, NY: McGraw Hill; 2013.

Evaluation/Tests	Clinical diagnosis.
Treatment	Topical corticosteroids for limited disease. If vitiligo is extensive, UV light therapy can be a treatment option.
Discussion	Depigmentation can occur anywhere, but it is commonly seen on the face, around the genitals, and on the hands. Depigmentation is believed to be secondary to autoimmune destruction of melanocytes. Vitiligo has been associated with autoimmune diseases such as type 1 diabetes, Graves's disease, and Hashimoto's thyroiditis. **Tinea versicolor** is caused by yeast (*Malassezia furfur*) in hot, sweaty conditions. Patches vary in color, typically occur on the back/chest, and can be hyperpigmented/pink/yellow or hypopigmented with associated scale.
Additional Considerations	**Albinism** is a genetic disorder of decreased production of melanin due to decreased tyrosinase activity or defective tyrosine transport. Patients are at increased risk for skin cancer.

CASE 44 | Acanthosis Nigricans

A 54-year-old obese woman with T2DM presents with skin darkening on some parts of her body for several years. Lesions are not painful or itchy, but they have become more noticeable with time. On exam, there is dark velvety discoloration noted in the folds of her neck and axilla.

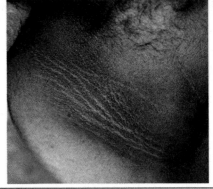

Acanthosis nigricans. Hyperpigmented, velvet-like plaques on lateral neck of a patient with diabetes mellitus.
Reproduced with permission from Soutor C, Hordinsky MK: Clinical Dermatology. New York, NY: McGraw Hill; 2013.

Evaluation/Tests	Clinical diagnosis.
Treatment	Weight loss and improved blood glucose control.
Discussion	Acanthosis nigricans is common in obese patients (due to insulin resistance without frank diabetes) and in diabetic patients. Acanthosis nigricans in a nondiabetic or obese patient can be associated with an underlying adenocarcinoma, usually in the GI or GU tract. **Candidiasis** occurs in skin folds, usually a moist environment such as underneath breasts or between the leg creases. The rash is erythematous (not hyperpigmented) and scaly, and it can be itchy and sometimes painful.
Additional Considerations	**Melasma**, also known as chloasma or mask of pregnancy, is an acquired hyperpigmentation on sun-exposed areas, often limited to the face, primarily in women. It has an increased incidence in pregnancy and with oral contraceptive pill (OCP) use. **Postinflammatory hyperpigmentation** is skin darkening in the area of a prior rash/lesion (such as a pimple) and can occur anywhere on the body.

BLISTERS

The differential diagnosis for blisters or bullae includes bullous pemphigoid, pemphigus vulgaris, Stevens-Johnson syndrome (SJS), and toxic epidermal necrolysis (TEN). The history will most often involve a newly started medication. Bullous pemphigoid occurs in older patients. Pemphigus vulgaris can be paraneoplastic, and there is shearing when pushing on the skin adjacent to the bullae (Nikolsky sign). SJS and TEN are a spectrum of the same disease that are determined by the amount of body surface involved. They will have macules, papules, and skin sloughing/peeling with systemic symptoms and involvement of the oral mucosa preceding the skin lesions.

CASE 45 | Bullous Pemphigoid

A 72-year-old man with hypertension presents for evaluation of a blistering rash. When the lesions first started, they were itchy; now they are tender to touch. He was recently started on furosemide for his blood pressure. On exam, he is afebrile and appears uncomfortable. He has large, tense blisters, and bullae over his bilateral legs, thighs, groin, and abdomen. When the skin surrounding the lesion is pulled laterally, there is no separation of the epidermis or creation of an erosion (negative Nikolsky sign). No lesions are noted on the palate or buccal mucosa.

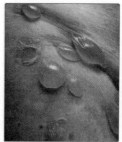 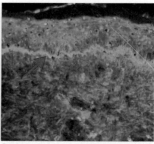

Bullous pemphigoid. A, Large, tense bullae, some of which are denuded on the upper leg.
A. Reproduced with permission from Kang S, Amagai M, Bruckner AL, et al: Fitzpatrick's Dermatology, 9th ed. New York, NY: McGraw Hill; 2019. B, Used with permission from Emmanuelm/Wikimedia Commons.

A   B

Evaluation/Tests	Skin biopsy shows subepidermal bulla with increased eosinophils and lymphocytes in the papillary dermis. Immunofluorescence staining shows a linear pattern at the epidermal–dermal junction.
Treatment	Remove the offending agent and start corticosteroids.
Discussion	Bullous pemphigoid is an autoimmune bullous disorder involving IgG antibodies against hemidesmosomes (epidermal basement membrane) and is a type II hypersensitivity reaction. It usually presents in older adults with comorbid conditions (e.g., T2DM, HTN), and blisters may be precipitated by a new drug (e.g., furosemide, NSAIDs, penicillin). Oral mucosa is often spared. **Pemphigus vulgaris** also presents in older adults and is also a type II hypersensitivity reaction. However, oropharyngeal lesions and a positive Nikolsky sign are seen. Triggers include ACE-I, phenobarbital, and penicillamine. It is caused by antibodies against desmoglein (responsible for keratinocyte adhesion). Skin biopsy shows intraepidermal vesicle formation due to loss of cohesion between epidermal cells (i.e., acantholytic lesions). Direct immunofluorescence microscopy shows IgG deposition on keratinocytes. Antibodies to desmoglein 1 and/or 3 are present.
Additional Considerations	**Erythema multiforme** presents with multiple types of lesions (macules, papules, target lesions) and can be associated with drugs (sulfa, B-lactams, phenytoin), infections (HSV, *Mycoplasma* pneumonia), autoimmune disease, or cancer. **Dermatitis herpetiformis** has smaller blisters (papules or vesicles) in groups (usually on elbows), is intensely itchy, and is seen in patients with celiac disease. 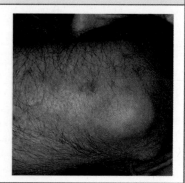 Dermatitis herpetiformis. Excoriated erosions on elbow and forearm. Reproduced with permission from Soutor C, Hordinsky MK: Clinical Dermatology. New York, NY: McGraw Hill; 2013.

CASE 46 | Stevens-Johnson Syndrome (SJS)

A 25-year-old man presents with fever and a progressively worsening, painful, blistering rash over his trunk and lips. He also reports fatigue, burning eyes, and a sore throat and mouth. He was started on lamotrigine for seizures about 3 weeks ago. The patient's temperature is 37.8°C, pulse is 115/min, blood pressure is100/65 mmHg, respirations are16/min, and O_2 saturation is 96% on room air. Skin exam shows erythematous macules, papules, and some targetoid lesions on the face, trunk, and back that are sloughing. When the skin surrounding the lesion is pulled laterally, there is separation of the epidermis and creation of an erosion (positive Nikolsky sign). There are hemorrhagic crusting lesions on the lips, and bullae and erosions are noted on the oral and genital mucosa. The lesions are tender to palpation. Bilateral conjunctivitis is noted. Less than 10% of her body surface area is affected.

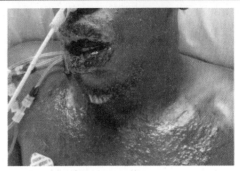

Stevens-Johnson syndrome (SJS).
Reproduced with permission from Jameson JL, Fauci AS, Kasper DL, et al: Harrison's Principles of Internal Medicine, 20th ed. New York, NY: McGraw Hill; 2018.

Evaluation/Tests	Clinical diagnosis. Biopsy can be done to confirm the diagnosis or rule out other causes. Depending on the stage of illness, a biopsy may show T-cell-mediated apoptosis of keratinocytes of the basal layer of the epidermis to full-thickness necrosis of the epidermis.
Treatment	Admit to the hospital and initiate aggressive supportive care, potentially in a burn unit
Discussion	Stevens-Johnson syndrome (SJS) is a severe, life-threatening, blistering mucocutaneous syndrome involving at least two mucous membranes. TEN is a more extensive form of SJS where >30% of the body surface area is affected. Both are usually associated with an adverse drug reaction (e.g., NSAIDs, antiepileptics, sulfa drugs, penicillin), exposure to which can occur 7–28 days from the onset of rash. **Staphylococcal scalded skin syndrome (SSSS)** is characterized by fever and an erythematous rash with sloughing of the upper layers of the epidermis and +Nikolsky sign. Biopsy shows destruction of keratinocyte attachments in the stratum granulosum. **Drug reaction with eosinophilia and systemic symptoms (DRESS)** is a hypersensitivity syndrome that is drug-induced and presents with systemic symptoms and at times eosinophilia. Patients may present with a morbilliform rash, high fever, lymphadenopathy, eosinophilia, LFT abnormalities, and inflammation of one or more internal organs. It typically presents 2–8 weeks after starting the responsible medication (e.g., carbamazepine, phenobarbital, phenytoin, allopurinol, olanzapine, and sulfa drugs).
Additional Considerations	**Erythema multiforme** presents with macules, papules, vesicles, and target lesions (rings with dusky red center) in a symmetric pattern on the distal extremities. It is associated most commonly with infections (e.g., mycoplasma, HSV). Other causes include drugs (e.g., sulfa drugs, beta-lactams, phenytoin), cancer, or autoimmune disease, and Nikolsky sign is negative.

RASH WITH FEVER

Drug reactions can lead to a maculopapular rash and a fever, often 7–10 days after the start of a medication. Bacterial infections can also present with a fever and rash. Impetigo is highly contagious, common around the mouths of kids, and causes sores with honey-colored crusting. Cellulitis involves the deep dermis and subcutaneous fat, in comparison to erysipelas, which involves the upper dermis and lymphatics, causing lymphangitic streaking and a more definite border on exam. Necrotizing fasciitis involves the deep soft tissues, including the muscles and subcutaneous fat, and clinically gives "pain out of proportion to their exam," as well as systemic symptoms and sepsis. Abscesses are painful, warm, and fluctuant, with surrounding erythema and purulence.

CASE 47 | Cellulitis

A 52-year-old woman with T2DM presents with worsening erythema of her right foot and leg for the past 2 days. Her symptoms started after she scraped her foot against a table. Patient's temperature is 38.3°C, pulse is 90/min, and blood pressure is 128/70 mmHg. Her right foot is warm, tender, swollen, and erythematous with poorly demarcated margins.

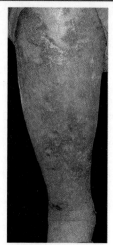

Cellulitis on leg of diabetic patient. Warm tender areas of erythema on foot and leg.
Reproduced with permission from Soutor C, Hordinsky MK: Clinical Dermatology. New York, NY: McGraw Hill; 2013.

Evaluation/Tests	Clinical diagnosis.
Treatment	Antibiotics targeting *Staph.* and *Strep.* species with consideration for community-acquired MRSA.
Discussion	Cellulitis is an infection of the skin that involves the deeper dermis and subcutaneous tissue. Common pathogens include *S. pyogenes* and *S. aureus*. Risk factors include DM, peripheral vascular disease, venous insufficiency, and breaks in the skin from trauma, bites, or tinea pedis. **Stasis dermatitis** is a noninfectious inflammation of the skin of the lower legs caused by chronic venous insufficiency, so it should occur without fever and with signs of chronic venous stasis, such as hyperpigmentation. **DVT** often presents with more diffuse redness, pain, and unilateral swelling without systemic signs of infection. **Necrotizing fasciitis** is characterized by pain out of proportion to exam, signs of necrosis, rapid progression, and systemic signs. **Contact dermatitis** is due to an exposure. **Erysipelas** is usually confined to superficial layers of skin with more distinct demarcation.
Additional Considerations	**Abscesses** are collections of pus within deeper layers of skin tissue, most often due to *S. aureus* infection. Abscesses arise from the dermis or subcutaneous tissue. Risk factors for developing an abscess include a break in the skin barrier, peripheral vascular disease, and diabetes. Labs may show nonspecific findings such as leukocytosis. Ultrasound may be helpful to determine if an abscess is present. Treatment is incision and drainage with culture of the purulent material to guide antibiotic therapy if warranted. If cultures are not available, prescribed antibiotics should cover methicillin-resistant *S. aureus* (MRSA). **Impetigo** is a contagious superficial skin infection and is often treated with topical mupirocin. If the infection is extensive, add oral antibiotics to cover common skin pathogens (*S. aureus* and *S. pyogenes*). Impetigo. Reproduced with permission from Stern S, Cifu AS, Altkorn D: Symptom to Diagnosis: An Evidence-Based Guide, 4th ed. New York, NY: McGraw Hill; 2020. **Bullous impetigo** has bullae and is usually due to staphylococcus, and it can progress to staphylococcal scalded skin syndrome.

CASE 48 | Necrotizing Fasciitis

A 63-year-old man with T2DM and alcohol abuse presents with severe foot pain and redness of his foot after stepping on a nail. Initially, he had severe pain followed by rapidly spreading redness. Though his pain has improved slightly, he now has numbness and fevers. He received his tetanus shot last year. Temperature is 38.9°C, pulse is 110/min, and blood pressure is 90/50 mmHg. The patient is not fully alert and is writhing in pain. His foot and leg are erythematous and swollen with a dusky purplish appearance near the puncture site. He also has blisters, decreased sensation, and crepitus on palpation of the leg. His pain appears to be out of proportion to exam findings.

Evaluation/Tests	WBC, ESR/CRP, CPK, and lactic acid are elevated.
Treatment	Treatment includes broad-spectrum antibiotics that cover gram positive, gram negative, and anaerobic bacterial—such as piperacillin-tazobactam and vancomycin—and prompt surgical exploration and debridement of necrotic tissues.
Discussion	Necrotizing fasciitis is an infection involving deeper tissue along the muscle fascial plane. It is a surgical emergency and is fatal if untreated. It can be polymicrobial or secondary to beta-hemolytic streptococcus. Risk factors include trauma, recent surgery, immunosuppression, DM, alcohol abuse, or IV drug abuse. Patients can have physical exam findings similar to cellulitis (e.g., erythema without a discrete border, pain, edema, warmth) of the affected body part. Compared to cellulitis, pain is initially out of proportion to the skin exam. However, the patient is more likely to have systemic signs and symptoms (e.g., fever/chills, altered mental status, hypotension), and skin changes can rapidly evolve and become bullous and necrotic. Crepitus and gas may be seen or palpated secondary to methane and CO_2 production. Decreased sensation can occur due to nerve destruction. Diagnosis is made clinically, but lab findings such as elevated WBC, ESR/CRP, CPK, and lactic acid can be helpful. It is important to obtain blood cultures to determine the causative bacteria and tailor antibiotic coverage. Imaging can be helpful, but the definitive diagnosis is made via surgical exploration, which should not be delayed for testing if necrotizing fasciitis is strongly suspected.

RASH WITHOUT FEVER

Rashes without fever can be due to bug bites such as scabies, tinea infections, or inflammatory dermatoses. Atopic dermatitis (eczema) is a chronic type 1 hypersensitivity reaction that causes erythematous, scaling, itching papules on flexor surfaces. Allergic contact dermatitis is a type 4 hypersensitivity reaction to substances such as poison ivy or nickel, while irritant contact dermatitis is nonimmunologic. Seborrheic dermatitis is commonly characterized by redness and greasy scaling in areas where the sebaceous glands are most active. Psoriasis causes recurrent silvery scaling papules and plaques on extensor surfaces. It can be associated with arthritis, Koebner phenomenon (new lesions on site of injured skin), and Auspitz sign (pinpoint bleeding when scales are scraped off). Lichen planus gives the 4 Ps—purple, polygonal, pruritic, papules—found on the flexural arms and legs and the mucus membranes. Pityriasis rosea starts with an erythematous single large herald patch followed by smaller erythematous scaling patches that are itchy and appear classically in a "Christmas tree" pattern. It tends to spare the face or legs distal to the knees. Secondary syphilis causes a rash that classically includes erythema on the palms and soles.

CASE 49 | Atopic Dermatitis (Eczema)

A 14-year-old boy with a history of asthma and seasonal allergies presents for evaluation of a recurring pruritic rash on his neck, arms, and legs. He has had this rash intermittently since 9 months of age. His mother has a history of asthma, allergic rhinitis, and eczema. He denies any new products or known exposures. On exam, he has thickened skin with hyperpigmented, scaly patches at the flexor surface of his elbows and knees.

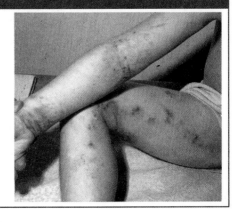

Atopic dermatitis, childhood presentation. Erythematous, scaly, excoriated plaques on the volar wrist and flexural extremities, most prominent in the antecubital and popliteal fossae.
Reproduced with permission from Soutor C, Hordinsky MK: Clinical Dermatology. New York, NY: McGraw Hill; 2013.

CASE 49 | Atopic Dermatitis (Eczema) *(continued)*

Evaluation/Tests	Clinical diagnosis.
Treatment	Skin moisturization with emollients and topical corticosteroids during flares.
Discussion	**Atopic dermatitis**, or **eczema**, is an inflammatory skin disease from hyperreactivity to an environmental stimulus. A history of atopic disease (such as asthma or allergic rhinitis) is a strong risk factor. Dry skin (xerosis) and intense pruritus, leading to scratching and excoriation or eventual thickened skin patches (lichenification), are common clinical features. This chronic relapsing condition most often involves the flexor surfaces such as the antecubital and popliteal fossae, as well as the face and neck, and increased IgE levels support the diagnosis. **Tinea corporis** (commonly from *Trichophyton rubrum*) can present with pruritic, scaling, and red patches, and a KOH prep can be ordered to rule that out. **Allergic contact dermatitis** is a type IV hypersensitivity reaction to a particular allergen that results in a localized skin reaction at the site of exposure. Common allergens include metals (nickel), fragrances, poison ivy, and topical antibiotics (e.g., neomycin). Treatment includes avoidance of the allergen and topical steroids. Acute allergic contact dermatitis from poison ivy on hand. Linear streaks of erythema and vesicles at sites of direct contact with urushiol. Reproduced with permission from Soutor C, Hordinsky MK: Clinical Dermatology. New York, NY: McGraw Hill; 2013.
Other Considerations	**Seborrheic dermatitis** occurs in areas that are abundant with sebaceous glands such as the scalp, face, nasolabial folds, and intertriginous regions. There may also be associated dryness, pruritus, and erythema. Seborrheic dermatitis may be more common in patients with HIV or Parkinson's disease, and it is associated with *Malassezia* species. Treatment includes keratolytic shampoos (selenium sulfide, zinc pyrithione) or topical antifungals (ketoconazole, ciclopirox), and the addition of topical steroids may be helpful. Infants can present with a cradle cap or diaper rash, which can be treated with regular bathing and emollients. **Psoriasis** is a chronic skin condition characterized by erythematous "silvery-scaled" plaques on extensor surfaces and may be associated with arthritis, which tends to involve the DIP joints. Topical corticosteroids and emollients may help in limited plaque psoriasis, whereas phototherapy and/or biologic immune agents may be necessary in more advanced cases.

CASE 50 | Pityriasis Rosea

A 23-year-old man presents with a rash on his trunk. He reports having had cold-like symptoms accompanied by headache and malaise 10 days ago. His partner noted a rose-colored solitary oval lesion on his back about 1 week ago. The lesion gradually enlarged, and this morning he developed multiple smaller lesions. The patient is sexually active but denies a history of STIs, and he uses condoms consistently. On exam, there is a 3-cm well-demarcated salmon-colored lesion on his lower back, as well as multiple small erythematous plaques with collarette scales in a "Christmas tree" distribution on his trunk. No lesions were noted on his palms or soles.

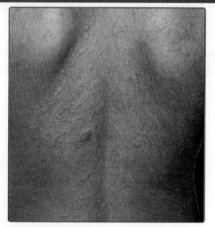

Vesicular pityriasis rosea, showing typical primary plaque and secondary papulovesicles. Note Christmas tree distribution.
Reproduced with permission from Kang S, Amagai M, Bruckner AL, et al: Fitzpatrick's Dermatology, 9th ed. New York, NY: McGraw Hill; 2019.

CASE 50 | Pityriasis Rosea *(continued)*

Evaluation/ Tests	Clinical diagnosis.
Treatment	No treatment is necessary as pityriasis self-resolves within 6 weeks. Topical corticosteroids can help control itching.
Discussion	Pityriasis rosea is a self-limited skin eruption that is often preceded by a viral syndrome. It classically begins with a solitary "herald patch." The well-demarcated spherical lesion with central clearing closely resembles tinea corporis. Days to weeks later, multiple smaller lesions with peripheral collar-like scales (collarette) emerge on the trunk, neck, and limbs. **Tinea corporis** is a single lesion, and a KOH prep would demonstrate segmented fungal hyphae. **Tinea versicolor** (typically caused by *Malassezia*) lesions share a similar distribution to pityriasis rosea but are hypopigmented as opposed to scaly. Hyperpigmented macules on the palms and soles are more typical of **secondary syphilis**.

CASE 51 | Lichen Planus

A 50-year-old woman with a history of hepatitis C presents with pruritic bumps on her wrist for several weeks. She denies any medications or new skin products. On exam, vitals are normal, and she has lacy (reticular) whitish lines on the buccal mucosa of her mouth. On the flexor surface of her wrists and forearms and legs, there are grouped pink-purplish, polygonal, flat-topped (planar), pruritic papules and plaques.

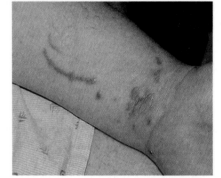

Lichen planus. Linear streaks of papules demonstrating the Koebner response.
Reproduced with permission from Soutor C, Hordinsky MK: Clinical Dermatology. New York, NY: McGraw Hill; 2013.

Evaluation/Tests	Clinical diagnosis.
Treatment	Mild cases can be treated with antihistamines and topical steroids, and more severe cases with oral steroids and light therapy.
Discussion	Lichen planus is a recurrent, T-cell-mediated, chronic inflammatory condition affecting the oral mucosa, genitalia, and skin. Risk factors include hepatitis C, medications (e.g., NSAIDs, ACE-I, thiazides), and stress. The 6 Ps are used to describe the typical lesions that are found on flexor surfaces (including the wrists, shins, lower back, genitals): planar (flat-topped), pruritic, purple, polygonal, papules, and plaques. Oral mucosal lesions are lacy-reticular whitish lines (Wickham's striae). Diagnosis is made clinically, but biopsy can confirm. The biopsy shows sawtooth infiltrate of lymphocytes at the dermal–epidermal junction. **Lichenoid drug reaction** or contact dermatitis should be considered in patients taking new medications or using a new product.

12

Neurology and Special Senses

Neelofer Shafi, MD
Saba Ahmad, MD
Ananya Gangopadhyaya, MD
R. Deepa Yohannan, MD
Javaneh Abbasian, MD
Azizur Rahman, MD

...mon causes for patients to seek medical attention and may require evaluation and management ... settings. In approaching a patient with a headache, obtaining a detailed history identifying key ... with categorization of headaches into primary or secondary causes and will guide you toward ...on and treatment. Primary headaches are common presentations in the outpatient setting. ...her etiologies, including space-occupying lesions (e.g., tumors, hematomas, hydrocephalus), ...matic injury, and infection (e.g., meningitis, encephalitis). Space-occupying lesions will also ...ial pressure, which can present with additional findings such as papilledema, nausea and ... Cushing reflex with irregular breathing, increased blood pressure, and bradycardia. Several ...cutely, and these can be life-threatening emergencies. ...of the key diagnoses to be familiar with and an approach to patients presenting with ...eadaches.

Differential Diagnoses for Headache

Primary Headache	Secondary Headache			
Tension-type Migraine with or 　without aura Cluster	*Infections* Sinusitis Meningitis Encephalitis Sepsis *Space-occupying lesions* Tumors Hematomas Hydrocephalous	*Vascular* Subarachnoid 　hemorrhage (SAH) Acute stroke Vascular malformation Giant cell arteritis 　(temporal arteritis) Cerebral venous sinus 　thrombosis Severe (arterial) 　hypertension	*Referred from:* Neck, ears, nose, 　teeth, mouth, eyes 　(e.g., glaucoma, 　optic neuritis) 　or nerves (e.g., 　trigeminal 　neuralgia)	*Other* Medication overuse 　headaches Trauma Idiopathic intracranial 　hypertension 　(pseudotumor cerebri) Substance use or 　withdrawal Hypoxia Hypercapnia Hypoglycemia Chiari malformations

Key Clinical Features of Common Primary Headaches

Primary Headaches	Key Clinical Features
Migraine	POUND: Pulsatile character, One-day duration, Unilateral location, Nausea, and Disability Ask about associated aura, photophobia, phonophobia More common in women than men
Tension-type	Squeezing pain in a band-like distribution around the head Usually lasts less than a day May be associated with neck pain, scalp tenderness More common in women than men
Cluster headache	Sharp, piercing unilateral retro-orbital pain Usually lasts 20 minutes to several hours Can be associated with ipsilateral conjunctival injection, rhinorrhea, lacrimation, or 　Horner's syndrome More common in men than women

Questions to Ask When Screening for Secondary Causes of Headaches

Screening for Secondary Headaches
New headaches >55 years
Sudden onset (e.g., thunderclap headache)
Systemic signs and disorders (e.g., Fevers, myalgias, weakness, known malignancy or immune compromised)
Neurologic symptoms or signs (e.g., visual changes, focal weakness, paresthesias, mental status changes)
Pulsatile tinnitus, positional provocation, precipitated by exercise

The patient's physical exam can help rule out secondary causes, but it often will not confirm a primary headache. Key portions of the exam will include vital signs, BMI, general appearance, and a full neurological exam, including fundoscopic exam. Exam findings of papilledema or focal neurological deficits would indicate a need for urgent imaging.

Lab testing is rarely needed for diagnosis of a primary headache, but it may be needed prior to initiating therapy. For example, it would be important to have a urine pregnancy test prior to initiating certain migraine therapies that could be teratogenic in a patient. Lab testing may be needed for evaluation of secondary headaches. For example, consider ESR for giant cell arteritis, lumbar punctures for idiopathic intracranial hypertension to assess opening pressure, and urgent cerebrospinal fluid analysis with cell count and gram stain for meningitis.

If there is an acute presentation with either head injury, papilledema, or a focal neurological deficit with concern for a possible bleed, then a CT scan of the head without contrast is indicated. Otherwise, an MRI is a more appropriate approach. For evaluation of a venous sinus thrombosis, MR venography may be indicated.

The management of headache often requires close follow-up visits in the outpatient setting to assess the patient's response to therapy. The use of a headache diary to monitor symptoms is helpful. Shared decision making plays a key role in choosing preventative medications for migraine management, as well as in tapering and stopping medications in suspected medication overuse headaches.

CASE 1 | Migraine

A 20-year-old woman presents with several episodes of a severe unilateral headache for the past three days. She reports seeing multiple small spots that look like "fireworks" before headaches start. Pain is on the right side of her head, behind the eyeball, and pulsating. She endorses photophobia and nausea/vomiting. She has tried ibuprofen with minimal relief. She reports no fevers, blurred vision, neck stiffness, vomiting, or lightheadedness. She has had similar headaches in the last few years around the same time as her menses. Her vital signs are normal, and there is no neck stiffness (nuchal rigidity). Fundoscopic and neurologic exams are normal.

Evaluation/Tests	Clinical diagnosis.
Treatment	NSAIDs (ketorolac), triptans, and/or antiemetics (metoclopramide) as abortive treatment as soon as the migraines start. Lifestyle modification (e.g., good sleep hygiene, avoiding dehydration and triggers) will help decrease the frequency of migraines. If migraines are not palliated with these measures or occur frequently, prophylaxis with an antiepileptic (i.e., topiramate, zonisamide, valproic acid), tricyclic antidepressant, or beta-blocker can be initiated.
Discussion	Migraines are the most common reason for patients to seek outpatient care of a headache. Key clinical features can be remembered with the POUND mnemonic: Pulsatile character, One-day duration, Unilateral, Nausea, and Disability. Up to one-third of patients have an aura such as scintillating scotoma, diplopia, sensory or auditory changes, vertigo, and rarely hemiplegia. There is usually a positive family history, and triggers may include menstruation and foods containing tyramine and monosodium glutamate (MSG). The physical exam has a key role in ruling out other concerning etiologies for headache. Imaging is only indicated if there are concerning features for a secondary headache.
Additional Considerations	**Tension headache** is the most common type of primary headache. The pain is usually mild to modest ("dull," "pressure," or "head fullness"), bilateral ("band-like"), and nonthrobbing. A tension headache can be precipitated by stress, and it usually occurs in the afternoon after long stressful work or school hours. It can also result from sleep deprivation or eye strain. Physical exam is usually normal, although scalp and neck tenderness may be noted. Treatment focuses on lifestyle modifications such as good sleep hygiene, proper posture, and acetaminophen or NSAIDs as needed.

CASE 2 | Cluster Headache

A 35-year-old man who is a heavy smoker presents with an excruciating unilateral headache. He is tearful and describes his headache as sudden onset and lasting for 15–20 minutes. He has a runny nose and watering of his right eye. These episodes have occurred every day for the past week. His vital signs are normal. He has a normal neurological, eye, and fundoscopic exam.

Evaluation/Tests	Clinical diagnosis; confirmed if the headache improves with 100% oxygen.
Treatment	The patient should be given high-flow oxygen and triptans (sumatriptan or zolmitriptan) for acute management. To prevent further cluster headaches, the patient should quit smoking. If necessary, verapamil can be given as prophylaxis.

CASE 2 | Cluster Headache *(continued)*

Discussion	Cluster headaches are a form of primary headache characterized by severe headaches that recur in clusters. On average, a cluster of daily attacks occurs for 6 to 12 weeks followed by a period of remission (up to 12 months or longer). Pain occurs on one side of the head, typically around the eye, and accompanies autonomic symptoms such as ptosis, miosis, lacrimation, conjunctival injection, rhinorrhea, and nasal congestion on the same side as the pain. Pain is severe and lasts 15–180 minutes when untreated, and patients may be agitated or active in behavior during headaches. Risk factors include male gender, tobacco use, and a positive family history. **Trigeminal neuralgia (tic douloureux)** does not accompany autonomic symptoms and involves repetitive, unilateral, shooting pain in the distribution of CN V (typically V1 and/or V2) that can be triggered by chewing, talking, or touching parts of the face. Patients with trigeminal neuralgia should be treated with carbamazepine.

CASE 3 | Idiopathic Intracranial Hypertension

A 28-year-old woman with morbid obesity presents with daily headaches for the last month. The headaches are frontal, described as intense pressure and throbbing, and last for about a day at a time. She associates nausea, light sensitivity, and occasional blurred vision with the headaches. She has tried acetaminophen, ibuprofen, and a combination analgesic (aspirin, acetaminophen, caffeine) without relief. She has no prior history of similar headaches. Her only prescription medications are isotretinoin for cystic acne and oral combined contraceptives. Her fundoscopic exam shows bilateral papilledema. Her neurological exam is within normal limits.

Evaluation/Tests	MRI and MRV appear normal. Lumbar puncture reveals elevated opening pressure and provides a brief period of relief.
Treatment	Treatment options include acetazolamide, weight loss, topiramate, and, in advanced cases, a lumbar-peritoneal (LP) shunt.
Discussion	Idiopathic intracranial hypertension, formerly known as pseudotumor cerebri, is a disorder characterized by increased intracranial pressure with no specific cause on neuroimaging or other evaluations. This condition is commonly seen in young women. Headaches are generalized, and they are typically worse in the morning. Coughing, sneezing, and other activities that further increase the intracranial pressure may worsen the headache. Some patients have pulsatile tinnitus. The increased pressure leads to compression and traction of the cranial nerves especially the optic and abducens nerves; therefore, decreased visual field and acuity and diplopia are warning signs. Increased pressure on lumbar puncture and the presence of papilledema are diagnostic. Risk factors include high-dose vitamin A, long-term tetracycline antibiotics (i.e., in acne), hormonal contraceptives, and obesity. Patients who demonstrate signs of increased intracranial pressure, such as papilledema and increased opening pressures on lumbar puncture, should receive imaging to rule out other causes such as tumors, hydrocephalus, or **cerebral venous sinus thrombosis (CVST)**. CVST is the formation of a blood clot in the dural venous sinuses. While a worsening headache may be the only symptom, many patients also have signs of stroke (e.g., aphasia, hemiplegia) and seizures. Most patients have at least one of the following risk factors: hypercoagulable states (pregnancy, use of a contraceptive drug, factor V Leiden mutation, as well as other abnormalities in hypercoagulability panel), thrombophilia, nephrotic syndrome (due to protein loss), chronic inflammatory disease (e.g., lupus, Bechet's disease), sickle cell disease, polycythemia vera, homocystinuria, direct injury to the venous sinuses, meningitis, local infection such as mastoiditis and sinusitis, and/or dehydration. Magnetic resonance venogram (MRV) would show a filling defect in the venous sinus. Patients with CVST should be treated with anticoagulation.

CASE 4 | Subarachnoid Hemorrhage (SAH)

A 45-year-old woman with a history of hypertension and smoking presents with acute onset of the worst headache of her life while lifting a heavy object at home an hour ago. Her headache was soon followed by several bouts of emesis and lethargy. She has no history of recurrent or chronic headaches, and she denies recent trauma, fevers, or chills. Her family history is notable for the sudden death of her father at age 58. The patient's temperature is 37°C, pulse is 68/min, respirations are 14/min, and blood pressure is 145/110 mmHg. The patient requires stimulation to open her eyes, but she will briefly regard and follow commands when aroused. Neck stiffness is also noted.

CASE 4 | Subarachnoid Hemorrhage (SAH) *(continued)*

Evaluation/Tests	Noncontrast head CT shows hyperintensities in the basal cistern, suggestive of blood in the subarachnoid space. If CT is negative, lumbar puncture should be considered, and it would show an elevated erythrocyte count, elevated opening pressure, and yellowish discoloration (xanthochromia). Angiography shows a ruptured aneurysm arising from the anterior communicating (ACom) artery. 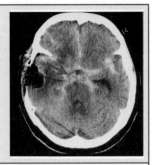 Reproduced with permission from Hakan T, Türk CC, Celik H. Intra-operative real time intracranial subarachnoid haemorrhage during glial tumour resection: A case report, Cases J 2008 Nov 11;1(1):306.
Treatment	The patient should be stabilized and referred to neurosurgery for endovascular coiling or surgical clipping. The calcium channel blocker nimodipine should also be given for prophylaxis of delayed cerebral vasospasm and ischemia.
Discussion	Subarachnoid hemorrhage (SAH) accounts for approximately 5–10% of all strokes. The majority of SAH are caused by ruptured saccular (berry) aneurysms, most commonly in the anterior circulation of the circle of Willis, with the most common location being branchpoints of the ACom (as in this case). SAH can also be caused by traumatic injury and arteriovenous malformations. The classic presentation includes acute onset of a severe "worst of life" thunderclap headache. Additional findings include symptoms related to increased intracranial pressure (nausea, vomiting, and impaired consciousness), meningeal irritation (neck stiffness), and focal neurologic deficits. ACom aneurysms may present with bitemporal hemianopsia due to proximity to the optic chiasm. Some patients may experience prodromal "sentinel headaches" in the days or weeks prior to the aneurysm rupture. Risk factors for SAH include hypertension, smoking, Ehlers-Danlos syndrome or other extracellular matrix disorders, and autosomal dominant polycystic kidney disease. Aneurysmal rupture leads to release of blood directly into the subarachnoid space, which can result in hydrocephalus, elevated intracranial pressure, and cerebral vasospasm. Xanthochromia is visible on lumbar puncture due to the presence of bilirubin from breakdown of RBCs. Acutely the greatest risk is rebleeding from the aneurysm; thus, neurosurgical securing of the aneurysm is the primary goal. Subacutely, the greatest risk to morbidity and mortality becomes delayed cerebral vasospasm and ischemia, which classically develop 3–10 days after SAH. Give nimodipine to help prevent vasospasm, and give an antiepileptic for seizure prophylaxis (e.g., levetiracetam). **Intracerebral hemorrhage (ICH)** is the most common cause of hemorrhagic stroke, and it is typically caused by systemic hypertension that leads to vasculopathy. Other causes include cerebral amyloid angiopathy, vascular malformations, coagulopathy, and hemorrhagic conversion of ischemic infarcts. Clinical presentation depends on the location of hemorrhage, and it may mimic ischemic strokes. The most common locations for typical hypertensive hemorrhages include the basal ganglia, thalamus, brainstem, and cerebellum. Chronic hypertension within lenticulostriate vessels can cause arteriolar hyalinization and fibrinoid necrosis, driving the formation of Charcot-Bouchard microaneurysms, which are prone to rupture and affect deep brain structures. Noncontrast head CT would show a circumscribed area of hyperdensity in the affected area. 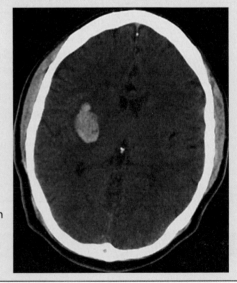 CT scan of a patient with sudden onset left hemiplegia shows an intracerebral hemorrhage in the right basal ganglia. Reproduced with permission from Walter LC, Chang A, Chen P, et al: Current Diagnosis & Treatment Geriatrics, 3rd ed. New York, NY: McGraw Hill; 2021.

CASE 4 | Subarachnoid hemorrhage (SAH) *(continued)*

| Discussion | **Epidural hematoma (EDH)** is commonly a consequence of traumatic injury to the pterion that causes tearing of the middle meningeal artery, resulting in hemorrhage into the potential space between the dura and the skull. Rupture of a high-pressure artery results in a balloon-like hematoma with a biconvex (lentiform) shape on CT. Patients often present with trauma associated with brief loss of consciousness, a return to consciousness (known as a "lucid interval"), followed by deteriorating exam associated with headache, nausea/vomiting, and decreased level of consciousness due to the rapid increase in intracranial pressure from the arterial bleed. Additional findings can include CN III palsy or transtentorial herniation. Patients with significant elevated ICP can present with the Cushing triad, where elevated ICP results in increased systolic BP, bradycardia, and irregular breathing. Noncontrast head CT would show a biconvex-shaped hyperdensity along the inner skull that does not cross suture lines with an associated skull fracture. | 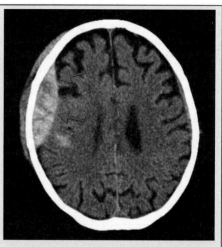
Used with permission from Hellerhoff/Wikimedia Commons. |

CASE 5 | Subdural Hemorrhage (SDH)

A 78-year-old man with a history of chronic alcohol abuse presents with gradual-onset headache for the past 5 days. The patient reports increasing difficulty walking and frequent falls over the last several weeks, with no history of trauma. The patient lives alone, but his family checks on him frequently. On exam, he is lethargic but arousable to voice, and he is oriented only to person and place. He has some mild right-sided weakness with right upper extremity drift.

Evaluation/Tests	His labs demonstrate an AST/ALT ratio of 2:1. Noncontrast head CT shows a crescent-shaped hyperintensity in the left hemisphere (red arrow) that crosses suture lines, with additional evidence of midline shift (yellow arrow). 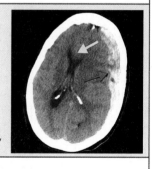 Used with permission from James Heilman, MD/Wikimedia Commons.
Treatment	Refer to neurosurgery for urgent surgical hematoma evacuation.
Discussion	Subdural hemorrhage (SDH) or subdural hematoma typically results from head trauma in elderly patients (often from falls), causing tearing of the bridging veins and bleeding into the potential space between the dura and arachnoid meninges. It can also be seen in chronic alcoholics, patients with underlying cerebral atrophy, or in shaken babies. Since it is a venous bleed, patients typically present with more subacute or chronic symptoms (as opposed to arterial bleeds like SAH and EDH, which present acutely). Symptoms can include headache, gait abnormalities, somnolence, and confusion. These can often be confused with other diagnoses, allowing SDH to go undiagnosed for some time. Head CT typically reveals a concave, crescent-shaped hemorrhage that crosses suture lines because it is below the point where the dura fuses to the periosteum. **Subarachnoid hemorrhage** and **intracerebral hemorrhage** may occur after trauma, but imaging appears different. **Ischemic stroke** to the brainstem or cerebellum may cause ataxia and falls, but this presents acutely as sudden onset. **Normal pressure hydrocephalus** presents with the characteristic triad of dementia, ataxia, and urinary incontinence ("wacky, wobbly, and wet") with no focal weakness or lethargy. **Wernicke's encephalopathy** typically presents with altered mental status, ophthalmoplegia, and ataxia, usually with no focal weakness. **Traumatic brain injury** without underlying hematoma may present with headache, nausea, vomiting, and drowsiness after head trauma, but CT is typically negative for hemorrhage.

CASE 6 | Chiari I Malformation

A 22-year-old man with a history of headaches, particularly worsened with coughing or bowel movements, presents for tingling of the hands and dropping things over the last 3 months. His symptoms have progressively worsened, and he has been having pain in his upper back and lower neck. He has no history of trauma. On exam, he has nystagmus in all gaze directions; his pupils are reactive to light and accommodation bilaterally. His biceps, triceps, and grip strength are decreased bilaterally, and he has diminished sensation to temperature and pinprick in both upper extremities and his upper back in a cape-like distribution. Findings in his lower extremities are normal. Reflexes are decreased in the upper extremities and normal in the lower extremities.

Evaluation/Tests	MRI of brain and spine reveal low-lying cerebellar tonsils (red arrow), extending below the foramen magnum and into the vertebral canal, as well as evidence of a cystic cavity at C8-T1 (yellow arrows). Used with permission from Dr. Frank Gaillard/Radiopaedia.
Treatment	Surgery to decompress the Chiari I malformation and syrinx.
Discussion	Chiari malformations are a group of congenital disorders caused by abnormal development of the cerebellum in the posterior fossa. In particular, this man is presenting with a **Chiari I malformation with syringomyelia**. Chiari I malformations are the most common type and involve protrusion of the cerebellar tonsils 5–10 mm through foramen magnum into the spinal canal without herniation of other cerebellar structures. Chiari I malformations are often asymptomatic, but they can manifest in adolescence or adulthood with headaches (especially with Valsalva maneuver) and cerebellar symptoms. It is also commonly associated with **syringomyelia**, a CSF-filled cystic cavity within the central canal of the spinal cord, often in the cervical region. Expansion of the syrinx can lead to compression of nearby structures, resulting in diminished pain and temperature sensation (spinothalamic tract crossing anterior white commissure) in a "cape-like" distribution and later lower motor neuron signs (ventral horn).
Additional Considerations	**Chiari II malformations** are more severe and present much earlier in life (i.e., in neonates just after birth) with herniation of tonsils and the cerebellar vermis, which can result in compression of the medulla and aqueductal stenosis (obstructive hydrocephalus). Chiari II malformation can also be seen in patients with lumbosacral meningomyelocele, which is associated with an incomplete neural tube closure and inadequate folate intake during early pregnancy. **Meningomyelocele** is obvious at birth, but hydrocephalus may not be overtly symptomatic due to open fontanelles and accommodative skulls.

BRAIN TUMORS

The most common etiology of brain tumors are metastases (lung, breast, kidney, etc.); however, there are more than 30 different kinds of primary central nervous system (CNS) tumors. Primary CNS tumors rarely metastasize, and they can be benign or malignant. Malignant tumors include glioblastoma multiforma (GBM), CNS lymphoma, and oligodendroglioma. Benign tumors include meningioma, hemangioblastoma, and schwannoma. Brain tumors typically present with headache, seizure, and other focal neurologic symptoms. Symptoms depend on the location of the mass, and most primary brain tumors are supratentorial in adults.

The primary treatment for most brain tumors is resection. Slow growing, benign tumors such as **meningiomas** and **schwannomas** may not be symptomatic for years. They are often found incidentally, requiring observation only. When symptoms do arise, they are due to local compressive effects that can range from tinnitus (schwannomas) to headache and seizure (meningiomas).

Brain Tumors and Key Associated Findings

Key Findings	Diagnosis
- Most common primary brain tumor in adults (age 50–60) - Tumor crosses the corpus callosum ("butterfly glioma") - Central necrosis surrounded by "pseudopalisading" pleomorphic tumor cells, which are positive for glial fibrillary acidic protein (GFAP) staining	Glioblastoma multiforme (GBM)
- Finely branching capillaries that appear as "chicken-wire" - "Fried egg" cells—round nuclei with clear cytoplasm - IDH mutations and 1p/19q codeletion	Oligodendroglioma
- Spindle cells concentrically arranged in a whorled pattern; psammoma bodies may be present - Most common benign CNS tumor in adults (rarely malignant) - Extra axial (outside the brain parenchyma) with dural tail	Meningioma
- Tumor of blood vessels mostly located in the cerebellum - Produces erythropoietin resulting in secondary polycythemia	Hemangioblastoma
- Benign tumor involving cranial and spinal nerves (Cerebellopontine angle tumors can affect CN VII resulting in facial paralysis and CN VIII resulting in tinnitus, hearing loss, and central vertigo) - Bilateral vestibular tumors found in neurofibromatosis type 2	Schwannoma
- Lumbar puncture shows pleocytosis in 80% of the patients - High-dose methotrexate containing regimens with or without radiation are used for treatment (no surgical resection needed)	Primary CNS lymphomas

CASE 7 | Glioblastoma Multiforme (GBM)

A 66-year-old man presents with 3–4 weeks of left-sided weakness and a worsening headache. His wife reports that the patient has had intermittent headaches for the last month. She also reports that he has had increasing difficulty raising his arm and leg on his left side over the last few weeks. On exam, he has left-sided hemiparesis with intact sensation. His right side has normal motor and sensory function.

Evaluation/Tests	Brain MRI or head CT with contrast shows a heterogeneously enhancing mass in the right hemisphere that extends across the corpus callosum toward the left side. A brain biopsy shows GFAP+ pseudopalisading tumor cells as well as central areas of necrosis, hemorrhage, and microvascular proliferation.

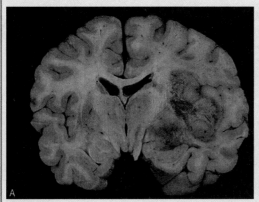 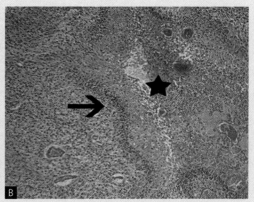

Glioblastoma multiforme (GBM). A, The right cerebral hemisphere is expanded by an irregularly contoured mass containing areas of necrosis (yellow) and small areas of hemorrhage. Although this lesion appears fairly well demarcated in this gross photograph, GBMs are aggressive astrocytic neoplasms that widely infiltrate the surrounding brain. B, The distinction between the various grades of infiltrating astrocytic neoplasms is based upon four histologic features: nuclear pleomorphism, mitotic figures, endothelial proliferation, and necrosis. GBMs, by definition, contain at least three of these four histologic features. In this section, the necrosis is apparent (star). As is characteristic for GBMs, this tumor has palisading of neoplastic cells at the edge of the necrosis (arrow). Hematoxylin and eosin, 100×.
Reproduced with permission from Kemp WL, Burns DK, Travis Brown TG. Pathology: The Big Picture. New York, NY: McGraw Hill; 2008.

CASE 7 | Glioblastoma Multiforme (GBM) (continued)

Treatment	Treat with a combination of surgical resection, chemotherapy, and adjuvant radiation therapy.
Discussion	This patient is presenting with glioblastoma multiforme (GBM), a grade IV astrocytoma, and the most common primary brain tumor in adults. GBM is highly malignant with poor survival rate (median survival is 10–12 months). Astrocytomas arise from astrocytes (GFAP+); they are usually found within the cerebral hemispheres; and they may show a characteristic "butterfly glioma" phenotype on imaging where the tumor crosses the corpus callosum. The tumor may cause mass effect symptoms and damage local structures. Patients often present with focal neurological symptoms such as weakness (as in this patient) in addition to headache, seizure, or altered mental status. Imaging and biopsy are key to differentiate between various tumor types.
Additional Considerations	Unlike primary brain tumors, **metastases** typically present as more than one lesion. Ischemic and hemorrhagic **strokes** typically present with acute **symptoms**. Used with permission from Jmarchn/Wikimedia Commons.

After leukemia, brain tumors are the second most common cause of pediatric cancers (approximately 20% of all pediatric cancers). Most pediatric brain tumors are primary in nature and most commonly arise infratentorially. The one exception is craniopharyngiomas, which are supratentorial. Symptoms depend on the location of the tumor and how rapidly it is growing.

CASE 8 | Pilocytic Astrocytoma

A 4-year-old girl is brought for evaluation of morning headaches for the past 3 weeks. Her parents brought her to the emergency department as she started vomiting this morning. She has had normal developmental milestones. On exam, the patient is lethargic with bilateral CN VI palsy. She demonstrates dysmetria on nose-finger test, and her gait is wide based and unstable.

Evaluation/Tests	Brain MRI or head CT with contrast show an enhancing lesion with solid and cystic components in the posterior fossa near the cerebellum. Spinal MRI shows no evidence of drop metastases. A brain biopsy shows long bipolar (hair-like) tumor cells that are strongly immunoreactive to glial fibrillary acidic protein (GFAP) and the presence of eosinophilic, corkscrew (Rosenthal) fibers. Reproduced with permission from Hafez RF. Stereotaxic gamma knife surgery in treatment of critically located pilocytic astrocytoma: preliminary result, World J Surg Oncol 2007 Mar 29;5:39.
Treatment	Treat with dexamethasone (to control edema), resection, and chemotherapy.
Discussion	Pilocytic astrocytoma is one of the most common pediatric brain tumors. In children, morning headache and vomiting are classic signs for increased intracranial pressure that is associated with a CNS mass lesion. Bilateral abducens nerve palsies suggest increased intracranial pressure as a result of obstructive hydrocephalus. It is a medical emergency because it can cause brain herniation. Childhood primary brain tumors are typically infratentorial (below level of tentorium cerebelli). Common locations include the cerebellum, 4th ventricle, brain stem, hypothalamus, or the optic chiasm; however, they may also occur in any brain region, including the cerebral hemispheres and the spinal cord. Pilocytic astrocytoma is low grade and considered benign because the progression tends to be slower than more aggressive tumors such as medulloblastoma or ependymoma. Clinical symptoms depend on the location of the tumor. Total resection can be curative.

CASE 8 | **Pilocytic Astrocytoma** *(continued)*

Discussion	**Medulloblastoma** is the most common malignant brain tumor in children, and it typically involves the cerebellum and 4th ventricle. Signs and symptoms of the tumor are related to increased intracranial pressure and cerebellar dysfunction. Neurologic exam may reveal papilledema, nystagmus, ataxia, and cranial nerve abnormalities. Medulloblastomas can cause "drop metastases" to the spinal cord, which is associated with a poor prognosis. Treatment is often a combination of surgery, radiation therapy, and chemotherapy. **Ependymomas** are rare but morbid tumors commonly found in the 4th ventricle, but they can also involve the spinal cord and can cause hydrocephalus.

CASE 9 | Craniopharyngioma

A 5-year-old boy is brought to clinic by his mother due to persistent headaches over the past 6 weeks. She reports that ibuprofen provides little relief of symptoms. She also notes that he has had several episodes of emesis since yesterday. On review of his growth chart, he has only grown 1.5 cm over the past year. Funduscopic examination reveals swelling of the optic disc. Confrontation testing demonstrates absence of the outer half of both the right and left visual fields.

Evaluation/Tests	CT scan shows characteristic calcifications and a mass in the sellar region. MRI shows a solid tumor with cystic structures containing fluid of intermediate density. IGF-1 level is decreased. 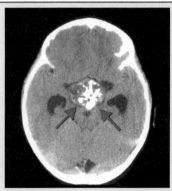 Reproduced with permission from Garnett MR, Puget S, Grill J, et al: Craniopharyngioma, Orphanet J Rare Dis 2007 Apr 10;2:18.
Treatment	Surgical resection.
Discussion	Craniopharyngiomas are the most common childhood supratentorial tumors. They are extra-axial and histologically benign. They derive embryologically from two main components: Rathke pouch (an upward invagination of ectoderm from the primitive oral cavity) or the infundibulum (a downward invagination of neuroectoderm from the diencephalon). Calcification on CT and cholesterol crystals in "motor-oil" like fluid within the tumor are seen on pathology. Patients present with symptoms of mass effect such as headache and visual disturbances. On physical exam, there may be optic pallor due to compression of the optic pathway or signs of increased intracranial pressure such as swollen optic discs or papilledema. Visual field testing may reveal bitemporal hemianopsia due to the tumor arising in the suprasellar region and compressing the optic chiasm. Other findings may include signs of hypopituitarism (hypothyroidism, adrenal insufficiency, growth hormone deficiency). Labs should be done for evaluation of pituitary hormone function (TSH, Free T4, cortisol, IGF-1). Sodium, serum osmolality, and urine osmolality should also be done to screen for diabetes insipidus (absence of vasopressin). The treatment of choice for craniopharyngioma is gross total resection. It can often be confused with **pituitary adenoma** because both cause bitemporal hemianopsia. Craniopharyngiomas are usually nonsecreting, whereas pituitary adenoma may secrete hormones like prolactin. 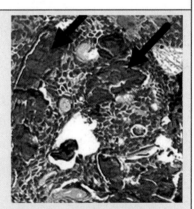 Used with permission from Nephron/Wikimedia Commons.
Additional Considerations	**Pinealomas** are tumors of the pineal gland, and they can result in Parinaud syndrome (vertical gaze palsy, obstructive hydrocephalus through compression of the cerebral aqueduct, and precocious puberty in males via β-hCG production).

WEAKNESS

When approaching a patient with weakness, it is important to determine whether the weakness is from a neurological cause or originating from another organ system and whether it is acute or progressively worsening. Non-neurological weakness is most often a generalized weakness due to medical conditions such as electrolyte abnormalities, infection, anemia, thyroid disease, or depression. Neurological weakness can further be delineated into central or peripheral origin. For the purposes of this discussion, the central nervous system (CNS) comprises brain and spinal cord, and the peripheral nervous system (PNS) encompasses neuromuscular junction, spinal nerve root, and peripheral nerves.

Differential Diagnoses of Weakness: Central vs. Peripheral

Central	Peripheral
Ischemic stroke	Guillain-Barré syndrome
Intracerebral hemorrhage (ICH)	Peripheral neuropathy (e.g., diabetic, alcoholic, B12/folate deficiency)
Primary brain tumor	
Brain metastasis	Compression neuropathies
Spinal cord tumor	Inherited neuropathies
Postictal paralysis	Myasthenia gravis
Multiple sclerosis	Amyotrophic lateral sclerosis
Hemiplegic migraine	Myopathy
Spinal muscular atrophy	
Poliomyelitis	

Distribution of Weakness

Affected Area	Localization
Hemiparesis of face, arm, and/or leg (Paresis is partial paralysis. Hemiparesis is partial paralysis of unilateral arm/leg.)	CNS (brain)
Paraparesis (partial paralysis of bilateral lower extremities)	CNS (thoracic or lumbar spinal cord)
Quadriparesis (partial paralysis of all four extremities)	CNS (cervical spinal cord)
Isolated extremity	PNS
Proximal muscles	PNS
Distal muscles	PNS

Key Features Helpful in Determining Central vs. Peripheral Localization

Key Associated Findings	Localization
Aphasia (loss of ability to express and/or understand speech)	CNS (brain)
Altered mental status (a general change in brain function leading to impaired consciousness, orientation, or cognition)	CNS (brain)
Seizures	CNS (brain)
Visual abnormalities	CNS (brain)
Headache	CNS (brain)
Bowel/bladder dysfunction	CNS (spinal cord)
Spasticity (continuous contraction of a muscle)	CNS (brain or spinal cord)
Hyperreflexia (increased/brisk reflexes)	CNS (brain or spinal cord)
Sensory abnormality	CNS or PNS
Areflexia (absent reflexes)	PNS
Myalgias (pain originating from muscles)	PNS
Atrophy (loss of bulk of a muscle)	PNS
Ataxia (unsteadiness or incoordination of gait, trunk, or extremity)	CNS or PNS

CASE 10 | Middle Cerebral Artery (MCA) Stroke

A 67-year-old man with diabetes, hyperlipidemia, and hypertension was giving a speech 1 hour earlier when he suddenly had word-finding difficulty and slow, effortful speech. He was holding a champagne glass up in his right hand, which he suddenly dropped. He was rushed immediately to the hospital. On exam, the patient's speech is effortful, slurred, and he speaks in short phrases. He has a right facial droop and right upper extremity weakness. His left arm and both lower extremities display full strength. He has sensory loss over the right arm and face.

Evaluations/Tests	A noncontrast head CT is negative for hemorrhage.
Treatment	The patient should be treated with tPA (tissue plasminogen activator) or mechanical thrombectomy. Once the source is treated, his risk of future strokes can be reduced with aspirin and/or clopidogrel, blood pressure control, and tight control of diabetes and hyperlipidemia.
Discussion	This patient is presenting with an **ischemic stroke**, an acute blockage of vessels that disrupts blood flow, leading to ischemia and liquefactive necrosis. In particular, this patient's stroke is a **left middle cerebral artery (MCA) stroke** involving Broca's area and the left frontal lobe. Acute onset neurological symptoms affecting language (aphasia) with right-sided face and arm weakness sparing the leg are suggestive of a left MCA stroke because the MCA supplies the face and upper extremity. The patient has aphasia, which is a disorder of language that localizes to the dominant hemisphere. He has a motor/expressive aphasia, given his intact comprehension with difficulty with repetition and fluency. Diabetes, hypertension, and hyperlipidemia are important risk factors. Other conditions that increase risk of stroke include atrial fibrillation and carotid artery stenosis. Patients presenting less than 4.5 hours since their last known well time, should be treated with tPA (tissue plasminogen activator). Patients may also be considered for mechanical thrombectomy even after 4.5 hours and up to 24 hours from their last known well time, if they have large vessel occlusion and evidence of salvageable tissue. **Hemorrhagic stroke** (i.e., ICH) can also cause similar symptoms and signs, thus a stat noncontrast CT should be ordered to rule out hemorrhage prior to initiation of IV tPA or endovascular therapy.

CASE 11 | Lateral Medullary Stroke (Wallenberg Syndrome)

A 64-year-old woman presents with vertigo and vomiting for the past hour. When the sensation began, she tried to drink some ginger ale to quell her nausea, but she had difficulty swallowing, and she has been hiccupping since. She also reports double vision and feeling that the room is spinning. Cardiac auscultation reveals an irregularly irregular heartbeat. Neurologic exam reveals a left eyelid droop and a left pupil that is smaller compared to right. She has persistent vertical nystagmus as well as decreased pain and temperature sensation in her right arm and leg compared to the left. Her strength is full in all extremities.

Evaluation/Tests	ECG shows an erratic baseline, no discrete P waves, and irregularly spaced QRS complex (atrial fibrillation). A noncontrast head CT is negative for hemorrhage. A brain MRI with and without contrast reveals a small brainstem infarct in the lateral medulla.
Treatment	The patient is a potential candidate for tPA therapy as less than 4.5 hours has passed since the onset of symptoms. In the long term, optimum control of blood pressure, glucose, and lipids is important. The underlying atrial fibrillation should be treated with anticoagulation, rate and rhythm control, and/or cardioversion.
Discussion	Lateral medullary stroke/syndrome, also known as Wallenberg syndrome, is caused by impaired function of the lateral medulla. Commonly, it is caused by infarction of the posterior inferior cerebellar artery (PICA) or its parent vessel, the vertebral artery. Clinical manifestations correlate with the neuroanatomy of the lateral medulla, and they commonly include only a subset of symptoms from all of the structures that can possibly be involved. Potential structures affected can include the vestibular nuclei (vertigo, vomiting, nystagmus), the nucleus ambiguus (dysphagia, hoarseness, impaired gag reflex, hiccupping), the spinal trigeminal nucleus (ipsilateral decreased face pain/temperature sensation), the lateral spinothalamic tract (contralateral body decreased pain/temperature sensation), sympathetic fibers (ipsilateral Horner syndrome), or the inferior cerebellar peduncle (ipsilateral ataxia, dysmetria). Classically, the patient has no motor weakness; this is one of the most important features to distinguish lateral medullary syndrome from other stroke syndromes. Another distinguishing feature is involvement of the nucleus ambiguous (CN IX, X, and XI), which is specific to PICA lesions. While **benign paroxysmal positional vertigo** (**BPPV**) would also present with nausea, vomiting, and vertigo, these symptoms would not be accompanied by unequal pupils and loss of sensation. Additionally, the nystagmus would resolve after a brief period rather than persisting as it did in this patient.

CASE 12 | Myasthenia Gravis

A 35-year-old woman presents with intermittent slurred speech and double vision for the past 3 months. She has noticed droopiness of her eyelids that worsens through the day. She also reports constant fatigue and shortness of breath. On exam, she has bilateral ptosis; binocular double vision upon sustained upgaze; and weakness in her eye closure, cheek puff, tongue protrusion, and neck flexion. Sensory exam is normal, and deep tendon reflexes are intact.

Evaluation/Tests	A chest CT reveals a mass in the anterior mediastinum consistent with thymoma. An edrophonium (tensilon) test shows improvement in ptosis. Electromyography (EMG) testing with repetitive nerve stimulation shows decreased muscle action potential responses. Serum testing for acetylcholine receptor (AChR) antibodies is positive.
Treatment	This patient should be treated with pyridostigmine (acetylcholinesterase inhibitor) and immunomodulation therapy. Patients with a concomitant thymoma may have improvement in symptoms following thymectomy.
Discussion	Myasthenia gravis is an autoimmune disorder, and it is the most common disorder affecting the neuromuscular junction (NMJ). It is characterized by the formation of autoantibodies to the postsynaptic AChR, which bind to the receptors and cause their endocytosis and loss from the NMJ. Hallmarks of myasthenia gravis include ptosis, diplopia, and weakness that worsens with increased muscle use. Patients may report feeling better in the morning and feeling worse by the end of the day. Involvement of respiratory muscles can lead to dyspnea. A proportion of patients present with predominantly ocular muscle involvement. A more common generalized form involves bulbar, limb, neck, and/or respiratory muscles and presents with fatigability of chewing, swallowing, slurred speech, shortness of breath, and proximal limb weakness. A unique feature often seen in myasthenia gravis is thymic hyperplasia or formation of a thymoma, likely due to an autoimmune response to thymic epitopes similar to those seen in the NMJ. The goal of treatment is to increase available ACh in the NMJ cleft, which can overcome the autoantibodies. Thus use of the acetylcholinesterase inhibitor pyridostigmine is first line. In contrast to myasthenia gravis, **Lambert-Eaton myasthenic syndrome** presents with weakness that improves with repeated use. The weakness is predominantly in proximal muscles and impacts the legs in particular. Acetylcholinesterase inhibitor administration does little to improve the symptoms. Lambert-Eaton myasthenic syndrome is typically a paraneoplastic syndrome associated with small cell lung cancer.

CASE 13 | Amyotrophic Lateral Sclerosis (ALS)

A 62-year-old man presents with painless asymmetric weakness that has progressed over the last 9 months. He first noticed changes in his handwriting, which progressed to difficulty picking small objects up with the right hand. Subsequently he developed noticeably slurred speech. At times, food got stuck in his throat, and he notes muscle twitches in his arms and legs. His wife also noticed difficulty rising from the chair. The patient denies numbness, tingling, or bowel or bladder dysfunction. He is alert and oriented to person, place, and time, but he has slurred speech and a hyperactive jaw jerk. He has fasciculations in his tongue and in several arm and leg muscles. He has asymmetric muscle atrophy in distal hand muscles and weakness in his right-hand intrinsic muscles, left arm abduction, and bilateral hip flexion. He has a positive Babinski sign on the right side and hyperreflexia in the arms. His sensory exam is normal.

Evaluation/Tests	MRI of the brain shows atrophy of the precentral gyrus. MRI of the cervical spine shows atrophy within the anterior horns. Electromyography (EMG) demonstrates motor neuronopathy with denervation and fibrillation.
Treatment	The patient should be treated with riluzole (PO), edaravone (IV), and supportive therapy.
Discussion	Amyotrophic lateral sclerosis (ALS), also known as Lou Gehrig disease, is a neurodegenerative disorder that affects motor neurons in the anterior horn of the spinal cord, brain stem, and motor cortex. About 90% of ALS is sporadic, and only 10% is familial. Approximately 20% of familial cases have a defect in the enzyme superoxide dismutase 1 (SOD1). Sporadic ALS affects men more than women and peaks in the sixth to seventh decades of life (earlier in familial cases). The hallmark of ALS is evidence of both upper motor neuron (UMN) signs (hyperreflexia, jaw jerk, positive Babinski sign, spasticity, increased tone) and lower motor neuron (LMN) signs (atrophy, weakness, fasciculations in the tongue, trunk, limbs) in the absence of sensory or autonomic abnormalities. Clinical presentation varies, but usually begins with focal muscle weakness in the limbs, and spreads to involve contiguous regions. A common presenting sign is weakness in the hands (dropping objects, handwriting, etc.). About a third of patients present with bulbar symptoms, such as dysarthria or dysphagia (bulbar-onset ALS), which is associated with more rapid progression of disease. ALS is progressive and fatal, and patients typically succumb due to complications of respiratory failure.

CASE 14 | Bell's Palsy (Facial Nerve Palsy)

A 48-year-old man presents with sudden onset of right facial weakness. In the morning, he noticed droopiness in the right corner of his mouth. By the end of the day, he could not raise his right eyebrow. The following morning, he woke up with dry eyes and increased sensitivity to sound in the right ear. He does have a history of mouth sores that resurface periodically. Upon exam, he has weakness in right eye closure and cheek puff, and he is unable to raise the corner of his mouth on the right side. Finger rub sounds more prominent in the right ear. No rashes or lesions were noted in the ear or mouth or on the skin.

Evaluation/Tests	Serologic testing for Lyme disease is negative. MRI brain with and without contrast is normal.
Treatment	The patient should be treated with eye protection (lubricants, patch at night). Prednisone (PO), and valacyclovir can be used if severe.
Discussion	Bell's (facial nerve) palsy, also known as idiopathic facial paralysis, is a clinical syndrome that describes acute peripheral facial nerve (CN VII) palsy of unknown etiology. Peripheral facial palsy has many causes, and herpes simplex virus (HSV) activation is the most common cause, followed by herpes zoster virus (VZV). Patients typically present with rapidly progressive unilateral facial paralysis over several hours. Characteristic features include facial droop, flattening of the nasolabial fold, and weakness or inability to close the eye. Given that the facial nerve has both motor, sensory and autonomic components, patients may also experience decreased tears/dry eye (parasympathetic innervation of the lacrimal gland), hyperacusis (stapedius muscle), and loss of taste sensation over the anterior 2/3 of the tongue (chorda tympani nerve). Most patients show gradual recovery of function. Bell's palsy is a diagnosis of exclusion. Other causes such as **Lyme disease** (particularly if the facial paralysis is bilateral), vestibular schwannoma, and Guillain-Barré should be ruled out before diagnosing this as Bell's palsy. **Herpes zoster oticus**, or **Ramsay Hunt Syndrome**, results from reactivation of the *Varicella zoster* virus along cranial nerves VII and/or VIII. It's characterized by a vesicular rash in the external auditory canal. Other features include unilateral facial palsy, loss of taste sensation (chorda tympani), and ear pain. It should be treated with acyclovir or valacyclovir and prednisone; otherwise, hearing loss and/or facial paralysis can be permanent.

CASE 15 | Poliomyelitis

A 34-year-old man born in India who recently moved to the United States presents for evaluation of chronic atrophy and weakness of the right leg. His symptoms developed in early childhood after a flu-like episode. He does not have an exact recollection of his symptoms, but he remembers that he initially developed weakness in his legs that then moved to his arms, resulting in hospitalization. With rehabilitation, he was able to gain strength in most of his limbs except for his right leg. He is able to ambulate with a cane. On exam, he has atrophy in his right leg muscles proximally and distally, decreased tone in the right leg, and absent deep tendon reflexes in the right leg. He did not have weakness in other limbs, and his sensory exam was normal.

Evaluation/Tests	Electrodiagnostic testing demonstrates chronic denervation on needle EMG. Lumbar puncture shows normal opening pressure and glucose, elevated protein, and lymphocytic pleocytosis. PCR serology is positive for poliovirus.
Treatment	Supportive therapy including monitoring of respiratory and swallow function, pain relief, and physical rehabilitation.
Discussion	Poliomyelitis is a poliovirus infection of the lower motor neurons (LMNs) in the anterior horn of the spinal cord. Poliovirus is an RNA virus and member of the *Picorniviridae* family enteroviruses. It is transmitted by oral-fecal contamination. While poliovirus has been eradicated in most developed countries with the help of polio vaccine, poliovirus still exists in small endemic areas of Africa and Asia. About 90–95% of patients infected with poliovirus are asymptomatic or have flu-like symptoms. Only 0.1% of patients infected with poliovirus develop paralysis. Asymmetric weakness typically starts in one limb, and it can progress to quadriplegia and respiratory failure within days. Other LMN signs such as hypotonia, flaccid paralysis, fasciculations, hyporeflexia, and muscle atrophy may be present. Legs are more commonly affected than arms, and proximal muscle groups are more affected than distal groups. About two-thirds of patients are left with residual weakness. Some patients may develop postpolio syndrome decades after initial onset, likely due to premature aging of the remaining motor neurons. **West Nile virus** can present as meningitis, encephalitis, or meningoencephalitis with confusion, headache, stiff neck, fever/chills, and decreased level of consciousness. Chronic denervation on EMG would not be present as in this patient.

SENSORY ABNORMALITIES

Sensory abnormalities can present as loss or absence of sensation (numbness or hypoesthesia), increased sensation (hyperesthesia), or abnormalities/alteration of sensation (paresthesia). Like other neurological symptoms, it is initially helpful to approach abnormalities of sensation by attempting to localize the lesion. Once localized to CNS or PNS, further characterization can be done. Primary modalities of sensation are usually checked first: touch, pain, and temperature through the spinothalamic tracts and vibration and proprioception through the dorsal columns. If primary modalities of sensation are mostly intact, and the patient is suspected to have a cortical abnormality (meaning originating from the brain), then higher cortical sensations can be examined, namely extinction, two-point discrimination, graphesthesia, and stereognosis.

Localizing the Source of Sensory Abnormalities Based on Anatomical Loss of Sensation

Affected Area	Localization
Unilateral face and/or leg	CNS (contralateral brain)
Trunk and extremities	CNS (spinal cord)
Distal extremities (stocking-glove pattern)	PNS
Single extremity	PNS

The affected modalities can help further localize the lesion. For example, lesions of the dorsal column tend to disproportionately affect vibration and proprioception.

Localizing the Source of Sensory Abnormalities Based on the Type of Sensory Defect

Modality Affected	Localization
Touch	Spinothalamic tract
Pain	Spinothalamic tract
Temperature	Spinothalamic tract
Vibration	Dorsal column
Proprioception (joint position sense)	Dorsal column
Two-point discrimination (the ability to discern that two close objects touching the skin are two distinct points, not one)	Contralateral sensory cortex
Graphesthesia (the ability to recognize writing on the skin purely by the sensation of touch)	Contralateral parietal lobe
Stereognosis (the ability to perceive the form of solid objects by touch)	Contralateral parietal lobe
Extinction (the inability to perceive multiple stimuli of the same type simultaneously, such as perceiving touch on both arms at the same time)	Contralateral sensory cortex

CASE 16 | Multiple Sclerosis (Predominantly Sensory Symptoms)

A 27-year-old woman noticed progressive graying of the center of the visual field of her left eye while out hiking on a hot summer day. She reported seeing "sparkles" in "the corners of her vision," and she had pain when she moved her left eye. Later that day, she started to feel shooting electrical pain down her neck that radiated into both her arms. The pain was so severe that she was taken to a local emergency department. In a darkened room, when a penlight is shone in her right eye, both eyes constrict; however, when it is then quickly shone in the left eye, her pupils dilate (left afferent pupillary defect). She reports pain with extraocular movements. She reports loss of color vision, particularly the color red. On exam, she has 5/5 strength in all extremities but loss of light touch and pinprick sensation below the T10 dermatome. When her neck is flexed, she reports an electric shock-like sensation radiating down her spine (positive Lhermitte's sign).

Evaluations/Tests	A T2-weighted MRI brain with and without contrast demonstrates periventricular plaques ("Dawson's fingers"). An MRI of the cervical and thoracic spine with and without contrast show additional areas of demyelination. Lumbar puncture shows increased IgG level and myelin basic protein in CSF as well as oligoclonal bands.

CASE 16 | Multiple Sclerosis (Predominantly Sensory Symptoms) *(continued)*

Treatment	The patient should be treated with high-dose glucocorticoids for acute flares. To slow progression and reduce relapses, the patient can take disease-modifying agents, such as beta-interferon, glatiramer acetate, fingolimod, or natalizumab. Her symptoms can be managed with baclofen for spasticity, antimuscarinic agents for bladder dysfunction, and TCAs or anticonvulsants for pain.
Discussion	**Multiple sclerosis (MS)** is an autoimmune-mediated inflammatory disease of the CNS, characterized by multifocal areas of demyelination *separated in space and time* with loss of oligodendrocytes and astroglial scarring. Most cases follow a relapsing-remitting course with periods of demyelination followed by remyelination. Over time, this can exhaust repair mechanisms, and the disease becomes secondarily progressive. Some can be primary progressive from the onset without remission. Patients typically present as young adults. This patient is presenting with MS with predominantly sensory symptoms and an episode of **acute optic neuritis**, a painful unilateral visual loss associated with afferent pupillary defect and a characteristic symptom of MS. Patients often have photopsia or "sparkles or shimmers in their peripheral visual fields," and they may have pain with extraocular movements because of optic nerve inflammation. **Lhermitte's sign** is the sensation of shooting electrical pain elicited by neck flexion that radiates down the body ("barber chair phenomenon"). **Uhthoff phenomenon** is the unmasking of symptoms of multiple sclerosis by a hot environment. This could include weather, exercise, fever, and hot showers. This phenomenon occurs as heat slows the conduction velocity of already demyelinated fibers, making symptoms more apparent. The patient has a sensory level at T10, indicating a spinal cord lesion that localizes above that level. Additional features of MS include cerebellar dysfunction, bowel and bladder dysfunction, fatigue, or spasticity. **Neuromyelitis optica** is another autoimmune demyelinating disorder that exclusively affects the optic nerve and spinal cord but usually not the brain. It is caused by autoimmune reactions to aquaporin-4 (AQP4) proteins found in astrocytic end feet.

CASE 17 | Guillain-Barré Syndrome (GBS)

A 42-year-old woman developed numbness and paresthesias in the feet upon awakening yesterday. Throughout the day, symptoms progressed upward toward her thighs. The following day, she noticed progression of symptoms to her hands and difficulty with balance and ambulation. She also noted dyspnea upon exertion. A couple of weeks ago, she had diarrhea for 5 days, which has since resolved. On exam, she has decreased sensation to pinprick, and she feels vibration in her legs up to the knees and in her arms up to the wrists. Her deep tendon reflexes are absent in the legs, and they are diminished in the arms. She has distal weakness in her legs, including foot dorsiflexors and plantar flexors, and her gait is wide based.

Evaluation/Tests	A lumbar puncture shows an elevated CSF protein and normal CSF cell count (cytoalbuminologic dissociation). EMG nerve conduction studies demonstrate demyelinating polyradiculopathy.
Treatment	The patient should be treated with intravenous immunoglobulin therapy (IVIG) or plasmapheresis.
Discussion	Guillain-Barré Syndrome (GBS) is an acute inflammatory demyelinating polyradiculoneuropathy (AIDP) that typically presents with rapid, progressive, ascending, **sensorimotor paralysis**. It is typically preceded by a respiratory or gastrointestinal illness (*Campylobacter jejuni*) a few weeks prior to onset of neurologic symptoms. The typical clinical presentation begins with sensory symptoms such as numbness and paresthesia in the feet, ascending to the proximal legs and the upper extremities. This is followed by distal ascending weakness, poor balance, respiratory involvement, and bulbar weakness. Involvement of the autonomic nervous system and respiratory failure may progress to life-threatening complications. Unlike **multiple sclerosis**, GBS is a single event rather than multiple neurological deficits at various times. GBS also has different CSF findings than MS (cytoalbuminologic dissociation rather than oligoclonal bands). **Botulism** is caused by toxins from bacteria called *Clostridium botulinum*. It can be acquired from canned food, wound infection, or in infants (usually who are less than 1 year old after ingesting honey). Unlike the ascending paralysis seen in GBS, botulism presents with descending paralysis characterized by difficulty swallowing, facial weakness, diplopia, respiratory failure, and paralysis.

CASE 18 | Charcot-Marie-Tooth (CMT) Disease

A 22-year-old man presents with slowly progressive bilateral foot and hand weakness. He recalls that as a child, he was always the slowest runner and that he could never balance himself on roller skates. In his young adulthood, he started to stumble and fall. He also noticed difficulty with buttoning shirts and manipulating small objects and has also had numbness in his feet. He recalls that his father had thin legs and required ankle braces for ambulation. He has one younger sister who is unaffected. On exam, the patient has absent deep tendon reflexes in all extremities. He lacks sensation up to his knees. He has a high steppage gait with pes cavus and hammer toes bilaterally.

CASE 18 | Charcot-Marie-Tooth (CMT) Disease *(continued)*

Evaluation/Tests	EMG shows slow nerve conduction velocities in the common peroneal and median nerves, indicating a demyelinating polyneuropathy. Genetic testing shows a gene duplication in the *PMP22* gene.
Treatment	Treat the patient with supportive management, such as occupational and physical therapy. Patients benefit from foot orthotics to improve gait stability.
Discussion	Charcot-Marie-Tooth (CMT) disease is a group of hereditary motor and sensory neuropathies (HMSN) caused by mutations in genes encoding for proteins expressed on myelin and axons of peripheral nerves. The most common mutation is *PMP22* duplication that causes CMT1A, a demyelinating sensorimotor polyneuropathy with an autosomal dominant mode of inheritance. CMT subtypes are typically classified based on clinical characteristics, mode of inheritance, electrodiagnostic features, and genetic mutation. There is a wide spectrum of disease presentation, severity, and mode of inheritance. Patients with CMT1A typically present in childhood with mild symptoms such as delayed walking, difficulties with running and balance. Over time, patients develop more disabling features such as characteristic foot deformities (pes cavus, hammer toes) as well as hand and foot weakness (foot drop), requiring mobility devices and orthotics to help with ambulation and activities of daily living. While the patient could have polyneuropathy due to other causes, the family history and confirmatory genetic testing indicate that this patient has CMT.

CASE 19 | Brown-Séquard Syndrome

A 29-year-old man who suffered a gunshot wound (GSW) to his abdomen awakens in the hospital and is unable to move his left leg. He also states that his right leg feels numb. Physical examination confirms that the patient cannot move his left leg, and he lacks sensation to light touch and proprioception in his left leg and left toes, respectively. He lacks sensation to temperature or pinprick in the right leg. He has no sensation to light touch beginning at the level of the umbilicus. His cranial nerves and upper extremity motor/sensory exams are normal. His bowel and bladder function are normal.

Evaluations/Tests	An MRI of the spine shows hyperintensity of the entire left spinal cord at the level of T10–T11, along with bony damage in the area likely secondary to the GSW.
Treatment	Treat underlying cause and consider high-dose steroids. The patient should also be treated with supportive care and physical therapy.
Discussion	Brown-Séquard syndrome is a constellation of findings caused by hemisection of the spinal cord. Typical causes include trauma (blunt or penetrating), severe disc herniation, spinal hematomas, transverse myelitis, tumors, and vertebral artery dissection. Injury to the corticospinal tract will cause ipsilateral UMN signs, including weakness below the level of the lesion as these UMN axons travel to more inferior destinations in the spinal cord. Injury to the anterior horn will cause ipsilateral LMN signs such as flaccid paralysis at the level of the lesion because these motor neurons exit the spinal cord and synapse with muscles at neuromuscular junctions. Injury to the dorsal column will result in ipsilateral loss of vibration, proprioception, and light touch below the level of the lesion. Injury to the spinothalamic tract will result in contralateral loss of pain, temperature, and crude touch below the lesion. This particular sensory loss is contralateral as the spinothalamic tract decussates early within the anterior white commissure of the spinal cord before ascending superiorly. However, the dorsal column pathway does not decussate until it reaches the level of the medulla within the brainstem. Therefore, these deficits will remain ipsilateral. Note that there will be ipsilateral loss of all sensory modalities at the level of the lesion. If the lesion occurs above the level of T1, damage to the oculosympathetic pathway may result in an ipsilateral Horner syndrome.

Loss of all sensation

LMN signs

UMN signs

Impaired pain and temperature sensation

Impaired proprioception, vibration, 2-point discrimination, and joint and position sensation

Reproduced with permission from Waxman SG: Clinical Neuroanatomy, 28th ed. New York, NY: McGraw Hill; 2017.

ALTERED MENTAL STATUS (AMS)

Disorders of the mental state are broad and numerous. Mental status is the first element tested in the neurological exam because it dictates the patient's ability to participate in the rest of the exam. Disorders of mental status include delirium, dementia, and alterations in levels of consciousness. The term "delirium" is synonymous with encephalopathy or acute confusional state. The causes of delirium are many, and delirium can coexist with other causes of cerebral dysfunction, such as dementia or stroke, thus making diagnosis potentially challenging. The presence or absence of other neurological symptoms, as well as the time course of onset, helps differentiate delirium from other disorders of mental status.

Differential Diagnoses for Altered Mental Status (AMS)

Neurological Causes	Infections	Metabolic
Cerebrovascular accident	Brain abscess	Hypo-/hypernatremia
Transient ischemic attack	Meningitis	Hypo-/hyperglycemia
Intracranial hemorrhage	Encephalitis	Hypo-/hyperthyroidism
Tumors	Endocarditis	Hypercalcemia
Seizures/postictal state	Sepsis	Hypoxia (e.g., pneumonia, pulmonary embolus)
		Hypercapnia
	Cardiovascular	Uremic or hepatic encephalopathy
	Myocardial infarction	Wernicke encephalopathy
	Heart failure	Drug or alcohol intoxication/withdrawal
	Arrhythmias	
	Hypertensive encephalopathy	**Other** (especially elderly or debilitated patients)
	Vasculitis	Medication side effects
		Fecal impaction
		Vitamin/nutritional deficiencies

Key Findings and AMS Differential Diagnosis

AMS with Key Associated Findings	Diagnoses
Slowly progressive	Dementia
Acute onset	Delirium or other organic etiology (stroke, seizure, meningitis, tumor, ICH, metabolic encephalopathy)
Fluctuating levels of consciousness	Delirium
Identifiable inciting factors (metabolic abnormalities, drug use, infection)	Delirium
Asterixis (jerking movements especially of the hands, associated with metabolic abnormalities)	Delirium
Tonic-clonic movements	Seizure
Focal neurologic deficits	Stroke, seizure, tumor, meningitis, or ICH
Ataxia, oculomotor dysfunction (eye movement abnormalities)	Wernicke's encephalopathy
Rapidly progressive, myoclonus (quick, involuntary muscle jerk)	Creutzfeldt-Jakob disease (CJD)
Visual hallucinations	Lewy body dementia
Disinhibition, socially inappropriate behavior, apathy	Frontotemporal dementia

CASE 20 | Alzheimer's Disease

An 86-year-old woman is brought in by her daughter who is concerned about her mother's increasing confusion and inability to care for herself over the last year. She has been having memory difficulties, and she has been dependent on family to help her with her finances for at least a year. Increasingly, she has been unable to cook or care for her household. More recently, she was found wandering by a neighbor several blocks from her home. She is alert and oriented only to person. She can answer simple questions and follow simple commands, but she has difficulty with attention and concentration, executive functions, memory, language, conceptual thinking, calculations, and orientation. The remainder of her exam is unremarkable.

CASE 20 | Alzheimer's Disease *(continued)*

Evaluations/Tests	An MRI brain shows nonspecific cortical atrophy out of proportion for her age. Basic blood tests, including TSH and B12, are normal, and HIV and RPR are negative.
Treatment	Treat with acetylcholinesterase inhibitors (donepezil, galantamine, or rivastigmine) and N-methyl-D-aspartate (NMDA) receptor antagonist (memantine).
Discussion	Alzheimer's dementia (AD) is the most common cause of dementia in the elderly, and its prevalence increases with age. AD is estimated to affect 20–50% of people greater than 85 years old. Similar to other neurodegenerative diseases, AD can be sporadic (90% of cases) or familial (10%), with familial cases typically showing an earlier onset. Progression is gradual. Early-onset AD is seen in familial AD with inherited mutations in amyloid precursor protein (APP), presenilin-1, or presenilin-2. In familial AD, there is an association with apolipoprotein E 4 (ApoE4). AD is characterized predominately by early memory loss, and it is progressive from mild cognitive impairment (disability in some normal daily activities) to moderate stage (difficulties with language, basic daily activities, and sometimes delusional thinking) to severe dementia (requiring assistance with all activities of daily living). Urinary and bowel incontinence, aphasia, agnosia, and apraxia develop at these later stages. There are no widely used biomarkers of AD, and it is considered a diagnosis of exclusion. Nonspecific findings include cortical atrophy, narrowing of gyri, and widening of sulci that is widespread but particularly involves the hippocampus. Definitive diagnosis is only possible at autopsy. Brain autopsy will reveal senile plaques composed of extracellular amyloid-beta and intracellular neurofibrillary tangles composed of hyperphosphorylated tau protein within gray matter. Evaluation is used to rule out other causes of dementia, especially reversible causes (thyroid disorder, syphilis, HIV, vitamin B12 deficiency, depression). There is no preventative treatment or therapy available to cure Alzheimer's disease. Treatment focuses on stalling intellectual decline and has modest effect. Abrupt cognitive, behavioral, and neurological deterioration in a patient with Alzheimer's disease (and other types of dementia) can result from infection, medication, or other reversible causes, and these should be medically evaluated. A B A, Neurofibrillary tangle (NFT). A bright red, elongated NFT partially fills the cell body of a large neuron (center of field) in the cerebral cortex of a patient with Alzheimer disease. B, Senile plaque. A brown-staining senile plaque with a central core of beta-amyloid protein is in the cerebral cortex of a patient with Alzheimer disease. Reproduced with permission from Reisner H. Pathology: A Modern Case Study, 2nd ed. New York, NY: McGraw Hill; 2020. The second most common cause of dementia in the elderly is **vascular dementia**, which has wide overlap with AD but shows a characteristic stepwise decline compared to progressive deterioration.
Additional Considerations	**Toxic-metabolic encephalopathy** is an organic brain disorder typically caused by the accumulation of toxic substances or waste products in the blood that can cross the blood-brain barrier and lead to neuronal damage. Causes of metabolic encephalopathy can include kidney failure causing uremia, liver failure causing hepatic encephalopathy, severe hypothyroidism, infection, or CO_2 poisoning.

CASE 21 | Frontotemporal Dementia

A 58-year-old man presents with behavioral and personality changes over the last 2 months. His wife reports that the patient has become much more impulsive, such as making insulting remarks and gestures that he never would have made before. She also describes that he is less motivated to go to the gym and to see his grandchildren, which he used to do regularly. He is also less engaged in general conversation. He has become preoccupied with watching the clock at the top of every hour, which is very unusual for him. He has no focal deficits on neurologic examination.

CASE 21 | Frontotemporal Dementia (continued)

Evaluation/Tests	An MRI of the brain shows focal atrophy of the frontal and temporal lobes. Neuropsychologic testing is consistent with cognitive impairment.
Treatment	Treatment is aimed at supportive care, particularly for the behavioral symptoms. Nonpharmacologic interventions can include an exercise program; physical, occupational, and speech therapy; and behavioral modification techniques.
Discussion	Frontotemporal dementia (FTD) is a neurodegenerative disorder and a common cause of early-onset (midlife) dementia. The gross pathology of FTD includes symmetrical or asymmetrical atrophy in the frontal lobe that can progress to include the temporal lobes. The time course of symptoms is important to differentiate FTD from Alzheimer's disease. In FTD, patients often demonstrate early changes in behavior or personality (behavioral variant) or altered speech/aphasia; these patients later develop neurocognitive deficits including memory loss. Changes in personality or behavior can include inappropriateness in social settings, compulsive behavior, loss of empathy, hyperorality, and disinhibition. Symptoms also typically appear in younger patients compared to AD, with FTD symptoms appearing in the fifth through seventh decade of life. Patients may also have associated movement disorders, with features of parkinsonism. Histology will show neuronal loss, with inclusions of hyperphosphorylated tau (Pick bodies), and/or ubiquitinated TDP-43. The predominantly behavioral symptoms, early onset, and location of the atrophy differentiates FTD from Alzheimer's disease.

CASE 22 | Normal Pressure Hydrocephalus (NPH)

An 82-year-old man presents to the emergency department after a fall. His wife is concerned that he has been having difficulty walking, memory loss, progressive difficulty caring for himself independently, and urinary incontinence over the past year. The patient is alert and oriented to name and place, but he incorrectly identifies the date. His gait is notable for small shuffling steps with difficulty turning.

Evaluations/Tests	MRI brain shows ventriculomegaly. Gait improvements are noted following high-volume lumbar puncture.
Treatment	Treat with ventriculoperitoneal shunting.
Discussion	Normal pressure hydrocephalus (NPH) is a form of communicating hydrocephalus commonly seen in elderly patients. It is characterized by a triad of gait apraxia, dementia, and urinary incontinence ("wobbly, wacky, and wet"). Gait disturbance is the most pronounced feature and is often described as a magnetic or "glue foot" gait. Patients move slowly with a wide base and difficulty turning. Diagnosis is challenging because the symptoms associated with NPH are nonspecific, they occur in many forms of dementia, and there is no universally accepted approach for diagnosis. However, it is important to evaluate for NPH because it is a potentially reversible disorder compared to other forms of irreversible dementia. Pathogenesis likely involves gradual reduction in the ability of arachnoid villi to reabsorb CSF, resulting in a gradual increase in CSF volume over time. Neuroimaging shows symmetric ventriculomegaly that is disproportionate to the amount of cortical atrophy. Gradual distention of fibers surrounding the ventricles such as those in the corona radiata results in decreased function. Confirmatory testing includes high-volume lumbar puncture that demonstrates improvement in gait speed, stride length, or number of steps required to turn. Definitive treatment is surgical implantation of a ventriculoperitoneal shunt to lower CSF volume. However, response rate to shunting is variable, and there is more likely to be an improvement in gait rather than in dementia. The improvement in the patient's gait following high-volume lumbar puncture makes **Parkinson's disease** less likely as Parkinson's would not improve following this procedure. Additionally, this patient's movement disorder primarily affects his gait as opposed to Parkinson's, which often affects movement of other extremities as well.

CASE 23 | Progressive Multifocal Leukoencephalopathy (PML)

A 38-year-old female with HIV was brought in for evaluation by a friend who is concerned about progressive confusion, slurred speech, and difficulty walking over the past 2 months. The patient does not see a physician regularly and takes no medications. She is only oriented to person. Cognitive testing demonstrates decreased attention and concentration, memory, calculations, and orientation. Her speech is slurred, and her gait is wide based.

CASE 23 | **Progressive Multifocal Leukoencephalopathy (PML)** (continued)

Evaluations/Tests	CD4 count is 17. MRI shows multifocal areas of periventricular white matter demyelination without contrast enhancement or surrounding edema, predominantly in the parietal and occipital lobes. CSF PCR is positive for the JC virus.
Treatment	Treat HIV with highly active antiretroviral therapy (HAART). Treatment for PML is supportive.
Discussion	Progressive multifocal leukoencephalopathy (PML) is an often fatal, rapidly progressive demyelinating disease caused by reactivation of a latent JC virus infection in immunosuppressed individuals. It mainly affects people with HIV/AIDS who are not on HAART, who are noncompliant with medications, and who have CD4 counts less than 200. It may also affect individuals with hematologic malignancies and those on immunomodulatory drugs like natalizumab and rituximab. JC virus is a polyomavirus that, upon reactivation, results in destruction of oligodendrocytes. PML usually manifests with subacute variable neurologic manifestations including altered mental status, motor dysfunction, gait disorder, and visual changes. Seizures may occur. Brain MRI can show symmetric or asymmetric white matter lesions that do not conform to a vascular territory or enhance with contrast. Brain biopsy is the gold standard for diagnosis; however, it carries significant risks. Therefore, the diagnosis may be established with CSF studies that show JC virus PCR positivity. There is no specific treatment for PML, so treatment is aimed at restoring the host immune response by optimizing HAART therapy in individuals with HIV, withdrawing immunosuppressive medications in patients without HIV-associated PML, and starting plasma exchange in natalizumab-associated PML. PML should be distinguished from **HIV-associated dementia** with a lumbar puncture. HIV-associated dementia would not be PCR positive for the JC virus. Brain imaging can also help distinguish the two etiologies. PML will have areas of demyelination, whereas HIV-associated dementia will show areas of cortical atrophy without demyelination.

CASE 24 | **Creutzfeldt-Jakob Disease**

A 67-year-old woman who works as a journalist has a 3-month history of progressive cognitive decline. She had a corneal transplant a year ago, and she initially had difficulty with concentrating, word finding, and meeting deadlines. Her colleagues became concerned about her cognitive changes, unsteady gait, and new erratic mood and behavior. A coworker slammed a door at work, and the patient jumped from her seat and had myoclonic jerking of her extremities. On exam, the patient is apathetic and only oriented to self. She has startle myoclonus and myoclonic jerks at rest.

Evaluations/Tests	MRI brain shows cortical ribboning (ribbon-like signal hyperintensity of the cortical gyri) and bilateral basal ganglia hyperintensities seen on diffusion-weighted imaging sequences. Lumbar puncture is positive for 14-3-3 protein, elevated tau protein, and positive real-time quaking-induced conversion (RT-QuIC) test. EEG shows periodic sharp wave complexes.
Treatment	Treatment is focused on supportive care. There is no cure.
Discussion	This patient is presenting with Creutzeldt-Jakob disease (CJD), a form of prion disease characterized by a rapidly progressive dementia with myoclonus and ataxia. Prion proteins (PrP) are naturally occurring proteins in neurons that can become misfolded from an alpha helix to a beta pleated sheet secondary structure when the host is exposed to pathogenic prion protein. Although there are heritable prion diseases, exposure to the protein itself causes CJD and, as such, is considered infectious. The pathogenic proteins are heat and protease resistant, so typical procedures to sterilize medical equipment will not prevent spread. Patients with CJD typically demonstrate myoclonus, which is a sudden muscle contraction. This can occur at rest or in response to sudden stimulation (startle myoclonus). Most transmitted cases are iatrogenic, and risk factors include those undergoing corneal transplants (as in this case), brain surgery, or personnel who work with brains. Other forms of prion disease include scrapie (in sheep), bovine spongiform encephalopathy (in cows), and kuru (in human cannibals). There is usually a long incubation period before rapid progression of symptoms. **PML** can cause rapidly progressive cognitive decline, but the patient does not have any risk factors for PML. The time course for her dementia is much more rapid than the typical course for **Alzheimer's disease**, making it less likely when compared to CJD. **Subacute sclerosing panencephalitis (SSPE)** is a progressive degenerative disease of the CNS that is often fatal, and it often occurs several years after measles infection. It is characterized by progressive dementia, myoclonus, and eventual autonomic dysfunction. CSF would have antimeasles antibody and elevated protein levels. EEG would demonstrate characteristic high-voltage bursts followed by delta waves with a flat pattern between these bursts.

MOVEMENT DISORDERS

Patients presenting with movement disorders may have a range of symptoms from acute onset to chronic progressive presentations, and the clinical evaluation and management are highly dependent on how a patient presents. Movement disorders comprise a group of conditions that cause abnormal involuntary movements/postures, slowness, or difficulty initiating movement. They are not the result of weakness, spasticity, or sensory disturbances. These disorders result from problems of the subcortical systems involved in movement planning, execution, and coordination. Careful observation and characterization of the movements help classify the movement disorder, and this is helpful in considering the possible etiology.

Tremor

Tremor is a rhythmic, involuntary, oscillating movement. The broad categories of tremor are resting tremor and action tremor. Resting tremor occurs in a body part that is not activated and completely supported against gravity. It is most commonly seen in Parkinson's disease, but it can also be seen in other parkinsonian syndromes. Action tremor is produced by a voluntary contraction of muscles and includes postural, intention, or task-specific tremor. These can be enhanced physiologic tremors (that can get worse with caffeine and stress), essential tremor, and drug-induced action tremors. Tremors can be primary or symptomatic. Symptomatic tremor is generally caused by disorders (tumors, strokes) affecting the cortico-striato-pallido-thalamic or cerebellar-thalamic pathways.

Parkinsonism

Parkinsonism is characterized by four cardinal features: resting tremor, bradykinesia or akinesia, rigidity (increased muscle tone), and postural instability. It is the second most common hyperkinetic movement disorder, and can be divided into primary and secondary types. Primary parkinsonism is seen in Parkinson's disease. Secondary causes include drug-induced parkinsonism from chronic dopamine antagonists (e.g., antipsychotics) or secondary to acute structural lesions of the frontal lobes, substantia nigra, basal ganglia, or thalamus.

Dystonia

Dystonia is an involuntary abnormal posture of a limb, trunk, or face that may be accompanied by twisting or repetitive movements. It can be limited to a single body part or can be more diffuse. Dystonic movements often resolve in sleep. Some patients obtain temporary relief from sensory stimuli (called a sensory trick). Acute dystonia can be seen shortly after initiating dopamine receptor antagonist medications such as antipsychotics/neuroleptics. Dystonic reactions most commonly involve the muscles of the head and neck (eyes, face, tongue, etc.) and less commonly the limbs and trunk. The resulting sustained muscle contractions can be quite severe and painful. Life-threatening concerns are seen with oral, cervical, or laryngeal dystonia due to potential involvement of respiratory muscles, presenting with stridor or aspiration. An oculogyric crisis is an acute dystonic reaction of the extraocular muscles, resulting in forced eye deviation and blurred vision. Treatment of acute dystonia involves anticholinergics (e.g., benztropine) or antihistamines (e.g., diphenhydramine), and most resolve over time. Tetanus can mimic dystonia, and delayed diagnosis can be fatal.

Chorea, Athetosis, and Ballismus

Chorea involves quick, involuntary, non-rhythmic movements of the limbs, face, or torso that occur in multiple directions. Athetosis involves slower, writhing-like movements in a more continuous fashion compared to chorea. Finally, ballismus involves large, random, flailing movements commonly involving the shoulder or hip, and often unilateral (in the case of hemiballismus).

CASE 25 | Parkinson's Disease

A 70-year-old right-handed man presents with a 2-year history of hand shaking. The patient first noticed an intermittent tremor of the right hand, but it has gradually become persistent. He also reports right shoulder pain for the past 6 months, and he is having difficulty getting out of a deep-seated chair. He denies any history of trauma, substance use, medication use, or toxin exposure. The patient is noted to have a right-hand resting tremor and little to no facial expression. He has mild cogwheel rigidity in the right arm. He walks with small, shuffling steps with a reduced right arm swing.

Evaluation/Tests	Clinical diagnosis.
Treatment	Treat with levodopa-carbidopa.

CASE 25 | Parkinson's Disease (continued)

Discussion	Parkinson's disease (PD) is a neurodegenerative disease characterized by loss of dopaminergic neurons within the substantia nigra pars compacta. The substantia nigra plays an important role in the nigrostriatal pathway to the basal ganglia, where it is involved in the initiation of movement. Loss of these neurons results in motor dysfunction. The four cardinal signs of PD include (1) resting tremor, often a "pill-rolling tremor," (2) rigidity, often described as "cogwheel," (3) akinesia or bradykinesia, and (4) postural instability, which may manifest as a shuffling gait. PD typically starts unilaterally and progresses to the contralateral side over time. Diagnosis of PD is clinical and requires presence of bradykinesia in addition to at least one of the following: rigidity, resting tremor, or postural instability in the absence of other causes (toxin exposure, cognitive decline, vertical gaze palsy, etc.). Other clinical features of PD include lack of facial expression ("masked face"), micrographia, stooped posture, and requiring many small movements to perform a normal motor function. Later in the course of the disease, patients may develop cognitive dysfunction. There is no diagnostic test for PD, but tests should be performed to rule out other causes of motor dysfunction. Loss of dopaminergic neurons results in a classic depigmentation of the substantia nigra pars compacta, and, on histology, Lewy bodies composed of misfolded alpha-synuclein are present (black arrow in histological image below). There are many therapeutic options to treat PD, most of which are based on increasing dopaminergic tone or decreasing cholinergic tone within the basal ganglia. The first-line treatment is levodopa (L-DOPA), which can be converted to dopamine within the CNS. To limit peripheral side effects, this is typically given with the peripheral DOPA decarboxylase inhibitor carbidopa. Long-term treatment with levodopa may result in a characteristic "on-off phenomenon" whereby patients experience fluctuations in symptoms. Similar symptoms can be seen in drug- (i.e., neuroleptics) or toxin- (i.e., MPTP) induced parkinsonism.

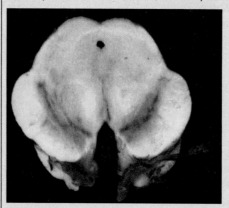 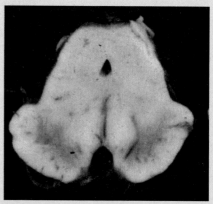

Pathologic specimens from a patient with Parkinson's disease (PD) compared to a normal control demonstrating reduction of pigment in SNc in PD (right) versus control (left).
Reproduced with permission from Jameson JL, Fauci AS, Kasper DL, et al: Harrison's Principles of Internal Medicine, 20th ed. New York, NY: McGraw Hill; 2018.

Lewy body dementia is similar to PD, but it typically presents with earlier cognitive deficits, visual hallucinations, sleep disorders, and intracellular Lewy bodies observed throughout the cortex.

Essential tremor is usually limited to particular regions of the body (i.e., just hands, head), whereas PD affects the whole body and has a characteristic gait. Essential tremor is a high-frequency action tremor that is classically observed with movement and/or sustained posture (e.g., outstretched arms), unlike the resting tremor seen in PD. Patients can be treated with propranolol (beta-blocker) or primidone (anticonvulsant).

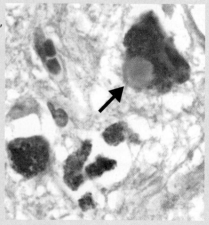

Reproduced with permission from Werner CJ, Heyny-von Haussen R, Mall G, et al: Proteome analysis of human substantia nigra in Parkinson's disease, Proteome Sci 2008 Feb 14;6:8.

CASE 26 | Huntington's Disease

A 34-year-old man with a history of depression is brought to the clinic accompanied by his mother for evaluation of abnormal movements. She has witnessed strange spontaneous writhing and dance-like movements with intermittent uncontrolled grimacing and grunting. His father died at the age of 41 from "dementia." On exam, the patient is noted to have rapid dance-like movements of all extremities. He cannot keep his tongue protruded and has a "milk-maids grasp" with alternating squeezing and releasing of the examiner's hand.

Evaluation/Tests	MRI or CT brain shows atrophy of the caudate and putamen, with flattening of the head of the caudate near the lateralventricle. Genetic testing shows CAG repeats on chromosome 4. 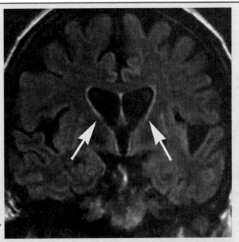 Huntington's disease. Coronal FLAIR images demonstrate bilateral symmetric abnormal high signal in the caudate and putamen. Reproduced with permission from Jameson JL, Fauci AS, Kasper DL, et al: Harrison's Principles of Internal Medicine, 20th ed. New York, NY: McGraw Hill; 2018
Treatment	The patient should receive symptomatic treatment with antidopaminergic agents (such as atypical antipsychotics and tetrabenazine).
Discussion	Huntington's disease (HD) is an autosomal dominant progressive neurodegenerative disease characterized by chorea, behavioral disturbances, and dementia. HD is a trinucleotide repeat disorder resulting from expansion of CAG repeats in the huntingtin (HTT) gene on chromosome 4. Chorea is a rapid, irregular, involuntary jerky movement that moves randomly from one body part to another in an unpredictable manner. Behavioral or neuropsychiatric symptoms often precede movement disturbances and can include aggression, depression, and suicidal ideation. Symptoms typically manifest between ages 20 and 50, and age of onset is mainly determined by the number of CAG repeats. Genetic anticipation is a phenomenon that results from expansion of CAG repeats during gametogenesis, resulting in offspring receiving a larger number of repeats. Increased repeats in the DNA promotes instability, resulting in earlier onset and increased severity of disease. A classic feature seen on imaging is atrophy of the caudate, which may manifest as a flattening of the normal convex head of the caudate adjacent to the lateral ventricle. HD is fatal within 10–20 years of onset of symptoms, and there is no cure. **Sydenham chorea** consists of involuntary, irregular, writhing, or "dance-like" movements seen in patients following streptococcal pharyngitis (strep throat) or scarlet fever. It is the most common movement disorder associated with bacterial infection and is thought to be due to *Streptococcus*-induced antibodies that cross-react with central nervous system antigens (molecular mimicry).

CASE 27 | Wilson's Disease (Hepatolenticular Degeneration)

A 20-year-old woman presents with 6 months of nervousness, postural tremor, and cramping and twisting of her feet and toes. Recently, she has also noted some trouble concentrating. Hepatomegaly is noted on exam. She also has a wing-beating tremor of her arms. Slit-lamp exam reveals fine brown dust-like ring around the edge of the limbus of the cornea in both of her eyes (Kayser-Fleischer rings).

Evaluation/Tests	Her serum copper is normal, but her ceruloplasmin is reduced; 24-hour urine sample shows increased copper excretion. MRI brain shows increased signal on T2-weighted images in the caudate, putamen, midbrain, and thalamus.
Treatment	Treat with D-penicillamine or trientine dihydrochloride in addition to zinc supplement and low copper diet. In patients with severe liver disease, liver transplant is indicated and is also curative.
Discussion	This patient is presenting with Wilson's disease (hepatolenticular degeneration), an autosomal recessive disorder of copper metabolism resulting from mutations in hepatocyte copper-transporting P-type ATPase (*ATP7B* gene on chromosome 13). Defects in this ATPase enzyme leads to inability to excrete copper

CASE 27 | Wilson's Disease (Hepatolenticular Degeneration) *(continued)*

Discussion	from the liver into bile, leading to copper accumulation. Wing-beating tremor and Kayser-Fleischer rings in the cornea are two classical signs in patients with Wilson's disease. In children, the disorder may present as liver disease. However, some patients may present as late as 40 years of age with abnormal movements or psychiatric symptoms. Abnormal movements include parkinsonism, tremor, ataxia, and dystonia. Tremor is classically proximal and high amplitude, giving the appearance of "wing beating" when the arms are abducted and elbows flexed. Diagnosis is made by looking at serum ceruloplasmin and urine copper levels. Serum copper may be misleadingly normal, reduced, or elevated. **Hereditary dystonia** and **Huntington's disease** do not present with hepatomegaly or Kayser-Fleischer rings.	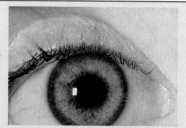 Reproduced with permission from Usatine RP, Smith MA, Mayeaux EJ, et al: The Color Atlas and Synopsis of Family Medicine, 3rd ed. New York, NY: McGraw Hill; 2019. Photo contributor: Marc Solioz, University of Berne.

CASE 28 | Malignant Hyperthermia

A 30-year-old man with no past medical history was taken to the operating room for debridement and open fixation of a femur fracture after a motor vehicle accident. He was placed under inhaled anesthesia, and about 45 minutes into the surgery, he became tachycardic to 120, and his blood pressure became labile up to 150/120 mmHg. His temperature increased to 40°C, and he became rigid and diaphoretic.

Evaluation/Tests	An arterial blood gas shows a PO_2 70 mmHg, PCO_2 55 mmHg, and a pH 7.30. His labs are significant for an elevated potassium and highly elevated CK. Urinalysis shows myoglobinuria.
Treatment	The patient's anesthesia should immediately be discontinued, and he should be given dantrolene. He should also be provided with ventilatory support, adequate oxygenation, and intravenous fluids.
Discussion	Malignant hyperthermia is a rare, life-threatening metabolic response to potent inhalational anesthetics and/or succinylcholine. Susceptibility to malignant hyperthermia is inherited in an autosomal dominant pattern, although it shows variable penetrance (not all patients with the mutation will display the disease). Mutations occur in the voltage-sensitive ryanodine receptor (*RYR1* gene), which is involved in calcium release from the myocyte sarcoplasmic reticulum. Mutations result in excess release of calcium, which causes increased ATP uptake and consumption, in turn generating heat and muscle damage. The earliest signs of a malignant hyperthermia episode include tachycardia and increased end-tidal CO_2 that does not improve with increases in minute ventilation. Muscle rigidity may be an early sign, but it is not always present. Hyperthermia, altered consciousness, and autonomic instability may occur. It can further lead to rhabdomyolysis, hyperkalemia, renal failure, ventricular fibrillation, and sudden cardiac arrest. **Neuroleptic malignant syndrome** presents similarly, but it occurs in patients receiving antipsychotic medications; they will also present with acute mental status changes. **Serotonin syndrome** is seen in drugs that increase serotonin (SSRI, SNRI, MAO inhibitors, TCAs, etc.) when taken in combination or at high dose and that result in neuromuscular hyperactivity, agitation, and autonomic stimulation.

ATAXIA

Ataxia is a neurological sign involving inaccurate or uncoordinated volitional movements. It often results from disease of the cerebellum or the tracts connecting the cerebellum to the rest of the nervous system. Other symptoms include dysmetria, gait unsteadiness with a wide base, dysarthria, and trunk titubation. Dysmetria is characterized by repeated over- or under-shooting of corrected movements and can be tested using the "finger-to-nose" and "heel-shin" test, as the affected limbs approach their target. Titubation is wavering movement and postural instability of the trunk. Primary ataxia is often genetic and typically progresses slowly over time; primary ataxias include the spinocerebellar ataxias, ataxia-telangiectasia, and Friedreich's ataxia. Causes of secondary ataxia include intoxication (alcohol, benzodiazepines, anticonvulsants), cerebellitis, metabolic disorders, encephalitis, Wilson's disease, thiamine deficiency, and acute focal cerebellar lesions (demyelination, tumor, stroke). These conditions are often accompanied by other neurologic signs with localization to the posterior fossa including cranial nerve palsies, nausea, emesis, and headache.

CASE 29	Tabes Dorsalis (Neurosyphilis)
	A 55-year-old man with diabetes, hypertension, and genital herpes presents with shooting pains down his spine and a tingling, prickling sensation in his hands and feet. He also notes intermittent sudden pain in his eye with tearing. His wife reports that he is more confused and that he seems unbalanced when walking. On exam, he has small pupils that do not constrict to light, but accommodation is intact. Sensation is diminished to light touch and vibration in all extremities, and he has a positive Romberg sign. Deep tendon reflexes are absent.
Evaluation/Tests	RPR and/or VDRL tests and FTA-Abs are positive. Lumbar puncture shows elevated CSF protein and leukocytes. HIV is negative. B12 and blood glucose are normal.
Treatment	Treat with intravenous penicillin.
Discussion	Tabes dorsalis is a complication of tertiary syphilis and a form of **neurosyphilis** caused by the destruction of the dorsal columns and dorsal roots of the spinal cord. Most commonly, it occurs when syphilis is undiagnosed and therefore untreated. Damage results in loss of proprioception and vibration sense. Patients will experience ataxia with a positive Romberg sign and a wide-based "tabetic gait" where their feet will slap the ground heavily. Patients may also experience sudden lancinating pain and anesthesia going down the spine, extremities, or ocular nerves, resulting in lacrimation. Patients also classically present with **Argyll Robertson pupil**, a pupil that accommodates but does not react to light. Other manifestations of tertiary syphilis include dementia, deafness, vision loss, and aortitis. There is increased incidence of neurosyphilis in patients who are also infected with HIV. **Diabetic neuropathy** is a great mimicker because it can attack various parts of the nervous system and present in numerous ways. Most commonly, it presents as neuropathic pain in the lower extremities with decreased sensation in the distal lower extremities. It typically does not present with confusion. **Subacute combined degeneration (SCD)** is a neurologic manifestation of **vitamin B12 deficiency** characterized by demyelination of the spinocerebellar tracts, lateral corticospinal tracts, and dorsal columns of the spinal cord. Patients present with loss of proprioception, vibration, and fine touch (dorsal columns), UMN signs (lateral corticospinal tracts), ataxia (spinocerebellar tracts), and numbness, lancinating pains, and paresthesias (peripheral nerves). Vitamin B12 deficiency can present in patients on a strict vegetarian diet or patients with a history of pernicious anemia, inflammatory bowel disease, bariatric surgery, or chronic use of metformin or proton pump inhibitors. Vitamin B12 deficiency results in a macrocytic, megaloblastic anemia.

SEIZURES

A **seizure** is defined as abnormal, hypersynchronous electrical activity of the brain. A clinical seizure can take many forms depending on the area of the brain affected. The most common seizure is a convulsive seizure where there is rhythmic or tonic muscle involvement of any or all limbs and trunk.

In clinical practice, seizures are classified based on their onset/initial manifestation. They can be focal (originating in one part of the brain) or generalized (originating in the whole brain all at once). Focal (previously called partial) seizures are classified based on the level of awareness as focal aware (intact consciousness, previously called simple seizure) or focal with impaired awareness (loss of consciousness, previously called complex seizure). Additionally, focal seizures are classified according to the presence or absence of motor symptoms (e.g., automatism). Focal onset seizures can spread and evolve to bilateral tonic-clonic seizures. Generalized seizures are classified based on having motor or nonmotor manifestation. Motor manifestation includes tonic, clonic, myoclonic, and tonic-clonic seizures. Nonmotor seizures are usually absence seizures.

Epilepsy is a chronic condition characterized by spontaneous seizures (2 or more unprovoked seizures >24 hours apart or by 1 unprovoked seizure with a probability of >60% of having a 2nd seizure over the next 10 years). Epilepsy can be classified as focal, generalized, combined generalized and focal, and unknown epilepsy. The etiology of epilepsy can be divided into six categories: structural, infectious, genetic, immune, metabolic, and unknown. Some of these etiologies can overlap; for example, a patient may have a structural lesion because of a genetic condition.

In a patient presenting with a first-time seizure, prompt evaluation is warranted to determine if a cause or reversible factors can be identified. Workup of a first-time, unprovoked seizure also includes electroencephalogram (EEG) and MRI brain to determine the risk of a recurrent seizure. If epileptiform activity is seen on EEG or a lesion is noted on MRI, this increases the risk of a 2nd seizure and thus changes patient management. EEG can also be a helpful diagnostic tool to confirm diagnosis, to localize the seizure onset, and to determine etiology in certain epilepsy syndromes and the likelihood of response to treatment. It is important to note that a normal EEG does not rule out epilepsy.

CASE 30 | Absence Seizure (Childhood Absence Epilepsy)

A 7-year-old girl with no prior medical history is brought for evaluation of episodic staring off into space. Her spells last 5–10 seconds. She has had a recent decline in school performance over the last 8–10 months. During the mental status exam, the child stops midsentence and stares with blinking and right-hand picking movements, lasting about 10 seconds. After the spell is over, she immediately finishes her sentence.

Evaluation/Tests	Bedside hyperventilation for 3 minutes triggers similar staring spells. Routine scalp EEG shows 3-Hz spike-wave discharges diffusely throughout the brain.
Treatment	Treat with ethosuximide (first line), valproic acid, or lamotrigine (certain medication such as carbamazepine and phenytoin can worsen absence epilepsy).
Discussion	Childhood absence epilepsy (CAE) is a generalized nonconvulsive epilepsy syndrome common in childhood that manifests as generalized nonmotor seizures like staring spells with a blank stare. Onset typically occurs between the ages of 4 and 10 with a slight female predominance. These seizures tend to be brief and self-limited, often lasting less than 20 seconds, and there is typically no postictal cognitive slowing seen. Patients may also have automatisms such as eye fluttering, lip smacking, and even unilateral picking, though any focal symptoms should prompt consideration of a focal seizure (complex partial seizures). Absence seizures can be brought about by hyperventilation at the bedside. On EEG, the hallmark is the 3-Hz generalized spike-slow wave discharges. Patients with childhood absence epilepsy can have ten to hundreds of seizures a day. Rarely, patients can have generalized tonic-clonic seizures. CAE is a self-limited epilepsy where prognosis is good—with 95% of patients outgrowing their seizures by puberty. **Focal seizures with impaired awareness** (also known as complex partial seizures) that manifest as staring will not be brought out by hyperventilation. However, such seizures should be considered in any patient with staring spells, particularly if the staring events are prolonged (greater than 30 seconds) or if they are followed by postictal confusion and tiredness.
Additional Considerations	**Juvenile myoclonic epilepsy (JME)** is a form of idiopathic generalized epilepsy that presents most commonly in the adolescent or young adult age groups with onset between ages 8 and 28. The clinical hallmark is the myoclonic seizure, which are quick motor jerks typically of the upper extremities and head that occur most often in the mornings shortly after awakening and with intact consciousness. Patients may also have generalized convulsive seizures, and they rarely can have absence seizures. EEG is characterized by 4- to 6-Hz generalized polyspike and slow-wave discharges. Seizures in JME are often exacerbated by alcohol consumption and sleep deprivation. Unlike CAE, JME is not usually self-limiting and usually requires lifelong antiseizure medication.

CASE 31 | Focal Seizure (Temporal Lobe Epilepsy)

A 35-year-old woman presents with her partner for evaluation of odd "spells." She reports intermittent episodes of an odd feeling in her stomach. She describes the sensation as equivalent to feeling she is in an elevator going down rapidly. With some of these events, symptoms evolve where she stares and does not answer questions, and her partner reports that she has picking movements of her left hand. Sometimes, he also notes that her eyes go off to the left, she lets out a loud cry, and then her whole-body starts shaking. After these events, she is usually confused and disoriented. Her exam is unremarkable.

Evaluation/Tests	Her CBC, CMP, blood alcohol level, and urine toxicology screen are all within normal limits. Brain MRI with and without contrast shows reduced right hippocampal volume with increased T2 signal suggestive of mesial temporal sclerosis
Treatment	The patient should be treated with an antiseizure medication.
Discussion	Temporal lobe epilepsy is the most common cause of focal epilepsy. Classically, temporal lobe seizures may present with "auras." Auras can include an unusual odor, a rising epigastric sensation (as just described) that can be likened to nausea, a feeling of déjà vu, or a strong emotion such as fear due to the proximity of the amygdala. Sometimes the seizures can be more limited focal seizures such as staring

CASE 31 | Focal Seizure (Temporal Lobe Epilepsy) *(continued)*

Discussion	and unresponsiveness, which is why it should be considered when working up absence epilepsy in children. There is frequently secondary generalization, which is now called focal to bilateral tonic-clonic seizures based on newer seizure classification with impaired awareness. Following a seizure, the brain may enter a postictal state characterized clinically by confusion, disorientation, decreased consciousness, and general slowing or suppression on EEG. Mesial temporal sclerosis is a common finding in temporal lobe epilepsy with neuronal cell death, gliosis, and sclerosis and can be visualized on MRI with reduced hippocampal volume and/or increased T2 signal
Additional Considerations	Postictal focal paralysis (known as **Todd's paralysis**) can be seen following different types of seizures. **Status epilepticus** is a neurological and medical emergency defined as continuous seizures lasting ≥5 min or more than one seizure without recovery between events. Convulsive status epilepticus is the most severe form, causing both neuronal dysfunction and systemic derangements such as rhabdomyolysis. Patients must be treated quickly with IV benzodiazepines and careful monitoring of airway and hemodynamic status. Patients are also treated with an "urgent control" antiseizure medication such as phenytoin and levetiracetam.

CASE 32 | Infantile Spasm (Tuberous Sclerosis)

A 7-month-old boy is brought for evaluation of brief episodes of twitching arms that occur multiple times every day. In a recent clinic visit, his pediatrician noted that he had not been sitting up and had a rash on the lower back with a leathery texture. His cardiac exam is significant for a holosystolic, high-pitched "blowing" murmur heard loudest at the apex and radiating toward the axilla. During the exam, the child thrusts his arms out numerous times.

Evaluation/Tests	ECG and echocardiogram confirm mitral regurgitation and presence of a mass in the heart. Abdominal MRI reveals an additional mass in the right kidney. Brain MRI with and without contrast shows presence of multiple cortical tubers throughout the cortex. EEG confirms seizure-like activity with periodic frequent epileptiform discharges. Genetic testing reveals mutations in the *TSC1* gene on chromosome 9.
Treatment	Treat with vigabatrin, ACTH, and a high-dose steroid. Additionally, patient should be referred to appropriate specialist for treatment of other findings and conditions.
Discussion	Tuberous sclerosis complex (TSC) is a multiorgan disease and one of several neurocutaneous disorders. It is caused by autosomal dominant mutations in one of two tumor suppressor genes: *TSC1* gene on chromosome 9 (encodes hamartin) or the *TSC2* gene on chromosome 16 (encodes tuberin). These mutations result in the growth of hamartomas in various organs throughout the body, notably the skin and CNS. TSC is the most common genetic cause of infantile spasm, which presents as 1- to 2-second seizures where the baby thrusts out his arm or bends forward with stiff extremities. Other neurologic manifestations are due to formation of cortical tubers, subependymal giant cell astrocytoma, and nodules. They also can include seizures, intellectual disabilities, and autistic behaviors. Dermatologic findings include facial angiofibroma, Shagreen patches, and hypomelanotic macules ("ash leaf spots"). Rhabdomyomas may be present in the fetal heart, which typically regresses after birth. Other features include angiomyolipomas (AML) in the kidney and lymphangioleiomyomatosis (LAM) in the lung. Conventionally, ACTH or high-dose steroid has been a treatment option. Vigabatrin is specifically indicated in infantile spasm associated with TSC. Another neurocutaneous disorder that can present with seizures is **Sturge-Weber syndrome** (encephalotrigeminal angiomatosis), a noninherited developmental anomaly of neural crest cell derivatives that affects small blood vessels. It presents with a port wine stain on the face in the cranial nerve V1 or V2 distribution, leptomeningeal angiomas, and episcleral hemangiomas.

OPHTHALMOLOGY

Ophthalmology is the subspecialty of medicine that deals with medical and surgical management of eye disorders. The eye is broadly divided into three main layers: (1) **sclera**—the white, nontransparent, structure that is continuous with the cornea in the front of the eye; (2) **uvea**—includes the iris, ciliary body, and choroid; and (3) **retina**—the innermost layer composed of rod and cone photoreceptors, retinal ganglion cells with axons giving rise to the optic nerve, and other cell types involved in converting light signals to electrochemical signals. Aqueous humor is produced in the ciliary body, and it flows between the iris and lens into the anterior chamber, where it is mostly reabsorbed at the iridocorneal angle through the trabecular meshwork into the canal of Schlemm. Dysregulation of the production, flow, or drainage of aqueous humor can result in elevated intraocular pressure and cause glaucoma.

The retina is part of the central nervous system and an extension of the diencephalon of the developing brain. As such, the eye serves as a unique window into various neurologic disorders. These include neurologic injuries resulting in increased intracranial pressure (which will manifest as papilledema), demyelinating disorders (which may present as optic neuritis, internuclear ophthalmoplegia, etc.), or injuries to cranial nerves involved in extraocular muscles, corneal sensation, or autonomic innervation (CN III, IV, V1, or VI).

Diabetes mellitus, long-standing hypertension, allergic hypersensitivity reactions, infections, vasculitides, and many more systemic diseases also have ophthalmologic manifestations. These conditions may lead to disruption of normal vasculature, formation of deposits, and neovascularization that result in formation of leaky vessels.

The ophthalmologist's basic tool is the slit lamp microscope, which allows observation of any of the three layers of the eye. The ophthalmoscope (or fundoscope) allows for visualization of the retina, including the macula, optic disc, and blood supply. When assessing changes in vision, both eyes must be assessed. Vison is documented using denotation based on Latin terminology: OS for the left eye, OD for the right eye, and OU for both eyes. Visual acuity is measured at a 20-foot distance, with 20/20 vision indicating that a patient can clearly see objects that are normally visible from 20 feet away. Higher denominators indicate worse vision. For example, 20/40 vision indicates that, at a distance of 20 feet, the patient can see objects that others can see from 40 feet.

EYE REDNESS

Red, or "bloodshot," eyes are a common concern. Clinically, this may be referred to as conjunctival injection or hyperemia, and it represents enlargement of the blood vessels within the conjunctiva. The various causes of conjunctival injection include infections, allergic hypersensitivity reactions, and autoimmune reactions.

CASE 33	Bacterial Conjunctivitis
A 40-year-old man with a history of contact lens use for myopia presents with unilateral red eye with an occasional burning sensation. He reports difficulty opening his eyes in the morning due to a thick crust on the lids. Exam shows intense redness of the right eye (hyperemia) with a thick, mucopurulent, yellow-green discharge and matted eyelids with notable crusting.	
Evaluations/Tests	Clinical diagnosis.
Treatment	Prescribe broad-spectrum topical antibiotics.
Discussion	This patient is experiencing conjunctivitis, which is inflammation of the conjunctiva, the thin tissue lining the outer surface of the eye and inner surface of the eyelid. Conjunctivitis can be bacterial (as in this case), viral, or allergic in etiology. The history of contact lens use increases risk for bacterial conjunctivitis. Unilateral symptoms and a classic thick discharge are more typical in bacterial conjunctivitis compared to allergic and viral conjunctivitis. A history of crusting can make it difficult to distinguish from viral conjunctivitis. Common pathogens include *Streptococcus pneumoniae*, *Staphylococcus aureus*, *Haemophilus influenzae*, and chlamydial and gonococcal sexually transmitted infections. The diagnosis is clinical, but it is important to examine the cornea to ensure there is no epithelial defect or ulcer. **Allergic conjunctivitis** typically presents with bilateral itchy eyes in patients with a history of atopy (asthma, seasonal allergies, eczema). It is typically mild and may have a classic clear stringy discharge. Treatment includes artificial tears, antihistamines, and avoidance of allergens. **Viral conjunctivitis** is the most common form of conjunctivitis, and it may be preceded by systemic or upper respiratory symptoms. Adenovirus is the most common viral cause. Viral conjunctivitis is characterized by sparse discharge and may have swollen preauricular lymph nodes. It is typically self-resolving.

CASE 34	Neonatal Gonococcal Conjunctivitis
A 2-day-old neonate is brought for evaluation of bilateral red eyes with discharge. Her mother did not receive any prenatal care and has a history of sexually transmitted infections (STI). Exam shows profuse bilateral purulent discharge from the eyes with diffusely injected conjunctiva.	
Evaluations/Tests	Gram stain and culture of eye discharge reveal Gram-negative intracellular diplococci.
Treatment	The patient should be admitted for evaluation for disseminated infection, and she should be treated with intramuscular ceftriaxone. Eye irrigation with saline should be used until the discharge clears.

CASE 34 | Neonatal Gonococcal Conjunctivitis *(continued)*

Discussion	This infant has **neonatal gonococcal conjunctivitis**. The physical exam, time of presentation (day 2 of life), and history of her mother (lack of prenatal care with history of STI) all make gonococcal conjunctivitis most likely. Additionally, the Gram stain is pathognomonic for *Neisseria gonorrhoeae*. The patient is also at risk for chlamydial conjunctivitis, and she should be treated for this as well. **Chlamydial conjunctivitis** can present similarly or with milder conjunctival injection, tearing, and mucoid discharge. Unlike gonococcal conjunctivitis, chlamydial conjunctivitis typically presents between 7 and 14 days of life. **Chemical conjunctivitis** occurs within hours of placing prophylactic silver nitrate eye drops in infants at birth; however, it is rarely seen now that erythromycin is used routinely.

CASE 35 | Viral Keratitis

A 55-year-old man presents with right eye pain, redness, photophobia, tearing, and decreased visual acuity. He has had similar symptoms in the past, along with a history of "cold sores." Exam of the right eye shows conjunctival injection (hyperemia).

Evaluations/Tests	Slit-lamp exam with fluorescein staining shows a thin, linear branching epithelial ulceration.
Treatment	The patient should be treated with valacyclovir and aggressive ocular lubrication.
Discussion	This patient is presenting with the classic symptoms of a **corneal ulcer due to HSV keratitis**. The hallmark of this disease is corneal dendrites seen with fluorescein on slit-lamp exam. The history of cold sores (herpes labialis) indicates a history of symptomatic HSV. HSV can be differentiated from **VZV** by the lack of a vesicular facial rash in the V1 dermatome on the ipsilateral side. **Bacterial keratitis** is often accompanied with mucopurulent discharge, and it is common in patients who wear contact lenses overnight.

ACUTE VISION LOSS

Timely diagnosis and treatment in cases of sudden or acute vision loss may help limit the extent of permanent visual disturbance. Many causes of acute vision loss are ophthalmologic emergencies and may be due to underlying life-threatening systemic diseases that require prompt treatment and management. Most patients will present hours to days after the onset of symptoms, and time is of the essence in some of the following entities.

Key Findings and Acute Vision Loss Differential Diagnoses

Acute Vision Loss and Key Associated Findings	Diagnoses
Pain	Acute angle closure glaucoma, optic neuritis, giant cell arteritis (headache)
Painless	Central retinal artery occlusion, retinal detachment
Associated neurologic symptoms	Optic neuritis
History of trauma	Retinal detachment
Systemic symptoms	Giant cell arteritis, central retinal artery occlusion
History of high myopia	Retinal detachment
History of high hyperopia	Acute angle closure glaucoma

CASE 36 | Retinal Detachment

A 25-year-old man with a history of high myopia presents with sudden onset of "flickering lights" in the temporal field of his right eye. Direct ophthalmoscopy demonstrates an orange and white corrugated appearance.

Evaluation/Tests	A full dilated eye exam reveals pigmented vitreous cells in the anterior segment and a white, fibrous ring (Weiss ring) on fundoscopic exam.
Treatment	The patient should be treated with urgent surgical repair if the macula is threatened.

CASE 36 | Retinal Detachment (continued)

Discussion	Retinal detachment is an ophthalmologic emergency involving the detachment of the neurosensory layer of the retina from the outermost pigmented epithelium, resulting in degeneration of photoreceptors. It has many etiologies, including predisposing retinal break, trauma, inflammation, diabetic retinopathy, medication side effects, and various infectious etiologies. Detachment is more common in patients with high myopia, or "nearsightedness." Symptoms often include flashes of light or floaters in the eye, a "drawn-down curtain" over the field of vision, and monocular vision loss. Immediate referral to an ophthalmologist for surgical evaluation and repair is the standard of care. **Ocular migraines** are more likely to present with repeated attacks of similar symptoms including temporary blindness that resolves after an hour. Ocular migraines are not likely to include vitreous debris and Weiss ring on ophthalmologic exam. **Vitritis** is uveitis that localizes to the vitreous cavity and may extend to the peripheral retina. Presenting features include redness, eye pain, blurry vision, floaters, and photophobia. **Retinitis** involves inflammation of the retina and can result in permanent damage and blindness if untreated. Infection is often the cause. It causes blurred vision, flashes, floaters, and side vision in the affected eye.

CASE 37 | Central Retinal Artery Occlusion

A 51-year-old woman with a history of systemic lupus erythematosus (SLE) and high cholesterol presents with sudden onset painless vision loss in the left eye. On exam, when a penlight is shone in her right eye, both eyes constrict; however, when it is then quickly shone in the left eye, her pupils dilate (left afferent pupillary defect). Her extraocular movements are intact. Fundoscopic exam reveals macular whitening with red foveal sparing ("cherry-red spot").

Evaluation/Tests	Serum antibody testing is positive for ANA, as well as anticardiolipin and anti-beta-2 glycoproteins antibodies confirming the diagnosis of SLE. CRAO is diagnosed based on history and fundoscopic exam alone.
Treatment	Ocular massage, hyperventilation, anterior chamber paracentesis, and topical antihypertensive drops can be used within 90 minutes of the occlusive event, but there is no known effective treatment.
Discussion	Central retinal artery occlusion (CRAO) presents with unilateral, painless vision loss. CRAO is often caused by emboli including cholesterol or platelet fibrin emboli from the carotids or calcium emboli from cardiac valves; this should be suspected in patients with cardiovascular risk factors. CRAO can also be caused by collagen vascular disease (SLE, polyarteritis nodosa), hypercoagulable disorders (antiphospholipid syndrome), or giant cell arteritis (GCA). The patient in this case has a hypercoagulable state due to her known diagnosis of SLE and her positive antiphospholipid antibody tests. Prognosis for CRAO is poor, and neovascular sequelae can occur; ophthalmologic evaluation is indicated within a month of onset. Patients with **retinal vein occlusion** can be asymptomatic, or they can present with a visual field defect and painless blurred or grayed vision. The fundoscopic exam would show retinal hemorrhages, venous engorgement, and edema in the affected area. **Optic neuritis** is a demyelinating inflammation of the optic nerve. It is most often associated with multiple sclerosis patients who present with sudden loss of vision and pain on movement of the affected eye. It can be an idiopathic inflammation or associated with infections (syphilis, tuberculosis, or in children typically related to viral etiologies) or inflammatory disorders (sarcoidosis). **Giant cell arteritis (GCA)** is an inflammatory disease of large blood vessels. Symptoms include headache, pain over temples, difficulty opening the mouth, fever, and body aches.

CASE 38 | Giant Cell Arteritis

An 83-year-old woman with a past medical history of polymyalgia rheumatica presents with vision loss in the right eye for the last 24 hours. The patient denies eye pain but endorses intermittent headache and low-grade fever over the last week. Her headache is throbbing and limited to the right side. She also reports pain in her jaw while chewing and notes malaise and generalized myalgias for the past 2 weeks. She denies diplopia, nausea, vomiting, or fevers or chills. She is tender to palpation over her left temporal artery, which is noted to be "cord-like." She has a normal gait, but difficulty is noted with her get-up-and-go testing.

Evaluation/Tests	ESR and CRP are elevated.
Treatment	Immediate steroid therapy should be initiated to prevent blindness, followed quickly by temporal artery biopsy to assess for focal granulomatous inflammation.

CASE 38 | Giant Cell Arteritis *(continued)*

Discussion	Giant cell (temporal) arteritis is an ophthalmologic emergency occurring in patients >55 years old resulting from large-vessel vasculitis affecting branches of the carotid artery, commonly the temporal artery. In addition to acute unilateral vision loss and headache, typical systemic symptoms include jaw claudication, weight loss, and low-grade fever. It is commonly associated with polymyalgia rheumatica, which is characterized by pain and stiffness without weakness in proximal muscles. In cases with moderate to high suspicion, systemic steroids should be given immediately—prior to the return of lab results—because delay in diagnosis can lead to blindness or involvement of the other eye. Steroid treatment should then be quickly followed by biopsy for confirmation. Prolonged treatment with steroids may produce false negative biopsy results. **Trigeminal neuralgia** similarly presents with facial pain. Patients can have sudden shock-like pain on one side of the face lasting seconds to a few minutes along the trigeminal nerve division of the face. **Optic neuritis** causes eye pain, and it is associated with vision loss. A **compressive optic nerve tumor** stemming from a pituitary adenoma leads to decreased visual acuity and bitemporal hemianopsia.

MOTILITY AND PUPIL ABNORMALITIES

The pupil and motility exams are an important diagnostic tool to uncover emergent underlying disease such as dissections, giant cell arteritis, uncontrolled diabetes, and tumors of the orbit. The pupil exam looks closely at the size and shape of the pupil, and its symmetry in size and shape with the neighboring eye. The afferent system can be assessed by comparing the response to light in each eye, to determine if an abnormality exists in one eye as compared to the other. In addition, the motility exam can uncover cranial nerve palsies, which may be isolated, congenital, or sequelae from an acute systemic issue.

CASE 39 | Horner Syndrome

A 56-year-old man presents with a "droopy right eyelid" for the last 3 days. He denies any pain or change in vision. He is a heavy smoker and drinker, but he denies a history of trauma. He has had a cough for the past several months, and he has lost some weight. On exam, he has ptosis on the right and anisocoria that worsens in dim light. He has full extraocular motility in both eyes and normal red reflexes. He also has supraclavicular lymphadenopathy, and pulmonary exam reveals wheezing and dullness to percussion over the right upper lobe.

Evaluation/Tests	CT chest reveals a mass at the apex of the right lung. MR angiogram (MRA) of the neck is normal.
Treatment	Treat the underlying cause of Horner's syndrome (in this case, the patient's lung cancer).
Discussion	Horner's syndrome is a disruption of the sympathetic chain innervating the face, leading to a classic triad of ptosis (drooping of eyelid), miosis (pupil constriction), and anhidrosis (absence of sweating, often with flushing). While there are many causes depending on the location of the lesion along the sympathetic chain, urgent workup of potential life-threatening etiologies is essential. Pancoast (superior sulcus) tumors are carcinomas found in the apex of the lung that can compress regional structures, including the stellate ganglion, that result in Horner's syndrome. MRA should be performed if there is high suspicion of a **carotid dissection**. Other causes include brain or spinal cord lesions (above T1). Pharmacological miosis occurs when a patient is using a cholinergic agonist such as pilocarpine, while physiologic anisocoria is a benign condition typically presenting as a 1-mm difference in pupil size irrespective of lighting.

CASE 40 | Marcus Gunn Pupil

A 25-year-old man presents with gradual decreased vision in the left eye. He denies any pain and reports normal vision of the right eye. When light is shined in the right eye, both pupils constrict. When swung to the left eye, both pupils dilate (left afferent pupillary defect).

Evaluation/Tests	CBC, RPR, and FTA-Abs tests are normal. MRI of the brain and orbits with and without contrast reveal a mass along the optic nerve.
Treatment	The patient should be assessed for possible surgical intervention.

CASE 40 | Marcus Gunn Pupil *(continued)*

Discussion	The swinging flashlight test is used to demonstrate a Marcus Gunn Pupil or a relative afferent pupillary defect (rAPD). In this test, the light shined in the normal eye shows constriction of the ipsilateral and contralateral pupil due to the direct and consensual reflexes, respectively. When light is shined in the affected eye, there is an impaired signal; in this case, it is due to cell death from an optic nerve glioma. The pupils in both eyes, therefore, dilate when light is shined in the affected eye. A Marcus Gunn pupil indicates an optic nerve lesion or severe retinal disease, significantly reducing signal input from the affected eye as compared to the unaffected eye. Causes include retinal infection (CMV, herpes, syphilis), retinal detachment, optic neuritis, optic damage (from tumor, trauma, severe glaucoma), or ischemic optic/retinal disease. Any impairment of one optic nerve compared to the other can cause Marcus Gunn pupil; increased intracranial pressure can cause unilateral or asymmetric optic atrophy, which would cause this relative afferent pupillary defect.

CASE 41 | Abducens Nerve (CN VI) Palsy

A 67-year-old woman with hypertension, hyperlipidemia, and poorly controlled diabetes presents with sudden onset of painless and horizontal double vision. She has no history of trauma or other symptoms. Her pupils are equal and reactive. Examination of extraocular movements reveals a complete lack of abduction in the left eye with a large left esotropia (eye turned inward).

Evaluation/Tests	Clinical diagnosis.
Treatment	Symptomatic patients should be treated with an eye patch.
Discussion	This patient is experiencing abducens (CN VI) nerve palsy. The abducens nerve innervates the lateral rectus muscle, so damage to this nerve causes an inability to abduct the eye that causes a medially displaced eye. Patients with uncontrolled diabetes or hypertension can manifest with ocular motility issues from cranial nerve palsies. An important distinction between CN VI palsies caused by microvascular changes and those caused by increased intracranial pressure is the evidence of diabetic changes in the eye (macular edema, diabetic retinopathy) and the absence of optic nerve changes indicating increased intracranial pressure (optic nerve pallor or edema). In any equivocal cases, an MRI of the brain and orbits should be ordered to rule out intracranial pathology. Often in ischemic CN VI palsy, there is partial or total resolution within 3 months; if resolution is not complete, prism glasses or strabismus surgery may be indicated. **Thyroid eye disease** is a chronic condition that can cause esotropia. Accompanying findings include proptosis, eyelid retraction, and dry eye disease. While **myasthenia gravis** should also be considered, this is often a fluctuating strabismus with fatigability and ptosis. **Cavernous sinus thrombosis** typically involves multiple cranial nerves.

CASE 42 | Trochlear Nerve (CN IV) Palsy

A 2-year-old child is brought for evaluation. His parents note that the child always tilts the head to the left and has done so since he was able to sit up at 6 months. On exam, the right eye appears higher than the left eye when the patient looks straight ahead. The child maintains a left tilt of his head at rest. With forced tilt to the right, his right eye is dramatically elevated compared to the left.

Evaluation/Tests	Clinical diagnosis.
Treatment	The patient should be treated with an eye patch and monitored for development of amblyopia.
Discussion	This patient is experiencing a trochlear (CN IV) nerve palsy. The trochlear nerve innervates the superior oblique muscle, which responsible for depression of the eye when adducted (intorsion of eye toward nose). Damage to this nerve limits the ability to depress the eye in an adducted position, as when going down stairs or reading a book. Fourth nerve palsies result in a hyperdeviation of the affected eye; most patients experience vertical binocular diplopia. To compensate for this, the patient will tilt the head to the contralateral side to achieve binocularity. In older patients, this is often a result of trauma or intracranial pathology, and MRI should be considered in a patient with new vertical diplopia. In children, a congenital 4th nerve palsy will manifest with a head tilt. **Torticollis** refers to acquired twisting of the neck due to spasm of the sternocleidomastoid muscle. It is treated with physical therapy.

CASE 43 | Oculomotor Nerve (CN III) Palsy

A 56-year-old woman presents with acute lowering of her right upper eyelid and vague periorbital pain and headache that started a few hours ago. On exam, there is complete ptosis of the right upper eyelid. Her right pupil is fixed and minimally reactive to light. Her left pupil is more constricted, and it is briskly reactive to light.

Evaluation/Tests	MRI/MRA brain reveals a saccular aneurysm of the posterior communicating (PCom) artery on the right side.
Treatment	Treat with microsurgical clipping or endovascular coiling of the unruptured aneurysm.
Discussion	This patient is experiencing an oculomotor (CN III) nerve palsy. The oculomotor nerve innervates a majority of the extraocular muscles, including the superior rectus, medial rectus, inferior rectus, and inferior oblique muscles. CN III palsy should be considered an emergency; it is critical to obtain imaging looking for aneurysm or tumor, including a mass causing uncal herniation. CN III has both motor (central) and parasympathetic (peripheral) components. Depending on the nerve fibers affected, initial symptoms and signs may differ. Motor (central) components tend to be affected primarily by vascular disease such as diabetes and hypertension, while parasympathetic (peripheral) components are first affected by compression, often by aneurysms or uncal herniation. In this case, the CN III nerve palsy is a consequence of compression from an **aneurysm of the posterior communicating artery**. **Internuclear ophthalmoplegia** is a purely horizontal motility issue, whereas a CN III palsy can involve vertical muscles as well as the eyelid. **Giant cell arteritis** should be considered in any elderly patient with accompanying headache or temporal pain.

CASE 44 | Internuclear Ophthalmoplegia (INO)

A 35-year-old woman presents with acute horizontal, binocular double vision. She denies pain or other neurologic issues. She is able to partially resolve the diplopia with convergence. On exam, she has a relative afferent pupillary defect present in her left eye. The right eye extraocular movements are intact. The left eye shows limited adduction. There are a few beats of jerk nystagmus in the right eye with abduction.

Evaluation/Tests	Brain MRI with and without gadolinium shows a white matter lesion in midbrain.
Treatment	Treat the underlying cause.
Discussion	Internuclear ophthalmoplegia (INO) is a horizontal gaze abnormality resulting from damage to the medial longitudinal fasciculus (MLF). The MLF is a heavily myelinated tract in the brainstem that coordinates crosstalk between CN III and CN VI nuclei, allowing both eyes to simultaneously move in the same horizontal direction. Damage to one or both MLFs can present with unilateral or bilateral adduction deficits in addition to horizontal nystagmus of the contralateral eye on abduction. Unique to INO, convergence movements are preserved. In younger adults, especially women of reproductive age, INO is often caused by demyelination secondary to multiple sclerosis. In older adults, INO can be caused by ischemic conditions such as stroke. Treatment is aimed at the underlying cause. An INO is a purely horizontal motility issue, whereas a primary **CN III palsy** can involve vertical muscles as well as the eyelid. By contrast, **myasthenia graves** and **thyroid eye disease** are chronic and dynamic motility disorders.

CHRONIC VISION LOSS

As opposed to sudden or acute vision loss, chronic vision loss takes months, years, or even decades to develop, and it is often painless. Risk factors for chronic vision loss include older age, systemic diseases such as hypertension and diabetes mellitus, or the presence of other cardiovascular risk factors. Family history and genetic predisposition are also important to consider for disorders of chronic vision loss. While age is an important risk factor, some inherited forms of vision loss may present earlier in life (adolescence or early adulthood).

Worsening visual acuity in older age may be normal. For example, presbyopia is an age-related impairment in lens accommodation due to decreased elasticity, changes in the curvature of the lens, and decreased strength of ciliary muscles. Presbyopia can be corrected with the use of magnifying reading glasses.

CASE 45 | Cataract

A 75-year-old woman with diabetes reports difficulty reading the newspaper. Her vision has worsened over the past year, and she has increased trouble driving at night. Her corrective lenses have not helped. She denies any eye pain. On slit-lamp exam, a grayish opacification of the lens is noted in both eyes.

CASE 45 | Cataract *(continued)*

Evaluation/Tests	Clinical diagnosis.
Treatment	Cataract surgery.
Discussion	This patient is presenting with cataracts, a painless opacification of the lens that results in impaired vision. The lens is surrounded by a basement membrane. Lens epithelial cells differentiate throughout life and form new lens fibers, which infoliate into the lens over time. These eventually may form protein aggregates, which lead to opacity within the lens and scatter light. Patients present with painless glare and vision loss, especially at night. Aging is the most significant risk factor for development of cataracts. Additional risk factors include excess alcohol use, excess sunlight, prolonged corticosteroid use, diabetes mellitus, trauma, or infection. Cataracts can also be seen in congenital conditions related to a number of underlying diseases including disorders of galactose metabolism, trisomies, congenital infections (e.g., Rubella), Marfan syndrome, Alport syndrome, myotonic dystrophy, and neurofibromatosis type 2. There is no medical treatment for cataracts, and surgical correction is warranted if severe. Reproduced with permission from Roshan M, Vijaya PH, Lavanya GR, et al: A novel human CRYGD mutation in a juvenile autosomal dominant cataract, Mol Vis 2010 May 22;16:887–96. **Presbyopia**, or age-related farsightedness, occurs with aging and leads to difficulty reading. **Diabetic retinopathy** and **hypertensive retinopathy** occur in patients with uncontrolled diabetes and hypertension, respectively. Patients presents with generally decreased vision and are diagnosed with a dilated eye exam of the retina.

CASE 46 | Open-Angle Glaucoma

A 68-year-old man with diabetes notes difficulty seeing out of both eyes. His vision has progressively worsened over the last year, and he especially has difficulty seeing objects directly in front of him. He wears corrective lenses for nearsightedness. He has no pain. Other than decreased visual acuity, his ophthalmic exam is normal.

Evaluation/Tests	Intraocular pressure (IOP) is elevated. Fundoscopy reveals a pale optic disc with thinning of the outer rim of the optic nerve head. The optic cup is enlarged, with optic cup:disc ratio >0.6 (see the image). Gonioscopy shows a normal anterior segment and drainage angle. Glaucoma results in "cupping" as the neural rim is destroyed and the central cup becomes enlarged and excavated. The cup-to-disc ratio is about 0.8 in this patient. Reproduced with permission from Jameson JL, Fauci AS, Kasper DL, et al: Harrison's Principles of Internal Medicine, 20th ed. New York, NY: McGraw Hill; 2018.
Treatment	Treat with prostaglandin agonist (latanoprost) eyedrops.
Discussion	This patient is presenting with signs and symptoms concerning for open-angle glaucoma, an ocular disease resulting from gradual elevation in intraocular pressure that causes neuropathy and atrophy of the optic nerve head within the retina. Patients with progressive loss of retinal ganglion cell axons present with a characteristic appearance on fundoscopy: pale, atrophied optic disc with an enlarged optic cup. Risk factors include age, family history, diabetes, and myopia (nearsightedness). Most cases

CASE 46 | Open-Angle Glaucoma *(continued)*

Discussion	are idiopathic, but secondary causes are due to blockages of the trabecular meshwork, which normally drains aqueous humor. Examples of secondary causes of open-angle glaucoma include uveitis, vitreous hemorrhage, and retinal detachment. Goal of therapy for open-angle glaucoma is lowering the intraocular pressure by using agents that either decrease the production of or increase the outflow of aqueous humor. Topical prostaglandin eye drops (e.g., latanoprost) are often first line to increase outflow. Additional therapeutic strategies focusing on decreasing production of aqueous humor include beta-blockers (timolol, betaxolol), alpha adrenergic agonists (brimonidine), and carbonic anhydrase inhibitors (dorzolamide, acetazolamide). If these do not work, laser therapy may be indicated. **Acute angle glaucoma** presents with acute changes in vision, and it must be managed emergently to prevent vision loss.

CASE 47 | Age-Related Macular Degeneration

A 70-year-old woman with a past medical history of hypertension, hyperlipidemia, and smoking presents with distorted vision and difficulty seeing. She notes that her peripheral vision is okay, but that seeing directly in front of her is difficult. She denies pain or injury. She began noticing this years ago, but it has finally reached a point where she decided to seek medical attention. On exam, a blind spot (scotoma) is noted in the central field of vision.

Evaluation/Tests	Fundoscopy shows deposition of yellowish material within the retina without signs of edema or hemorrhage and atrophy of retinal pigment epithelium.
Treatment	Treat with a multivitamin, antioxidants, zinc, and smoking.
Discussion	This patient is presenting with age-related macular degeneration (AMD) resulting from degeneration of the macula in the central retina. This results in vision loss, particularly in central vision (scotomas) and in distortion of vision (metamorphopsia). The macula contains the highest concentration of cone photoreceptors in the retina, particularly in the fovea centralis. Risk factors for AMD include age, smoking, other cardiovascular risk factors, and family history. AMD is further divided into two types: dry (>80% of cases) and wet (10–15%). Dry AMD results from subretinal inflammation and oxidative damage, which lead to the formation of drusen deposits, which are yellowish extracellular material that deposit near retinal pigment epithelium. This results in atrophy and loss of vital nutrients for photoreceptors. Vision loss in dry AMD is gradual, and it occurs over years or decades. Wet AMD is less common, but vision loss may be more rapid. As drusen deposits and other abnormal extracellular matrix proteins deposit within the retina, this creates a hypoxic environment that promotes the development of new leaky vessels (neovascularization). Neovascularization within the retina can promote hemorrhage leading to gray or green discoloration of the retina). In addition to these treatments, wet AMD may also be treated with injections of anti-VEGF antibodies such as bevacizumab to limit neovascularization. Unlike **open-angle glaucoma**, which presents with loss of peripheral vision initially, macular degeneration presents with loss of central vision first.

CASE 48 | Diabetic Retinopathy

A 45-year-old man with poorly controlled diabetes mellitus presents with blurry vision, floaters, and decreased night vision. Fundoscopy reveals retinal edema, hard exudates, and dot and blot hemorrhages within close proximity of the foveal avascular zone.

Evaluation/Tests	Advanced testing reveals capillary microaneurysms and vitreous hemorrhage with evidence of neovascularization.
Treatment	Optimize blood glucose control and treat with intravitreal anti-vascular endothelial growth factor (VEGF) medications (i.e., bevacizumab) and with surgery if edema and retinopathy are significant.
Discussion	Diabetic retinopathy is caused by the effects of chronic hyperglycemia on the retina. Glycosylation of tissue proteins results in intracellular sorbitol accumulation within the basement membrane of retinal capillaries. This drives thickening of the basement membrane and damage to pericytes and endothelial cells. Patients present with decreased night vision and decreased color vision. There are two forms

CASE 48 | Diabetic Retinopathy *(continued)*

Discussion	of diabetic retinopathy: nonproliferative and proliferative. The nonproliferative form occurs first and it involves the leak of lipids and fluid from damaged capillaries into the retina. Examination reveals hemorrhages, macular edema, hard exudates, and capillary microaneurysms. Decreased blood delivery to the retina establishes a state of chronic hypoxia, which then drives the proliferative form of diabetic retinopathy. This form is characterized by the formation of new blood vessels in response to chronic hypoxia (neovascularization). Newly formed vessels are particularly leaky, and this can lead to vitreous hemorrhage and put traction on the retina that could lead to retinal detachment. **Hypertensive retinopathy** similarly presents with microaneurysms and hemorrhage; however, additional findings include arteriovenous nicking, cotton-wool spots, and occasionally presence of papilledema.

CASE 49 | Retinitis Pigmentosa

A 15-year-old boy presents with difficulty navigating in poorly illuminated rooms. He also notes poor peripheral vision but denies eye pain or redness. On exam, he has impairment in his peripheral vision with an afferent pupillary defect in both eyes. Dilated funduscopic exam is significant for retinal bone spicule-shaped deposits around the macula and hyperpigmentation.

Evaluation/Tests	ERG (electroretinogram) reveals decreased electrical activity, predominantly in the periphery (rod photoreceptors) compared to center (cone photoreceptors).
Treatment	There is no cure. Treatment is supportive.
Discussion	This patient is presenting with retinitis pigmentosa, a progressive inherited disease involving retinal degeneration. Multiple forms of inheritance exist including autosomal dominant and autosomal recessive forms. Symptoms often appear early in life, commonly in children or adolescents, but they may also appear in adulthood. Degeneration initially affects peripheral rod photoreceptors, causing symptoms such as night blindness, decreased peripheral vision with intact central vision, and glare sensitivities. Eventually degeneration will affect central cone photoreceptors, resulting in blindness. It is important to rule out reversible causes of retinal degeneration including drug toxicity or infection.

VISUAL FIELD DEFECTS

When light enters the eye, it is refracted by the cornea, focused by the lens, and it ultimately converges on the retina. The retina contains a complex histologic architecture with 10 layers. The innermost layer is the retinal pigment epithelium, which provides nutrients to photoreceptors. Rods and cones form the next layer and use opsins (rhodopsin and photopsin/iodopsin, respectively) to convert photons to electrochemical signals in the form of the neurotransmitter glutamate. Additional layers contain second-order neurons and supporting glial cells, but ultimately these signals converge on the third-order retinal ganglion cells, which project toward the brain forming the optic nerve (CN II).

It is important to understand the neuroanatomy of how vision is transmitted from the retina to its ultimate destination in the primary visual cortex of the occipital lobe (see image). Lesions at various points along this pathway can result in a multitude of visual field defects that, when understood, can be used to localize the neuroanatomic location of the insult. As signals are conveyed along the optic nerve, the fibers from the nasal retina (portraying vision from the temporal field) in each eye decussate at the level of the optic chiasm, ensuring that the entire left or right visual field ends up in a single lateral geniculate nucleus of the thalamus on the contralateral side. Generally, lesions before the level of the optic chiasm result in unilateral or monocular visual field defects, while lesions at or past the level of the optic chiasm result in bilateral visual field defects. As signals are then conveyed from the lateral geniculate nucleus to the primary visual cortex along the optic radiations, they are further separated into superior and inferior visual fields. When an image finally converges on the primary visual cortex, it is upside-down and left-right reversed.

Optic Pathway Lesions and Associated Field Defects

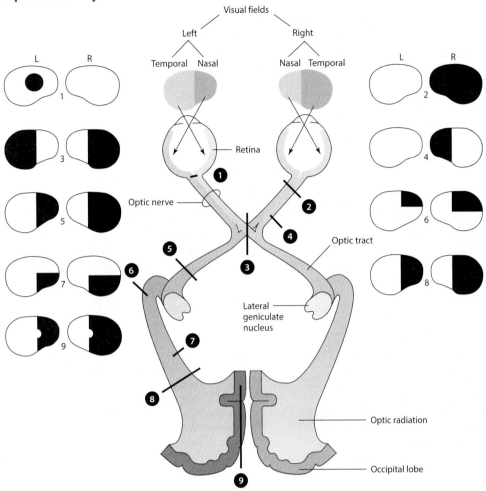

Common visual field defects and their anatomic bases. 1. Central scotoma caused by inflammation of the optic disk (optic neuritis) or optic nerve (retrobulbar neuritis). 2. Total blindness of the right eye from a complete lesion of the right optic nerve. 3. Bitemporal hemianopia caused by pressure exerted on the optic chiasm by a pituitary tumor. 4. Right nasal hemianopia caused by a perichiasmal lesion (e.g., calcified internal carotid artery). 5. Right homonymous hemianopia from a lesion of the left optic tract. 6. Right homonymous superior quadrantanopia caused by partial involvement of the optic radiation by a lesion in the left temporal lobe (Meyer loop). 7. Right homonymous inferior quadrantanopia caused by partial involvement of the optic radiation by a lesion in the left parietal lobe. 8. Right homonymous hemianopia from a complete lesion of the left optic radiation. (A similar defect may also result from lesion 9.) 9. Right homonymous hemianopia (with macular sparing) resulting from posterior cerebral artery occlusion. Defects are shown in black.

Reproduced with permission from Greenberg DA, Aminoff MJ, Simon RP: Clinical Neurology, 11th ed. New York, NY: McGraw Hill; 2021.

CASE 50	Bitemporal Hemianopia (Optic Chiasm Lesion)
	A 28-year-old man presents with progressive loss of vision. He noted that it is especially poor while driving because he has difficulty seeing out of the periphery of both eyes. He reports that his vision is slightly worse on the right. He also has a dull headache that has progressively worsened along with his vision. He and his wife have been trying to have children, but they have not been able to conceive. On exam, he can read only the nasal half of letters on the Snellen eye chart.
Evaluation/Tests	Serum prolactin levels are elevated. MRI of the brain and orbits reveals a pituitary mass compressing the optic chiasm.
Treatment	Treat medically in the early stages with bromocriptine. If ineffective, surgical resection is appropriate.

CASE 50 | Bitemporal Hemianopia (Optic Chiasm Lesion) *(continued)*

Discussion	This patient is presenting with a bitemporal hemianopsia, a visual field defect due to compression or damage of the optic chiasm leading to loss of temporal visual fields in both eyes. The optic chiasm is the X-shaped structure formed by the decussation of optic nerve fibers from the nasal hemiretina that conveys information from the temporal visual field. The optic chiasm is located anatomically in the suprasellar region, just rostral to the sella turcica housing the pituitary gland. Pituitary tumors such as a **prolactinoma** (as in this case) can compress the medial optic chiasm, resulting in loss of temporal visual fields in both eyes in addition to mass effect leading to headaches. Nasal visual fields are initially unaffected as the fibers from the temporal hemiretina do not cross in the optic chiasm and remain ipsilateral. Lesions to the lateral aspect of the optic chiasm (i.e., from **ICA aneurysm**) may result in an ipsilateral nasal hemianopia. Glioma of optic nerve involving the optic chiasm can also lead to vision loss. **Craniopharyngioma** is a rare type of brain tumor that may present with bitemporal inferior temporal quadrantanopia or bitemporal hemianopsia. **Strokes** occurring in the occipital cortex can lead to hemianopia and quadrantanopia.

CASE 51 | Homonymous Hemianopia (Optic Tract Lesion)

A 70-year-old man with hypertension, hyperlipidemia, and atrial fibrillation presents with blurred vision for the last 3 hours. His vision is especially bad when looking to his left. He wears prescription glasses, but these do not help correct his visual deficit. On exam, he has loss of the left visual field in each eye and irregular cardiac rhythm.

Evaluation/Tests	ECG shows irregularly spaced QRS complexes with absent P waves (atrial fibrillation). MRI of brain and orbit with and without contrast show a small area of ischemia surrounding the right optic chiasm.
Treatment	Treat underlying stroke. Consider tPA or mechanical thrombectomy.
Discussion	This patient is experiencing a homonymous hemianopia caused by damage to the optic tract due to ischemia. The optic tract conveys the nerve fibers from the optic nerve and chiasm to the lateral geniculate nucleus (LGN) of the thalamus. Due to the decussation of nasal hemiretina fibers in the optic chiasm, the optic tracts carry the visual hemifield for the contralateral side. Therefore, damage to the right optic tract, as seen in this patient, manifests as a contralateral homonymous hemianopia, where the left visual field in both eyes is defective. Causes include ischemia, malignancy, or demyelinating disease like multiple sclerosis.

CASE 52 | Inferior Quadrantanopia (Parietal Lobe Lesion)

A 55-year-old woman presents to her ophthalmologist for a routine glaucoma follow-up. During this visit, she was unable to perform visual field testing due to an inability to focus. She was able to focus in her previous exams. She was also having difficulty writing her name. On exam, she has decreased vision in the lower portion of the right visual field bilaterally. Color motility and dilated eye exam are within normal limits.

Evaluation/Tests	CT/MRI of brain with and without contrast reveals a poorly circumscribed mass in the left parietal lobe that extends across the corpus callosum.
Treatment	The patient should be evaluated for chemotherapy, radiation, and/or surgical resection.
Discussion	This patient is presenting with an inferior quadrantanopia, caused by compression or damage to the superior optic radiations in the parietal lobe. In this case, her visual field defect is caused by a tumor of the parietal lobe, such as an astrocytoma or glioblastoma multiforme. Other causes include stroke (e.g., MCA infarct). The superior optic radiations convey information from the LGN to the visual cortex in the occipital lobe. Nerves are conveying information from the contralateral lower visual field of both eyes; therefore, damage results in an inferior quadrantanopia ("pie on the floor" defect). Additional parietal symptoms may include hemispatial neglect, agraphia, acalculia, finger agnosia, and left-right disorientation. The inferior optic radiations travel within the temporal lobe and convey information from the contralateral upper visual field of both eyes; therefore, damage would result in a **superior quadrantanopia** ("pie in the sky" defect). Additional temporal symptoms could include memory deficits, hallucinations, or seizures.

CASE 53	Homonymous Hemianopia with Macular Sparing (Occipital Lobe Lesion)
	A 70-year-old man with diabetes and severe unstable angina reports blurred vision for the last 2 hours. He had a CABG (coronary artery bypass grafting) surgery 2 days ago for severe left main stem artery stenosis. His vision change is mainly on the right visual field in both eyes. Further visual field testing revealed a right homonymous hemianopia; however, his central vision was unaffected (macular sparing).
Evaluation/Tests	Noncontrast CT shows no sign of hemorrhage. MRI of the brain demonstrates an acute infarct of the left occipital lobe in the distribution of the posterior cerebral artery (PCA).
Treatment	The patient should be considered for tPA or mechanical thrombectomy.
Discussion	This patient is experiencing a homonymous hemianopia with macular sparing caused by damage to the occipital lobe. The occipital lobe is the location of the primary visual cortex, and each side receives nerve inputs from the entire contralateral visual field. Damage to one side of the occipital lobe (as seen in this patient with a left PCA stroke) results in a contralateral homonymous hemianopia. The central visual field may be unaffected (macular sparing) due to the collateral blood supply for this region of the visual cortex from branches of the PCA and MCA. Given the large number of cone photoreceptors concentrated in the macula, it has a large representation within the occipital cortex, and it requires blood supply from multiple sources.
	If damage to the occipital lobe occurred bilaterally, macular sparing would not be found, and the patient would experience full cortical blindness.
	Lesions of the occipital lobe can be distinguished from lesions of the **optic tract** by determining whether the patient has macular sparing. Macular sparing is present in occipital lobe lesions but not in optic tract lesions.

OTOLARYNGOLOGY

Otolaryngology is the subspecialty of medicine that deals with medical and surgical management of diseases of the head and neck, including the ear, nose, and throat. Because otolaryngology is a broad field covering multiple disciplines and organ systems, various chief concerns are spread throughout this book. Here, we will discuss neurological symptoms related to the ear, including auditory and vestibular function.

HEARING LOSS

The general approach to hearing loss initially involves differentiating between conductive and sensorineural hearing loss. Conductive hearing loss is caused by impairment in the ability of sound waves reaching the cochlear apparatus in the inner ear (external auditory canal → tympanic membrane → ossicles → oval window). Sensorineural hearing loss involves defects in neuronal transmission from the hair cells of the inner ear to the central nervous system. It can affect any structures along that path, including the vestibulocochlear nerve (cranial nerve VIII) and brainstem nuclei.

A detailed exam, including performance of Weber and Rinne tests using tuning forks, is important. The Weber test involves placing a vibrating tuning fork on the middle forehead to determine the lateralization of hearing loss. Lateralization is indicative of unilateral hearing loss; no lateralization can be normal or indicate bilateral hearing loss. The Rinne test involves placing a vibrating tuning fork on the mastoid process and then holding it in front of the ear. This test evaluates air vs. bone conduction. Air conduction, which relies on the patent ear canal, intact tympanic membrane, and the amplifying characteristics of the ossicular chain (malleus, incus, and stapes), is normally greater than bone conduction. With bone conduction, vibrations surpass the amplification of the ossicular chain and transmit directly through bone to the cochlea. While these tests are often helpful in the initial evaluation of hearing loss, audiometry is the gold standard in elucidating sensorineural vs. conductive hearing loss. It can also assess the tympanic membrane and middle ear function.

For conductive hearing loss, the general approach is to identify where there is a physical obstruction of the sound waves between the external auditory canal and the oval window. Look for cerumen impaction of the auditory canal, perforations in the tympanic membrane, or fluid in the middle ear space. Imaging of the middle ear space can be used to evaluate for cholesteatoma, otosclerosis, or discontinuity of ossicular chain. Treatment of conductive hearing loss depends on the principal problem, and it can include cerumen disimpaction, removal of middle ear fluid, and surgical corrections to the tympanic membrane or other structures. Sound amplification devices or bone-anchored hearing aids may also be helpful. For sensorineural hearing loss, the primary goal is to determine whether the cause is easily reversible. Reversible causes include use of ototoxic drugs such as loop diuretics, aminoglycosides, aspirin, or cisplatin. Also assess for nonreversible causes such as age- or noise-related hearing loss, structural damage to CN VIII, or CNS lesions such as vestibular schwannomas. Nonreversible causes can be treated with sound amplification devices or cochlear implants.

Differential Diagnosis for Conductive vs. Sensorineural Hearing Loss

Conductive Hearing Loss	Sensorineural Hearing Loss
Cerumen impaction Tympanic membrane perforation Otosclerosis (can result in a fixed, immobile stapes footplate) Cholesteatoma Middle ear effusion (fluid buildup such as from otitis media)	Presbycusis (bilateral, progressive, elderly) Noise-induced hearing loss Meniere's disease Ototoxic medications (aspirin, NSAIDs, aminoglycosides, etc.) Vestibular schwannoma Stroke Meningitis Syphilis (rare)

CASE 54 | Conductive Hearing Loss (Cholesteatoma)

A 40-year-old woman with a history of multiple ear infections presents with gradual painless loss of hearing in her right ear. She has also noticed chronic drainage from that ear. She denies fever and dizziness. On exam, she has decreased hearing on the right side. Weber tuning fork test localizes to the right ear, and the Rinne test demonstrates bone conduction greater than air conduction on the right. The left ear has air conduction greater than bone conduction. The right tympanic membrane has a small perforation and deep retraction pocket with accumulation of keratinized squamous debris.

Evaluation/Tests	Audiometry demonstrates conductive hearing loss.
Treatment	The patient should be evaluated for surgical intervention.
Discussion	This is a typical presentation of conductive hearing loss due to a cholesteatoma. The patient has classic signs of unilateral hearing loss, a history of chronic otitis media infections, and painless otorrhea. Cholesteatomas are benign lesions made of a keratinized, desquamated epithelial collection in the middle ear, which may lead to erosion of the ossicles or mastoid air cells. Hearing loss from cholesteatoma is typically conductive. Primary cholesteatomas result from chronic negative pressure in the middle ear, which leads to the formation of retraction pockets and cysts filled with keratinized debris. Secondary cholesteatomas are thought to be due to squamous epithelium migrating to the middle ear, so they are more likely to present with an intact tympanic membrane with a pearly mass behind the tympanic membrane. A CT of the temporal bones can be used to define the borders of the cholesteatoma, but otherwise the diagnosis is clinical. Chronic conductive hearing loss from **chronic otitis media** will present with persistent fluid in the middle ear space but will lack the keratinized debris of a cholesteatoma. **Tympanosclerosis**, or scarring of the tympanic membrane, also presents with conductive hearing loss. However, the tympanic membrane is more likely to appear thickened with decreased mobility rather than deeply retracted with squamous debris. Audiometry can also be used to help differentiate tympanosclerosis from cholesteatoma.

CASE 55 | Sensorineural Hearing Loss (Acoustic Neuroma)

A 55-year-old woman with neurofibromatosis type 2 presents with bilateral hearing loss, tinnitus, and unsteadiness with walking. She has noted gradual hearing loss over the last few years. On exam, she has decreased hearing on both sides. Weber test does not lateralize. Rinne demonstrates air greater than bone conduction bilaterally. Her external auditory canal and tympanic membranes appear normal.

Evaluation/Tests	MRI with gadolinium shows enhancing lesions bilaterally in the region of the internal auditory canal with variable extension into the cerebellopontine angle.
Treatment	Treat with hearing aids and evaluate for surgical resection of the vestibular schwannomas.
Discussion	This is a typical presentation of vestibular schwannoma (acoustic neuroma), a tumor of Schwann cell origin that can affect any peripheral nerve but often involves cranial nerve VIII. The patient has bilateral sensorineural hearing loss, tinnitus, and vestibular deficits. The patient's history of neurofibromatosis type 2 should place bilateral vestibular schwannomas high on the differential. Hearing loss is typically gradual and bilateral, but it can be both sudden and unilateral. Facial weakness, though not common, is possible due to proximity of the vestibulocochlear nerve to the facial nerve near the cerebellopontine angle. Over 100 congenital syndromes are associated with sensorineural hearing loss, including Alport syndrome.

CASE 55 | Sensorineural Hearing Loss (Acoustic Neuroma) *(continued)*

| Discussion | **Meniere's disease** leads to both vertigo and sensorineural hearing loss. It typically affects only one ear, and it may present similarly to a vestibular schwannoma.
Presbycusis is the most common type of sensorineural hearing loss, and it is caused by natural aging of the auditory system. Onset commonly occurs in fifties–sixties, and it progresses gradually, with ability to hear higher-frequency sounds often affected first due to hair cell damage at the cochlear base.
Noise-induced hearing loss also involves loss of high-frequency hearing first, and it may also be accompanied by tinnitus. Air and bone conduction can both be affected. Classic scenarios for noise-induced hearing loss include construction workers, aviation workers, and veterans.
Medications such as diuretics, aminoglycosides, aspirin, and cisplatin can be ototoxic as well. |

DIZZINESS AND VERTIGO

Dizziness is a common chief concern that is often challenging to interpret because many symptoms experienced by a patient may be described as dizziness. A detailed history is important to help determine if a patient's sensations of dizziness are consistent with vertigo. Symptoms that a patient may describe when discussing their dizziness may include lightheadedness, blacking out, unsteadiness, or mental fog. These symptoms are often caused by brief episodic cerebral hypoperfusion due to a myriad of possibilities, including but not limited to orthostatic hypotension, carotid or vertebral artery stenosis, and atrial fibrillation. If the patient describes a "room-spinning" sensation, this is more consistent with vertigo, which points toward a vestibular pathology, inner ear pathology, or neurologic phenomenon. These are also commonly accompanied by nystagmus, and they may involve hearing loss, tinnitus, and nausea. The main function of the vestibular system is to detect linear and angular acceleration of the head in coordination with the eyes and the rest of the body.

For symptoms of vertigo, the next step is to differentiate between peripheral and central vertigo. Peripheral vertigo is caused by pathologies affecting the vestibular apparatus in the inner ear (utricle, saccule, or semicircular canals) or cranial nerve VIII. Symptoms are often intermittent or positional, and they commonly stop with visual fixation. They may also be associated with hearing loss, tinnitus, or feelings of unsteadiness. Central vertigo is caused by pathologies affecting the brainstem nuclei, cerebellum, or other central pathways within the brain or spinal cord conveying vestibular information. Symptoms are often nonpositional, do not improve with visual fixation, and may be accompanied by central neurological deficits such as facial droops, dysarthria, and more.

CASE 56	Benign Paroxysmal Positional Vertigo (BPPV)	
A 52-year-old woman with no significant past medical history presents with sudden onset of a spinning sensation. Symptoms started when she got out of the bed this morning. The spinning sensation lasted less than a minute but recurred when she laid back down in the bed. Episodes present only on head movement. Her symptoms are associated with nausea. She denies weakness of arms or legs, and she has no hearing loss or tinnitus. She is not orthostatic, and she has no focal weakness or sensory deficits.		
Evaluation/Tests	Dix-Hallpike maneuver is positive: The patient begins upright in a seated position. The examiner turns the patient's head 45 degrees to the right or left and, while supporting the patient's head, lowers her to a supine position so that the head is hanging over the edge of the bed. The head should be extended backward by about 20 degrees. The eyes are observed for rhythmic oscillatory horizontal or vertical involuntary eye movements (nystagmus). Nystagmus is noted, and the patient reports both vertigo and nausea. When the maneuver is repeated with the head turned to the opposite side, no nystagmus is detected.	
Treatment	Treat with the Epley maneuver.	
Discussion	Benign paroxysmal positional vertigo (BPPV) is the most common cause of vertigo. Vertigo in BPPV is episodic and brief, with duration lasting anywhere from a few seconds to less than a minute. BPPV is caused by dislodged particles (otoliths) within the semicircular canals that disrupt the normal flow of endolymph and signaling of vestibular hair cells. Nystagmus is common toward the affected side and can be induced for diagnostic purposes using the Dix-Hallpike maneuver. The first-line treatment for BPPV is the Epley's maneuver, which can provide relief by tilting the head to an angle where the otoliths can move out of the semicircular canals.	

CASE 56 | Benign Paroxysmal Positional Vertigo (BPPV) *(continued)*

Discussion	While BPPV can present with episodic attacks of vertigo, these attacks are normally associated with changes in position and with the lack of additional findings of tinnitus and hearing loss, as seen in Meniere's.
	Meniere's disease is an idiopathic condition affecting the inner ear often due to impaired circulation and reabsorption of endolymph. Typical features include spontaneous episodic vertigo lasting minutes to hours, fluctuating sensorineural hearing loss, tinnitus, and ear fullness. Hearing loss commonly involves low-frequency hearing first, and patients may exhibit horizontal nystagmus. Vertigo is often severe, and it is associated with nausea and vomiting with disabling imbalance. Diuretics are thought to reduce attacks by decreasing the quantity of endolymph.
	Posterior circulation Stroke is a common cause of central vertigo, and it should be considered in any patient with vascular risk factors and focal neurological findings. The region supplied by the blocked artery will affect the presentation and constellation of symptoms.
	Patients with **vestibular neuritis** may have a preceding upper respiratory tract infection.

13
Psychiatry

Rachel Bernard, MD, MPH
Sean Blitzstein, MD

CHILD AND ADOLESCENT PSYCHIATRY

Childhood psychiatric diseases may manifest as difficulties with attention, language, or behavior. When evaluating these cases, it is important to assess how much the condition is affecting the child's social and school functioning. Generally, these diseases appear at a young age and are present throughout childhood. In practice, diagnosis and treatment of childhood psychiatric diseases often involve multidisciplinary teams. A main goal of treatment is to increase the child's functioning at school and at home, and care teams may include a psychiatrist and therapist or social worker.

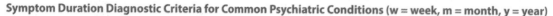

Symptom Duration Diagnostic Criteria for Common Psychiatric Conditions (w = week, m = month, y = year)

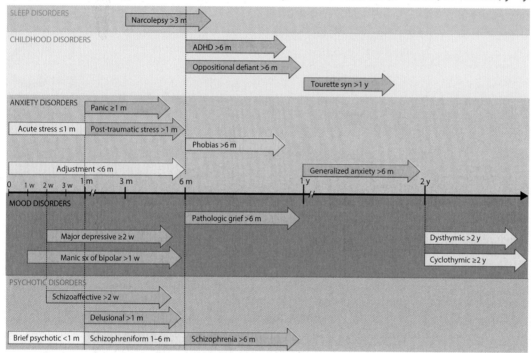

CASE 1	Attention-Deficit/Hyperactivity Disorder (ADHD)	
An 8-year-old boy is referred for psychiatric evaluation after displaying increasingly unruly behavior in school. His teachers report that he often makes careless mistakes; hands in incomplete, sloppy homework; speaks out of turn; and gets out of his seat without permission. The boy's mother notes he does not listen at home and is always running around. He has trouble following routines, like getting ready for school in the morning, because he is disorganized and forgetful. Exam reveals fidgety and social disinhibited behavior, with impaired concentration and loud, rapid speech.		
Evaluation/Tests	Clinical diagnosis.	
Treatment	First-line treatments include stimulants such as methylphenidate and amphetamines in combination with behavioral therapy (e.g., positive reinforcement). Other nonstimulant treatment options include atomoxetine and alpha-2 adrenergic agonists such as clonidine.	
Discussion	The diagnosis of ADHD involves having inattentive and/or hyperactive/impulsive symptoms in more than one setting, for 6 or more months, with presentation of some of these symptoms before age 12. Symptoms of inattention include careless mistakes, impaired attention, lack of follow-through in work, avoidance of tasks that take mental effort, distractibility, and forgetfulness. In addition, symptoms of hyperactivity/impulsivity include fidgetiness, restlessness, excessive talking, difficulty waiting turns, blurting out answers, interruption of others, and difficulty remaining seated. Rarely thyroid tests and electroencephalogram (EEG) are done to rule out thyroid problems or seizure activity.	
Additional Considerations	**Tourette syndrome** is a neurologic disorder most commonly seen in males and characterized by multiple motor (e.g., blinking and grimacing) and vocal (e.g., grunting and coprolalia) tics. To receive the diagnosis of Tourette syndrome, tics should be present for over 1 year, must have started before age 18, and must not be due to another medical or psychiatric condition. It is often associated with OCD and ADHD.	

CASE 2 | Autism Spectrum Disorder (ASD)

A 3-year-old boy is brought into clinic because of speech delay. His mother says he has failed to say any coherent words. She is also worried because he does not reciprocate affection, such as hugging her back. Regarding his behavior, she has noticed that he constantly lines up his trains and examines their wheels intently and becomes easily agitated with changes in routine. On exam, he does not respond to questioning and exhibits limited eye contact and occasionally rocks back and forth while seated.

Evaluation/Tests	Clinical diagnosis. Vision and hearing testing are normal, and lead levels are within normal limits.
Treatment	Treatment involves special education and behavioral management to target the core symptoms of ASD and requires a multidisciplinary approach.
Discussion	Autism spectrum disorder involves persistent impairment in socialization, communication, and restricted activities/interests beginning at an early age. Regarding social interaction, patients usually fail to develop or seek out peer relationships, lacking social reciprocity with impaired use of nonverbal communication. They tend to have problems with communication with language delays, poor eye contact, and trouble initiating and maintaining conversations. Patients with ASD have restricted and repetitive patterns of activities (i.e., inflexible routines with insistence on sameness), behaviors (e.g., rocking, hand flapping, spinning), and interests.

CASE 3 | Conduct Disorder

A 13-year-old boy is brought for evaluation due to disruptive behavior. His parents report that he has been suspended from school numerous times for initiating fights with other kids and stealing from them. They state that he is consistently disobedient, staying out late, and lying about what he has been doing. The other day they found him trying to put his hamster in the microwave. Physical exam is normal.

Evaluation/Tests	Clinical diagnosis.
Treatment	Treatment involves individual cognitive behavior therapy (CBT) and/or family therapy. In some cases, mood stabilizers or antipsychotic medications may be used.
Discussion	Conduct disorder usually presents in middle childhood to adolescence and is more commonly seen in males. It consists of a repetitive or persistent pattern of behavior in which the basic rights of others or societal norms/rules are violated. Behaviors may be aggressive (e.g., animal cruelty, rape, bullying, destruction of property) or nonaggressive (e.g., deceitfulness, theft, truancy). Conduct disorder may progress to antisocial personality disorder in adulthood. A urine toxicology screen may be helpful in ruling out substance abuse disorders. In contrast, **oppositional defiant disorder** involves defiant behavior toward authority figures, but it lacks the violation of societal norms that conduct disorder includes.

EGO DEFENSES

Ego defenses are psychological processes that help an individual to cope/deal with undesired feelings such as aggression, fear, or anxiety. These processes can be conscious or unconscious. Ego defenses can be sorted into "immature" and "mature" categories, with the vast majority of these defenses being "immature." Mature defenses include Sublimation, Altruism, Suppression, and Humor (remember, "Mature adults wear a 'S.A.S.H.'").

CASE 4 | Regression

A previously toilet-trained 6-year-old girl begins wetting the bed when her baby sister is born.

Evaluation/Tests	Clinical diagnosis.
Discussion	Regression is an immature ego defense mechanism involving the involuntary reversion to an earlier developmental stage in response to a stressor that creates tension or conflict. Regression only occurs after milestones have already been met. In contrast, if the 6-year-old girl failed to progress in school and social situations after the birth of her baby sister, this would qualify as **fixation**, in which the individual remains at a more immature level of development (e.g., if the girl had never been toilet-trained before the birth of her sister and subsequently was unable to progress in her toilet training).

CASE 5 | Suppression

A 24-year-old woman watches her favorite movie the night before her USMLE Step 1 exam to help her forget about her anxiety toward the test.

Evaluation/Tests	Clinical diagnosis.
Discussion	Suppression is a mature ego defense that temporarily and intentionally keeps emotions or ideas from conscious awareness, such as this example in which this medical student is temporarily suppressing her anxiety so that she can relax before Step 1. **Repression**, in contrast, is unconsciously withholding unwanted emotions or ideas from awareness. **Dissociation** is also temporary, but it involves a dramatic personality change to avoid this emotional stressor, and the individual has little to no memory of the event, such as if this student couldn't remember anything about sitting for Step 1 after she took it. **Isolation of affect** is when an individual separates emotion from their related events, such as if this student with anxiety toward Step 1 talked about it without an emotional response and with minimal affect. In this vignette, the student is not separating herself from her emotions; rather, she is temporarily suppressing them so that she can relax rather than detaching completely.

CASE 6 | Splitting

A 25-year old woman with a past psychiatric history of borderline personality disorder is currently on an inpatient floor being treated for suicidal ideation. During an interview, she states that all the male doctors have been "angels," but the female doctors are "evil."

Evaluation/Tests	Clinical diagnosis.
Discussion	Splitting is an immature ego defense mechanism that consists of an all-or-nothing appraisal system, usually concerning individuals or groups of people. The rigidity and extreme polarization involved allows the individual to attend to the information they believe best supports their current position or opinion. Splitting is commonly seen in borderline personality disorder. Individuals with this disorder believe that people are either all good or all bad at various times, which also contributes to their frequently unstable and tumultuous relationships. Splitting differs from **idealization** in that idealization focuses on only attributing exaggerated positive qualities. Calling all of the male doctors "angels" could be idealization, but the "evil female doctors" make this a case of splitting. In splitting, one day the female doctors may be "evil" and the next day "angels." In idealization, the idealized party tends to stay consistent (the male doctors are always "angels"). **Projection** is an immature defense mechanism in which one attributes their own unacceptable impulses, thoughts, or feelings to an external source. The projection of their unacceptable thoughts often mirrors their own internal impulse, such as a man accusing his wife of cheating when that is his desire. Even though this patient seems to project negative feelings toward herself onto the other women, the contrast with calling all the men "angels" makes splitting more likely. **Displacement** is an immature ego defense mechanism in which one redirects their own emotions or impulses onto a neutral object or person. Colloquially, we call this "taking out our feelings on someone else." Displacement differs from projection in that displacement redirects a conflict from the involved parties to a third, uninvolved party. In this vignette, displacement would be if the patient had a conflict with the female doctor, then berated the worker bringing her lunch.

CASE 7 | Reaction Formation

A 40-year-old woman who feels intense hatred toward her 16-year-old stepdaughter continually dotes on her and buys her anything she desires.

Evaluation/Tests	Clinical diagnosis.
Discussion	Reaction formation is an immature ego defense mechanism that involves an individual responding exactly opposite to their actual feelings or thoughts. Reaction formation is not necessarily gratifying for the individual, as opposed to **altruism**, in which the negative feelings are alleviated with the generosity. An example would be if this woman used volunteering for local service organizations to feel better about herself amidst this hatred for her stepdaughter.

CASE 7 | Reaction Formation (continued)

Discussion	**Sublimation** is a mature ego defense mechanism in which one channels unacceptable impulses into socially accepted and constructive behaviors that do not conflict with one's own value system. Sublimation in this case might look like the woman expressing her hatred through joining a boxing class to release her negative emotions. Sublimation differs from altruism in that sublimation refers to more "negative" behaviors (such as violence) that happen to have a socially acceptable context (like kickboxing or football).
	In contrast to sublimation, **acting out** involves expressing these emotions in a socially unacceptable way (like kicking a stranger on the street).
	Reaction formation goes beyond **suppression** because the individual is replacing the negative emotions with an opposing *action* rather than simply (and consciously) suppressing these emotions.

CASE 8 | Denial

A 49-year-old man with newly diagnosed lung cancer skips his oncology appointments because he doesn't believe that he is sick.

Evaluation/Tests	Clinical diagnosis.
Discussion	Denial is an immature ego defense in which a person unconsciously blocks external events or facts from their conscious awareness. By doing so, an individual can avoid recognition of a painful reality. In this case, the patient convinces himself that he doesn't really have cancer and subsequently doesn't believe he needs to attend his doctor's appointments.
	Rationalization is an immature ego defense mechanism in which one justifies their own unacceptable attitudes, beliefs, or behaviors through logical reasoning to reduce their anxiety. With rationalization, he is not ignoring the reality; rather, he is minimizing the pain of the reality. By doing this, an individual can avoid difficult truths and self-blame. Rationalization uses logic to decrease stress, whereas intellectualization ignores the stress altogether. In this example, rationalization might be the patient convincing himself that he should not go to his appointment because the office is "too far out of the way."
	Intellectualization would be if the patient tried to distance himself from his diagnosis by focusing on medical literature and statistics about survival rather than dealing with the emotional weight of this diagnosis.
	Isolation of affect involves separating an individual's feelings from the events causing them, such as this patient describing their cancer prognosis and therapy without an emotional response.

AMNESIA, DISSOCIATION, AND DELIRIUM

Amnesia is a loss of memory and can be anterograde (inability to form new memories) or retrograde (loss of memories that occurred prior to the event). In practice, many conditions cause both anterograde and retrograde amnesia. In diagnosing and treating memory disorders, it is important to assess and treat for reversible causes (e.g., vitamin deficiencies, endocrine disorders, or chronic infection such as neurosyphilis). Neuropsychological evaluation can help determine if individuals are impaired in one (e.g., memory) or multiple areas (e.g., memory, visual spatial reasoning, and language skills) and help inform strategies for dealing with the deficit(s).

Dissociation involves feelings of detachment and estrangement from the self. This can be seen in "dissociative amnesia," which is when individuals lose ability to recall important personal information, often due to trauma. Dissociation also includes dissociative identity disorder, which was previously known as "multiple personality disorder"; however, this condition is quite rare.

Delirium is commonly encountered on inpatient medical and surgical wards. This condition is characterized by a "waxing and waning" level of consciousness. Delirium is always a result of another condition, such as infection, ischemia, medications, or metabolic disturbance. Hyperactive delirious patients are usually easy to identify as they may be yelling, agitated, or otherwise disruptive. Hypoactive delirious patients are more common but harder to recognize, as they are withdrawn and have subtle disorientation. Delirium is by definition reversible, but it may take months to fully resolve.

CASE 9 | Wernicke-Korsakoff Syndrome

A 68-year-old man with a long history of alcohol use is brought in by the police after being found wandering in the streets. He reluctantly admits that he got lost but claims some of the street names have changed. When asked his address, he describes his house and neighborhood but avoids directly answering the question. He is disheveled and has an ataxic gait. The rest of the physical exam is normal.

CASE 9 | Wernicke-Korsakoff Syndrome *(continued)*

Evaluation/Tests	BMP and CBC are within normal limits. Blood alcohol level (BAL) is 0, and urine toxicology screen is negative. Thiamine level is low. AST and ALT are elevated at 130 and 65, respectively. MRI brain shows mamillary body atrophy.
Treatment	Treatment should include thiamine supplementation, alcohol cessation, and referral to a rehabilitation program.
Discussion	**Korsakoff syndrome** is a chronic amnestic syndrome caused by thiamine (vitamin B1) deficiency due to prolonged alcohol use. It is characterized by impaired recent memory, anterograde amnesia, and confabulation (unconsciously making up answers when memory has failed). Even with thiamine repletion, it is reversible in only about 20% of patients. **Wernicke encephalopathy** categorizes the early stages of this syndrome and is characterized by confusion, ophthalmoplegia, and ataxia. It can then progress to Korsakoff syndrome, which includes irreversible memory loss, confabulation, and personality changes. It is associated with necrosis of the mammillary bodies and periventricular hemorrhage.

CASE 10 | Dissociative Identity Disorder

A 23-year-old woman is brought to clinic for evaluation for "memory issues." The patient recently visited her family for the holidays. Her boyfriend states that she had to interact with her abusive, alcoholic father and seems like someone else ever since. The patient speaks in a childlike singsong voice and asks to be called by a name different than what is listed on her driver's license. She states she does not recognize her boyfriend despite their dating for 10 months. Vital signs are normal, and she is cooperative but childlike in attitude and not oriented to her name.

Evaluation/Tests	Clinical diagnosis. BMP, CBC, LFTs, and TSH are normal. BAL is 0. Urine toxicology screen is negative. MRI is normal.
Treatment	Psychotherapy is the treatment of choice and traumatic memories are directly addressed. The goals of treatment include maintenance of safety, stabilization, identity integration, and symptom reduction. Pharmacotherapy can be used to treat any comorbid conditions (e.g., MDD, PTSD). Pharmacotherapy can be used to treat any comorbid conditions (e.g., MDD, PTSD).
Discussion	Dissociative identity disorder is characterized by a disruption of identity manifested by at least two distinct personality states dominating at different times, associated with extensive memory lapses in autobiographical information, daily occurrences, or traumatic events, which causes significant distress or impairment in functioning and is not due to the effects of a substance or medication. It moves beyond **dissociative amnesia** in which the patient cannot remember basic personal information. Instead, in dissociative identity disorder, the patient has more than one distinct identity, asking to be referred to by a different name rather than simply forgetting one's name.

CASE 11 | Delirium

A 79-year-old woman with no psychiatric history is sent from her nursing home for erratic behavior for the past 3 days. Nursing home staff report that for some parts of the day she appears completely at baseline, but for the past few nights she has appeared confused, aggressive, and restless. She has been receiving lorazepam for agitation. She was recently diagnosed with a UTI and started on treatment. When interviewed, she reports she has been kidnapped and someone is stealing all her money and starts yelling for help. Her mental status is waxing and waning, and she is unable to pay attention during the interview. On exam, she appears confused and pulls out her IV line. Her vital signs and oxygenation are normal. She has no focal neurologic deficits or other abnormal findings on physical exam.

Evaluation/Tests	Clinical diagnosis. CBC, BMP, LFTs, and TSH are normal. ECG and chest X-ray are normal. Urinalysis is positive for nitrites and WBCs. Urine culture is pending.
Treatment	Treat the underlying cause of the delirium, in this case, most likely a UTI. In addition, discontinue any medications that may cause or contribute to delirium, such as lorazepam (which may need to be weaned depending on the length and dose of treatment). Frequently reorient the patient to their surroundings, and mobilize and stimulate the patient. Avoid restraints if possible.
Discussion	This patient's presentation is consistent with delirium given the sudden change in baseline cognition with waxing and waning mental status that is worse at night (sundowning). Diagnostic criteria include (1) disturbance of attention and awareness (2) that develops over a short time period, fluctuates throughout the day, and is a change from baseline, and (3) additional disturbance in another area of cognition such as memory, orientation, language. These disturbances should not be better explained by

CASE 11 | Delirium *(continued)*

Discussion	another neurocognitive or medical condition. There should also be some evidence of an underlying cause or causes, such as the UTI in this patient. Delirium is associated with increased morbidity and mortality and can present as hyperactive or hypoactive delirium. This case illustrates hyperactive delirium. In contrast, **hypoactive delirium** could present with more subtle characteristics, such as a patient "acting strangely," being more withdrawn than usual, or talking to oneself. Hypoactive delirium is more common in the elderly and is also more difficult to detect.

PSYCHOSIS

Psychosis refers to a dysfunctional perception of reality. Psychosis can be seen in many psychiatric illnesses, including psychotic disorders, mood disorders, substance use disorders, neurocognitive disorders, or other medical conditions such as delirium.

The foundation of psychosis is a combination of the following symptom categories: delusions, hallucinations, disorganized speech, and disorganized behavior.

If psychosis is present, it is important to identify the length of symptoms, the severity of symptoms, and whether the symptoms are caused by another condition (such as delirium or drug intoxication) as this will help define the diagnosis.

Timeline	<1 month	1–6 months	>6 months
Diagnosis	Brief psychotic disorder/episode	Schizophreniform disorder	Schizophrenia

**CASE 12	Schizophrenia**	
A 21-year-old man presents with 2 months of paranoia and odd behavior. He reports that someone planted a microchip in his brain and his thoughts are being intercepted. He hears their voices for most of the day and believes the voices are CIA officers. His college counselor says that he has isolated himself from others and has not been attending class for weeks. His family reports that the odd behavior started 7 months ago, which they thought was due to school stress. On physical exam, he is paranoid, disheveled, malodorous, nervous, and has flat affect. His thoughts are illogical and disorganized with thought blocking.	
Evaluation/Tests	Clinical diagnosis. CBC, BMP, TSH, and head CT are normal. Urine toxicology and blood alcohol level (BAL) are negative.
Treatment	The patient should be admitted to the psychiatric unit for safety, and a typical or atypical antipsychotic should be offered. Typical (first-generation) antipsychotics have higher risk of extrapyramidal symptoms, while atypical (second-generation) antipsychotics have higher risk of metabolic syndrome. The most efficacious antipsychotic is clozapine, which carries a risk of agranulocytosis and requires weekly blood draws; it is therefore a third-line medication.
Discussion	Schizophrenia is a lifelong illness present in <1% of the general population, with initial onset usually in young adulthood. This patient presents with several common features of schizophrenia, namely paranoid delusions and auditory hallucinations, as well as classic abnormalities in hygiene, odd behavior, disorganized thought process, and flat affect. In order to meet the diagnostic criteria for schizophrenia, the patient must have two (or more) of the following symptoms present for a significant portion of time during a 1 month period: (1) delusions, (2) hallucinations, (3) disorganized speech, (4) grossly disorganized or catatonic behavior, or (5) negative symptoms. At least one feature must include delusions, hallucinations or disorganized speech. These symptoms must cause a significant disturbance in occupational or social functioning, and some symptoms must be present for at least 6 months, which may include a prodromal period. Additionally, other psychiatric, substance, or medical disorders must be ruled out for a diagnosis of schizophrenia to be made. **Brief psychotic disorder** is characterized by a period of 1 day to 1 month of 1 or more symptoms of (1) delusions, (2) hallucinations, or (3) disorganized speech +/− grossly disorganized or catatonic behavior, with full return of premorbid functioning. **Schizophreniform** disorder is characterized by presence of symptoms for 1–6 months, while **schizophrenia** is for greater than 6 months. History taking and collateral information can be used to confirm the time course and rule out a primary mood disorder (e.g., **major depressive disorder with psychotic features, Bipolar I**) or other primary psychotic disorder.

CASE 12 | Schizophrenia (continued)

Additional Considerations	Although many patients with schizophrenia present with positive symptoms (delusions, hallucinations, disorganization), many also suffer from **negative symptoms**, characterized by flat affect, poverty of speech and/or thought, anhedonia, amotivation, apathy, and lack of self-care. Whereas positive symptoms are treated successfully with antipsychotics, negative symptoms are more difficult to treat. A nonpharmacologic treatment that can be efficacious is social skills training.

CASE 13 | Schizoaffective Disorder

A 28-year-old man presents with suicidal thoughts for the last 2 weeks. Patient states that voices have been telling him to "kill himself" and "finish it". He believes that these voices are part of a conspiracy at work to get him to leave his job. According to him, he first noticed his coworkers were starting to plot against him 7 months ago when they started to blame him for work that wasn't done. He started to hear voices 2 months after that. He has also been feeling very sad since the voices started and now feels depressed most days. Two weeks ago, he started to seriously think about suicide and developed a plan to hang himself but then decided to come seek help. On physical exam, he has restricted affect and is tearful at times. He has suicidal ideation, auditory hallucinations and appears to be responding to internal stimuli (looks over his shoulder, saying, "Stop").

Evaluation/Tests	Clinical diagnosis. Urine toxicology is negative. CBC, BMP, LFTs, TSH are normal, blood alcohol level (BAL) normal.
Treatment	Begin an antipsychotic, and consider additional treatment for the mood component as well (e.g., SSRI if depression symptoms, lithium if manic symptoms).
Discussion	Schizoaffective disorder, depressed type, can easily be confused for schizophrenia or MDD with psychotic features. Obtaining a good history of both the mood and psychotic symptoms from the patient and collateral sources is important. Schizoaffective disorder has about 1/3 the prevalence of schizophrenia, with typical onset in early adulthood. Similar to schizophrenia, schizoaffective disorder has a significant lifetime risk for suicide. The diagnostic criterion of schizoaffective disorder requires: 1. Uninterrupted period of illness during which there is major mood disorder along with symptoms of schizophrenia (two or more symptoms of (a) delusions, (b) hallucinations, (c) disorganized speech, (d) negative symptoms, or (e) disorganized/catatonic behavior). 2. Delusions/hallucinations for two or more weeks without major mood episodes. 3. Symptoms of major mood disorder present for the majority of the total duration of illness. **Delusional disorder** diagnosis requires the presence of one or more delusions for over 1 month without meeting criteria for schizophrenia and is not attributable to effects of substance use or another medical condition or mental disorder. The delusions may be associated with hallucinations that are related to the delusional theme. There is not usually a significant mood component, functioning is not markedly impaired, and behavior is not obviously bizarre outside of the delusional theme.

MOOD DISORDERS

Mood disorders are characterized by a primary disturbance in mood. The primary mood disturbance is generally mania or depression. In order to meet criteria for a mood disorder, the symptoms have to be persistent (>1 week for a manic episode and >2 weeks for a depressive episode).

In the setting of a **manic episode**, a diagnosis of **Bipolar I** is made if no other psychiatric or medical cause of episode is found.

Bipolar II disorder is characterized by a hypomanic episode (i.e., manic symptoms for several days but no psychotic symptoms and no significantly impaired functioning or hospitalization required) and the absence of a previous manic episode.

Major depressive disorder (MDD) is when a patient has a major depressive episode (>5 symptoms for >2 weeks) that is not caused by another medical or psychiatric condition.

Persistent depressive disorder (dysthymia) is a persistent state of depressive symptoms lasting for >2 years. Dysthymia often presents with milder symptoms than a major depressive episode, but symptoms consistent with major depression could be present during the entire 2-year period.

Both bipolar disorder and MDD can present with psychotic features. It may be difficult to determine whether a patient has a mood disorder with psychotic features or primary psychotic disorder (e.g., schizophrenia, schizoaffective disorder). Note that patients with primary psychotic disorders have psychotic symptoms in the *absence* of mood symptoms.

Therapy for mood disorders often includes a combination of medications and cognitive behavioral therapy (CBT). CBT involves teaching patients how to recognize negative thought patterns and retrain their responses to these thoughts. Both are effective individually, but the combination is more effective than medication or CBT alone.

CASE 14	Bipolar Disorder, Type I

A 24-year-old man presents with 2 weeks of irritability and uncontrolled energy. He reports that he has recently become aware that he has been chosen by God to be the next great poker champion. He is proud that he has been training for 22 hours a day, requiring little sleep. He reports that he has had to take a break from practicing in the casino as he lost all of his earnings last weekend but reports that he has a plan on how to win it all back so he can earn his title. On physical exam, he is pacing around the room, has very quick speech, and is hyperverbal and distractible.

Evaluation/Tests	Clinical diagnosis. Urine toxicology test for drugs of abuse (specifically cocaine or other stimulants) is negative.
Treatment	Treat with a mood stabilizer such as lithium or valproate.
Discussion	In order to receive a diagnosis of bipolar I, a patient must exhibit a manic episode that is not due to substance abuse or other medical or psychiatric conditions. An additional depressive episode is not necessary to diagnose bipolar I if the patient has already exhibited a manic episode. The definition of a manic episode includes: 1. Elevated/irritable mood for >1 week; 2. Three of the following 7 symptoms: (a) inflated self-esteem, (b) decreased need for sleep, (c) pressured speech, (d) flight of ideas, (e) distractibility, (f) increase in goal-directed activity or psychomotor agitation, and (g) excessive involvement in risky activities; 3. Symptoms that are severe enough to interfere with occupation or social functioning; and 4. Symptoms that are not attributable to drugs or medical conditions. The major differentiation between hypomania in **bipolar II** and mania in bipolar I is impairment of normal functioning. With bipolar II, the impairment is not significant enough to lead to major distress and does not require hospitalization. Psychotic symptoms (e.g., hallucinations, delusions) are also only seen with mania in bipolar I disorder. The diagnosis of bipolar II disorder requires at least one episode of hypomania in addition to one episode of major depression. A hypomanic episode requires: 1. Abnormal and persistently elevated, expansive, or irritable mood in addition to persistently increased energy for at least 4 days in a row; 2. Three or more symptoms of grandiosity, decreased need for sleep, more talkative/pressured speech, flight of ideas/racing thoughts, distractibility, increased goal-directed behavior, increased risky behaviors; 3. A change in functioning of the patient but not severe enough to require hospitalization; 4. Absence of psychotic features; otherwise it is considered a manic episode. The severity of symptoms in this case is consistent with bipolar I, specifically the delusions and significant interference with functioning.

CASE 15	Major Depressive Disorder (MDD)

A 45-year-old woman presents with 4 weeks of feeling very sad and hopeless about the future. She reports that she used to walk her dog every day, but lately she hasn't been feeling up to it. She thinks this may be because she has been having trouble sleeping through the night. She says that she has no energy to take care of her house or family, but even if she did have the energy, she doesn't think it would make any difference. She denies suicidal ideation or plan. On physical exam, she has had a 15-pound weight loss since her last visit. She has slow speech and does not make eye contact.

Evaluation/Tests	Clinical diagnosis. Urine toxicology and BAL are negative, and TSH is normal.
Treatment	Assess for immediate danger to self or others (suicidality or homicidality). Begin treatment with SSRIs and CBT.
Discussion	The diagnosis of MDD requires a 2-week period of at least 5 of the following: (1) depressed mood, (2) diminished interest or pleasure (anhedonia), (3) appetite change/significant weight loss or weight gain, (4) insomnia, (5) psychomotor agitation/retardation, (6) fatigue/low energy, (7) worthlessness/guilt, (8) reduced concentration/indecisiveness, (9) recurrent thoughts of death. The pneumonic "SIG E CAPS" is often used to help remember these symptoms (Sleep disturbance, loss of Interest, Guilt, Energy loss,

CASE 15 | Major Depressive Disorder (MDD) *(continued)*

Discussion	Concentration problems, Appetite changes, Psychomotor retardation, Suicidal ideation). Symptoms must cause distress and not be due to another psychiatric or medical condition. If a patient demonstrated previous manic episodes, consider a diagnosis of either **bipolar I** or **II** rather than MDD. **Persistent depressive disorder (dysthymia)** consists of chronic depression most of the time (no more than 2 months without symptoms) for at least 2 years, associated with at least 2 of the following: poor concentration, feelings of hopelessness, insomnia/hypersomnia, appetite changes, low energy, and low self-esteem. The individual may have major depressive episodes or meet criteria for major depression continuously.
Additional Considerations	**Grief/bereavement** is a normal process that people go through and can include hearing the voice of a loved one or wishing they died instead of the loved one. This becomes more concerning if they continue to have a significant degree of impairment >12 months after the death of the loved one. This impairment would include one of the following: persistent yearning/longing for the deceased, intense sorrow/emotional pain, preoccupation with the deceased, or preoccupation on the circumstances of the death, in addition to significant symptoms of mood and distress relating to the death of the loved one.

POSTPARTUM DISORDERS

Postpartum mood disturbances are common. Most women with symptoms will have **postpartum blues**, which describes a depressed affect that starts shortly after delivery and resolves within 1–2 weeks (this is not considered a psychiatric diagnosis). **Postpartum depression** is defined by symptoms within 4 weeks of delivering a child that are severe enough to meet criteria for a major depressive episode (severe symptoms >2 weeks). **Postpartum psychosis** is much rarer; however, it can be incredibly dangerous to the patient and infant. Patients with a history of mood disorder or psychotic disorder are most susceptible to this disease.

CASE 16 | Postpartum Psychosis

A 29-year-old woman and her 2-week old child are brought for evaluation by the husband. He is worried that she is acting bizarre and is worried about her ability to care for their baby. The patient refuses to talk to the doctors but stares at the corner of the room and mutters to herself. Per the husband, she has been worried about someone kidnapping and replacing their baby. During this time, she has not been sleeping, is struggling with concentration, and has not been eating or showering. Earlier in the evening, he witnessed her hovering over the crib holding a pillow above the crying infant, so he rushed them in for an evaluation. His wife does not have a past psychiatric history, but he notes that she was very depressed for 4 months after she miscarried 2 years ago. On physical exam, she has a healing C section wound and appears distracted and suspicious.

Evaluation/Tests	Clinical diagnosis. CBC, BMP, TSH are normal. Urine toxicology is negative.
Treatment	The patient should be admitted to inpatient psychiatry, and antipsychotics should be initiated. The safety of the infant must be ensured; the baby must not be left alone with the mother.
Discussion	Postpartum psychosis is a psychiatric emergency and necessitates quick identification and intervention. Although an uncommon diagnosis, the risk for suicide in this disorder is increased in the first year with rare but increased risk of infanticide. The onset of symptoms typically is rapid and include hallucinations, delusions, bizarre behavior, and/or disorganization. Typically, the women have a history of psychiatric illness and symptoms may present in those who stop psychiatric medications during pregnancy. However, it can occur in women without previously diagnosed disorders. Patients should be admitted, evaluated, and treated for any primary psychiatric disorders including bipolar I (most common etiology), schizophrenia, or schizoaffective disorder. **Postpartum blues** describe a period of days to 1 week of mild symptoms of depression that do not meet criteria for a major depressive episode. **Postpartum depression** is characterized by more severe symptoms that meet criteria for a major depressive episode in the first 4 weeks postpartum and should be treated with an antidepressant. Breast-feeding mothers should be educated on the risks of transmission of an antidepressant into the breast milk and the effects on an infant.

ANXIETY SPECTRUM DISORDERS

Anxiety disorders are characterized by excessive fear or worry. There is a spectrum of anxiety-related disease, ranging from generalized anxiety disorder to very specific phobias (e.g., flying). These diseases are characterized by a fear that is out of proportion to the exposure, persistent, associated with additional symptoms, and causes significant distress or interferes with functioning. These disorders, particularly obsessive-compulsive disorder, may be referred to as ego-dystonic conditions. This means that the patients afflicted with these disorders find the symptoms distressing and at odds with their ideal self-concept. These fears interfere with patients' lives in a way that's distressing for them. Anxiety spectrum disorders are generally best treated with SSRIs/SNRIs and/or cognitive-behavioral therapy.

CASE 17 | Panic Disorder

A 35-year-old woman presents with chest pain. She states that it started about 2 hours ago while she was on the phone with her sister. She had sudden onset of chest pain, heart palpitations, shortness of breath, numbness/tingling around mouth and on tips of fingers, and a sense of impending doom. The symptoms lasted for 20 minutes before resolving. This is her fourth presentation with the same cluster of symptoms in the last 5 months. Despite previous evaluations and reassurances, she remains concerned about these symptoms.

Evaluation/Tests	Clinical diagnosis. ECG shows normal sinus rhythm, Troponin is normal ×2. Previous recent tests including CBC, TSH, BMP, CT chest, and stress test have been normal.
Treatment	Consider SSRI and/or cognitive behavioral therapy. PRN anxiety medications, such as benzodiazepines, can be considered for the short term.
Discussion	Diagnosis of panic disorder requires an abrupt and intense fear/discomfort that peaks within minutes and has 4 or more symptoms of: palpitations/tachycardia, sweating, trembling, SOB/smothering sensation, chest pain, nausea, dizziness/lightheadedness, hot/cold chills, paresthesias, derealization/depersonalization, fear of losing control, fear of dying. In addition to these symptoms, there must also be worry about having panic attacks or maladaptive behavioral changes related to attacks (e.g., avoidance) for at least 1 month. Panic attacks are characteristically unprovoked (out of the blue) but can also be triggered by known events or stimuli. When panic attacks are triggered, patients often try to avoid the situations by minimizing travel or even not leaving their home. Risk factors for developing panic disorder are a history of sexual/physical abuse, smoking, recent onset of stressors, and respiratory problems (asthma). It is also important to screen for other psychiatric disorders, as panic disorder is often associated with other anxiety and mood disorders. Of note, agoraphobia is often seen with panic disorder.

CASE 18 | Specific Phobia

A 33-year-old woman presents with worry about an upcoming flight. The patient states she has to fly to her sister's wedding and is terrified. She has tried to visit her sister three other times in the past, but she has panicked right before takeoff and gotten off the plane. On physical exam, she has a euthymic affect but is in notable distress when talking about flying.

Evaluation/Tests	Clinical diagnosis.
Treatment	Exposure therapy, a form of cognitive behavioral therapy, can help decrease the patient's fear response. As-needed benzodiazepines can also be used short term for a known, planned exposure (e.g., a flight).
Discussion	Specific phobia is an extreme, persistent fear/anxiety about a specific object/event (the stimulus) that is out of proportion to the actual danger it poses. The stimulus almost always provokes immediate fear and is actively avoided or endured with great distress. The phobia is generally persistent for more than 6 months. Around 75% of patients who have a phobia typically have more than one fear. Phobias sometimes develop after a traumatic event (e.g., plane crash) but can also occur without this history. Onset of a phobia typically begins in childhood and is more common in women.

CASE 19 | Generalized Anxiety Disorder (GAD)

A 26-year-old man presents with anxiety. He is concerned about how his anxiety is impacting his performance at a high-pressure job. He worries that people are judging his work poorly, despite never having a bad job performance evaluation. He also is concerned about his boyfriend's health, worrying that he will crash his car or become sick. The worrying impacts his efficiency and concentration at work, but he still functions well in his job despite it being so distressful. He also reports fatigue, difficulty sleeping due to worry, and muscle tensions. At times of increased stress, he notes nausea, diarrhea, and increased sweating. This has been going on since college, but it has gotten worse since starting this job 2 years ago. On physical exam, his affect is anxious at times but otherwise normal.

Evaluation/Tests	Clinical diagnosis. TSH is normal, and urine toxicology is negative.
Treatment	The treatment includes an SSRI and/or cognitive behavioral therapy.

CASE 19 | **Generalized Anxiety Disorder (GAD)** *(continued)*

Discussion	For the diagnosis of GAD, the patient must have symptoms of worry/anxiety about multiple topics happening most days for at least 6 months, associated with 3 or more symptoms of restlessness, fatigue, difficulty concentrating, irritability, muscle tensions, or sleep disturbance. Many patients with GAD also have somatic symptoms such as sweating, nausea, diarrhea, trembling, and muscle tension. This anxiety disorder responds well to cognitive behavioral therapy and/or medications (the first line is SSRIs). For **adjustment disorder**, symptoms must occur within 3 months of the onset of a stressor and not persist more than 6 months after the stressor has resolved. Symptoms must cause marked distress that is out of proportion to the stressor, or the patient must have a significant impairment in functioning. The patient must not meet criteria for a major depressive episode. Symptoms of adjustment disorder can include depression, anxiety, and/or disturbance of conduct and are treated with supportive psychotherapy.

CASE 20 | Obsessive-Compulsive Disorder (OCD)

A 26-year-old man is referred to his dermatologist for severely chapped skin on his hands bilaterally. He reports vigorously washing his hands in scalding hot water dozens of times daily in response to uncontrollable and intrusive fears that his hands are dirty and contaminated. He realizes this is unrealistic but feels a great deal of anxiety when he is unable to wash them. These difficulties have occurred for many years, but he was recently encouraged to seek help because it has affected his work as a waiter. On physical exam, he has erythematous, chapped hands bilaterally, and is anxious appearing.

Evaluation/Tests	Clinical diagnosis.
Treatment	A combination of therapy (CBT) and medications (SSRIs) is most effective.
Discussion	OCD is characterized by obsessions and/or compulsions that are distressing, impairing, and time-consuming. Obsessions are undesired thoughts that are recurrent, intrusive, and increase anxiety. Compulsions (repetitive behaviors or mental rituals) are performed in order to relieve the anxiety, and may increase when a patient resists acting on them. Unlike **obsessive-compulsive personality disorder**, OCD is ego-dystonic, which means that the patient is distressed by the obsessions and is frustrated by them but performs the compulsions anyway (see OCPD case).

CASE 21 | Post-Traumatic Stress Disorder (PTSD)

A 25-year-old man who was recently discharged from the military presents with nightmares for the past 3 months. He states that he watched a tank get blown up by an improvised explosive device, and one of his friends who was on the tank died. He reports often thinking about this event in places where it "sneaks up on him," sometimes at work or at church. He reports having frequent nightmares. He has been unable to drive his car since returning home. He also describes being on edge and is easily startled by loud noises, and he feels guilty that he survived and his friend didn't.

Evaluation/Tests	Clinical diagnosis. Urine toxicology test is negative.
Treatment	A combination of CBT and pharmacotherapy, specifically an SSRI, is most effective.
Discussion	PTSD diagnosis requires an exposure to a traumatic event, as well as six additional symptoms from four other clusters of symptoms: 1. Intrusions (distressing memories, dreams/nightmares, flashbacks) 2. Avoidance (avoiding memories or triggers for the memories) 3. Negative mood/thinking (negative thoughts, distortions, negative mood, guilt, shame, diminished interest or participation, detachment) 4. Alteration in arousal (irritability, recklessness, hypervigilance, concentration or sleep issues, exaggerated startle) Symptoms must be disturbing, not attributed to substance use or another condition, and be present for >1 month. In contrast, **acute stress disorder** is similar to PTSD, but the symptoms are present for less than a month. PTSD can be distinguished from **depression** by the presence of avoidance, intrusive symptoms, and an aroused state. The avoidance of driving and sensitivity to loud noises due to the trauma leads to a PTSD

CASE 21 | Post-Traumatic Stress Disorder (PTSD) *(continued)*

Discussion	diagnosis in this case, whereas a similar patient could be diagnosed with depression if he had the same feelings of guilt and sleep disturbances but also symptoms like loss of interest/concentration, depressed mood, and suicidality. PTSD can be distinguished from **anxiety disorders** by the presence of a traumatic event, nightmares/flashbacks, and hypervigilance.

PERSONALITY DISORDERS

Personality disorders are defined by persistent patterns of behavior that deviate from expectations of that individual's culture and are manifested by disturbances in cognition, affectivity, interpersonal relationships, and impulse control. By definition, personality disorders are ego-syntonic, which means that the beliefs and thought patterns from these disorders are in line with the patient's self-image and do not produce personal distress. They are fundamental to the patient's personality and in line with their values. This makes personality disorders difficult to treat, for physicians often have difficulty convincing patients that they have a problem. In contrast, ego-dystonic disorders, such as OCD, are distressing to patients, so they are more likely to be interested in treatment. As in multiple other psychiatric diagnoses, diagnosis requires that the symptoms lead to clinically significant distress or impairment in social, occupational, or interpersonal functioning. The mainstay of treatment for most personality disorders is psychotherapy.

These disorders are grouped into clusters, which are often remembered with the mnemonic "weird (Cluster A), wild (Cluster B), worried (Cluster C)." **Cluster A** personality disorders are characterized by difficulty forming meaningful relationships and have a genetic link to schizophrenia, but they lack overt psychosis. Cluster A includes paranoid, schizoid, and schizotypal personality disorders. **Cluster B** personality disorders are antisocial, borderline, histrionic, and narcissistic personality disorders. They are considered dramatic and erratic, and they have a genetic association with substance use and mood disorders. **Cluster C** personality disorders are avoidant, obsessive-compulsive, and dependent personality disorders. These patients are anxious and fearful, and there is a genetic association with anxiety disorders.

CASE 22	Schizoid Personality Disorder
\multicolumn{2}{l}{A 21-year-old man presents for a work physical. He is doing a work-from-home job because his last job required him to "interact with too many people". He is quiet and only answers direct questions. He has been living in his mother's basement, and his mother states that he stays in the basement around 22 hours per day. He is not sexually active, does not "have much of a social life," but reports being content with his space and is satisfied with the work that he does. He is quiet, has a restricted affect, but other physical exam findings are normal.}
Evaluation/Tests	Clinical diagnosis. Depression screening is negative.
Treatment	Psychotherapy.
Discussion	**Schizoid personality disorder** is characterized by detachment from others and restricted expression of emotions and the presence of at least four of the following: 1. No desire for close relationships 2. Proclivity for solitary activities 3. Low interest in sexual experiences with others 4. Takes pleasure in few activities 5. Lacks close friends 6. Appears indifferent to praise 7. Shows flat affect or detachment Schizoid personality disorder cannot be diagnosed in the presence of schizophrenia or a mood disorder with psychotic features. Unlike avoidant personality disorder, patients with schizoid personality disorder don't mind being alone and are not distressed with their detachment from society. Patients with **avoidant personality disorder** are distressed by being alone and have four of the following characteristics: 1. Avoids occupational activities requiring interpersonal contact 2. Unwilling to get involved with people unless certain will be liked 3. Restraint in intimate relationships due to fear or shame or ridicule 4. Preoccupied with being criticized in social situations 5. Inhibited in interpersonal situations due to feelings of inadequacy

CASE 22 | Schizoid Personality Disorder *(continued)*

Discussion	6. Views self as inept/unappealing/inferior
	7. Unusually reluctant to take personal risks due to fear of embarrassment.
	Avoidant personality disorder entails a sense of inadequacy and social inhibition due to fears of criticism. Note: This is a Cluster C personality disorder, characterized more by "worries" than "weirdness."
Additional Considerations	**Paranoid personality disorder** is characterized by the presence of at least four of the following:
	1. Suspects that others are trying to harm them
	2. Preoccupied with loyalty
	3. Reluctant to confide in others due to fear
	4. Reads threats into benign comments
	5. Bears grudges
	6. Perceives attacks on character that are not apparent to others and is quick to counterattack
	7. Has recurrent suspicions regarding fidelity of sexual partner
	By definition, someone does not have paranoid personality disorder if they are diagnosed with schizophrenia, bipolar, or depression with psychotic features. This condition is not characterized by hallucinations.
	A patient with a **delusional disorder** may have a delusion that their coworkers are colluding against them. This contrasts with paranoid personality disorder, where the paranoia spans into multiple areas of the person's life, pervading into multiple relationships and interactions.

CASE 23 | Antisocial Personality Disorder

A 24-year-old man presents to urgent care following a physical encounter with a neighbor. He states that the neighbor "looked at him too many times" and "deserves what he got". He then states, "I didn't hurt him as bad as the guy last month; he was in the hospital for a week!". He smiles during the entire encounter and is eager to share more details. On review of his chart, it's noted that the animal humane society was called in the past due to concern for abuse of his pet dog. When he was 15, he spent the night in jail after assaulting a peer, which he happily discusses. Physical exam findings are normal.

Evaluation/Tests	Clinical diagnosis. Urine toxicology is negative.
Treatment	Psychotherapy.
Discussion	Antisocial personality disorder is characterized by disregard for others and violations of the rights of others and at least 3 or more of the following:
	1. Failure to conform to legal norms
	2. Deceitfulness or manipulating others
	3. Impulsivity
	4. Irritability and recklessness, physical fights
	5. Reckless disregard for safety of others
	6. Irresponsibility or inconsistent work behavior
	7. Lack of remorse
	Antisocial personality disorder is only diagnosed in adults but requires evidence of **conduct disorder** in the individual as an adolescent.

CASE 24 | Borderline Personality Disorder

A 36-year-old woman presents for a routine exam. She reports that she was recently arrested for shoplifting cosmetics. She states that her boyfriend "blew up at her" for getting arrested again. She says, "I should just kill myself. That will show him!". She admits that he sometimes physically abuses her, but she stays with him because no one else cares about her. At the end of the visit, she thanks the doctor profusely for being so much better than the last doctor … and angrily states, "He didn't care about me at all!". She is talkative, but all other physical exam findings are normal.

| Evaluation/Tests | Clinical diagnosis. Urine toxicology is negative. |
| Treatment | Dialectical behavioral therapy. |

CASE 24 | Borderline Personality Disorder *(continued)*

Discussion	Borderline personality disorder is characterized by unstable interpersonal relationships and unstable sense of self and at least five of the following:
	1. Frantic efforts to avoid real or imagined abandonment 2. Pattern of unstable or intense relationships 3. Unstable self-image 4. Impulsivity—spending, sex, substances, etc. 5. Recurrent suicidal threats or self-harm 6. Marked mood reactivity 7. Chronic feelings of emptiness 8. Inappropriate or intense anger 9. Transient, stress-related paranoid ideation or dissociative symptoms
	Impulsivity or dangerous behaviors are often noted. It can be associated with splitting, in which the patient believes people/groups are all good or all bad. Patient should be assessed for suicidal ideation and methods of self-harm (e.g., self-mutilation) as both are common in patients with borderline personality disorder.

CASE 25 | Histrionic Personality Disorder

A 46-year-old woman presents for a routine exam at a doctor's office. She stands up several times during the visit to check herself in the mirror and asks if her new dress is pretty. On exam, she is wearing revealing clothing and jumps up dramatically, yelling that the stethoscope is "too cold!". At the end of the visit, she starts tearing up and says that no doctor has ever been so attentive previously.

Evaluation/Tests	Clinical diagnosis.
Treatment	Psychotherapy.
Discussion	Histrionic personality disorder is characterized by attention-seeking behavior, excessive emotional behavior, and inappropriate sexuality or intimacy and at least five of the following:
	1. Uncomfortable when not center of attention 2. Inappropriately sexual or provocative 3. Rapidly shifting and shallow emotions 4. Uses physical appearance to draw attention 5. Speech is excessively impressionistic (not detailed) 6. Theatrical or exaggerated emotions 7. Suggestible 8. Overestimates intimacy of relationships
	This can often appear similar to dependent personality disorder in which individuals have an excessive need for support and affirmation. However, histrionic patients perform their behavior to seek attention more than the affirmation, and their excessive emotionality and concern with their appearance will highlight this distinction. In contrast, **dependent personality disorder** entails excessive need to be taken care of and fears of separation, which makes patients prone to being in abusive relationships. They struggle to make decisions themselves and have low self-esteem, causing them to seek constant support from others. It is characterized by five or more of the following:
	1. Difficulty making everyday decisions without excessive reassurance 2. Needs others to assume responsibility for major areas of life 3. Difficulty expressing disagreement with others due to fear of loss of support 4. Difficulty initiating projects due to lack of confidence 5. Goes to excessive lengths to obtain support from others 6. Feels uncomfortable or helpless when alone 7. Urgently seeks another relationship as a source of care when a close relationship ends 8. Unrealistically preoccupied with fears of being left to take care of themselves
	Note: Dependent personality disorder is a Cluster C personality disorder, as it is most characterized by the "worry" that they cannot exist on their own.

CASE 26 | Narcissistic Personality Disorder

A 43-year-old man is seen in clinic after making a scene in the waiting room for being asked to wait 10 minutes for his appointment. He is annoyed that he had to wait while "regular people got to see the doctor". He explains that he has a "very important job" and should not have to wait at all for his appointments as it is very burdensome to leave his job even for a few minutes. He explains that he got his job due to his "superior intellect" and "unprecedented business acumen". He explains that he is "constantly needed" at his work and that his coworkers are jealous of his superiority. Physical exam findings are normal.

Evaluation/Tests	Clinical diagnosis.
Treatment	Psychotherapy.
Discussion	Narcissistic personality disorder entails a sense of grandiosity, unreasonable expectations of others due to sense of entitlement, and lack of empathy for others. They also react poorly to criticism and think they know best. It is characterized by five or more of the following: 1. Grandiose sense of self-importance 2. Preoccupied with fantasies of unlimited success/power/intelligence 3. Believes they are "special" and should have only "special" peers 4. Requires excessive admiration 5. Sense of entitlement 6. Interpersonally exploitative 7. Lacks empathy 8. Envious of others or believes others are envious 9. Arrogant or haughty

CASE 27 | Obsessive-Compulsive Personality Disorder (OCPD)

A 54-year-old woman presents for a routine exam. She states it has taken her 2 years to find a doctor because she was looking for someone who met a list of her criteria, which included making sure the doctor's medical school was in a state that did not have the death penalty. She is an attorney and explains that she has been staying late at the office every night because she does not trust that her staff can format her work in the best way or proofread her documents as well as she can. She reports not engaging in social activities or hobbies as her reports "could always be made a little bit better". She has missed some work deadlines as her reports were "not quite right yet".

Evaluation/Tests	Clinical diagnosis.
Treatment	Psychotherapy.
Discussion	Obsessive-compulsive personality disorder is characterized by four or more of the following: 1. Preoccupation with details/rules/order to the extent that the major point of the activity is lost 2. Perfectionism that interferes with task completion 3. Excessive devotion to work at the expense of leisure activities and relationships 4. Overconscientiousness or inflexibility in matters or morality, ethics, or values 5. Inability to discard worthless objects 6. Reluctance to delegate tasks 7. Miserly spending attitude 8. Rigidness and stubbornness OCPD entails preoccupation, perfectionism, and lack of flexibility. These patients, however, do not see a problem with their perfectionism (ego-syntonic) as opposed to **OCD patients**, who are distressed with their obsessive thoughts. OCPD patients are preoccupied with perfectionism and control rather than with admiration (narcissistic personality disorder), and their sometimes unusual beliefs are consequences of this perfectionism and need for control. Individuals with **schizotypal personality disorder**, however, have fantastical beliefs that are not necessarily oriented toward perfection and control as with OCPD individuals.
Additional Considerations	**Schizotypal personality disorder** is characterized by interpersonal deficits as well as eccentric behavior and at least five of the following: 1. Ideas of reference (over-reading significance into everyday events) 2. Odd beliefs or magical thinking 3. Unusual perceptual experiences, including bodily illusions

CASE 27 | Obsessive-Compulsive Personality Disorder (OCPD) *(continued)*

Additional Considerations	4. Odd thinking and speech
	5. Suspiciousness or paranoid ideation
	6. Inappropriate or constricted affect
	7. Behavior or appearance that is odd, eccentric, or peculiar
	8. Lack of close friends
	9. Excessive social anxiety
	It cannot be diagnosed in the presence of schizophrenia or a mood disorder with psychotic features. This magical thinking is not delusional or centered on a particular delusion, but the beliefs may be odd and lead to unusual behaviors.
	Schizoid vs. schizotypal mnemonic: "Schiz-oid likes to av-oid others."

FACTITIOUS AND SOMATIC DISORDERS

Factitious and somatic disorders may be unconscious (somatic symptoms) or conscious (malingering/factitious disorder). Motivations may be for obvious external gain (malingering) or not (factitious disorder). Chief concerns may be subjective (somatic symptom disorder), health diagnoses (illness anxiety disorder) or neurological (conversion disorder).

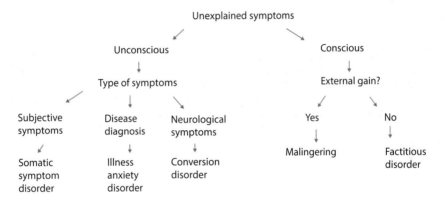

CASE 28 | Factitious Disorder

A 45-year-old woman without past medical history presents to the emergency room with confusion, dizziness, sweating, "shakiness," and blurred vision. She denies any alcohol or illicit drug use. She is subsequently admitted to the medical service for severe hypoglycemia. On physical exam, she is tachycardic and hypertensive. She has pale skin with needle marks and is diaphoretic, tremulous, and anxious.

Evaluation/Tests	BMP is normal except for glucose of 50. BAL is 0, urine toxicology is negative. CBC, LFTs, TSH, and HbA1c are normal. She has elevated insulin levels and low C-peptide levels. Collect collateral information from the family
Treatment	Address the test results and diagnosis in a nonjudgmental, nonthreatening manner.
Discussion	Factitious disorder is characterized by falsification of psychological or physical signs or symptoms or induction of disease or injury, associated with identified deception, without clear external rewards (e.g., avoiding military/work/jail or monetary gain). The motivation is to assume the sick role. The behavior is not due to another mental disorder. Repeated and long-term hospitalizations are common. In this case, the patient's symptoms, needle marks, low C-peptide, and lack of past medical history suggest that she injected herself with insulin, leading to her medical encounter. This diagnosis should also be considered when faced with an unusual presentation of a common disorder (e.g., a skin abscess that speciates with enteric bacteria rather than the usual *Staphylococcus aureus* or *Streptococcus pyogenes*).
	Malingering describes an intentional production of false or exaggerated symptoms for secondary gain or an external incentive. Malingering should be suspected in any patient who is inconsistent in reporting, does not cooperate with the interview, discusses impending legal proceedings, or has a history of antisocial personality disorder. In this case, malingering might be suspected if the patient mentioned that she missed a mandatory court date due to being in the hospital.

CASE 29 | Functional Neurological Symptom (Conversion) Disorder

A 27-year-old wheelchair-bound woman comes to the hospital for six days of leg weakness. Four years ago, she had a traumatic stillbirth and since then has had difficulty walking. She has seen six neurologists, and none can find a physiological reason for her weakness. She worries that doctors may think she is faking her symptoms because nothing on the repeated examinations explains her weakness. She says she would love to walk so she can travel by airplane to be there for her sister who just gave birth to her first son. On exam, she is sitting comfortably in a wheelchair, is smiling, and seems unaffected by her condition. Her weakness is lessened when distracted.

Evaluation/Tests	Clinical diagnosis.
Treatment	Validate the patient's experience of symptoms. Treatment should include a multidisciplinary approach with reassurance, education, physical therapy, psychotherapy, cognitive behavioral therapy, antidepressants if appropriate, and exercise.
Discussion	Functional neurological symptom disorder (conversion disorder) is classified by abnormal neurological symptoms that: 1. are not consistent with a recognized neurological condition, 2. cause significant distress and impairment, 3. are not better explained by another medical or mental disorder. "Functional" refers to the symptoms resulting from a failure of the functioning of the nervous system, as opposed to a structural lesion or pathology. Psychological factors are not required for diagnosis but are often associated with this disorder. This disorder should be considered when neurological symptoms are incompatible with known disease or are inconsistent throughout the examination.

EATING DISORDERS

Eating disorders can develop in any gender at any age, although they are significantly more frequent in females. It is important to distinguish an eating disorder from people who engage in intense/odd diets or exercise regimens but do not have a diagnosable eating disorder. Like many other psychiatric illnesses, eating disorders must include a component of psychological disturbance, i.e., the condition causes significant physical or psychological distress. Anorexia nervosa can sometimes be confused with bulimia nervosa. Anorexia by definition requires a significantly low body weight, whereas other eating disorders do not. Bulimia is characterized by binge eating episodes with any compensatory behavior, whether purging, exercise, fasting, or laxatives.

CASE 30 | Bulimia Nervosa

A 15-year-old girl presents for a routine appointment. She describes problems at school with social situations, wanting to fit in with the popular crowd and be thinner. She struggles to lose weight but describes feeling out of control with food for the past 6 months, where she eats large amounts of food, such as an entire pizza and gallon of ice cream. She quickly feels guilty afterward, and then makes herself throw up by sticking her fingers down her throat. These episodes occur at least 2–3 times per week. Her vital signs are normal, her height is 5 feet 2 inches, and she weighs 135 pounds. Her BMI is 27.5. She has sialadenosis (salivary gland enlargement), dental caries, and abrasions on the dorsum of her right hand (Russell's sign).

Evaluation/Tests	Labs show hypochloremic, hypokalemic alkalosis, with compensatory elevation in bicarbonate. Amylase is elevated.
Treatment	Nutritional education should be combined with CBT and an SSRI.
Discussion	In this case, the purging behavior is consistent with a diagnosis of bulimia. Bulimia is characterized by the following: 1. Recurrent episodes of binge eating and recurrent attempts to lose weight and compensate for overeating (e.g., vomiting, fasting, diuretics, laxative abuse, or excessive exercise) at least once a week for 3 months 2. Perception of self-worth is excessively influenced by body shape and weight 3. Does not occur exclusively during an episode of anorexia nervosa If the patient's BMI is <18.5 kg/m^2, then the diagnosis is **anorexia nervosa** even if the patient presents with frequent purging. Diagnosis of anorexia nervosa is made when there is the following: restriction of energy intake relative to requirements, leading to significantly low body weight; intense fear of gaining weight or becoming fat or persistent behaviors that prevent weight gain; disturbed body image, undue influence of weight or shape on self-evaluation; or denial of the seriousness of the current low body weight.

CASE 30 | Bulimia Nervosa *(continued)*

Discussion	**Binge-eating disorder** is characterized by recurrent episodes of binge eating (eating an excessive amount of food in a 2-hour period associated with a lack of control), with at least three of the following behaviors: eating very rapidly, eating until uncomfortably full, eating large amounts when not hungry, eating alone due to embarrassment or feeling disgusted, depressed, or guilty after eating. The binge eating occurs at least weekly for 3 months, causes severe distress, and doesn't occur exclusively during the course of anorexia or bulimia. Treatment encompasses a multimodal approach, with CBT or interpersonal psychotherapy, a strict diet/exercise program coordinated by a dietician, and potentially an SSRI.

PSYCHIATRIC PHARMACOLOGY AND DRUG EMERGENCIES

Psychiatric medications can have potentially dangerous side effects when taken incorrectly or because of drug–drug interactions. This may result in hemodynamic instability, which is why the first step in caring for these patients is assessing and supporting vital signs. After ensuring the patient is stable, the offending medication can be determined through careful history taking and medication reconciliation, as well as physical exam findings. It is important to immediately stop the responsible medication(s) and to administer an antidote or other stabilizing medication as needed.

CASE 31 | Neuroleptic Malignant Syndrome (NMS)

A 22-year-old man is admitted to the psychiatric floor for observation after presenting with acute psychosis and agitation and receiving several doses of intramuscular haloperidol. The next day the patient appears confused and on physical exam is diaphoretic with generalized lead pipe muscle rigidity. His vital signs are significant for a temperature of 40°C, pulse is 112/min, respirations are 32/min, and blood pressure is 150/96 mmHg.

Evaluation/Tests	Creatine kinase is elevated to >1000 international units/L. CBC shows leukocytosis, elevated ALT and AST, and metabolic acidosis on basic metabolic panel. MRI, CT, and CSF analyses are normal.
Treatment	The causative agent should be stopped and supportive measures including administration of IV fluids should be initiated. Treatment may include benzodiazepines and dantrolene, followed by the addition of bromocriptine or amantadine in more severe cases.
Discussion	Neuroleptic malignant syndrome is associated with the use of medications including antipsychotics (neuroleptics) and antiemetics. It is characterized by changes in mental status with reduced or fluctuating level of consciousness, lead pipe rigidity, myoglobinuria, fever, and autonomic dysfunction (tachycardia, elevated or labile blood pressure, and tachypnea). It presents almost identically to **malignant hyperthermia**, which also has rigidity and myoglobinuria, but malignant hyperthermia occurs after induction with fluranes, halothane, or succinylcholine rather than after administration of antipsychotics. Both NMS and malignant hyperthermia will present with metabolic acidosis, but malignant hyperthermia will have significant hypercarbia unlike NMS. NMS also presents similarly to **serotonin syndrome** in that they both have fever, hypertension, diaphoresis, and confusion, but NMS has the characteristic lead pipe rigidity and significantly elevated creatine kinase. Serotonin syndrome would instead have clonus, hyperreflexia, and tremor. Context will help differentiate these as well. NMS is from antipsychotics; serotonin syndrome is from a number of serotonergic drugs, particularly in combination; and malignant hyperthermia is from anesthetics.

CASE 32 | Serotonin Syndrome

A 55-year-old woman is admitted to the hospital for 3 days of emesis. She is started on ondansetron to control the nausea and continued on her home medications, which include fluoxetine for her major depressive disorder and amitriptyline for migraine prophylaxis. During her stay, she begins to experience increased agitation and confusion. She is febrile to 38.3°C, pulse is 115/min, and blood pressure is 164/96 mmHg. She is diaphoretic and exhibits myoclonus with 4+ DTRs.

Evaluation/Tests	CK is elevated, CBC shows leukocytosis, and BMP shows decreased serum bicarbonate. CT head is normal. Urinalysis and CSF analysis by lumbar puncture are also normal.

CASE 32 | Serotonin Syndrome *(continued)*

Treatment	All serotonergic agents should be discontinued and supportive measures initiated to normalize vital signs. Benzodiazepines may be used for sedation.
Discussion	Serotonin syndrome is associated with increased serotoninergic activity in the CNS caused either by an interaction between multiple serotonergic drugs or intentional overdose of a serotonergic medication. The syndrome is characterized by: – Mental status changes—confusion, restlessness, and delirium; – Autonomic dysregulation—diaphoresis, hyperthermia, tachycardia, hypertension; – GI disturbance—diarrhea and vomiting; – Neuromuscular hyperactivity—myoclonus, hyperreflexia, and bilateral Babinski sign. When differentiating serotonin syndrome from **neuroleptic malignant syndrome (NMS)** or **malignant hyperthermia**, the context of the case (i.e., the presence of serotonergic drugs rather than antipsychotics or anesthesia) will be particularly useful. Additionally, the neuromuscular hyperactivity with tremor and hyperreflexia differentiates serotonin syndrome from NMS and malignant hyperthermia (both present with rigidity).

CASE 33 | Lithium Toxicity

A 40-year-old woman with a past psychiatric history of bipolar disorder presents with confusion and lethargy. Her husband reports that over the past few days, she has been vomiting and experiencing profuse diarrhea. Besides her psychiatric medications (lithium), her husband reports that she was recently started on hydrochlorothiazide for newly diagnosed hypertension. On exam, she has bilateral hand tremors and uncoordinated limb movements.

Evaluation/Tests	Lithium level is elevated. BMP, urinalysis, and toxicology screen are normal.
Treatment	Treat with IV fluids and, if necessary, dialysis.
Discussion	Lithium is used as a treatment for various psychiatric conditions, most notably bipolar disorder. It has a narrow therapeutic index, with toxicity occurring at levels >1.5 mEq/L. As lithium is excreted almost entirely by the kidneys, volume depletion, renal impairment, and drugs that alter renal function (e.g., NSAIDs, ACE inhibitors, or thiazides) can cause an increase in lithium reabsorption. In acute intoxication, patients can present with nausea, vomiting, and diarrhea. Neurologic sequelae develop later and manifest as confusion, lethargy, ataxia, coarse tremors/fasciculations, and hyperreflexia.

CASE 34 | Tricyclic Antidepressant (TCA) Toxicity

A 32-year-old man with a history of major depressive disorder is brought to the ED after he was found unresponsive following an apparent suicide attempt by drug overdose. En route to the hospital, he has a tonic-clonic seizure. His temperature is 38.8°C, pulse is 105/minute, respirations are 8/min, and blood pressure is 82/48 mmHg. His skin is warm and flushed, mucus membranes are dry, and pupils are dilated.

Evaluation/Tests	Urine and blood toxicology tests and alcohol level are negative. ECG monitoring shows widened QRS and frequent ventricular arrhythmias. Chart review confirms that he was prescribed TCAs for his depression.
Treatment	Treat with sodium bicarbonate to prevent arrhythmias. For this patient, manage side effects: IV fluids for hypotension and benzodiazepines for seizure protection.
Discussion	Tricyclic antidepressants are now rarely used in the treatment of depression, anxiety, and obsessive-compulsive disorder but are still used to treat migraines and neuralgic pain. Tricyclic antidepressant (TCA) toxicity can acutely manifest with vital sign abnormalities such as hyperthermia, tachycardia, hypotension, and respiratory depression. TCAs also have central and peripheral anticholinergic effects, which can cause dilated pupils, flushing, dry mucus membranes, urinary retention, and ileus. Patients may also exhibit CNS effects ranging from decreased level of consciousness to seizures. Other complications include prolonged QRS and ventricular arrhythmias. Because of these serious side effects and potential lethality in overdose, TCAs are generally not used first-line for psychiatric conditions.

DRUG INTOXICATION AND WITHDRAWAL

Substance intoxication or withdrawal can present in dramatic ways and can mimic other psychiatric illness such as mania, psychosis, panic attacks, or depression. A good history and physical are key to determining the proper diagnosis when dealing with substance intoxication or substance withdrawal. Patients may be delirious or obtunded, making it more difficult to determine the substance involved. Other times, patients with substance use may not be forthcoming about their use, so the history and physical may need to be supplemented with some detective work. Hypertension and tachycardia, along with anxiety, agitation, or tremor, could be from sedative withdrawal or stimulant intoxication. Sedation can be seen in stimulant withdrawal or sedative intoxication. If sedation is accompanied by hypotension, bradycardia, or hypoxia, sedative intoxication is more likely than stimulant withdrawal. Agitation can occur with intoxication or withdrawal of stimulants or sedatives.

Other clues can be collected from a thorough physical exam in cases where substance use is suspected. Jaundice may lead to consideration of alcohol use. Needle or track marks may be clues to opioid use. The smell of alcohol or marijuana may also be a clue. Pinpoint pupils can be a sign of opioid use. Nystagmus may lead one to consider PCP. Alcohol levels and toxicology screens can be helpful, as well as collateral from EMS, police, family, and friends. Finally, the location where the patient was found, as well as substances or paraphernalia on or near the patient, can be helpful. For substance intoxication and withdrawal, hemodynamic stability is always the number one focus.

CASE 35 | Alcohol Withdrawal and Delirium Tremens

A 47-year-old man who had a surgical procedure 4 days ago suddenly becomes somnolent. He is a successful businessman who reportedly takes very good care of his health. This afternoon, he reported to a nurse that he saw faces moving on the walls, and he appeared tremulous. He then became somnolent and was difficult to arouse. He has no known psychiatric history. Patient's temperature is 38.5°C, pulse is 130/min, respirations are 20/min, and blood pressure is 160/92 mmHg. He appears diaphoretic, minimally responsive, and is groaning.

Evaluation/Tests	CBC, TSH are normal. Urine toxicology is negative. ECG, head CT, and chest X-ray are normal. Collateral history from wife confirms he drinks heavily on a regular basis.
Treatment	Treat with benzodiazepines and symptomatic management. Consider thiamine if the patient has a long history of heavy alcohol use.
Discussion	Alcohol withdrawal is the result of the sudden decrease or abstinence of alcohol use resulting in anxiety, tremor, insomnia, gastrointestinal upset, transient hallucinations, and seizures that cause impairment in functioning. Alcohol increases activation at the gamma-aminobutyric acid type A (GABA-A) receptor. Chronic use results in downregulation of GABA receptors. The sudden decrease in GABA-A stimulation from the lack of alcohol results in withdrawal symptoms that typically begin with anxiety and tremor within 6–8 hours, hallucinations within 8–12 hours, seizures at 24–48 hours, and the potentially fatal delirium tremens (DTs) within 3–5 days. Delirium tremens describes the disturbance in cognition from alcohol withdrawal that is associated with autonomic abnormalities and has a mortality up to 20% if untreated. A key feature of DTs is the presence of delirium with unstable vital signs, and the condition requires frequent monitoring.
Additional Considerations	**Alcohol intoxication** presents in early stages with mood lability, memory/coordination impairment, slurred speech, and can progress to lethargy, coma, and respiratory depression depending on the amount consumed as well as the patient's alcohol use history and tolerance. Intoxication can present with lethargy and coma above levels of 250 mg/dL among those who are not heavy drinkers and can be tolerated without lethargy or respiratory depression in those with a high level of use and tolerance.

CASE 36 | Opioid Intoxication

A 22-year-old woman is found minimally responsive, lying on the sidewalk. She is picked up by EMS and brought to the Emergency Room. On exam, her temperature is 36.3°C, blood pressure is 95/65 mmHg, pulse is 65/min, respirations are 5/min, and O_2 saturation is 88%. She is minimally responsive to sternal rub and has trace emesis on her shirt. She is thin and her pupils are miotic and slow, and shallow breathing is noted. The rest of her exam is unremarkable.

Evaluation/Tests	Urine toxicology is positive for opiates. BMP, CBC, TSH, CK, blood glucose, and ABG are normal. CT head, ECG, CXR are normal, BAL is 0, and acetaminophen level is normal.
Treatment	Naloxone and supportive care including IV fluids, oxygen and airway protection.

CASE 36 | Opioid Intoxication (*continued*)

Discussion	Opioid intoxication can present with sedation and respiratory depression; opiate intoxication can be fatal if not recognized and treated with reversal agents and respiratory support. Clues to opiate intoxication include needle marks, lethargy, slow/shallow breathing, miotic pupils, and collateral history. Use of other sedatives such as alcohol and benzodiazepines with opiates will increase the risk of lethargy, respiratory depression, and death. Opioid overdose is treated with naloxone, an opioid receptor antagonist. Naloxone will send patients into opioid withdrawal, but opioid withdrawal is not life-threatening, whereas opioid overdose can be lethal.
	Opioid withdrawal is the constellation of symptoms after cessation or reduction of opioid use that is not life-threatening in an otherwise healthy patient. Symptoms include anxiety, piloerection, abdominal cramps, lacrimation, rhinorrhea, diaphoresis, yawning, and gastrointestinal distress. Treatment includes either symptomatic treatment such as ondansetron or promethazine for nausea, loperamide for diarrhea, and dicyclomine for abdominal cramps or treating with methadone or suboxone. Opioid addiction is often treated with methadone maintenance programs or suboxone (buprenorphine plus naloxone combination). Methadone is a long-acting opioid that will prevent withdrawal; its long half-life minimizes an acute high, so it does not lead to as much abuse as shorter-acting opioids.

CASE 37 | Benzodiazepine Intoxication

A 28-year-old woman with new onset panic disorder who was recently started on 10 mg escitalopram and 2 mg lorazepam as needed, presents with drowsiness and confusion. Vital signs are normal, but her speech is slurred and she has mild ataxia.

Evaluation/Tests	Blood glucose, CBC, BMP are normal. BAL and acetaminophen levels normal. CT head and ECG are normal. Urine toxicology is positive for benzodiazepines.
Treatment	Flumazenil.
Discussion	Benzodiazepine intoxication can present similarly to alcohol intoxication with mood lability, memory/coordination impairment, slurred speech, and ataxia. Although it is rarely fatal without coingestion of other sedatives, intoxication can progress to lethargy, coma, and respiratory depression, depending on the amount consumed and the patient's benzodiazepine use history and tolerance. Benzodiazepine intoxication is treated with flumazenil, which is a competitive antagonist that acts at the GABA receptor. If patients are treated with flumazenil, they should be observed for the symptoms of benzodiazepine withdrawal.
Additional Considerations	Just as benzodiazepine intoxication can mirror alcohol intoxication, **benzodiazepine withdrawal** presents similarly to withdrawal from alcohol. Patients present with tachycardia, tachypnea, hypertension, diaphoresis, anxiety, tremor, and, at its most severe, confusion, visual hallucinations, and generalized seizures. Similar to alcohol withdrawal, severe benzodiazepine withdrawal is treated with an IV benzodiazepine, such as diazepam.

CASE 38 | Cocaine Use Disorder

The parents of a 16-year-old boy bring him for evaluation of depression. They have received phone calls from school because over the past month his grades went from As to Cs. He has recently been spending more time with a new group of friends, quit the basketball team, and is not doing his chores at home. He has been fighting with his parents almost daily, and they note that he gets occasional nosebleeds. He feels his parents are overreacting because he is not depressed but just "growing up." On physical exam, his temperature is 37.5°C, blood pressure is 165/98 mmHg, pulse is 115/min, respirations are 22/min, and O_2 saturation is 98%. He is a thin, well appearing boy, with dilated pupils and psychomotor agitation.

Evaluation/Tests	Urine toxicology is positive for cocaine.
Treatment	Referral to rehabilitation programs.
Discussion	Cocaine use disorder describes a pattern of cocaine use that leads to clinically significant impairment and distress. It occurs within a 12 month period, and is characterized by at least two of the following: (1) taking more cocaine than intended, or for longer than intended; (2) having difficulty cutting down use despite efforts; (3) spending a great deal of time using or recovering from use; (4) cravings; (5) failure to fulfill major role obligations at home, work, or school; (6) continued use despite these problems; (7) giving up important occupational/social/recreational activities because of cocaine use; (8) use threatening physical safety; (9) use persisting despite knowledge of physical or psychological problems from cocaine. Use may also be marked by development of tolerance (the need for larger amounts of cocaine to achieve desired intoxication and/or diminished response to the same amount) or withdrawal. Similar to intoxication with other stimulants, physical symptoms include irritability, psychomotor agitation, insomnia, tachycardia, hypertension, and dilated pupils.

CASE 39 | Stimulant Withdrawal

A 21-year-old man presents with depressed mood and suicidal ideation that began abruptly yesterday. He denies previous history of depression, mania, psychosis, or anxiety and cannot identify any triggering events. He notes increased sleep, dysphoria with irritability, anhedonia, and increased appetite. He denies family history of mental illness. He denies substance abuse or trauma history. He is a single undergraduate student who is applying for medical school and lives in an apartment. He denies homicidal ideation or hallucinations but endorses suicidal ideation without plan or intent. His speech is normal, but he replies with short answers. On physical exam, his temperature is 37.6°C, blood pressure is 155/95 mmHg, pulse is 110/min, respirations are 21, and O$_2$ saturation is 99%. He appears lethargic, has depressed mood and congruent affect with irritability noted and a linear thought process.

Evaluation/Tests	CBC, BMP, TFTs are normal. BAL is 0, but urine toxicology screen is positive for amphetamines.
Treatment	Referral to substance rehabilitation programs.
Discussion	Stimulant withdrawal can present with two phases: an acute phase lasting 1–3 days, manifested by depressed mood, irritability, low energy, increased sleep and increased appetite; and a second phase with similar but milder symptoms lasting for days to weeks. Stimulant drugs such as amphetamines are used to treat ADHD but may also be abused (i.e., MDMA and methamphetamine).

CASE 40 | Phencyclidine (PCP) Intoxication

A 22-year-old man is brought into the hospital for attempting to assault a police officer. He screams at the nursing staff that he is going to kill everyone if he isn't allowed to leave because the police are framing him. He is placed in soft restraints because he attempted to hit a safety aide. His friend says he has never acted this way before and has no known psychiatric diagnoses. On physical exam, temperature is 37.3°C, blood pressure is 160/95 mmHg, pulse is 118/min, respirations are 20/min, and O$_2$ saturation is 98%. He is agitated, kicking his feet and clenching his fists. He has vertical nystagmus, and his pupils are normal in size.

Evaluation/Tests	Urine toxicology is positive for PCP, BAL is negative.
Treatment	Reassurance and a supportive environment. Consider administering an antipsychotic or benzodiazepine to calm the patient.
Discussion	Phencyclidine intoxication is characterized by erratic, hostile, and often violent behavior that can also be associated with psychosis. After PCP ingestion, patients can demonstrate physical signs of nystagmus, vital sign abnormalities such as hypertension or tachycardia, slurred speech, muscle rigidity, and seizures. Ensuring the safety of the patient and staff is imperative, and if necessary, use of restraints or antipsychotics may be used to maintain a safe environment.
Additional Considerations	Intoxication from **lysergic acid diethylamide (LSD)** can mimic other hallucinogens and usually improves over 6–12 hours. Patients present with a variety of symptoms such as hallucinations and visual disturbances. These may include seeing moving patterns of bright colors on people and objects, visualizing geometric images within larger images, and seeing trails behind moving objects or halos around objects. Individuals may also experience synesthesia, which is mixing of sensory perceptions, such that the individual may "see" sounds or "feel" colors. Other symptoms include depersonalization, difficulty expressing thoughts, distorted perception of time, extremes of emotion, and "bad trips" with panic attacks. **Cannabis intoxication** can cause distress when consumed in higher doses. This is seen more often with edible cannabis and in cannabis-naïve patients. The presentation can include anxiety, paranoia, sedation, slowed responses and thought, palpitations, injected sclera, tachycardia, hypertension, nausea, dry mouth, increased appetite, attention, and short-term memory deficits. Symptoms generally resolve within a few hours. **3,4-methylenedioxymethamphetamine (MDMA)** (also known as ecstasy or molly) intoxication can present with changes in mental status, seizures, anxiety, confusion, paranoia, euphoria, psychomotor agitation, restlessness, hyperthermia, vision changes, palpitations, dry mouth, nausea, abdominal cramping, sweating, bruxism, mydriasis, and/or tachycardia. MDMA use can also cause serotonin syndrome with fever, muscle rigidity, hypertension, tachycardia, agitation, and elevated CK. It can further lead to hyponatremia when individuals overconsume water in order to reduce hyperthermia.

14
Renal

Natalia Litbarg, MD
Claudia Lora, MD
Manpreet Samra, MD
Samuel Ohlander, MD

RENAL FUNCTION AND RENAL FAILURE

The three major manifestations of kidney disease are decreased glomerular filtration rate* (GFR), proteinuria, and hematuria. Serum creatinine (Cr), which is measured routinely by ordering a basic metabolic panel, is most often used to estimate GFR. The normal ranges of Cr range from 0.5 to 1.0 mg/dL for women and 0.7 to 1.2 mg/dL for men; however, these levels depend on the patient's muscle mass, from which creatinine is derived. Therefore, serum Cr may be misleading at extremes of muscle mass. A patient must be in steady state for an accurate measurement of Cr. Proteinuria and hematuria are discussed later in the chapter.

Afferent arteriolar vasoconstriction or efferent arteriolar vasodilation will decrease GFR. Afferent arteriole vasoconstriction can be caused by renal hypoperfusion, intravascular volume depletion, hepatorenal syndrome, sepsis, nephrotic syndrome, congestive heart failure (CHF), and use of nonsteroidal anti-inflammatory drugs (NSAIDs). Efferent arteriole vasodilation can be caused by angiotensin II blockade (angiotensin-converting enzyme (ACE)-inhibitors and angiotensin receptor blockers (ARBs)). These hemodynamic changes will frequently cause reversible decreases in GFR, causing reversible acute kidney injury (AKI). In cases of severe or prolonged compromises of GFR, chronic renal damage can ensue, leading to chronic kidney disease (CKD).

---

*Estimated or measured GFR and/or creatinine clearance (CrCl) are the tools used to estimate kidney function. These tools have their limitations because of the kidney's capacity for compensation by hyperfiltration and hypertrophy at the level of a single nephron. This is why GFR does not always directly correlate with the amount of functional nephrons and hence is limited in detecting and estimating the severity of kidney disease and monitoring its progression.

ACUTE KIDNEY INJURY (AKI)

The etiology of AKI can be divided into three main categories based on the anatomical location of the lesion: prerenal, intrarenal, or postrenal (see tables). To establish the etiology of AKI, a thorough history, physical examination, and laboratory and radiological findings must be obtained. When obtaining the history, try to elicit possible causes of volume depletion such as blood loss, nausea/vomiting, decreased oral intake, polyuria, or increased loss of insensible fluids (those lost through skin or respiration) such as from heat shock. Look for evidence of hypotensive episodes either documented (e.g., intraoperative) or suggested by the patient's symptoms (e.g., dizziness, lightheadedness, syncope). Carefully elicit history of exposure to nephrotoxic agents such as IV contrast dyes or medications (particularly NSAIDs, antibiotics, proton pump inhibitors (PPI), chemotherapy agents). Careful history of urinary symptoms such as dysuria, urinary frequency, polyuria, hematuria, and decreased urine output might suggest complete or partial urinary obstruction from kidney stones, benign prostatic hyperplasia, or other causes. Symptoms of extrarenal manifestations of systemic diseases such as systemic lupus erythematosus (SLE) and vasculitis (e.g., history of skin rashes, joint pain, hemoptysis, neurological abnormalities) should also be sought when suspecting AKI related to glomerulonephritis. Abnormal laboratory tests including urinalysis (UA), serum blood urea nitrogen (BUN), creatinine (Cr), and electrolytes can be helpful in identifying the cause of AKI. In patients with oliguria (defined as less than 400 mL urine per day, or less than 0.5 mL/kg/hour), the fractional excretion of sodium (FeNa) can help differentiate between a prerenal state and intrinsic renal damage. A FeNa < 1% generally indicates a prerenal state. Examining the urinary sediment is helpful to distinguish between glomerular and tubulointerstitial lesions causing AKI (see tables). Lastly, a renal ultrasound may help diagnose a postrenal cause (e.g., obstruction).

Differential Diagnosis for AKI

Prerenal	Intrarenal	Drugs
True total body volume depletion: (Hemorrhage, over-diuresis, vomiting, diarrhea, decreased oral intake, increased insensible fluid losses, diabetic ketoacidosis)	Glomerular diseases (e.g., glomerulonephritis (GN)) Vascular diseases Tubulo-interstitial diseases (e.g., acute interstitial nephritis (AIN), acute tubular necrosis (ATN)) Vasculitis SLE	ACE-I (prerenal, ATN) ARBs (prerenal, ATN) NSAIDs (AIN, ATN) Iodinated contrast dye (ATN) Antibiotics (AIN, ATN) Chemotherapy agents PPIs (AIN) Antiretrovirals Diuretics (prerenal, AIN)
Intravascular volume depletion with interstitial edema/third spacing: (severe hypoalbuminemia with decreased oncotic pressure (e.g., nephrotic syndrome, CHF, pancreatitis, burns, hepatorenal syndrome)		

(continued)

Differential Diagnosis for AKI (*continued*)

Prerenal	Intrarenal	Drugs
Hemodynamic changes—vasoconstriction of afferent arteriole: (sepsis, NSAIDs, hypercalcemia, contrast dye, nephrotic syndrome, hepatorenal syndrome, rhabdomyolysis, CHF)	Rhabdomyolysis Sarcoidosis **Postrenal** Urinary tract obstruction (prostate enlargement, bilateral kidney stones, tumor)	Phosphate-containing bowel preps Hydralazine (GN)

Key Associated Findings and Acute Kidney Injury (AKI) Differential Diagnoses

Acute Kidney Injury (AKI) with Key Associated Findings	Diagnoses
Severe volume depletion or hypotension (e.g., dehydration, diarrhea, hemorrhage, medication-induced, sepsis, intraoperative complications) Dry mucous membranes, orthostatic hypotension, decreased urine output, decreased skin turgor, or absent axillary sweat	Prerenal; consider ATN (if prolonged volume depletion)
Volume overload (e.g., CHF, burns, nephrotic syndrome, pancreatitis, or cirrhosis) S3 heart sound, elevated JVP, heart murmurs, pedal edema, ascites, or anasarca	Prerenal, ATN (due to prolonged hypoperfusion)
Cirrhosis, enlarged liver, ascites, jaundice	Prerenal, ATN, hepatorenal syndrome
Rash, fever, or eosinophiluria after drug exposure (e.g., antibiotics, NSAIDs)	Acute interstitial nephritis (AIN)
Hemoptysis, upper respiratory tract involvement (sinusitis)	GN secondary to vasculitis, Goodpasture's syndrome
Severe hypertension, livedo reticularis, absent pulses	Thrombotic microangiopathy (TMA)
Fever, mental status changes, diarrhea	Hemolytic uremic syndrome (HUS), thrombotic thrombocytopenic purpura (TTP)
Pregnancy-related emergency	Preeclampsia, ATN, cortical necrosis, HELLP syndrome, TMA
RBC casts, dysmorphic RBCs ("active" urinary sediment)	Glomerulonephritis (GN)
Low complements and active urinary sediment	Glomerulonephritis secondary to SLE, MPGN, endocarditis, poststreptococcal, hepatitis C, cryoglobulinemia
Normal complements and active urinary sediment	Glomerulonephritis secondary to vasculitis, anti-GBM, IgA nephropathy, TMA
Decreased urine output, sudden onset anuria, hematuria, urinary frequency, inability to empty bladder	Genitourinary (GU) obstruction

Urinary Sediment	
Cast Type	**Significance**
RBC cast ("active urinary sediment")	Glomerulonephritis
WBC cast	Acute interstitial nephritis, infection, glomerulonephritis
Muddy brown cast or granular cast	Acute tubular necrosis
Hyaline cast	Benign

Simplified approach to a patient with AKI

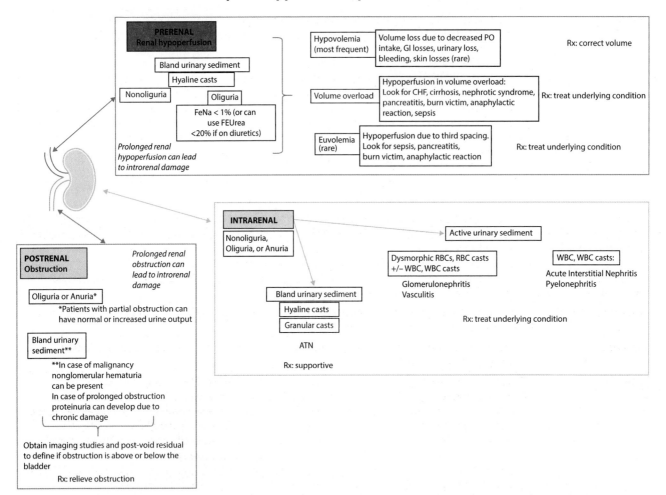

CASE 1 | Prerenal AKI

A 69-year-old woman with a history of hypertension is brought to clinic for evaluation of extreme weakness and lethargy. She returned from a trip to Mexico the day before and reported watery diarrhea, anorexia, and extreme weakness for the past 2 days. She is taking all her prescribed medications including lisinopril and chlorthalidone. She reports poor food and water intake and has noted decreased urine output. She denies any pain, dysuria, frequency, or hematuria. On exam, she is somnolent but arousable. Her vital signs are temperature 37.5°C, blood pressure 88/52 mmHg, and pulse 107/min. She is unable to stand up for an orthostatic blood pressure check, but her systolic blood pressure drops into the 70s, and heart rate increases to 120s when sitting up from a reclining position. The rest of the exam is notable for dry mucous membranes, decreased skin turgor, and absence of axillary sweat. Foley catheter is placed and urine output is about 50 ml after 2 hours.

Evaluation/Tests	BUN is 74 mg/dL, serum creatinine is 2.84 mg/dL (up from 0.98 mg/dL from a few months ago), and urinalysis demonstrates specific gravity 1.030, trace proteinuria, and several hyaline casts but is negative for WBCs, RBCs, or granular or cellular casts. CBC and LFTs are normal, and calculated FeNa is 0.6%.
Treatment	Treat with IV fluids. PO fluids can be used in milder cases. Hold diuretics and ACE inhibitors until volume status and serum creatinine improve.
Discussion	This patient is presenting with prerenal AKI due to volume depletion from traveler's diarrhea. The history of traveler's diarrhea in the context of taking diuretics and decreased PO intake, orthostatic blood pressure and heart rate changes, increased BUN/Cr ratio (>20:1), and low FeNa (<1%) are all consistent with a prerenal presentation of AKI. The most sensitive diagnostic test would be administration of fluids. If fluids improve blood pressure, tachycardia, and creatinine level, the diagnosis of prerenal AKI is confirmed. Cases of straightforward prerenal AKI constitute about 50% of all cases of AKI. If serum creatinine continues worsening in spite of improved volume status, further workup is warranted. Bland urinary sediment (absence of cells or cellular casts) makes any diagnosis associated with inflammation (such as **AIN**, acute **GN**, pyelonephritis) highly unlikely. Hyaline casts are proteinaceous casts that can present in any state of slow urinary flow.

CASE 1 | Prerenal AKI *(continued)*

Discussion	Prerenal states can also be caused by intravascular volume depletion with interstitial edema/third spacing, resulting in kidney hypoperfusion (e.g., due to heart failure). Therefore, in **heart failure**, the treatment is aimed at improving cardiac output. Prolonged and severe prerenal states can lead to **ATN**. Prerenal states associated with **hepatorenal syndrome (HRS)**, sepsis, and severe nephrotic syndrome require treatment of the underlying condition. HRS occurs due to massive splanchnic vasodilation that is perceived by the body as central hypovolemia. This causes cardiac dysfunction, and the body responds with arteriolar vasoconstriction. With respect to renal function, HRS causes severely decreased hydrostatic glomerular pressure by vasoconstriction of the afferent arteriole. This causes a decrease in GFR and an increase in serum Cr levels. This hemodynamic defect is corrected rapidly with a functional liver transplantation.

CASE 2 | Postrenal AKI

A 78-year-old man with a history of hypertension and benign prostatic hyperplasia (BPH) is seen in clinic for lower abdominal pain. He has no fever, nausea, or vomiting, but he has had no urine output for 12 hours. His medications include amlodipine. On examination, vital signs are normal except for mild tachycardia and a palpable, tender mass in the suprapubic region. Digital rectal examination reveals enlarged, nontender, smooth prostate.

Evaluation/Tests	Creatinine is 1.98, up from a baseline of 0.79 mg/dL. UA shows 3–5 RBCs and is otherwise normal, there are no cellular casts present. CBC is normal.
Treatment	Insertion of the Foley catheter will be curative for most bladder outlet obstruction causes. Consult Urology and treat underlying BPH.
Discussion	This patient is presenting with postrenal obstructive AKI secondary to BPH. Suprapubic mass and tenderness in an elderly man is highly suggestive of bladder outlet obstruction from enlarged prostate. Patients frequently will give history suggestive of urinary obstructive symptoms such as urinary frequency, nocturia, weak urinary stream, dribbling, and incomplete emptying. Dysuria and hematuria might be present. Polyuria can be a symptom of partial obstruction. Immediate decompression of the bladder with a Foley catheter will resolve the AKI in an acute obstruction. Long-standing obstruction may result in permanent kidney damage. After Foley placement, patients can develop postobstructive diuresis. Fluid and electrolyte replacement will be needed in some cases of severe postobstructive diuresis.

CASE 3 | Intrarenal AKI: Acute Tubular Necrosis (ATN)

A 68-year-old man with a history of hypertension presents with fever, abdominal pain, and vomiting. Abdominal CT scan with contrast shows a strangulated hernia, and he is taken for exploratory laparotomy, bowel resection, and hernia repair. Postoperatively, his urine output decreases to 10 mL/hr. He is given empiric IV antibiotics and ibuprofen for pain control. His bladder volume after voiding (postvoid residual) is measured at 45 mL (normal is less than 50–100 mL). On examination, he is afebrile, blood pressure is 95/58 mmHg, pulse is 108/min, and his mucous membranes are dry. His bowel sounds are slightly decreased, and his abdomen is soft, slightly distended, and tender with deep palpation. His surgical incision is clean and dry, and there are no skin rashes.

Evaluation/Tests	Labs are notable for BUN 15 (baseline 9 mg/dL) and serum creatinine 1.41 (baseline 0.92 mg/dL), and urinalysis shows multiple granular or muddy brown casts. Renal ultrasound is normal, and his calculated FeNa is 2.8%.
Treatment	The treatment of intrarenal AKI/ATN consists of supportive measures, such as optimization of the patient's volume status, discontinuation of all nephrotoxins, adjusting medications per eGFR, treatment of underlying causes (e.g., infection), and providing renal replacement therapy with dialysis, when needed.
Discussion	This patient has acute tubular necrosis (ATN). ATN is likely multifactorial due to a combination of renal hypoperfusion and nephrotoxic exposures. This patient presented with abdominal pain and vomiting with likely volume depletion (prerenal state) and then received nephrotoxic contrast dye. Postoperatively he is given NSAIDs and antibiotics, which are also potential nephrotoxins. His prerenal state on presentation might have contributed to the severity of tubular injury as volume depletion predisposes to ATN. Decreased urine output, FeNa > 2%, normal BUN/Cr ratio (<20/1), and multiple granular casts in urine are all suggestive of tubular injury. Normal renal ultrasound and normal postvoid residual rule out **obstructive causes**. **AIN** cannot be excluded with certainty in this scenario due to exposure to antibiotics and NSAIDs, but urinalysis does not show eosinophilia. Additionally, AIN usually requires several days to manifest.

CASE 4	Intrarenal AKI: Acute Interstitial Nephritis (AIN)
	A 65-year-old man undergoes a total knee replacement, which is complicated by infection. He is being treated with nafcillin. On day 10 of antibiotic administration, he develops a low-grade fever and a pruritic rash on his chest and arms. He has no other medical conditions and takes no other medications, herbal preparations, or supplements. He denies dysuria, hematuria, or decreased urine output. His temperature is 38.9°C, and other vital signs are normal. On exam, he has an erythematous macular rash involving all the extremities and trunk.
Evaluation/Tests	Serum creatinine is increased to 2.06 mg/dL from normal baseline, and CBC is normal except for increased eosinophil count. UA is remarkable for 10–25 WBCs, and hyaline casts and urine eosinophils are detected by Hansel's stain.
Treatment	Stop offending agent (nafcillin).
Discussion	This is a classic presentation of acute interstitial nephritis (AIN) secondary to beta-lactam antibiotic use. AKI with fever, skin rash, and leukocyturia after a recent drug exposure is highly suggestive of AIN. However, the classical triad of rash, leukocyturia (and eosinophiluria), and fevers is seen in <10% of cases of AIN and is most commonly associated with beta-lactam antibiotic use. Production of antibodies to the offending medication may play a role in the inflammatory process leading to damage of the kidney interstitium. Some other drug classes commonly causing AIN include NSAIDs, antibiotics (e.g., trimethoprim-sulfamethoxazole, beta-lactams), and proton pump inhibitors. The majority (>70%) of AIN in adults is associated with drugs; however, various infections and systemic diseases such as SLE, Sjögren's syndrome, and sarcoidosis can cause acute interstitial inflammation of the kidneys. In this patient with normal baseline renal function and relatively short exposure, full recovery of renal function is expected upon discontinuation of the medication. In rare circumstances if there is no improvement, steroids can be tried. The clinical presentation can share features with **pyelonephritis** or **poststreptococcal glomerulonephritis (PSGN)**; however, the patient does not have an elevated WBC count, and the time course for PSGN is 2–3 weeks after initial URI symptoms. This patient's timeline is more consistent with exposure to beta-lactam antibiotic. A rash would not be expected in a **prerenal AKI**.

CHRONIC KIDNEY DISEASE (CKD)

Chronic kidney disease (CKD) is defined as the presence of kidney damage or decreased kidney function for 3 or more months. The staging of CKD is determined by the glomerular filtration rate (GFR, <90%) and amount of albuminuria (30 mg/g or higher). It is important to diagnose CKD early and to prevent its progression to end-stage renal disease (ESRD). The two most common causes of CKD are diabetes and hypertension. Diabetic kidney disease often occurs concurrently with diabetic neuropathy and diabetic retinopathy as a result of poorly controlled diabetes. Hypertensive nephrosclerosis occurs in the setting of poorly controlled hypertension for years. Independent of the cause of ESRD, patients with GFR <15 mL/min/1.73 m^2 and uremic manifestations, require renal replacement therapy (RRT), which may include hemodialysis, peritoneal dialysis, or kidney transplantation. Reasons for starting RRT include acidosis not responding to treatment, electrolyte imbalances (especially hyperkalemia that is difficult to control medically), fluid overload resistant to diuretics, and uremic symptoms (such as decreased appetite, nausea, vomiting, dysgeusia, fatigue, and lethargy). Uremic exam findings include hyperreflexia, asterixis, and pericardial friction rub.

One important complication of CKD includes secondary hyperparathyroidism. As CKD progresses, there is decreased calcium reabsorption and increased phosphate retention by the kidney. Hyperphosphatemia stimulates osteocytes and osteoclasts in bone to release fibroblast growth factor 23 (FGF23), which exerts negative feedback on phosphate reabsorption but also decreases vitamin D levels. Decreased vitamin D can worsen hypocalcemia, which stimulates secretion of parathyroid hormone. Individuals with CKD may also have anemia due to decreased erythropoietin. As eGFR decreases, these individuals develop acidosis, electrolyte abnormalities, and hypervolemia.

Stages of Kidney Disease

Stages	GFR (mL/min/1.73 m²)	Function
Stage 1	>90%	Normal
Stage 2	60–89%	Mildly decreased
Stage 3A	45–59%	Mild–moderately decreased
Stage 3B	30–44%	Moderately–severely decreased
Stage 4	15–29%	Severely decreased
Stage 5	<15%	Kidney failure

CASE 5 | Uremia

A 65-year-old man with hypertension, type 2 diabetes mellitus, hyperlipidemia, and chronic kidney disease presents for a 6-month follow-up appointment. He reports nausea, anorexia, and worsened shortness of breath and fatigue for the past 2 weeks. He reports no change in urination but does report pruritis and weight loss. His wife notes that the patient at times is lethargic and confused. On examination, vital signs are normal except blood pressure of 165/88 mmHg. He has conjunctival pallor, dry skin, a pericardial friction rub, bilateral basilar crackles, 2+ bilateral lower extremity edema, hyperreflexia, and asterixis.

Evaluation/Tests	His basic metabolic panel shows: sodium 134 mEq/L, potassium 5.9 mEq/L, bicarbonate 14 mEq/L, BUN 156 mEq/L, Cr 18.93 mg/dL, phosphate 9.7 mg/dL, calcium 7.8 mg/dL. CBC is notable for Hgb 7.6 g/dL, and his albumin is 2.3 g/dL. Chest X-ray shows bilateral pleural effusions and enlarged cardiac silhouette. Renal ultrasound shows bilateral kidneys around 8 cm in length without hydronephrosis.
Treatment	Renal replacement therapy is indicated for symptomatic uremia. Urgent renal replacement therapy is recommended for acidosis, severe electrolyte abnormalities, toxic ingestions, fluid overload that is refractory to diuresis, and symptomatic uremia. Either hemodialysis or peritoneal dialysis can be used as an initial treatment for uremia. Renal transplantation requires advanced planning and cannot be used to treat acute uremia.
Discussion	The patient is showing multiple classical symptoms and signs of uremia including GI (nausea, anorexia, weight loss), neurological (lethargy, fatigue, hyperreflexia, asterixis), and cardiac (pericardial rub of uremic pericarditis) findings in the setting of CKD. He also exhibits symptoms of uremic encephalopathy, which can manifest with spectrum from mild symptoms such as fatigue, lethargy, and confusion to severely altered mental status and seizures. Uremia typically develops in the setting of CKD but can be seen in AKI if there is rapid decline in renal function. Patients with uremia present with elevated urea in the blood and associated fluid, electrolyte, hormone, and metabolic abnormalities that develop as renal function deteriorates. Uremia also has toxic effects on many tissues, and severe complications may include seizure, cardiac arrest (from electrolyte abnormalities: hyperkalemia, hypocalcemia, or metabolic acidosis), spontaneous bleeding, and death. Severe pruritis is related to uremia and severe hyperphosphatemia.

ALBUMINURIA AND PROTEINURIA

An abnormal amount of protein or albumin in the urine (proteinuria or albuminuria) most frequently indicates the presence of kidney disease even if serum creatinine and glomerular filtration rate (GFR) are normal. Normally, protein excretion in the urine is less than 150 mg/day. The albumin fraction is about 20% of the total urinary protein and should be less than 30 mg/day. The other proteins normally excreted in the urine include tubular Tamm-Horsfall protein and various globulins also found in the blood (e.g., immunoglobulins). A rough measure of the 24-hour total protein excretion can be estimated by calculating a spot random urinary protein-to-creatinine ratio.

Ways to Detect Protein or Albumin in Urine

Urine dipstick	Detects urine albumin in semiquantitative fashion (does not detect other proteins)
24-hour urine collection for protein and/or albumin	Measured in grams or milligrams per day Most accurate but cumbersome Simultaneous creatinine collection should be performed to estimate accuracy of the urine collection
Spot urine albumin-to-creatinine or protein-to-creatinine ratios	Measured in grams or milligrams per gram of creatinine Quick, easy test to estimate 24 hours protein excretion This test is accurate if used in patients at a steady state (i.e., no AKI) with average muscle mass

Causes of proteinuria can be classified as:

- **Abnormalities of the glomerular filtration barrier**—Despite high concentration in blood, albumin normally does not pass into the urine. Damage to the glomerular filtration barrier, results in albuminuria, with albumin constituting >50–75% of total protein in urine.
- **Overflow proteinuria**—This can occur with significant increase in concentration of filtered serum protein. The most frequent cause is monoclonal light chain immunoglobulin such as Bence-Jones protein in multiple myeloma.
- **Tubular proteinuria**—This is due to tubular damage and inflammation; in this case, the predominant protein excreted in urine will be Tamm-Horsfall protein produced by the tubular cells.
- **Transient proteinuria**—This does not signify renal pathology. It can occur in congestive heart failure, heavy exercise, and fever.
- **Benign orthostatic proteinuria**—This is a rare condition of abnormal protein excretion when the patient is in an upright position.

Definitions of Proteinuria

Normal urine protein	<150 mg/day
Overt proteinuria*	>150 mg/day
Nephrotic range proteinuria	>3000 mg/day
Albuminuria ("microalbuminuria")**	>30 mg/day

*In pregnancy, urinary protein excretion can increase to up to 300 mg/day.
**Albuminuria or abnormal albumin in the urine (over 30 mg/day or over 30 mg/g) might be detected as the earliest manifestation of the glomerular filtration barrier abnormality, while total urinary protein still remains normal (below 150 mg/day). In fact, the measurements of albuminuria are used routinely in screening diabetic patients for developing diabetic nephropathy and in kidney donors for early detection of kidney disease.

Nephrotic Syndrome

Nephrotic syndrome is diagnosed in the presence of four clinical manifestations:

1. Nephrotic range proteinuria—defined as massive proteinuria (>3.5 g/day)
2. Edema
3. Hypoalbuminemia (serum albumin <3 g/dL)
4. Hyperlipidemia (hypercholesterolemia and hypertriglyceridemia)

Complications of nephrotic syndrome include increased infection risk, hypercoagulability, protein malnutrition, hypervolemia, and renal failure.

Evaluation of the Patient with Nephrotic Syndrome

Obtain a careful history to look for systemic disease including DM, SLE, malignancy, and infections. History of medication use, IV drug abuse, or smoking is very important to note. The following blood and urine tests should be obtained in any patient with significant proteinuria: serum creatinine and electrolytes including serum glucose level, serum albumin level, and lipid profile. The majority of nephrotic syndromes present with bland urinary sediments. Urinalysis with active urinary sediment is suggestive of nephritic syndrome even in the presence of nephrotic-range proteinuria. Additional laboratory workup includes hemoglobin A1c to screen for diabetes; ANA to screen for SLE; and hepatitis B and C, HIV, and syphilis serologies to screen for common infectious causes of glomerular disease. Complement C3 and C4 levels will help to identify idiopathic membranoproliferative glomerulonephritis (MPGN), and lupus- and postinfectious-associated GNs. Serum and urine protein electrophoresis, serum, and urine free light chains with ratios can help diagnose monoclonal gammopathy. More recently, testing for anti-PLA2R (anti-phospholipase A2 receptor antibody) is recommended to support diagnosis of idiopathic membranous nephropathy. In most cases, the diagnosis is confirmed with a kidney biopsy. The only exclusion is pediatric nephrotic syndrome, which is usually caused by minimal change disease (MCD) and responds very well to empiric treatment with steroids.

Differential Diagnosis

Nephrotic syndrome can be due to two categories of disease processes:

1. *Primary (idiopathic) glomerular disease*—Examples include minimal change disease, membranous nephropathy, and focal segmental glomerulosclerosis
2. *Systemic diseases*—Examples include endocrine (diabetes mellitus), autoimmune (SLE), infectious (hepatitis B, hepatitis C, HIV, syphilis, poststreptococcal glomerulonephritis), oncological (solid tumors), hematological (leukemia, lymphoma, amyloid, or myeloma).

In pediatric patients, hereditary nephropathies can be present, but they are rare. Secondary nephrotic syndrome or nephrotic-range proteinuria can develop due to obstructive nephropathy, sickle cell disease, chronic renal allograft rejection, obesity, or obstructive sleep apnea. Medications can also induce nephrotic-range proteinuria: NSAIDs in association with AIN; pamidronate and IVIG can cause collapsing FSGS; interferon, lithium, and sirolimus have been shown to cause severe proteinuria; and several antiangiogenesis and other chemotherapy agents have been associated with severe proteinuria and thrombotic microangiopathy. Tobacco use was shown to cause nephrotic-range proteinuria and nodular sclerosis glomerular lesions similar to diabetic nephropathy. Various drugs of abuse have been associated with significant proteinuria as well.

Differential Diagnoses for Proteinuria

Cardiovascular	Autoimmune	Idiopathic	Medication related
• HTN • Atheroembolic disease **Endocrine** • Diabetic nephropathy • Obesity-related FSGS **GU** • Chronic obstructive uropathy (secondary FSGS) **Infectious Disease** • HIV-associated nephropathy (collapsing FSGS) • Hepatitis B and C (membranous) • Syphilis (membranous) • PSGN	• Lupus (membranous) • AA amyloid • Rheumatoid arthritis • Scleroderma **Hematology/oncology** • Sickle cell anemia (FSGS) • Monoclonal gammopathy • (AL, AH amyloid, monoclonal immunoglobulin deposition disease) • Lymphoma (MCD) • Leukemia (MCD) • Adenocarcinoma (MN) • Bone marrow transplant/GVHD	• Membranous nephropathy (MN) • Minimal change disease (MCD) • FSGS • MPGN • IgA nephropathy **Congenital/Genetic** • Finnish type FSGS • Congenital anomalies of the kidney and urinary tract • Fabry's disease	• NSAID (AIN or MCD) • IVIG (collapsing FSGS) • Bisphosphonates (collapsing FSGS) • Anti-VEGF (TMA) • Gold, penicillamine (MN) **Drug abuse related** • Cocaine (TMA) • Smoking/tobacco-associated nephropathy

Key Associated Findings and Proteinuria Differential Diagnoses

Proteinuria with Key Associated Findings	Diagnoses
Diabetic with visual changes, neuropathic pains, or poor glycemic control	Diabetic nephropathy
Decreased urine output, frequency, enlarged prostate	Obstructive uropathy
Edema, weight gain, periorbital edema, anasarca	Nephrotic-range proteinuria/nephrotic syndrome (NS), heart failure, liver disease
Renal vein thrombosis	Membranous nephropathy
Hematuria	Vasculitis, IgA nephropathy
Skin/malar rash, joint pains	Lupus nephritis, vasculitis, Henoch Schönlein purpura (HSP)
Hemoptysis, epistaxis, joint pains	Anti-GBM, vasculitis
Flank pain, hematuria/AKI	Renal vein thrombosis, membranous nephropathy, or NS
Severe HTN, papillary edema, decreased pulses	Thrombotic microangiopathy
Weight loss, B symptoms (night sweats), malignancy	Membranous nephropathy, minimal change disease due to lymphoma or leukemia
Macroglossia, bruising, neuropathy	Amyloidosis
Distended bladder, increased postvoid residual	FSGS secondary to obstructive uropathy
Morbid obesity	FSGS secondary to OSA and/or obesity
Sickle cell	FSGS secondary to sickle cell disease

CASE 6 | Diabetic Nephropathy

A 30-year-old woman with type 1 diabetes mellitus, complicated by diabetic retinopathy and neuropathy, presents for evaluation of worsening renal function and leg swelling. She states she is consistently taking her insulin and metoprolol but had stopped her lisinopril several months ago due to a cough. She denies NSAID use or any other over-the-counter medications. She reports good glycemic control at home but states her blood pressure has increased in the last few months to 140–150/80–90 mmHg range. On physical exam, she is afebrile, blood pressure is 154/87 mmHg, pulse is 74/min, respirations are 18/min, SpO_2 is 98% on room air, and BMI is 28. Examination is significant for mild periorbital edema and 2+ bilateral lower extremity pitting edema.

Evaluation/Tests	CBC is normal. Her serum creatinine is 1.55 mg/dL, and BUN is 18 mg/dL. Albumin, lipids, and random serum glucose are normal. Urine analysis is notable for 4+ protein; spot urinary protein and creatinine are 210 mg/dL and 67 mg/dL, respectively; and her protein/creatinine ratio is calculated at 3.134 g/g, increased from measurements taken a few months ago.

CASE 6 | Diabetic Nephropathy *(continued)*

Treatment	Add angiotensin II receptor blockers (ARBs). ACE inhibitors (e.g., lisinopril) and ARBs have been shown to decrease proteinuria and delay kidney disease progression. Reduce blood pressure to <130/80 mmHg. If blood pressure is not at goal on the maximum dose of ACE-I or ARB, add diuretics given the patient's volume expansion.
Discussion	This patient has nephrotic-range proteinuria secondary to diabetic nephropathy but does not have nephrotic syndrome because of the absence of hyperlipidemia and hypoalbuminemia. Her nephrotic-range proteinuria is likely due to progression of her diabetic nephropathy despite her serum creatinine appearing stable. Diabetic nephropathy is one of the microvascular complications of both type I and type 2 DM. Hyperglycemia results in nonenzymatic glycation of proteins, resulting in mesangial expansion, thickening of the glomerular basement membrane (GBM), and increased proteinuria. Diabetic nephropathy initially presents with albuminuria, and, if not aggressively treated, will develop to progressive renal failure frequently accompanied by nephrotic range proteinuria. Classical nephrotic syndrome is not always present, and occasionally microhematuria is detected. In diabetic nephropathy, kidney biopsy shows mesangial expansion, GBM thickening, and—in more advanced cases— nodular glomerulosclerosis (Kimmelstiel-Wilson nodules see image). However, given the patient's history T1DM and documented microvascular diabetic end-organ damage (retinopathy, neuropathy), a kidney biopsy is not necessary for the diagnosis in this patient. Used with permission from Doc.mari/Wikimedia Commons.

CASE 7 | Minimal Change Disease (MCD)

A 15-year-old boy with no significant past medical history presents with bilateral lower extremity and facial swelling and frothy urine for 1 week. He denies any medications (including NSAIDs) or herbal supplement use. He does not smoke, drink alcohol, or use illicit drugs. He denies hematuria, dysuria, or any other urinary symptoms. Family history is negative for any kidney disease, diabetes, or hypertension. He has a temperature of 36.7°C, blood pressure 110/56 mmHg, pulse 66 bpm, respirations 18/min, and SaO_2 98% on room air. His BMI is 24. Physical examination is significant for periorbital edema and 3+ bilateral lower extremity pitting edema.

Evaluation/Tests	CBC and serum electrolytes and serum glucose are normal. BUN is 11 mg/dL, Cr is 0.91 mg/dL, and serum albumin is 1.8 g/dL. Urine analysis is notable for 4+ protein, and urine protein/creatinine ratio is 7.24 g/g. Lipid profile demonstrates triglycerides 280 mg/dL and total cholesterol 330 mg/dL.
Treatment	In pediatric populations, a rapid response to empiric corticosteroid treatment is both diagnostic and curative. In such cases, renal biopsy is not needed.
Discussion	The most likely diagnosis for this young and otherwise healthy patient without any evidence of any systemic disease or drug exposure and with abrupt onset of edema and nephrotic syndrome is primary (idiopathic) minimal change disease (MCD). Minimal change disease is the major cause of nephrotic syndrome in children (90% of cases of nephrotic syndrome) but is less common in adults (10–25% of cases of nephrotic syndrome in adults). MCD is often idiopathic but may be triggered by infection, immunization, or, rarely, secondary to lymphoma due to cytokine-mediated damage. The classic biopsy finding of MCD is normal glomeruli on light microscopy with effacement of the foot process on electron microscopy (red arrow). Diagram (A) and electron micrograph (B) of minimal change disease. Electron microscopic features of minimal change disease include effacement of podocyte foot processes in the absence of ultrastructural features of other diseases. Reproduced with permission from Reisner H. Pathology: A Modern Case Study, 2nd ed. New York, NY: McGraw Hill; 2020.

CASE 7 | Minimal Change Disease (MCD) *(continued)*

Additional Considerations	In **adults, MCD** can be secondary to a viral infection (hepatitis C) or malignancy (lymphoma or leukemia); therefore, laboratory workup and renal biopsy is almost always indicated prior to making a decision about treatment. As with other patients with nephrotic syndrome, treatment with ACE inhibitors (ACEIs) or angiotensin receptor blockers (ARBs) are strongly advocated for reduction of proteinuria and intraglomerular pressure. Frequently, the high blood pressure in patients with nephrotic-range proteinuria is due to volume expansion, so additional diuretic therapy may be warranted. Hyperlipidemia should also be treated.

CASE 8 | Focal Segmental Glomerulosclerosis (FSGS)

A 28-year-old man without significant past medical history presents with an 18-pound weight gain and bilateral leg swelling over the last 2 weeks. He denies a history of smoking, alcohol, or illicit drug use. He is not on any medications and denies any over-the-counter medications use, including NSAIDs. Family history is significant for hypertension. Vital signs are temperature 36.7°C, pulse 77/min, blood pressure 164/93 mmHg, respirations 18/min, and SaO_2 99% on room air. Examination is significant for 2+ lower extremity edema.

Evaluation/Tests	Labs show normal electrolytes, BUN 15 mg/dL, and serum creatinine 1.4 mg/dL. Serum albumin is 2.1 g/dL. Urinalysis reveals 4+ protein, no WBCs, 3–5 RBCs, no cellular casts. Urine protein/creatinine ratio is calculated at 8.345 g/g based on urine spot check. His HIV and hepatitis B and C tests are negative. Total cholesterol level is elevated, and triglycerides are 370 mg/dL. Renal biopsy reveals focal and segmental sclerosis on light microscopy.
Treatment	The treatment of primary FSGS is similar to that of other nephrotic syndromes and includes ACE-I or ARB treatment, blood pressure control, lipid control, and diuretics if volume overload is present. Depending on the severity and acuity of the presentation, a trial of glucocorticoid therapy may be indicated, although response is inconsistent.
Discussion	Focal segmental glomerulosclerosis (FSGS) is a common cause of nephrotic syndrome in adults. The classical pathologic lesion of FSGS on light microscopy is characterized by focal (some but not all glomeruli) and segmental (part of but not the entire glomerulus) sclerosis and hyalinosis. On electron microscopy, effacement of foot processes is observed similar to MCD. Nonspecific IgM and complement C1 and C3 deposits may be seen on immunofluorescent staining. FSGS can be primary (idiopathic) or secondary to other conditions including HIV, sickle cell disease, chronic obstructive uropathy, medications such as pamidronate or IVIG, drug abuse, and more. **Membranous and secondary nephrotic syndromes**, including MCD, FSGS, and MN, are part of the differential and can only be excluded on renal biopsy. FSGS can present similarly to MCD with acute onset of edema and nephrotic syndrome. However, compared to MCD, FSGS is more likely to present with renal insufficiency, microscopic hematuria, and hypertension, as in this young man. Also, unlike patients with MCD, patients with FSGS are less likely to respond to glucocorticoids and more likely to progress to ESRD. **HIV-associated nephropathy (HIVAN)** presents with nephrotic syndrome but has a different pathological appearance than classical forms of FSGS and is described as a collapsing form of FSGS.

Focal segmental glomerulosclerosis. Glomerulus with segmental sclerosis (PAS stain)

Reproduced with permission from Reisner H. Pathology: A Modern Case Study, 2nd ed. New York, NY: McGraw Hill; 2020.

CASE 9 | Primary Membranous Nephropathy

A 46-year-old man without significant past medical history is referred by his primary care physician for incidental finding of 3+ proteinuria on routine urinalysis. For some time, the patient reports noticing swelling of his legs in the evenings and his face is puffier in the mornings. He also reports low back pain. He denies smoking, alcohol, or drug use, and his family history is unremarkable. On exam, he is normotensive, mildly overweight, and has 2+ bilateral pitting pedal edema.

CASE 9 | Primary Membranous Nephropathy *(continued)*

Evaluation/Tests	Serum creatinine is at a baseline of 0.9 mg/dL, UA demonstrates 3+ protein with specific gravity 1.010, absence of cells or casts. Additional laboratory tests are remarkable for urine protein 9 g per 24 hours, serum albumin 1.2 g/dL, lipid panel with elevated LDL, total cholesterol, and triglycerides. The complement C3 and C4 are normal, and ANA is negative. Serum and urine electrophoresis do not demonstrate monoclonal spike. Hepatitis B and C, syphilis, and HIV serologies are negative. HgbA1c is 5.1%. Urine sediment examined under the microscope is notable for the presence of oval fat bodies and "Maltese cross–like" structures under polarized light. Renal ultrasound performed with color Doppler demonstrates left renal vein thrombosis. Serum anti-phospholipase A2 receptor (aPLA$_2$R) demonstrates significantly elevated titers. Renal biopsy shows diffuse capillary and GBM thickening in glomeruli on light microscopy (shown in image), "spike and dome" appearance of subepithelial electron-dense deposits on electron microscopy, and immunofluorescence staining shows diffuse granular glomerular basement membrane staining with IgG and C3. Membranous glomerulonephropathy. A hematoxylin and eosin stained section of kidney showing a glomerulus with thickening of the basement membrane of the glomerular capillary tuft, producing a "wire loop" pattern. Reproduced with permission from Kemp WL, Burns DK, Travis Brown TG. Pathology: The Big Picture. New York, NY: McGraw Hill; 2008.
Treatment	ACE inhibitors or ARBs are indicated in the majority of patients with nephrotic syndrome. Diuretics might benefit severe symptomatic edema and/or hypertension. Treatment of hyperlipidemia is indicated. Renal vein thrombosis is treated with anticoagulation. Corticosteroids and other immunosuppressive or cytotoxic drugs might be indicated in certain cases or with severe disease presentation; however, patients with primary membranous nephropathy often have poor response to corticosteroid treatment. Up to a quarter of patients with primary MN can have spontaneous remission within 5 years.
Discussion	This patient's proteinuria, lower extremity edema, hyperlipidemia, hypoalbuminemia, and renal vein thrombus seen on ultrasound are consistent with membranous nephropathy. The classic presentation of primary membranous nephropathy is renal failure with renal vein thrombosis along with symptoms such as lumbar spine pain. Typically, symptoms start gradually, or patients may present with asymptomatic proteinuria. MN can be primary (idiopathic) or secondary, where it is associated with other conditions like malignancy, infections, SLE, and medications (including NSAIDs and penicillamine). Serum levels of circulating aPLA$_2$R (an antibody against podocyte membrane glycoprotein) are elevated in 70–80% of patients with idiopathic membranous nephropathy, and normal in patients with other etiologies of nephrotic syndrome. The immunofluorescent stain for aPLA2R can be present in many cases of primary membranous nephropathy. **Membranous nephropathy** can often be **secondary to malignancy**. Therefore, malignancy should be actively sought by performing age-appropriate screening and medical history guided cancer workup. Given this patient's lack of symptoms concerning for malignancy, this is less likely in his case.

HEMATURIA

Hematuria can be classified as gross hematuria (visible to the naked eye) and microscopic hematuria (visible only on microscopic examination of the urinary sediment). Microscopic hematuria is defined as the presence of three or more erythrocytes per high power field on a spun urine sediment. When approaching a patient with microscopic hematuria, the first step is to determine whether the source of the RBCs is glomerular or extraglomerular. RBCs that arise from the glomerulus traverse the tubules and in doing so become sheared or may be trapped in protein, forming RBC casts. The presence of dysmorphic RBCs and RBC casts is often referred to as "active" urinary sediment. In contrast, RBCs that are extraglomerular in origin are smooth and biconcave, as they appear in plasma.

Differential Diagnoses for Hematuria

Noncancerous	Malignant
Renal/glomerular causes	Urothelial carcinoma of the kidney or ureter
Urinary tract infection	Urothelial carcinoma of the bladder
Nephrolithiasis	Squamous cell carcinoma
Bladder stone	Adenocarcinoma
Benign prostatic hyperplasia	Prostate cancer
Urethral stricture	
Acute urinary retention	
Recent urologic procedure	
Menorrhagia	
Genitourinary Trauma	

Likely causes of hematuria in adult patients vary by age and history. Nephrolithiasis is more common in younger patients, while older patients, especially those with smoking history, are at higher risk for renal, ureteral, or bladder cancer. In men, benign prostatic hyperplasia and prostate cancer should also be in the differential. Infection is another common cause of hematuria, particularly in women, though one should not delay a full hematuria evaluation under the assumption that an infection is the source of the bleeding. As noted, many findings on a UA may suggest a UTI, but these findings should not preclude further evaluation to identify alternative pathologies. The recommended evaluation for microhematuria or history of gross hematuria is to obtain upper urinary tract imaging and to perform cystoscopy to evaluate the urethra and bladder.

Common Test Findings for Hematuria and Differential Diagnoses

Test Finding	Diagnoses
Urinalysis	
RBC: $\geq$3 RBC/HPF	Microhematuria by definition
WBC: >10 WBC/HPF	UTI, inflammation, STI
Leukocyte esterase: positive	UTI
Nitrites: positive	UTI
Urine crystals: positive	Nephrolithiasis
Urine culture: >10^3 colony-forming units	UTI
CT abdomen/pelvis	
Hydronephrosis	Ureteral carcinoma, obstructive nephrolithiasis, extrinsic compression
Ureteral filling defect	Ureteral carcinoma, ureteral polyp, obstructive nephrolithiasis
Bone lesions	Metastatic cancer

The following section focuses on glomerular hematuria, which is the hallmark of nephritic syndromes.

Nephritic Syndrome

Nephritic syndrome is characterized by four main features:

1. "Active" urinary sediment with hematuria
2. Hypertension
3. Renal failure
4. Proteinuria (generally <3.5 g/day)

The approach to the patient with suspected nephritic syndrome should include a careful medical history, physical exam, and serologic workup. Nephritic syndromes can be divided into those that consume complement proteins (C3, C4) and those that do not (see table). Ultimately, the combination of history, serologic workup, and a kidney biopsy establishes the disease entity causing the nephritic syndrome.

Workup of Active Urinary Sediment

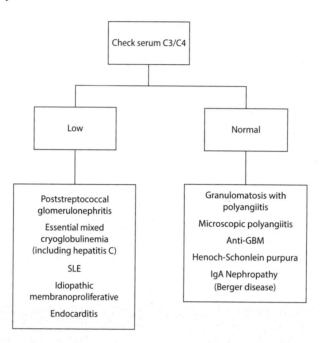

Renal and Glomerular Causes of Hematuria

| **Autoimmune**
• SLE
• Vasculitis (e.g., polyarteritis nodosa)
• Anti-GBM disease

Idiopathic
• Membranoproliferative glomerulonephritis (MPGN)
• IgA nephropathy (Berger disease)
• IgA vasculitis (Henoch-Schönlein purpura)
• Pauci-immune vasculitis
• TMA
• Anti-GBM disease | **Pulmonary-Renal Syndromes**
• Eosinophilic granulomatosis with polyangiitis (EGPA)
• Anti-GBM disease
• Granulomatosis with polyangiitis (GPA)
• C3 Glomerulonephritis

Endocrine
• DM (papillary necrosis) | **Hematology/Oncology**
• Sickle cell (papillary necrosis)
• Monoclonal gammopathy–induced dense deposit disease (DDD) or MPGN (rare)

Infectious
• Hepatitis C–associated MPGN
• Hepatitis B–associated polyarteritis nodosa
• Syphilis-associated MPGN
• HIV-associated TMA
• Bacterial/viral infection
• Poststreptococcal glomerulonephritis (PSGN)
• *E. coli* diarrhea (hemolytic uremic syndrome, HUS)
• Thrombotic thrombocytopenic purpura (TTP) | **Medications**
• Anti-VEGF drugs (TMA)
• Hydralazine (vasculitis)
• NSAIDs (papillary necrosis)

Congenital
• Autosomal dominant polycystic kidney disease (ADPKD)
• Autosomal recessive polycystic kidney disease (ARPKD)
• Alport's syndrome |

Key Associated Findings and Hematuria Differential Diagnosis

Hematuria with Key Associated Findings	Diagnoses
Back or flank pain radiating to groin pain, costovertebral angle tenderness	Nephrolithiasis, pyelonephritis, papillary necrosis (sickle cell crisis)
Suprapubic tenderness	UTI, urinary retention

(continued)

Key Associated Findings and Hematuria Differential Diagnosis (continued)

Hematuria with Key Associated Findings	Diagnoses
Dysuria, irritative voiding symptoms (frequency, urgency, nocturia)	UTI, bladder stone
Pinpoint urethral meatus, dysuria, irritative voiding symptoms, split urinary stream	Urethral stricture
Lower abdominal pain, tobacco history Irritative voiding symptoms	Bladder cancer
Lower urinary tract symptoms (slow stream, frequency, nocturia, incomplete emptying)	Benign prostatic hyperplasia
Gross hematuria, acute anuria	Obstructive uropathy
Nodular and firm prostate on digital rectal exam	Prostate cancer
Hematuria occurring concurrently with respiratory infection (synpharyngitic hematuria) Exercise-induced gross hematuria	IgA nephropathy (Berger disease)
Skin rashes, joint pains	SLE, vasculitis, HSP
Hemoptysis, epistaxis	Anti-GBM, vasculitis
Bloody diarrhea	*E. coli* hemolytic uremic syndrome (HUS)
Fever, mental status changes, low platelets	TTP
Post pharyngitis	Poststreptococcal glomerulonephritis (PSGN)

CASE 10 | Poststreptococcal Glomerulonephritis (PSGN)

A 12-year-old girl is brought to clinic by her parents after reporting seeing blood in her urine. She recently completed a course of antibiotics for Group A streptococcus pharyngitis. Her symptoms improved within a few days of starting antibiotics; however, about 2 weeks later she developed acute onset reddish urine, decreased urine output, and swelling of her legs. Vitals are normal except for blood pressure 150/90 mmHg, and she has 1+ lower extremity edema bilaterally.

Evaluation/Tests	Laboratory tests show creatinine of 1.6 mg/dL and BUN of 50 mg/dL. Urinalysis shows many RBCs, RBC casts, and 1+ protein. Urine protein to creatinine ratio is 0.8 g/g. Complement C3/C4 levels are low.
Treatment	Early treatment of Group A streptococcus infection with antibiotics can lessen the severity of the course of PSGN. If GN develops, treatment is supportive. Edema is managed with diuretics, and hypertension is managed with antihypertensive medications.
Discussion	This patient has poststreptococcal glomerulonephritis (PSGN), as evidenced by a Group A streptococcus infection with acute onset of hematuria a week or more after the infection. In a suspected case of PSGN, a recent diagnosis of Group A streptococcus via a positive throat or skin culture or serologic tests (antistreptolysin O or anti-DNAse B) showing an increase in antistreptococcal antibodies lends support to the diagnosis of PSGN. Complement levels, particularly C3, are usually low. Diagnosis is usually clinical. The symptoms present 1–4 weeks after the pharyngitis and include sudden-onset hematuria with oliguria, hypertension, edema, and RBCs, RBC casts, and protein in the urine. This glomerulonephritis is caused by immune complex deposition formed by antibodies and streptococcal antigen, which then trigger complement activation, endocapillary proliferation, and neutrophil infiltration. Most cases in children will resolve spontaneously with supportive treatment, but it may progress to renal insufficiency in adults. Biopsy is only obtained for cases with an unusual presentation or in rapidly progressive renal dysfunction. On light microscopy of the glomerulus, PSGN will show enlarged, hypercellular glomeruli with endocapillary proliferation and neutrophil infiltration. Immunofluorescence will show deposition of IgG, IgM, and C3 along the GBM and in the mesangium, with a diffuse, granular "starry sky" appearance. On electron microscopy, immune complex deposits are seen as subepithelial electron-dense "humps" and subendothelial deposits._x000D_
Though other nephritic conditions can present with similar symptoms, the clear history of a recent streptococcal infection makes other causes less likely. If hematuria occurs within less than 7 days of pharyngitis, it is referred to as "synpharyngitic." **IgA nephropathy** is synpharyngitic as it typically starts within 7 days of URI symptoms compared to PSGN, which is postpharyngitic.

CASE 11 | IgA Nephropathy (Berger Disease)

A 34-year-old man with no significant past medical history presents with episodic gross hematuria over the last few days. He also had associated "cold" symptoms of nasal and chest congestion and cough. He reports that he had a similar episode of dark brown urine 2 years ago. Vital signs are normal except for a blood pressure of 158/90 mmHg. Physical exam reveals trace lower extremity edema.

Evaluation/Tests	Laboratory tests are significant for a creatinine of 1.4 mg/dL, normal complement levels, and urinalysis showing hematuria and proteinuria. Urine protein to creatinine ratio of 2.4 g/g. A renal biopsy shows mesangial proliferation and predominance of IgA antigen–antibody complex deposition in the mesangium.
Treatment	Treat proteinuria with ACEI or ARB and with goal urine protein excretion <1 g/day. Hypertension should be managed with additional antihypertensive medication if needed for goal blood pressure <130/80 mmHg. Immunosuppressive therapy might be indicated for aggressive disease.
Discussion	This patient has a classic presentation of IgA nephropathy, an immune complex deposition disease diagnosed by renal biopsy. IgA nephropathy is the most common primary glomerulonephritis worldwide and most often occurs in Caucasian or Asian males. It often occurs concurrently with an upper respiratory ("synpharyngitic") or gastrointestinal infection, and the only symptom may be gross hematuria. It may also be associated with proteinuria, microscopic or gross hematuria, hypertension, and elevated creatinine. About 20–30% of patients with IgA nephropathy progress to end-stage renal disease in 20–30 years, but controlling hypertension and proteinuria can help prevent progression. It is important to note that mesangial IgA deposits on biopsy are pathologic findings in both IgA nephropathy and **IgA vasculitis** (also known as **Henoch-Schönlein purpura** or HSP), two conditions which are often associated with each other. IgA vasculitis is the most common childhood systemic vasculitis, typically follows a URI, and it can also present with palpable purpura on the buttocks and legs, arthralgias, and abdominal pain. Therefore, the two should be distinguished based on clinical presentation.

CASE 12 | Papillary Necrosis

An 18-year-old woman with sickle cell disease presents with right flank pain and gross hematuria. For the past 3 days, she has been treating herself for a vaso-occlusive pain crisis with NSAIDs, hydrocodone, and folic acid. She denies symptoms of an upper respiratory infection, dysuria, or fevers. The patient is afebrile, tachycardic, and in acute distress secondary to pain.

Evaluation/Tests	CBC is notable for Hgb 5.2 g/dL. UA shows numerous RBCs, and her BUN and Cr are slightly elevated from baseline. Renal ultrasound shows increased echogenicity of the right renal medulla. CT confirms papillary necrosis.
Treatment	Treatment is usually directed toward improving the renal hypoxia by adequate hydration and alkalization of urine. Exchange blood transfusion might be indicated in sickle cell crisis to lower the Hgb S proportion.
Discussion	This patient with a history of sickle cell disease, hematuria, and increased echogenicity findings on ultrasound most likely has renal papillary necrosis secondary to vaso-occlusive crisis. Renal papillary necrosis is a diagnosis of exclusion. CT findings may show papillary necrosis and sloughing. Pathologically, it is characterized by coagulative necrosis of medullary pyramids and papillae caused by any condition which affects medullary perfusion. A number of conditions can lead to medullary ischemia. Most important of these are diabetes mellitus (nonenzymatic glycosylation of renal vasculature), sickle cell disease (dysmorphic RBCs obstructing small renal vessels), chronic analgesics use such as NSAIDs (decreased prostaglandin synthesis resulting in vasoconstriction of afferent arteriole and renal hypoperfusion), renal transplant rejection, pyelonephritis, and urinary tract obstruction. In addition to hematuria, urinalysis may show proteinuria, pyuria, and low specific gravity. Urine cultures should be obtained to rule out pyelonephritis. Renal ultrasound is an appropriate first step in evaluation of any hematuria. CT scan is required for definitive diagnosis of papillary necrosis and is helpful in ruling out renal stones or renal vein thrombosis.

CASE 13 | Granulomatosis with Polyangiitis

A 55-year-old man presents with hemoptysis, shortness of breath, and hematuria. He reports worsening fatigue, arthralgias, chronic sinusitis with bloody nasal discharge, and a 10-pound weight loss over the last 1–2 months. Vital signs show a temperature of 38.3°C and a blood pressure of 165/95 mmHg. On exam, he has bilateral crackles in the lungs and mild bilateral pitting edema of both lower extremities.

Evaluation/Tests	Chest X-ray shows pulmonary nodules and cavities. UA shows many dysmorphic RBCs, RBC casts, and proteinuria. Labs notable for BUN 60 mg/dL and creatinine 2.1 mg/dL (previously normal) and positive PR3-ANCA (c-ANCA). Renal biopsy shows necrotizing vasculitis with crescents and granulomas. Immunofluorescence shows no immune deposits ("pauci-immune").
Treatment	Patients with Pauci-immune (or ANCA-positive) vasculitis are initially treated with either cyclophosphamide or rituximab, frequently with glucocorticoids.
Discussion	This patient with positive antibodies against PR3 (proteinase 3)-ANCA (c-ANCA), nasopharyngeal involvement, and hematuria likely has pauci-immune glomerulonephritis secondary to granulomatosis with polyangiitis (GPA) (formerly known as Wegener's granulomatosis). Pauci-immune refers to the lack of immunofluorescence seen on staining. Pulmonary manifestations of GPA include upper respiratory tract symptoms (nasal septum perforation, chronic sinusitis, otitis media, mastoiditis), lower respiratory tract symptoms (hemoptysis, cough, dyspnea), and renal findings including hematuria and RBC casts. GPA is a necrotizing small-vessel vasculitis that presents with granulomas in the lung and a necrotizing glomerulonephritis with crescents and granulomas. Other pauci-immune vasculitides are **eosinophilic granulomatosis with polyangiitis (EGPA)**, formerly known as Churg-Strauss syndrome, and microscopic polyangiitis (MPA). Both EGPA and MPA are positive for antibodies against MPO-ANCA (p-ANCA). EGPA is associated with asthma, sinusitis, skin nodules, and peripheral neuropathy but may also involve the heart, GI tract, or kidneys. It is a granulomatous necrotizing vasculitis with eosinophilia. IgE levels are often elevated in EGPA, and biopsy will show crescenteric glomeruli, granulomas, and eosinophilic infiltrates. **Microscopic polyangiitis** is a necrotizing vasculitis that involves lungs, kidneys, and skin (palpable purpura). It does not typically show nasopharyngeal involvement and does not present with granulomas. Biopsy will show crescents in glomeruli without granulomas or eosinophilic infiltrates. In all three diseases, immunofluorescence will show few or no immune deposits. GPA, EGPA, MPA most frequently present as **pulmonary-renal syndromes** and renal biopsy with minimal or absent immune deposits on immunofluorescence. Thus the clinical presentations and ANCA-positivity findings are key to distinguish the different diagnoses. There can be an overlap with **anti-GBM glomerulonephritis/Goodpasture syndrome**. However, anti-GBM complex antibodies would be present on immunofluorescence stain on renal biopsy, which is absent in pauci-immune glomerulonephritis.

CASE 14 | Anti-GBM Glomerulonephritis (Goodpasture Syndrome)

A 23-year-old man presents with hemoptysis and worsening shortness of breath for the past 3 days. On exam, he is afebrile, tachypneic, tachycardic with blood pressure 156/93 mmHg and SaO$_2$ 90% on room air. He has diffuse crackles on lung auscultation and mild bilateral lower extremity edema.

Evaluation/Tests	Chest X-ray shows pulmonary infiltrates concerning for alveolar hemorrhage. Labs show creatinine of 3.1 mg/dL from baseline of 0.8 a month ago, BUN 72 mg/dL, hemoglobin of 7.9 g/dL, and anti-GBM IgG antibodies are positive in the blood. Renal biopsy shows linear GBM deposits on immunofluorescence and necrotizing crescentic glomerular lesions.
Treatment	Treatment includes plasmapheresis as well as cyclophosphamide and corticosteroids.
Discussion	This is a classic presentation of **rapidly progressive (crescentic) glomerulonephritis (RPGN)** secondary to **Goodpasture syndrome**. This patient with hemoptysis, shortness of breath, and renal failure has anti-GBM glomerulonephritis, caused by autoantibodies to the alpha-3 chain of type IV collagen in the glomerular basement membrane. Anti-GBM disease can be renal-limited (called anti-GBM nephritis) or can manifest with both renal and pulmonary symptoms (Goodpasture syndrome). Light microscopy of the kidney biopsy typically demonstrates crescentic glomerular lesions. A smooth, linear pattern along the glomerular basement membrane on immunofluorescence staining confirms the diagnosis. Anti-GBM disease is usually rapidly progressing, with the majority of patients developing ESRD within a few months of presentation if untreated.

FLANK PAIN

The presenting symptom of flank pain stretches across multiple organ systems and pathologies. Though flank pain strongly suggests retroperitoneal pathology, this may be difficult to differentiate on the patient's initial presenting complaint. A good history is imperative to rule out traumatic and musculoskeletal etiologies. Acute presentation following physical exertion and associated with pain during specific movements suggests musculoskeletal etiology; pain with deep breathing and associated respiratory symptoms suggests pulmonary etiology. Ultimately, any mass, inflammation, or infection of a retroperitoneal or pelvic structure may result in flank pain.

Differential Diagnoses for Flank Pain

Renal	Reproductive	Gastrointestinal	Vascular
Renal/ureteral stone Pyelonephritis Renal cell carcinoma Transitional cell carcinoma Retroperitoneal fibrosis	Ovarian cyst Ectopic pregnancy	Colitis Gastroenteritis Small bowel obstruction	Abdominal aortic aneurysm
Musculoskeletal	**Other Malignancies**	**Skin**	**Pulmonary**
Broken rib Broken vertebrae Muscle strain Costochondritis Trauma	Adrenal carcinoma Hepatocellular carcinoma Colon cancer	Varicella zoster virus	Pleuritis Pneumonia

Renal causes of flank pain are less associated with specific movements. Renal colic associated with kidney stones is classically described as a unilateral flank pain that does not improve with body repositioning, often leading to frequent shifting in attempt to get comfortable. Flank pain from kidney stones (nephrolithiasis) is the result of urinary obstruction and is often described as the most severe pain a person has ever experienced. Obstructing stones cause acute, severe pain that comes in waves. The waves of pain are associated with ureteral peristalsis. Pain may shift toward the lower abdomen as the stone descends down the ureter, and there may be radiation down into the groin as the stone nears the bladder. Stones are more common in individuals with a family history of stones. If there is an underlying infection, systemic symptoms such as fever or chills may be present. Infected obstructing stones should be dealt with promptly given the possibility of progressing to pyelonephritis or sepsis. In the uninfected patient, tachycardia, nausea, and vomiting may be present secondary to pain. Stones are often associated with hematuria. Pyelonephritis can have many of the same presenting symptoms of an infected kidney stone, with the exception that there is rarely "colicky" pain in pyelonephritis. Instead, their flank pain is persistent and associated with fever, dysuria, and urinary frequency.

Renal masses are often taught using the "too late triad" of flank pain, hematuria, and palpable mass. This was historically due to the fact that many patients would initially present with these three symptoms secondary to advanced renal malignancy. However, in modern clinical practice with more routine imaging, renal masses rarely present in this fashion, but they should remain in the differential diagnosis.

Initial helpful tests include CBC to assess for leukocytosis or anemia, BMP to evaluate electrolytes and creatinine, and urinalysis and urine culture to assess for hematuria, proteinuria, and urinary tract infection. Renal ultrasound can be obtained to assess for hydronephrosis and ureteral dilation but is not as sensitive or accurate for diagnosing ureteral stones. Noncontrast abdominopelvic CT is fast, easy to read, and has a very high sensitivity for diagnosing kidney or ureteral stones.

Key Associated Findings and Flank Pain Differential Diagnoses

Flank Pain with Key Associated Findings	Diagnoses
Acute onset, unilateral, colicky pain radiating to groin, unable to find comfortable position Hematuria	Nephrolithiasis
Fever, chills, dysuria Costovertebral angle tenderness	Pyelonephritis, infected nephrolithiasis
Missed menses	Ectopic pregnancy
Associated with shortness of breath or cough	Consider pulmonary causes
Associated with specific movements, reproducible tenderness	Consider musculoskeletal causes
Changes in bowel habits	Consider GI cause
Burning, shooting, and tingling unilateral pain, rash	Varicella zoster virus (VZV), shingles

CASE 15 | Nephrolithiasis (Kidney Stones)

A 33-year-old man presents with sudden onset of sharp, severe left flank pain with radiation to the groin. He has associated nausea and vomiting. He denies dysuria, hematuria, fevers/chills, or any similar episodes in the past. He has tried acetaminophen with no improvement in the pain. His father has a history of recurrent kidney stones. He is in moderate distress, changing his body position frequently because he is unable to get comfortable. Temperature is 37.5°C, pulse 108/min, with mild costovertebral angle tenderness on the left. His abdomen is nondistended with mild tenderness to palpation in the left mid-lower quadrant. He has no spinal tenderness, his straight leg raise test is negative, and his genitourinary exam is unremarkable.

Evaluation/Tests	Urinalysis: positive RBCs. CT showed a 5-mm calcific density in the left proximal ureter with moderate hydronephrosis.
Treatment	IV hydration, pain control.
Discussion	Kidney stones are formed in the urine by stone-forming constituents: calcium, oxalate, and uric acid. Crystals, foreign bodies, or the renal papillary basement membrane itself can act as nidi, upon which ions from the supersaturated urine form microscopic crystalline structures. The size of urinary tract stones varies from gravel to staghorn calculi. The composition too varies based on presence of infection or other metabolic alterations. Most common are calcium oxalate stones in patients with hypercalciuria and normal calcium levels. This patient's presentation of lumbar pain with radiation and associated hematuria is most consistent with acute nephrolithiasis. The classic pain in nephrolithiasis is referred to as "renal colic," which results from the stone becoming impacted within the ureter as it passes toward the urinary bladder. Treatment is supportive care as most stones will pass on their own: IV hydration, NSAIDs, non-narcotic or narcotic analgesics, alpha blockers (tamsulosin, terazosin), and/or antiemetics (metoclopramide, ondansetron). Complications can include hydronephrosis and pyelonephritis and may warrant antibiotics and urologic intervention. Stones that are 7 mm and larger are unlikely to pass spontaneously and may require surgical intervention.

RENAL AND URINARY TRACT MASSES

Tumors of the urinary tract system are diagnosed and treated in multiple ways based on the individual location and histology of the tumor. Surgical resection is the primary treatment for most tumors, often followed by chemotherapy or active surveillance. There is no standard screening for tumors of the urinary tract. Risk factors for most urinary tract tumors include smoking and family history. These tumors primarily present in older adults, with the exception of Wilms's tumor, which presents in children.

Primary renal tumors include renal cell carcinomas (RCCs), benign oncocytomas, and Wilms's tumor, which is the most common renal malignancy of early childhood (years 2–4). **Renal cell carcinoma** occurs most commonly in older men aged 50s–70s. Clear cell carcinoma is the most common histological type of renal malignancy, but sarcomatoid histology can also be present and is more difficult to treat. Renal cell carcinoma has a strong association with von Hippel-Lindau (vHL) syndrome, and it is often associated with paraneoplastic syndromes such as ectopic EPO, ACTH, PTH-rp, and renin excretion. **Oncocytomas** may present similarly to RCCs, and even though they are benign, their treatment is often surgical resection to exclude malignancy. They arise from the collecting ducts of the nephron. In young children, **Wilms's tumor** also presents as a large, palpable, unilateral flank mass with hematuria. It may be part of several syndromes: WAGR complex (Wilms's tumor, aniridia, genitourinary malformations, mental retardation/intellectual disability), Denys-Drash syndrome (Wilms's tumor, early onset nephrotic syndrome, gonadal dysgenesis), and Beckwith-Weidemann syndrome (Wilms's tumor, macroglossia, organomegaly, and hemihyperplasia).

Bladder cancer is related to age and exposure to environmental carcinogens, specifically smoking. It can also be associated with chronic irritation and inflammation of the urinary tract and initially presents with painless hematuria. Tumors are most commonly derived from uroepithelium. There are several risk factors for bladder cancer (remember Pee SAC: P = phenacetin, S = smoking, A = aniline dyes, C = cyclophosphamide), but the most common is smoking. Bladder cancer can be evaluated with cystoscopy; tumor staging dictates the treatment of choice, which may include surgery, intravesical chemotherapy, or systemic therapy.

Diagnosis and Key Features of Renal Masses and Urinary Tract Cancers

Key Features	Diagnoses
Hematuria, palpable mass, flank pain, fever, weight loss Cells with clear cytoplasm and arranged in nests with intervening blood vessels: "clear cell carcinoma" subtype is most common Gene deletion on chromosome 3 (the deletion can be sporadic or inherited as in von Hippel-Lindau syndrome)	Renal cell carcinoma (RCC)

(continued)

Diagnosis and Key Features of Renal Masses and Urinary Tract Cancers (*continued*)

Key Features	Diagnoses
Benign epithelial cell tumors arising from the collecting ducts that present with hematuria, palpable mass, and flank pain	Oncocytomas
Child with a large, palpable, unilateral flank mass, and hematuria Loss of function mutation in tumor suppressor genes *WT1* or *WT2* on chromosome 11	Wilms's tumor
Arises from chronic irritation and inflammation of the urinary tract leading to squamous metaplasia, followed by dysplasia, then carcinoma Risk factors include: *Schistosoma haematobium* infection (Middle East), chronic cystitis, smoking, aniline dyes, cyclophosphamide exposure, and chronic nephrolithiasis	Bladder cancer

CASE 16 | Bladder Cancer

A 72-year-old man with a 50-pack/year history of smoking and hypertension presents for evaluation of intermittent blood in his urine for the last year. He has a history of chronic urinary tract infections but denies dysuria or fevers. Hematuria is painless, but he has frequent urges to urinate. He denies incontinence, malaise, vaginal bleeding, or spotting. He has no significant family history. On exam, he has no costovertebral angle tenderness or abdominal tenderness.

Evaluation/Tests	Urinalysis is positive for 3+ blood and several leukocytes. No bacteria are noted, and leukocyte esterase and nitrites are negative. Cystoscopy reveals a 3-cm irregular mass protruding from the bladder with urothelial cells showing a nested pattern of invasion.
Treatment	Depending on tumor staging, treatment may include intravesical chemotherapy, tumor resection, cystectomy, and systemic therapy.
Discussion	Bladder cancer is the fifth most common malignancy in the United States and the most common genitourinary malignancy in men and women, with the most common subtype being urothelial (transitional cell) carcinoma. Squamous cell carcinoma of the bladder is less common overall but more common in unindustrialized countries with exposure to the parasitic trematode *Schistosoma haematobium* endemic in the Middle East and East Africa. Most cases of urothelial carcinoma are attributable to smoking. Other risk factors include occupational exposure to aromatic amines (e.g., aniline dyes), aromatic hydrocarbons (e.g., coal tar), formaldehyde, or medications such as phenacetin and cyclophosphamide. Patients with noninvasive bladder cancer should undergo continued surveillance with regular cystoscopy, resection as needed, and intravesical chemotherapy. Invasive bladder cancer is treated with neoadjuvant chemotherapy and cystectomy. Painless hematuria always warrants workup for bladder cancer with cystoscopy. History of **chronic urinary tract infections** may increase the likelihood of a recurrent UTI, but the urinalysis is negative. **Renal stone** or **renal cancer** may have symptoms other than hematuria, such as pain, fever, and recurrent urinary tract infections.

CASE 17 | Renal Cell Carcinoma (RCC)

Vignette	A 60-year-old man presents with 3 weeks of left flank pain and recent onset of hematuria. He denies dysuria but has noticed some sweats and has lost 20 pounds over the last month. He also notes feeling more fatigued than usual. On exam, he is febrile, and there is fullness in his left flank.
Evaluation/Tests	CBC reveals a hemoglobin of 17 g/dL. Ultrasound demonstrates a complex left renal mass suspicious for RCC.
Treatment	Nephrectomy.
Discussion	The triad of flank pain, hematuria, and palpable mass is a classic presentation for renal cell carcinoma, although all three rarely occur together. Elevated hemoglobin is likely resulting from a paraneoplastic syndrome due to excess EPO production often found in RCC. Biopsy will reveal polygonal cells with clear cytoplasm arranged in nests with intervening blood vessels (A). On gross exam, the high lipid content of the tumor may give it a golden-yellow appearance (B). CT imaging of the abdomen and pelvis (C) or MRI should be done for better visualization. Treatment includes either partial or complete nephrectomy. Renal cell carcinoma may extend locally into the renal vein or inferior vena cava and may present with varicocele due to increased venous pressure within the pampiniform plexus. The acute development of a varicocele that does not reduce with lying down may prompt an evaluation for a large retroperitoneal mass, especially if unilateral and right-sided. Uniquely, RCC is one of the few carcinomas that tends to favor hematogenous metastases. A patient who presents with metastatic disease should receive systemic therapy.

CASE 17 | Renal Cell Carcinoma (RCC) *(continued)*

Discussion	
	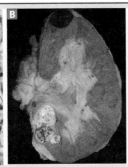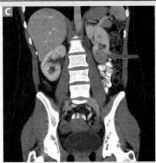

Part A used with permission from Dr. Yale Rosen/Flickr. Part B reproduced with permission from Reisner H. Pathology: A Modern Case Study, 2nd ed. New York, NY: McGraw Hill; 2020. Part C reproduced with permission from Behnes CL, Schlegel C, Shoukier M, et al: Hereditary papillary renal cell carcinoma primarily diagnosed in a cervical lymph node: a case report of a 30-year-old woman with multiple metastases, BMC Urol 2013 Jan 15;13:3.

RCC can cause fevers, so it can be difficult to distinguish from **pyelonephritis**. However, pyelonephritis would not present with a flank mass or polycythemia.

Simple **renal cysts** are benign growths in the kidney requiring no treatment; radiologic findings help clarify the diagnosis.

Bladder cancer also presents with hematuria, but it is classically painless. Bladder cancer also tends to arise in patients with exposure risk factors such as smoking or cyclophosphamide.

CONGENITAL URINARY TRACT ANOMALIES

Urinary tract anomalies are relatively common and represent approximately 1/3 of all congenital anomalies. While not inherently morbid, anomalies of the kidney and collecting system instead create an increased risk for disease and account for almost 50% of end-stage renal disease in children.

Renal	Collecting System	Bladder and Urethra
Renal agenesis Horseshoe kidney Ectopic kidney	Duplex kidney Nonobstructive mega-ureter Vesicoureteral reflux Ureteropelvic junction outlet obstruction Ectopic ureter	Posterior urethral valves (males only) Hypospadias Epispadias

In considering structural disease of the urinary tract, it is easiest to visualize a simple plumbing network with potential points for obstruction or leaking backflow valves. These faults lead to renal injury through either increased collecting system pressure (acute or chronic obstruction, reflux) or through recurrent pyelonephritis with renal scarring. These mechanisms are reinforcing in that urinary stasis increases the risk for recurrent infections.

Prenatal ultrasound screening may identify many patients with potential anomalies, while other patients will present with acute illness derived from their aberrant anatomy. Some patients may only be diagnosed incidentally as older children or adults. Nonetheless, imaging is the crux of diagnosing a GU anomaly.

The critical question in the setting of a renal anomaly is its potential implication for renal injury over time. The likelihood for intervention is often proportional to the severity of disease. For example, while 30% of pediatric UTI cases demonstrate vesicoureteral reflux (VUR), 80% of low-grade VUR cases will resolve spontaneously compared to 12% of high-grade cases.

Congenital Urinary Tract Anomalies and Imaging

Findings	Diagnosis
Ultrasound of kidney and bladder	
Hydronephrosis	Ureteral obstruction Vesicoureteral reflux Bladder outlet obstruction GI tract obstruction Posterior urethral valves (male infants)

(continued)

Congenital Urinary Tract Anomalies and Imaging (*continued*)

Findings	Diagnosis
Few to numerous large renal cysts, "bunch of grapes"	Autosomal dominant polycystic kidney disease (ADPKD) Multicystic dysplastic kidney disease
Numerous small renal cysts or diffuse echogenicity within kidney	Autosomal recessive polycystic kidney disease (ARPKD)
Hydroureter	Vesicoureteral reflux Bladder outlet obstruction (bilateral hydroureter) Megaureter (obstructive or primary)
CT abdominal/pelvis	
"Claw sign"	Wilms' tumor
Intratumor calcifications	Neuroblastoma

PEDIATRIC ABDOMINAL MASS

The presentation of an abdominal mass in a pediatric patient is highly variable. Patients may present in any clinical setting, the abdominal mass may be a primary symptom or an incidental finding, and its onset may be acute or insidious. Patient age is crucial as differing etiologies often present in an age-dependent manner. Abdominal masses in newborns are of urinary tract origin in approximately 2/3 of cases, with hydronephrosis or multicystic dysplastic kidney disease being the most common etiologies. Antenatal screening history is valuable as prenatal ultrasound may reveal genitourinary abnormalities. Symptom chronicity and associated symptoms also help to narrow the differential. An abdominal tumor may be insidious with slow growth and only noted incidentally, or it may present with acute bowel obstruction due to extrinsic compression on adjacent structures. Similarly, acute infection may reveal a chronic condition such as hydronephrosis due to outlet obstruction.

Critical exam components include mass location, mobility, tenderness, and evaluation of other intra-abdominal organs (the liver, spleen, and descending colon to assess stool burden). It is important to distinguish an abdominal mass from abdominal distension that may reflect a GI-related etiology (e.g., volvulus). Imaging is the crux of the evaluation for an abdominal mass. Ultrasound is used to avoid undue ionizing radiation exposure within the pediatric population. Neonate pathology is often evident on prenatal ultrasound, leading to early evaluation in the newborn period. Large bladders and hydronephrosis associated with oligohydramnios in a male patient suggest posterior urethral valves causing bladder outlet obstruction. Posterior urethral valves are an embryologic abnormality of male urethral development and not seen in females. CT or MRI is necessary for characterization and staging as well as for evaluation for resectable disease. With renal masses, attention must be paid to the contralateral side and possible syndromic disease. Biopsy of renal masses is generally discouraged in order to avoid tumor seeding or spillage.

Key Features: Wilms' Tumor vs. Neuroblastoma

	Wilms' Tumor	Neuroblastoma
Presentation	Asymptomatic, abdominal fullness or palpable mass	Irritable child, may note pain in extremities
Signs	WAGR syndrome (Wilms's tumor in 30%, Aniridia, Genitourinary abnormalities, mental Retardation (intellectual disability)) Aniridia Hemihypertrophy Macroglossia	Raccoon eyes Blue/purple rash like marks or nodules on the skin "blueberry muffin spots" Tender limbs
Abdominal exam	Displacing mass Does not cross midline	Fixed mass May cross midline
Imaging	Rarely calcified "Claw sign"—normal parenchyma wrapping around mass as it grows out from the kidney Well circumscribed May invade renal vein/IVC	Commonly calcified Poor margins Encases but does not invade vessels
Origin	Renal	Extrarenal (adrenal gland or paravertebral sympathetic ganglia)

CASE 18 | Wilms' Tumor (Nephroblastoma)

A 3-year-old boy is brought to clinic for evaluation of right abdominal swelling. He does not complain of any discomfort. His medical history is significant for surgical correction of an undescended right testicle when he was a year old. Vital signs and eye exam are normal. Abdominal exam is notable for a distinct large mass in his right flank and right upper abdomen that does not cross the midline and is nontender to palpation.

Evaluation/Tests	Ultrasound shows an abdominal mass originating from the right kidney. Abdominal/pelvic CT reveals preserved renal parenchyma wrapping around the mass as it grows out from the kidney ("claw sign").
Treatment	Radical nephrectomy with adjuvant chemotherapy.
Discussion	The patient's symptom of painless, flank mass is most concerning for a renal mass, and in children of this age, Wilms' tumor (nephroblastoma) is the most common solid renal malignancy of early childhood (ages 2–4). It is typically sporadic but can be congenital in 10% of cases. Loss of function of Wilms' tumor suppressor genes *WT1* or *WT2* on chromosome 11 can result in Wilms' tumor. Wilms' tumor is also a part of several syndromes, including WAGR syndrome (Wilms' tumor, Aniridia, Genitourinary abnormalities, mental Retardation/intellectual disability) due to a mutation in *WT1*; Denys-Drash syndrome (Wilms' tumor, diffuse mesangial sclerosis with early-onset nephrotic syndrome, gonadal dysgenesis), also caused by a mutation in *WT1*; and Beckwith-Wiedemann syndrome (Wilms' tumor, multiple growth abnormalities such as macroglossia, organomegaly, or hemihyperplasia). Patients may also present with hematuria, hypertension, cryptorchidism, or acquired von Willebrand disease. Compared to a Wilms' tumor, which may be displaced, **neuroblastoma** is fixed and unable to be displaced. Neuroblastoma would present with lesions in multiple organs, may cross the midline, and has a predilection for the adrenal glands.

RENAL CYSTIC DISEASE

Renal cysts arise primarily from the renal tubule epithelium. They can occur due to genetic or nongenetic processes and can be simple or complex. Simple cysts are very common, are typically asymptomatic, and filled with renal ultrafiltrate (anechoid on ultrasound imaging). Complex cysts have solid components on imaging and should be followed or removed due to risk of carcinoma. The most common ones are simple cysts. There is also polycystic kidney disease (PKD), which can be autosomal dominant (ADPKD), autosomal recessive (ARPKD) or acquired (due to age or chronic kidney disease). Their prevalence increases with age. Some unusual causes of renal cysts are von Hippel-Lindau (VHL) disease and tuberous sclerosis.

Renal Cyst Differential Diagnosis

Congenital	Acquired
Autosomal dominant polycystic kidney disease (ADPKD) Autosomal recessive polycystic kidney disease (ARPKD) VHL Tuberous sclerosis	Age-related CKD-induced

CASE 19 | Autosomal Dominant Polycystic Kidney Disease (ADPKD)

A 45-year-old man presents to the doctor's office with right-sided flank pain for 2 weeks. He has noticed blood-tinged urine twice in the past week. He has not seen a doctor in many years. Ten years ago, he was diagnosed with hypertension and started on amlodipine 10 mg daily, which he has been taking regularly. In the past 2 years, he has presented to urgent care multiple times for symptomatic UTIs. His family history is notable for ESRD in his father and a brother who died of a ruptured brain aneurysm at age 39. On exam, he is afebrile, his blood pressure is 142/100 mmHg, pulse is 98/min, and abdominal exam is notable for enlarged and palpable kidneys and bilateral flank tenderness.

Evaluation/Tests	Labs are notable for Cr of 1.8 mg/dL (10 years ago, it was 0.9 mg/dL). Urinalysis is remarkable for 150 RBC, 5 WBC, and 30+ protein. CT abdomen and pelvis shows bilateral enlarged kidneys with renal parenchyma mostly replaced by cysts. A 5-mm right ureteral stone and 3 liver cysts are noted as well.
Treatment	Treatment is supportive. Patients with ADPKD are encouraged to increase fluid intake (up to 3 L per day) and follow a low-sodium diet. ACE inhibitors and ARBs can be used to manage HTN or proteinuria if it develops. Recently, ADH antagonists like tolvaptan have been demonstrated to delay cyst growth and slow progression of kidney disease. Dialysis and renal transplantation are offered once ESRD ensues.

CASE 19 | Autosomal Dominant Polycystic Kidney Disease (ADPKD) *(continued)*

Discussion	Polycystic kidney disease (PKD) is an inherited disorder characterized by enlarging renal cysts leading to progressive kidney enlargement, renal insufficiency and various extrarenal manifestations. The disease can be inherited in an autosomal dominant or recessive form. ADPKD is most often due to a mutation in *PKD1* on chromosome 16 but can also be caused by a mutation in *PKD2* on chromosome 4. Renal failure typically occurs in 50–60 years of age. It is associated with liver cysts and intracranial berry aneurysms (which may lead to subarachnoid hemorrhage), mitral valve prolapse, and diverticulosis. Other manifestations of ADPKD include nephrolithiasis and urinary tract infections. ARPKD is most commonly caused by a mutation in *PKHD1* on chromosome 6, and it involves cystic dilation of collecting ducts, typically presenting in infancy. It is associated with other congenital abnormalities including hepatic fibrosis and Potter sequence.

URINARY INCONTINENCE

Incontinence results from derangements to the micturition cycle that impair the ability of the bladder to sufficiently empty or hold urine. An intact micturition cycle consists of (1) a filling phase wherein the bladder is relaxed while the sphincter is contracted, leading to low-pressure bladder filling, and (2) an emptying phase wherein the bladder contracts while the sphincter relaxes, resulting in sufficient emptying of the bladder. The average adult bladder capacity is 500 mL, and normal voiding frequency is every 3 to 4 hours during wakeful hours. Waking overnight once to void is also considered normal.

Urinary Incontinence types

Diagnosis	Etiology
Stress incontinence	Urinary sphincter weakness due to intrinsic weakness, denervation, or injury (e.g., following prostatectomy or vaginal delivery)
Urgency incontinence	Dysfunctional urinary storage due to detrusor muscle hyperactivity (e.g., bladder spasm, neurogenic bladder in multiple sclerosis)
Mixed incontinence	Shared stress and urge components, usually with a predominant symptom profile of one or the other
Overflow incontinence	Incomplete emptying due to bladder outlet obstruction (e.g., BPH, vaginal prolapse, constipation) or urine leaking from a distended, hypoactive bladder (e.g., neurogenic bladder due to peripheral nerve or spinal cord injury).
Nocturnal enuresis	Urinary incontinence while asleep; may be due to bladder spasm, overflow, or significant evening fluid intake

An effective differential diagnosis is possible based largely on patient history and a simple diagnostic evaluation. Patient symptoms may reveal specific failure points within the micturition cycle that lead to incontinence. Patient history is also critical and may point to simple or complex etiology (e.g., postoperative sphincter injury vs. diabetic neuropathy). A voiding diary is valuable as it provides insight to patient drinking and voiding behavior. Diagnostic studies are generally limited. Urinalysis and urine culture are helpful to assess for urinary tract infection or hematuria. A postvoid ultrasound of the bladder is critical to assess for significant volume of residual urine that indicates an inability to voluntarily empty the bladder. Interventional diagnostic studies include cystoscopy to evaluate for physical causes of bladder irritation (e.g., tumor) or urethral obstruction (e.g., stricture). Urodynamic studies provide a functional assessment of the bladder and sphincter during the micturition cycle. Complicated incontinence cases, notably those with mixed components or involving neurogenic etiology, merit urodynamic evaluation in order to better delineate pathophysiology prior to intervention.

Key Associated History Findings and Incontinence Differential Diagnosis

Incontinence with Key Associated History Findings	Diagnoses
Chronic constipation	Overflow incontinence due to neurogenic dysfunction or outlet obstruction
Incontinence with increased abdominal pressure (e.g., laugh, cough, sneeze)	Stress urinary incontinence, overflow incontinence
Urinary frequency and/or urgency	Overactive bladder, urgency incontinence, overflow incontinence
Small volume voids and/or weak urinary stream	Possible overflow incontinence due to outlet obstruction
History of prostatectomy or endoscopic urethral procedure	Stress incontinence due to sphincteric injury with insufficiency
History of diabetes or spinal cord injury or other neuropathy	Stress, urge, or mixed incontinence due to neurogenic bladder

Key Associated Exam Findings and Incontinence Differential Diagnosis

Incontinence with Key Associated Exam Findings	Diagnosis
Palpable bladder, abdominal fullness (constipation)	Overflow incontinence due to neurogenic dysfunction or outlet obstruction
Bladder or vaginal prolapse, urethral stenosis, hypertonic pelvic floor muscle tone	Overflow incontinence due to outlet obstruction
Hypotonic pelvic floor muscle tone	Possible stress incontinence or overflow incontinence due to neurogenic bladder

CASE 20 | Overactive Bladder

A 29-year-old woman presents with irritative voiding symptoms. She describes feeling an urge to urinate every 30–60 minutes, and she urinates 15 times per day. She denies dysuria, cloudy urine, or incontinence with cough. She wakes up 3 times per night to urinate. She drinks coffee throughout the day and has no history of frequent urinary tract infections or tobacco use. Physical exam is normal without evidence of generalized weakness or spinal deformity. Her external genital exam and pelvic floor tone on bimanual exam are normal.

Evaluation/Tests	Clinical diagnosis. Postvoid bladder ultrasound shows no retention. A voiding diary demonstrates significant daily fluid intake, urinary frequency, and urgency. Urodynamic studies may be performed for complex cases after medication therapy has failed or where diagnosis is in doubt.
Treatment	Treatment relies first on mitigating contributing behaviors and practicing proper bladder hygiene, such as cutting down on caffeinated products, regular scheduled voiding, etc. Pharmacotherapy may be initiated if behavioral modification fails. Anticholinergics are first-line medications.
Discussion	Overactive bladder (OAB) reflects a complex of lower urinary tract symptoms, primarily involving urinary urgency, with or without associated urge incontinence. Diagnosis is largely clinical with physical examination, and laboratory evaluation can rule out other morbid causes of these symptoms such as prolapse, infection, bladder stones, or bladder cancer. Urinalysis and culture are usually negative. Urodynamic studies may demonstrate detrusor instability. There are multiple conditions with a similar symptom profile, including bladder irritation from consumed irritants (e.g., caffeine), from infection, or from mechanical irritation (e.g., bladder stones, bladder cancer), or neurogenic bladder, polydipsia, or bladder outlet obstruction. If patients are not able to tolerate the anticholinergic side effects such as dry mouth, dry eye, or constipation, consider the use of beta-3 agonists (e.g., mirabegron). Procedural intervention with neuromodulation or intravesical botulinum toxin injection are reserved for cases refractory to medication. **Neurogenic bladder** is a dysfunction of the urinary bladder due to disease or injury of the central nervous system or peripheral nerves involved in the control of urination. Postvoid residual volumes will be elevated indicating urinary retention. Conditions associated with neurogenic bladder include spinal cord injury, multiple sclerosis, or stroke. The lesion location is associated with patient symptoms. For example, suprasacral lesions (e.g., demyelinating lesions in MS) may lead to bladder spasticity and urgency symptoms similar to OAB, while peripheral lesions lead to bladder atonia, urinary retention, and elevated postvoid bladder volumes.

ELECTROLYTE DISTURBANCES

Electrolytes regulate important physiological functions. Thus electrolyte imbalances can cause significant physiological disturbances and symptoms. Acute low levels are usually caused by loss of body fluids through prolonged vomiting, diarrhea, sweating, or high fever.

Differential Diagnosis for Electrolyte Disturbances

Hypophosphatemia: Renal wasting (e.g. Fanconi's) Severe malnourishment Alcoholism Chronic diarrhea Primary hyperparathyroidism Fibroblast growth factor 23 (FGF-23) excess **Hyperphosphatemia:** Vitamin D deficiency Renal failure Secondary hyperparathyroidism Tumor lysis syndrome Vitamin D intoxication Phosphate enemas Metabolic or respiratory acidosis Rhabdomyolysis	**Hypocalcemia:** Hypoparathyroidism Parathyroidectomy/hungry bone syndrome Renal wasting Vitamin D deficiency/rickets Hypomagnesemia **Hypercalcemia:** Primary or tertiary hypoparathyroidism Sarcoidosis Hypervitaminosis D Malignancy (breast, lung, bone, myeloma, metastatic disease) Tuberculosis Thiazide diuretics Paget's disease	**Hypokalemia:** Vomiting, diarrhea Diuretics Mineralocorticoid access Hyperaldosteronism Renal tubular acidosis Hypomagnesemia Low dietary intake, malabsorption Metabolic alkalosis Insulin Beta-2 adrenergic agonists Dialysis Liddle, Gitelman, or Bartter syndromes **Hyperkalemia:** Renal failure ACEI/ARB NSAIDS Cyclosporine, tacrolimus Metabolic and respiratory acidosis Hypoaldosteronism Burns/trauma Hemolysis Rhabdomyolysis Tumor lysis syndrome Hyperglycemia/DKA	**Hypomagnesemia:** Diuretics PPI Cisplatin Cyclosporine Malnourishment Alcoholism Chronic diarrhea Laxative use Gitelman or Bartter syndrome Pancreatitis **Hypermagnesemia:** Renal failure Magnesium containing laxatives/antacids Lithium toxicity Iatrogenic (treatment of preeclampsia) Aminoglycosides Amphotericin B

Electrolyte Abnormalities and Key Features

Key Feature(s) or Associated Symptom(s)	Electrolyte Abnormality
Volume depletion or overload Confusion, seizures, lethargy	Hyponatremia
Hyperglycemia, polyuria Diuretic medications Ileus, bladder dysfunction, hypoventilation ECG: prolonged PR, depressed ST, U wave	Hypokalemia
Metabolic acidosis ECG: peaked T waves, QRS widening, sine wave	Hyperkalemia
Moans, stones, groans, abdominal pain, constipation, decreased appetite, nausea, vomiting, peptic ulcer disease	Hypercalcemia
Conjunctival icterus, skin pruritus/eruptions	Hyperphosphatemia
Paralysis, weakness, paresthesia	Hyper- and hypokalemia, hypophosphatemia
Rhabdomyolysis, muscle pain	Hyperkalemia, hyperphosphatemia (hypophosphatemia can trigger rhabdomyolysis)
Tetany	Hypocalcemia, hypomagnesemia
ECG: torsade de pointes	Hypocalcemia, hypomagnesemia, hypokalemia

Disorders of Sodium Balance

When approaching patients with disorders of sodium balance, it is important to recognize that the serum sodium level is not a measure of total body sodium but rather of the relationship of water to sodium in the body. A patient with hypernatremia (Na > 145 mEq/L) has too little water in relation to sodium or is dehydrated. Conversely, a patient with hyponatremia (Na < 135 mEq/L) has too much water in relation to sodium.

Whether the kidneys are conserving or excreting water depends on the presence or absence of antidiuretic hormone (ADH). As its name implies, ADH causes the kidneys to conserve water (i.e., not diurese) by increasing the number of aquaporin-2 channels in the collecting tubule. Therefore, look for concentrated urine in order to determine if ADH is present. You can do so by comparing the urine osmolality to that of serum. If the urine osmolality is greater than the serum osmolality, it means the urine has been concentrated (water has been removed from it), which indicates that ADH is present. In the setting of hypernatremia, ADH should be present because the kidneys should be actively conserving water to correct the hypernatremia. In patients with hypernatremia and low urine osmolality, suspect diabetes insipidus (DI) that is either central (due to inability to excrete ADH) or nephrogenic (due to inability of the kidneys to respond to ADH). DI is characterized by polyuria, polydipsia, and nocturia. Indeed, polyuria and nocturia are usually the presenting complaints in DI. Hypernatremia develops if the patient with DI has limited access to fluids.

You can apply a similar rationale to the workup of hyponatremia. Under normal conditions, ADH is released from the posterior pituitary when osmoreceptors in the hypothalamus sense an increase in effective plasma osmolality. Therefore, ADH should not be released in the setting of hyponatremia and low serum osmolality. In other words, the kidney should be excreting water to correct the hyponatremia, and the urine osmolality should be lower than serum osmolality. If ADH is elevated in the presence of hyponatremia and low sodium osmolality, this finding may be pathologic, as in the case of the syndrome of inappropriate ADH (SIADH) or may be due to the presence of nonosmotic stimuli of ADH such as pain or nausea.

One important nonosmotic stimulus of ADH is hypoperfusion. When baroreceptors sense hypoperfusion, they activate the renin angiotensin aldosterone system (RAAS). When the hypoperfusion persists despite the activation of RAAS, ADH is secreted as a "backup" mechanism. Because the body sacrifices osmolality for the sake of perfusion, patients with hypoperfusion develop hyponatremia. Hypoperfusion may be caused by loss of volume (hypovolemia) due to diarrhea, vomiting, or bleeding. These patients have hypovolemic hyponatremia. The treatment of hypovolemic hyponatremia is volume resuscitation.

Hypoperfusion may also be a result of decreased effective circulating volume as in CHF, cirrhosis, or nephrotic syndrome. In these cases, the patient is volume overloaded as evidenced by edema, pulmonary congestion, and ascites; however, their intravascular volume is low. In the case of CHF, intravascular volume is low due to decreased ejection fraction. In cirrhosis, it is low due to splanchnic vasodilation and hypoalbuminemia. These patients develop hypervolemic hyponatremia. The treatment of hypervolemic hyponatremia is fluid restriction, diuretics, and sodium restriction. The latter may seem counterintuitive, but it is important to remember that in these cases of hypervolemic hyponatremia, the patient's low effective circulating volume leads to activation of the RAAS system. Therefore, these patients are retaining sodium, leading to worse edema, pulmonary congestion, and ascites. Note that hypervolemic hyponatremia can also be seen in advanced CKD when the kidneys have decreased capacity to dilute urine. When patients with advanced CKD drink an excess of fluids, they develop hyponatremia due to their impaired ability to dilute urine. In these cases, ADH is appropriately suppressed, and the urine osmolality will be low.

The differential diagnosis for euvolemic hyponatremia includes: hypothyroidism, adrenal insufficiency, nonosmotic stimuli of ADH (e.g., pain), SIADH, psychogenic polydipsia, "tea toast diet" or "beer potomania." SIADH is due to excessive, inappropriate release of ADH. There are many causes of SIADH including malignancy (particularly small cell carcinoma of the lung), CNS pathology (e.g., stroke), and lung pathology (e.g., pneumonia). Several medications are associated with inappropriate ADH release, including cyclophosphamide and SSRIs. Therefore, a careful medication history is important when assessing patients with hyponatremia. SIADH is a diagnosis of exclusion. Hypothyroidism and adrenal insufficiency need to be ruled out before establishing a diagnosis of SIADH. The treatment of SIADH includes free water restriction, diuretics, and salt tablets. In primary or psychogenic polydipsia, hyponatremia develops due to an intake of water that surpasses the dilutional capacity of normal kidneys. This disorder is mainly treated with water restriction. "Tea and toast diet" and "beer potomania" refer to a diet high in fluids and low in solutes (i.e., electrolytes). The kidneys depend on solutes to excrete free water. Therefore, diets low in solutes impair the kidneys' ability to excrete free water and lead to hyponatremia. This type of hyponatremia is treated by increasing solute intake.

Differential Diagnosis of Hypotonic Hyponatremia based on Volume Status

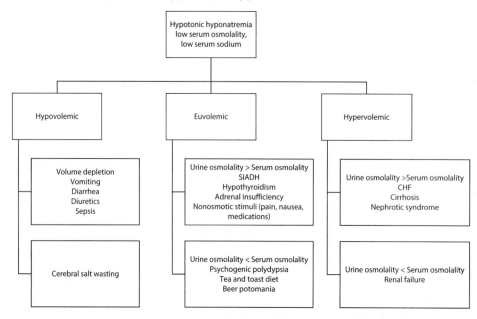

CASE 21	Nephrogenic Diabetes Insipidus

A 48-year-old woman with a history of bipolar disorder, who has been stable on lithium for 15 years, is admitted for emergent surgery after a biking accident. She is made NPO (nothing by mouth) for an orthopedic procedure the following morning; however, it gets postponed one more day, during which time she remains NPO. She reports increased thirst and ongoing polyuria. On exam, she is afebrile, has dry mucous membranes, pulse 105/min, and blood pressure 95/52 mmHg. On the day of her surgery, her urine output in a 24-hour period is 3 L and her serum sodium is 159 mEq/L.

Evaluation/Tests	Her labs are sodium 159 mEq/L, serum osmolality 325 mOsm/kg, urine osmolality 120 mOsm/kg, and urine specific gravity 1.005. Serum glucose is normal.
Treatment	During her hospitalization, her urine output should be matched with hypotonic IV fluids while NPO. After surgery, she should be allowed to drink ad libitum. If possible, lithium should be discontinued. Consider amiloride.
Discussion	Polyuria occurring despite fluid restriction should raise suspicion for **diabetes insipidus (DI)**, which can be central or nephrogenic. Lithium is one of the leading causes of **nephrogenic diabetes insipidus**. Lithium enters the distal tubule through the epithelial sodium (ENaC) channel and prevents ADH from inserting aquaporin channels on the luminal side of the cell, resulting in an aquaresis (excretion of water without electrolytes). Amiloride, a thiazide diuretic, blocks the ENaC channel and prevents lithium from entering the cell, allowing for water to be taken up by the collecting duct. Nephrogenic DI from chronic lithium use can be irreversible. The longer the patient has been on lithium, the less likely it is that her or his concentrating abilities will improve. This patient was on chronic lithium and likely had underlying nephrogenic DI. In diabetes insipidus, one would see a normal serum sodium level (in a person allowed to drink ad libitum) or hypernatremia (in a person undergoing fluid restriction, like our patient). With hypernatremia, the urine specific gravity should be high because the kidneys should be preserving water. In diabetes insipidus, specific gravity is low (<1.010) because of the kidneys' inability to concentrate urine. With hypernatremia, urine osmolality should normally be high. In diabetes insipidus, urine osmolality will be less than plasma osmolality but usually will be >100 mOsm/kg; urine osmolarity of <100 mOsm/kg is generally due to psychogenic polydipsia or "tea and toast" diet. **Central diabetes insipidus** is either idiopathic or occurs as a result of a head trauma, neurosurgery, or a brain tumor. Patients with **psychogenic polydipsia** (sometimes called primary polydipsia) are characterized by excessive water intake; this usually results in polyuria and low-normal serum sodium levels rather than high-normal sodium levels. A water deprivation test can be used to distinguish between **psychogenic polydipsia** and **diabetes insipidus**. In cases of psychogenic polydipsia, the urine osmolality will become concentrated, and serum sodium will normalize if water is withheld because these individuals have normal urine concentrating abilities in the kidneys. Administration of desmopressin (synthetic analog of ADH) can be used to distinguish between central and nephrogenic diabetes insipidus. A person with central diabetes insipidus will experience a rise in urine concentration (urine osmolality) if desmopressin is administered. A person with nephrogenic diabetes insipidus will continue to have dilute urine despite administration of desmopressin.

CASE 22 | Hypovolemic Hyponatremia

A 30-year-old woman with no past medical history presents to the emergency department with 5 days of nausea, vomiting, and diarrhea. She has been unable to keep anything down. Physical exam is notable for a woman who appears uncomfortable and in mild distress. Her orthostatic vitals are as follows: supine BP is 106/72 mmHg and pulse is 108/min; standing blood pressure is 83/60 mmHg, and pulse is 120/min.

Evaluation/Tests	Her labs are notable for serum Na: 128 mEq/L, FeNa < 1%, urine sodium: <10 mEq/L.
Treatment	Volume resuscitate with IV isotonic fluids such as normal saline or lactated ringer.
Discussion	This otherwise healthy patient with severe gastrointestinal distress and hyponatremia on labs is consistent with hypovolemic hyponatremia presentation. In cases of hyponatremia, it is important to evaluate volume status. Orthostatic vitals are helpful to assess for intravascular volume depletion. A basic metabolic panel can confirm low serum sodium, and urine electrolytes should show a low urine sodium <20, and F_eNa should be <1% in hypovolemic hyponatremia. This patient exhibits orthostatic hypotension, which is signified by a ≥20-mmHg drop in systolic blood pressure when standing or a drop in diastolic blood pressure by ≥10 mmHg when standing. Her urine sodium is appropriately low. This occurs because her intravascular volume depletion stimulates both RAAS activation and ADH. Increased aldosterone expression induces sodium retention by the kidney, hence decreasing urine sodium levels. Treatment involves resuscitation with IV normal saline (provides salt and water). For moderate to severe chronic hyponatremia (>48 hours or unknown duration), frequent monitoring of serum sodium is indicated to avoid correcting the serum sodium too quickly. Rapid correction of hyponatremia can lead to central pontine myelinolysis. **Salt-wasting nephropathy** leads to an erroneous excretion of sodium into the urine during a volume depleted state, which is usually a result of chemotherapeutic agents or head trauma. Thus urine sodium would be high. Her history and urine studies do not suggest **surreptitious diuretic abuse**; urine sodium would be elevated if loop diuretics had recently been ingested. In this case, diarrhea is leading to both sodium and water loss. However, the patient has become hyponatremic because more sodium is being lost *relative to* water.
Additional Considerations	**Hypervolemic hyponatremia** may be seen in patients with decompensated heart failure. Despite their hypervolemic state, they are often intravascularly depleted, which leads to RAAS activation and ADH stimulation. The elevated aldosterone levels lead to sodium reabsorption in the distal convoluted tubule and a low urine sodium, whereas increased ADH leads to excess water retention. Hypervolemic hyponatremia is generally due to cardiac, hepatic, or renal dysfunction. A good physical exam (to confirm hypervolemia) and urine sodium levels will help distinguish the etiology of hyponatremia. Aggressive diuresis typically improves this type of hyponatremia.

CASE 23 | Hyperkalemia

A 54-year-old man with hypertension, diabetes mellitus, and CKD presents for a follow-up blood pressure check after his lisinopril was increased from 10 mg to 20 mg daily. He has no complaints. His other medications include metoprolol XL 25 mg and insulin. On exam, his blood pressure is 121/78 mmHg, pulse is 64/min, and the rest of the exam is remarkable only for 1+ pedal edema.

Evaluation/Tests	Labs notable for K: 6.5 mEq/L (previously 4.8 mEq/L); eGFR: 35 mL/min/1.73 m2(at baseline level); bicarbonate: 24 mEq/L; and glucose: 130 mg/dL. ECG with peaked T waves.
Treatment	Given the peaked T waves on his ECG, calcium gluconate should be administered to stabilize his cardiac membranes to prevent arrhythmias. Additionally, administration of insulin, glucose, and albuterol is helpful in rapidly correcting his high potassium levels. These treatments are temporary as they simply help to shift potassium intracellularly. To truly decrease total body potassium, use a non-K-sparing diuretic such as a loop diuretic, potassium binders such as kayexalate or patiromer, or dialysis if kidney function is significantly decreased. Long term, this patient's ACE inhibitor should be decreased or discontinued. Addition of a diuretic and decreased dietary potassium intake is needed.
Discussion	This patient has marked hyperkalemia noted on labs along with ECG changes most likely due to his ACE inhibitor dose increase. The RAAS inhibition caused by lisinopril is most likely causing his hyperkalemia. Angiotensin-converting enzyme (ACE) inhibitors prevent the conversion of angiotensin I to angiotensin II, which is required for aldosterone production. Aldosterone stimulates potassium secretion by the principal cells in the distal collecting duct. Therefore, it is important to reduce the dose or stop the lisinopril. ARBs can also cause hyperkalemia. Hyperkalemia can present with muscle weakness and cardiac manifestations such as peaked T waves and lengthening of the PR interval and QRS duration. In severe cases, the P wave can disappear and the QRS can widen into a sine wave pattern. Severe hyperkalemia is life-threatening and should be considered a medical emergency.

CASE 23 | Hyperkalemia *(continued)*

Discussion	There are multiple other causes of hyperkalemia. **DKA** can cause hyperkalemia due to movement of intracellular potassium to the extracellular space, but it is unlikely given that this patient does not have severely elevated glucose levels and has a normal serum osmolarity. Beta-2 adrenergic activity drives potassium into cells and lowers serum potassium (hence albuterol can help). Use of **beta blockers** can counter this action. This is unlikely to be the cause of our patient's hyperkalemia because he had been using this medication prior to this recent lab finding, and the increased lisinopril dose is more likely to be the culprit. Lastly, given that his **decreased GFR** and CKD are at his baseline, this is unlikely to cause his current hyperkalemia.
Additional Considerations	Patients with **hypokalemia** can present with muscle weakness, respiratory failure, cardiac arrhythmias and ECG abnormalities such as flattening of the T wave, ST segment depression, presence of U waves, and prolonged QT interval. Potassium wasting diuretics can cause hypokalemia. Hypokalemia can be proarrhythmogenic, so potassium should be replaced quickly intravenously if there is severe potassium deficiency <3 mEq/dL. Causes of **hypophosphatemia** include medications (diuretics, insulin, phosphate binding antacids, theophylline, bisphosphonates, etc.), alcoholism, severe burns, chronic diarrhea, DKA, hyperparathyroidism, Fanconi syndrome, and hereditary hypophosphatemic rickets with hypercalciuria and X-linked familial hypophosphatemia. Severe complications of hypophosphatemia include arrhythmias, respiratory depression, rhabdomyolysis, hemolytic anemia, and death.

ACID–BASE DISORDERS

Acid–base disorders involve an abnormal number of hydrogen ions (H^+) circulating within the blood and are measured by arterial pH. The approach to the patient with an acid–base disturbance is as follows:

1. First, **determine the primary disorder** by examining the arterial blood gases (ABG) and comparing the bicarbonate (HCO_3^-) to the pH.

    The normal range of arterial pH should be 7.35–7.45.

    The Henderson-Hasselbalch equation can be summarized as: $pH \sim \dfrac{HCO_3^-}{pCO_2}$

    Therefore, blood pH is proportional to HCO_3^- (bicarbonate) and inversely proportional to pCO_2.

    If HCO_3^- decreases (<20 mEq/L), then the pH should lower. Therefore, if a change in HCO_3^- is driving the change in pH, the patient has a primary metabolic acidosis.

    If HCO_3^- increases (>28 mEq/L), then the pH should also increase and may reflect primary metabolic alkalosis.

    If the direction of change in HCO_3^- is not consistent with the direction of change in the pH, look at the pCO_2 because it is likely that your primary acid–base disturbance is respiratory in nature. Elevated pCO_2 (>44 mmHg) will lower pH, and this would be considered a primary respiratory acidosis. Conversely, decreased pCO_2 (<36 mmHg) will raise pH, and this would be considered a primary respiratory alkalosis.

    > Low pH due to low HCO_3^- → primary metabolic acidosis.
    > High pH due to high HCO_3^- → primary metabolic alkalosis.
    > Low pH due to high pCO_2 → primary respiratory acidosis.
    > High pH due to low pCO_2 → primary respiratory alkalosis.

2. Second, **determine whether there is a compensatory response** to the primary acid–base disturbance.

    Whenever there is a primary acid–base disturbance, the body's natural physiological response is to compensate either through altering reabsorption vs. excretion of HCO_3^- (renal compensation) or through hyperventilation vs. hypoventilation to adjust pCO_2 levels (respiratory compensation). For example, in metabolic acidosis, when the bicarbonate drops, the body compensates by decreasing the pCO_2 through hyperventilation in attempts to "blow off" excess acid and normalize arterial pH. Note that the primary disorder and compensation move in the same direction (i.e., if the primary disturbance involves a drop in HCO_3^-, the compensatory response will involve a drop in pCO_2).

3. Third (and most significant in the differential diagnosis of patients with metabolic acidosis), **calculate the anion gap** by using the formula:

$$\text{Anion gap} = Na^+ - (Cl^- + HCO_3^-)$$

The normal range of the anion gap is 8–12 mEq/L, and it is based on the difference between major cations (i.e., Na^+) and anions (i.e., Cl^- and HCO_3^-). The small, normal anion gap is due to the presence of unmeasured anions found normally in plasma, including citrate, phosphate, and negatively charged proteins. However, in cases of an increased anion gap, there are additional anions within the plasma such as lactate, formic acid, salicylates, oxalic acids, and ketoacids. Acutely, HCO_3^- drops as it has to buffer the extra acid, thus resulting in a drop in available HCO_3^-. Since these other acids are not included in the formula, the drop in HCO_3^- will result in a larger difference between measured cations and anions, causing an increased anion gap. If an anion gap is identified, a helpful mnemonic is "MUDPILES" to form a differential diagnosis:

M	Methanol (formic acid)
U	Uremia (uric acid)
D	Diabetic or alcoholic ketoacidosis (ketoacids)
P	Propylene glycol or paraldehydes
I	Iron, isoniazid, or isopropyl alcohol
L	Lactic acidosis (lactate)
E	Ethylene glycol (metabolized to glycolic acid and oxalic acid)
S	Salicylates (aspirin)

Metabolic acidosis can be divided into anion gap metabolic acidosis (AGMA) or nonanion or normal anion gap metabolic acidosis (NAGMA). In NAGMA, the loss of HCO_3^- is compensated for by an increase in Cl^- ions (hyperchloremic acidosis), so the anion gap remains normal. For consideration of the differential diagnosis for NAGMA, the mnemonic "HARDASS" is helpful:

H	Hyperalimentation
A	Addison disease
R	Renal tubular acidosis (kidney disease)
D	Diarrhea
A	Acetazolamide
S	Spironolactone
S	Saline infusion

4. **In the setting of NAGMA, calculation of the urinary anion gap (UAG)** may help distinguish between renal and GI losses by providing an estimate of urinary acid excretion in the form of ammonium (NH_4^+). The UAG is calculated as:

$$\text{UAG} = (\text{Urine } Na^+ + \text{Urine } K^+) - \text{Urine } Cl^-$$

Normally, the levels of Na^+ and K^+ in the urine, exceed that of Cl^-, resulting in a positive UAG in healthy patients. In the setting of metabolic acidosis, the kidneys generate NH_4^+ to excrete acid from the body; however, urine NH_4^+ is difficult to measure directly. Cl^- is the major anion excreted with NH_4^+ in urine, and urinary Cl^- can be used as an indirect measure of urinary NH_4^+ excretion. In metabolic acidosis, the urine should have high NH_4^+ and Cl^- levels because the kidneys should be excreting acid. Looking at the formula for UAG, you will see that, in the presence of metabolic acidosis, if the kidneys are responding correctly, the UAG should become negative (e.g., diarrhea (non-renal HCO_3^- loss)). In contrast, if the kidneys are not handling acid appropriately, as in the case of renal tubular acidosis (RTA), the UAG will remain positive. Since the two major causes of NAGMA are GI losses or RTA, a simple way to remember how to interpret the UAG is "neGUTive" with GI or non-renal bicarbonate losses.

CASE 24 | Nonanion Gap Metabolic Acidosis (NAGMA)

A 65-year-old man with a history of hypertension and CKD is noted to have a low bicarbonate during a routine clinical visit. His only medications include amlodipine. On physical examination, he is afebrile, blood pressure is 146/84 mmHg, pulse is 76/min, and respirations are 12/min. BMI is 28, and he has 1+ lower extremity edema.

Evaluation/Tests	Labs: Na^+ 136 mEq/L, K^+ 5.2 mEq/L, Cl^- 108 mEq/L, bicarbonate 17 mEq/L, creatinine 1.7 mg/dL, and glucose 98 mg/dL. Urinalysis specific gravity 1.018, pH 5.5, 30 protein, 0 RBC, and 0 WBC.
Treatment	Treatment is oral sodium bicarbonate.
Discussion	This patient has a nonanion gap metabolic acidosis (NAGMA) of renal etiology, in this case CKD. His calculated anion gap of 11 mEq/L is normal. The two main causes of NAGMA are renal or gastrointestinal losses of bicarbonate. Clues to GI losses would be history of diarrhea or laxative abuse. Another way to differentiate between these conditions is to calculate a urine anion gap using the following equation: $$\text{Urinary anion gap} = (U_{Na} + U_K) - U_{Cl}$$ A positive urine anion gap suggests a renal cause, and a negative urine anion gap is consistent with gastrointestinal bicarbonate loss.
Additional Considerations	Diabetic ketoacidosis (DKA) and lactic acidosis cause an **anion gap metabolic acidosis** (see Endocrinology Chapter). In DKA, ketone bodies are produced due to insulin deficiency and are responsible for the anion gap acidosis. Other causes of anion gap metabolic acidosis include uremia, salicylates, isoniazid, iron supplements, or ingestion of ethanol, ethylene glycol (antifreeze), methanol, or propylene glycol (see Pharmacology Chapter).

CASE 25 | Proximal Renal Tubular Acidosis (Type 2) (Fanconi Syndrome)

A 36-year-old man with a history of seizures presents for routine follow-up. His seizures have been well controlled with valproic acid for the past 10 years. He has no other complaints. On physical examination, he is afebrile, blood pressure 124/65 mmHg, pulse 78/min, and respirations 12/min. BMI is 23, and the rest of his examination is normal.

Evaluation/Tests	Labs include sodium 135 mEq/L, chloride 106 mEq/L, bicarbonate 20 mEq/L, potassium of 2.8 mEq/L, creatinine 1.1 mg/dL, glucose 96 mg/dL, and phosphate 1.9 mg/dL. Urinalysis demonstrates urine pH: 5.1, +1 protein, +2 glucose, no RBCs/WBCs, and no casts.
Treatment	Discontinue medications, which can cause Fanconi syndrome.
Discussion	This patient has type 2 (proximal) renal tubular acidosis (Fanconi syndrome) from long-term valproic acid use for seizure control. The combination of a nonanion gap metabolic acidosis (calculated anion gap of 9 mEq/L), hypokalemia, hypophosphatemia, low urine pH (<5.5), and glucosuria with normal serum glucose are consistent with proximal tubule dysfunction. Valproic acid is known to cause renal tubulointerstitial disease characterized by proximal tubular damage. Other common causes of proximal RTA include carbonic anhydrase inhibitors, tenofovir, aminoglycosides, multiple myeloma, and heavy metals. The defect in the proximal convoluted tubule impairs reabsorption of bicarbonate, leading to excess excretion in urine and a metabolic acidosis.
Additional Considerations	**Type 1 (distal) RTA** occurs due to a defect in urine acidification most commonly caused by decreased activity of the proton pump in the alpha intercalated cells in the collecting duct, which prevents secretion of H^+ in urine. Patients present with a nonanion gap metabolic acidosis and urinary pH > 5.5. Patients with type I RTA often present with hypokalemia and hypercalciuria. The latter can lead to nephrolithiasis. Type 1 RTA may be caused by autoimmune disorders like Sjögren's syndrome or SLE and medications such as amphotericin B. Treatment includes oral sodium bicarbonate and treating the underlying disorder(s).
	Type 4 (hyperkalemic) RTA is caused by renin deficiency and/or decreased aldosterone production (hypoaldosteronism or aldosterone resistance). This deficiency occurs most commonly in patients with advanced kidney disease due to tubulointerstitial damage such as in diabetes, systemic lupus erythematosus, obstruction, chronic NSAID use, or sickle cell disease. Drugs that impair renin or aldosterone production include NSAIDs, calcineurin inhibitors, and ACE inhibitors. Patients who have type IV RTA typically present with hyperkalemia, a normal anion gap metabolic acidosis, and impaired urine acidification. However, they still have the ability to maintain the urine pH to <5.5. Treatment of type IV RTA includes a low potassium diet, and diuresis to increase potassium excretion in urine. Other treatments include correction of the underlying cause and discontinuation of offending medications.

15

Reproductive and Urology

Catherine Wheatley, MD
Samuel Ohlander, MD
Nuzhath Hussain, MD
Nimmi Rajagopal, MD

OBSTETRICS AND GYNECOLOGY

An important dichotomy exists in the care of the patients that can become pregnant, both in the unique pathology attributable to the female reproductive system and to the temporary physiology that occurs during pregnancy. This section will briefly describe normal female reproductive physiology; however, the main focus will be on the recognition, management, and treatment of abnormal labor, obstetric emergencies, and gynecologic abnormalities.

NORMAL FEMALE REPRODUCTIVE PHYSIOLOGY

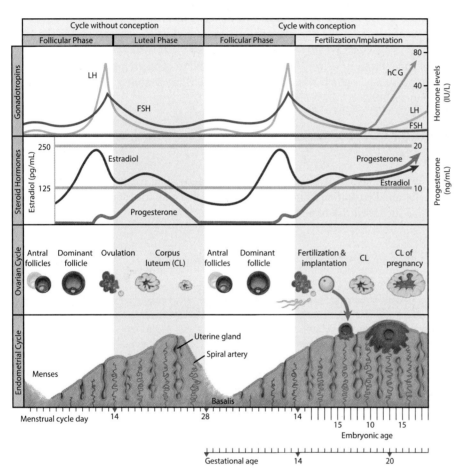

Gonadotropin control of the ovarian and endometrial cycles. The ovarian-endometrial cycle has been structured as a 28-day cycle. The follicular phase (days 1 to 14) is characterized by rising estrogen levels, endometrial thickening, and selection of the dominant "ovulatory" follicle. During the luteal phase (days 14 to 21), the corpus luteum (CL) produces estrogen and progesterone, which prepare the endometrium for implantation. If implantation occurs, the developing blastocyst begins to produce human chorionic gonadotropin (hCG) and rescues the corpus luteum, thus maintaining progesterone production. FSH = follicle-stimulating hormone; LH = luteinizing hormone.
Reproduced with permission from Cunningham G, Leveno KJ, Bloom SL, et al: Williams Obstetrics, 25th ed. New York, NY: McGraw Hill; 2018.

Normal Menstrual Cycle

Follicular Phase (Days 1–13)	Ovulation (Day 14)	Luteal Phase (Days 15–28)
Starts with menses	Release of mature ovum	Without luteinizing hormone (LH) or human chorionic gonadotropin (hCG) stimulation (as seen in pregnancy), the corpus luteum lasts from days 15 to 28, and then involutes.
Ends with ovulation/LH surge	Development of the corpus luteum	Corpus luteum produces progesterone and some estradiol.
Increase gonadotropin-releasing hormone (GnRH), follicle stimulating hormone (FSH), estrogen	Increase LH	Progesterone > estrogen
Proliferative phase of uterine lining		Secretory phase of uterine lining
Dominant follicle increases in size		If no fertilization or implantation, sloughing of endometrial lining

NORMAL PREGNANCY AND LABOR

The terms "gravida" and "para" are often used to describe people who are currently or have been pregnant. Gravida describes the number of times a patient has ever been pregnant, including a current pregnancy. This includes pregnancies that resulted in term deliveries, preterm deliveries, previable deliveries, miscarriages, induced abortions, molar and ectopic pregnancies. Para consists of four different categories and refers to the outcomes of each pregnancy. The four numbers are term pregnancies (37+ weeks gestational age), preterm pregnancies (20–36 + 6 weeks gestational age), early pregnancy losses (prior to 20 weeks gestational age), and living children (of any age). For example, a patient who has been pregnant five times, with two term deliveries, one preterm delivery, a first trimester miscarriage, an induced abortion at 15 weeks, and three living children would be a G5P2123.

Physical exam maneuvers typically performed to confirm or monitor pregnancy include measurement of the fundal height (generally not until after 20 weeks), assessment of fetal heart tones (typically heard starting at 10–12 weeks), and movement of the fetus (often starts around 18 weeks). After 24 weeks, the fundal height in centimeters will be approximately the same as the number of weeks of pregnancy.

Important tests to confirm pregnancy include serum or urine β-hCG and ultrasound to confirm intrauterine pregnancy and to rule out ectopic pregnancy and other pathology. In high-risk patients, chorionic villus sampling (CVS) or amniocenteses may be done to detect fetal genetic abnormalities.

NORMAL INFANT/CHILD MILESTONES

Newborn: The APGAR Score

APGAR scores are the "vital signs" of the newborn after delivery and higher scores indicate a better outcome. Points are given for Appearance, Pulse, Grimace, Activity, and Respiration 1 and 5 minutes after delivery. If the score is <7 at 5 minutes, further evaluation is needed as there can be an increased risk of neurologic damage.

Infant/Child Milestones

Developmental delay may be suggested if milestones are not met.

Age	Motor	Social	Verbal/Cognitive
Infant (0–12 mos.)	Primitive reflexes disappear Posture stronger Picks objects up Points to objects	Smile Stranger anxiety Separation anxiety	Orients Object permanence Oratory
Toddler (12–36 mos.)	Cruises Climbs Cube stacking Cutlery use Kicks ball	Recreation Rapprochement Realization	Words
Pre-school (3–5 years)	Drive 3 wheels Drawing Dexterity	Freedom Friends	Language Legends

Sexual Development

Genitalia, pubic hair, and breast development are assigned Tanner stages.

	Stage 1 (prepubertal)	Stage 2 (~8–11.5 yrs.)	Stage 3 (~11.5–13 yrs.)	Stage 4 (~13–15 yrs.)	Stage 5 (usually >15 years)
Both	No pubic hair	Pubic hair appearance (pubarche)	Pubic hair coarsens.	Pubic hair increases but spares thighs	Pubic hair crosses over to thigh
Female (menarche: 10–16 years)	Flat chest, raised nipple	Breast buds (thelarche)	Breast enlargement	Raised areola, increased breast enlargement	Adult breast contours, areola flattens
Male		Testicular enlargement	Penis size/length increases	Penis width/glans increase	Penis/testes adult size

CASE 1 | Pregnancy (Amenorrhea)

A 31-year-old G0 presents with missed menses for 2 months. She has been having vaginal intercourse with a male partner and she denies use of condoms or any other form of contraception. She has associated nausea, fatigue, and breast tenderness. Exam is unremarkable.

Evaluation/Tests	Pregnancy test is positive.
Treatment	Begin prenatal vitamins and discuss pregnancy options (prenatal care with OB/midwife/family medicine or abortion care services based on patient desires).
Discussion	Amenorrhea is a common presenting sign for pregnancy. When a patient presents with amenorrhea, a pregnancy test should be ordered if the patient is of reproductive age. Pregnancy tests rely on the detection of the beta subunit of human chorionic gonadotropin (β-hCG) in the urine; it appears in the urine relatively early in pregnancy. β-hCG helps maintain the corpus luteum (and progesterone levels) for the first 8–10 weeks of pregnancy. After 8–10 weeks, the placenta is able to synthesize estriol and progesterone on its own, and the corpus luteum degenerates. Increased progesterone throughout pregnancy prevents shedding of the endometrium of the uterus, so pregnant patients do not get menses. Several other physiologic adaptations occur in pregnancy, including increased glomerular filtration rate (GFR), increased cardiac output, physiologic mild anemia, hypercoagulability, hyperventilation, and increased fat utilization. Amenorrhea in nonpregnant patients can be due to many other conditions such as ovulatory or thyroid dysfunction.
Additional Considerations	**Normal labor** is characterized by repetitive uterine contractions that have sufficient frequency, intensity, and duration to cause progressive cervical dilation and effacement. Cervical effacement is the process of thinning of the cervix as it stretches in preparation for vaginal birth. The uterine contractions are coordinated, regular, and increase in frequency over the stages of labor. The fetus also has risk for potential complications of labor and delivery, including shoulder dystocia, nerve injuries, and hypoxic ischemic encephalopathy. Maternal complications can include postpartum hemorrhage, placental abruption, venous thromboembolism, etc. **Braxton-Hicks contractions** occur in the mid- to late third trimester, and they are self-limited. They involve uterine contractions without cervical thinning or effacement. **Multifetal gestations** should always be confirmed by ultrasound in order to determine the chorionicity, amnionicity, and number of fetuses as this will affect the management and delivery plan for the pregnancy. **Dichorionic twins** have different placentae (which may or may not be fused), whereas monochorionic twins share a placenta. This is noteworthy because **monochorionic twins** have the potential to develop twin-twin transfusion syndrome, in which blood flow is preferentially shunted toward one twin over another via arteriovenous anastomoses in the placenta. Amnionicity refers to the number of amniotic sacs that surround the pregnancy. Diamniotic twins have two separate amniotic sacs, while monoamniotic twins share an amniotic sac. Monoamniotic twins are quite rare (2% of all twin pregnancies), and they are at risk of cord entanglement in utero. Dichorionic-diamniotic twins are formed from either ovulation of two ova, cleavage of a single ovum before fertilization, or immediate cleavage of the blastomere. Monochorionic-diamniotic twins are formed from cleavage of the zygote (blastocyst stage) on days 4–8. Monochorionic-monoamniotic twins are formed from cleavage of the zygote on days 9–12.

ABNORMALITIES IN PREGNANCY

Abnormalities Specific to Pregnancy

Symptom or Sign	Differential Diagnosis
Abdominal pain	Preterm labor, labor, ectopic pregnancy, miscarriage (missed, incomplete, spontaneous), threatened miscarriage, placental abruption, uterine rupture, preeclampsia, eclampsia, acute fatty liver of pregnancy
Depressed mood	Postpartum blues, postpartum depression
Hypertension	Gestational hypertension, molar pregnancy, preeclampsia, eclampsia, HELLP syndrome
Nausea and/or vomiting	Normal pregnancy, hyperemesis gravidarum

(continued)

Abnormalities Specific to Pregnancy (*continued*)

Symptom or Sign	Differential Diagnosis
Postpartum hemorrhage	Endometritis, uterine atony, uterine rupture or trauma, retained placenta, morbidly adherent placenta, DIC
Uterine size less than dates	Incorrect dating, oligohydramnios, intrauterine growth retardation
Uterine size greater than dates	Incorrect dating, polyhydramnios, fetal macrosomia, molar pregnancy, multiple fetal gestation
Vaginal bleeding	Preterm labor, labor, implantation bleeding, ectopic pregnancy, molar pregnancy, miscarriage (missed, incomplete, spontaneous), threatened miscarriage, premature rupture of membranes, placental abruption, placenta previa, vasa previa

Abdominal Pain in Pregnancy

An important aspect of evaluation of any clinical symptom in a pregnant patient is to consider both obstetric and nonobstetric etiologies.

Diagnoses commonly found in pregnant people of nonobstetric origin include:

Abdominal Quadrant	Differential Diagnosis
Right upper quadrant	Cholelithiasis, cholecystitis, choledocholithiasis, acute fatty liver, lung infection, fibroid degeneration, bowel obstruction
Right lower quadrant	Appendicitis, nephrolithiasis, cystitis, ovarian cyst rupture/torsion, fibroid degeneration, bowel obstruction
Left upper quadrant/epigastric	Gastritis, GERD, pancreatitis, myocardial infarction, pericarditis, pneumonia/other lung infection, fibroid degeneration, bowel obstruction
Left lower quadrant	Nephrolithiasis, constipation, ovarian cyst rupture/torsion, fibroid degeneration, bowel obstruction

If the pain is obstetric in origin, one can further create a differential diagnosis based on trimester of presentation.

First Trimester (0–13 + 6 weeks)	Second Trimester (14–27 + 6 weeks)	Third Trimester (28 weeks and beyond)
Ectopic pregnancy	Miscarriage	Preterm labor or labor
Miscarriage	Preterm labor	Intra-amniotic infection
	Placental abruption	Placental abruption
	Uterine rupture	Uterine rupture
	Preeclampsia/eclampsia	Preeclampsia/eclampsia
	Acute fatty liver of pregnancy	Acute fatty liver of pregnancy

CASE 2 | Ectopic Pregnancy

A 38-year-old woman with a history of pelvic inflammatory disease (PID) and tobacco use presents with right lower quadrant pain, nausea, and vomiting. She reports that the pain started the night prior as a dull pain and has acutely worsened. She has a history of irregular menses, and her last menses was 8–10 weeks ago. She denies any vaginal discharge or bleeding. Her PID was treated 2 years ago. On exam, she has right lower quadrant tenderness with rebound and guarding. The pelvic exam is notable for dark red blood in the vagina and tenderness in the right adnexa.

Evaluation/Tests	Serum quantitative β-hCG test is positive. On transvaginal ultrasound, no intrauterine pregnancy is seen. A large mass is noted in the right adnexa, and significant free fluid is seen in the abdomen.

CASE 2 | Ectopic Pregnancy *(continued)*

Treatment	Surgery.
Discussion	Ectopic pregnancy is the leading cause of maternal death in the first trimester. Most ectopic pregnancies are implanted in the ampulla of the fallopian tube, but implantation can also occur in the abdomen, cervix, prior Cesarean scar, or any other location outside the uterus. Classic presentation is a history of amenorrhea followed by vaginal bleeding and abdominal/pelvic/adnexal pain. It can be clinically mistaken for appendicitis, so patients of reproductive age with symptoms and signs resembling appendicitis should also be evaluated for ectopic pregnancy. Risk factors include previous ectopic pregnancy, PID, tobacco use, infertility, advanced maternal age, ruptured appendix, and prior tubal surgery. Ectopic pregnancy can be a surgical emergency; therefore, prompt diagnosis is necessary. If the patient is stable, medical (methotrexate) or surgical therapies can be explored. **Spontaneous miscarriage/abortion** (loss of products of conception (POC)) typically occurs before 20 weeks due to various causes that can be attributed to fetal (anatomic or genetic malformations) or maternal factors (trauma, exposure to toxins/infections, antiphospholipid antibodies, diabetes). • *Complete* is characterized by POC expulsion, cessation of bleeding, closed cervical os, and ultrasound without any retained products. • *Threatened* is characterized by no POC expulsion, uterine bleeding with or without pain, cervical os closed, intact membranes, and viable embryo/fetus. Management involves pelvic rest and close monitoring. • *Incomplete* is characterized by partial POC loss, bleeding, mild cramping, cervical os open, and retained products. • *Missed* is characterized by embryonic or fetal demise without symptoms such as bleeding and cramping. Diagnosis is confirmed by ultrasound that shows an embryo or fetus without fetal cardiac activity. Management of an incomplete or missed miscarriage involves passage of tissue either by dilation and curettage, medical therapy like misoprostol, or expectant management.

Vaginal Bleeding in Pregnancy

Bleeding in pregnancy can have several etiologies, both obstetric and nonobstetric. The first step in evaluating a pregnant patient with bleeding is to assess vital signs and to hemodynamically stabilize the maternal patient. Once stabilized, determine gestational age for the pregnancy as etiologies of bleeding may differ based on trimester.

Obstetric Causes of Vaginal Bleeding

First Trimester	Second Trimester	Third Trimester	Postpartum
Ectopic pregnancy	Miscarriage (<20 weeks)	Preterm labor	Tone (uterine atony)
Threatened miscarriage	Preterm labor (>20 weeks)	Placental abruption	Trauma (lacerations, uterine rupture)
Incomplete miscarriage	Placental abruption	Premature rupture of membranes	Tissue (retained placenta)
Complete miscarriage	Premature rupture of membranes	Placenta previa	Thrombin (disseminated intravascular coagulopathy)
Molar pregnancy	Placenta previa	Vasa previa	Endometritis
Implantation bleeding	Vasa previa		Morbidly adherent placenta

CASE 3 | Hydatidiform Mole (Complete Mole)

A 30-year-old woman presents with vaginal bleeding, abdominal cramps, and pelvic pressure and pain. She also reports extreme nausea and vomiting. Her last menstrual period was 9 weeks ago. On exam, her blood pressure is 150/88 mmHg, pulse is 110/min, and her uterus is larger than expected for her last menstrual period (LMP).

Evaluation/Tests	Imaging and pelvic ultrasound show uterine cysts ("honeycombed" or "snowstorm" or "cluster of grapes") and no fetal parts. Quantitative β-hCG is very elevated. TSH is low, free T4 is high. No fetal heart tones detected.

CASE 3 | Hydatidiform Mole (Complete Mole) *(continued)*

Evaluation/Tests	Transverse sonographic view of a uterus with a complete hydatidiform mole. The classic "snowstorm" appearance is created by the multiple placental vesicles. The mole completely fills this uterine cavity, and calipers are placed on the outer uterine borders. Reproduced with permission from Hoffman BL, Schorge JO, Bradshaw KD, et al: Williams Gynecology, 3rd ed. New York, NY: McGraw Hill; 2016.
Treatment	Dilation and curettage. Serial monitoring of β-hCG to confirm resolution of the mole.
Discussion	This is the classic presentation of a hydatidiform molar pregnancy, which is caused by the abnormal proliferation of trophoblastic epithelium with the absence of a viable fetus. The patient typically presents with hypertension (before 20 weeks gestation), vaginal spotting or bleeding, and absent fetal heart tones. Hydatidiform moles can be divided into complete or partial moles. Complete molar pregnancies typically have an enlarged uterine size, and they are accompanied by elevated β-hCG levels. Sometimes, highly elevated β-hCG levels will manifest with symptoms of early preeclampsia, hyperemesis gravidarum, hyperthyroidism, and theca-lutein cysts. Ultrasound establishes the diagnosis. Treatment involves evacuation of the trophoblastic tissue and trending β-hCG levels to ensure resolution and to monitor small risk of progression to gestational trophoblastic neoplasia (including choriocarcinoma). At the genetic level, a complete mole is usually caused from a single sperm and an enucleated egg. The paternal DNA from the sperm is subsequently duplicated, so the karyotype of a complete mole is 46,XX or 46,XY. In contrast, a **partial mole** typically forms from two sperm and a nucleated egg, giving rise to a characteristic triploid karyotype of 69,XXX, 69,XXY, or 69,XYY. Partial moles will have elevated β-hCG, and they often show presence of fetal parts on imaging. It is important to distinguish a molar pregnancy from a normal intrauterine pregnancy or missed miscarriage. A **missed miscarriage** is a pregnancy loss that has not yet passed through the cervix. It can be managed expectantly, with medication, or with surgery.

CASE 4 | Placental Abruption

A 26-year-old G4P3003 at 39 weeks gestational age presents with abrupt vaginal bleeding accompanied with abdominal pain. She reports that the pain started about 1 hour ago and that she is not feeling her baby move regularly. The patient has a history of cocaine use disorder. On exam, the patient is irritable and diaphoretic with dilated pupils and elevated blood pressure. The patient's fundus is firm and tender. The cervix appears dilated to 2 cm, and brisk bleeding is noted.

Evaluation/Tests	Urine toxicology screen is positive for cocaine. Ultrasound reveals a 2-cm fluid collection at the inferior edge of the junction between the placenta and the uterine wall. Placenta is visualized posteriorly without evidence of previa. Fetal movements decreased.
Treatment	Emergent delivery.
Discussion	Approximately 1/3 of all antepartum bleeding is due to placental abruption. Placental abruption is the premature separation of a normally implanted placenta from the uterine wall due to maternal/uterine bleeding into the decidua basalis. Abruption may be complete or partial; bleeding may be concealed or apparent. Blood in the basalis layer can stimulate forceful uterine contractions, leading to ischemic abdominal pain. Risk factors include hypertension, advanced maternal age, multiparity, cocaine use, tobacco use, chorioamnionitis, and trauma. Complications include hemorrhagic shock, DIC, uterine atony, fetal hypoxia, and maternal and fetal death. Evaluation includes obtaining a toxicology screen, CBC, coagulation factors, fibrinogen level, and electronic fetal monitoring. If the patient is full-term and hemodynamically stable with a normal fetal heart rate, vaginal delivery is appropriate. A patient who is full-term and hemodynamically unstable should be resuscitated with fluids, packed red blood cells, fresh frozen plasma, and platelets if needed. Once the maternal patient is stable, they should undergo an emergent cesarean section. In **placenta previa**, the placenta attaches to the lower uterine segment over or <2 cm from the internal cervical os, causing painless bleeding in the third trimester.

CASE 5	Placenta Previa

A 30-year-old woman at 34 weeks gestation presents with bright red vaginal bleeding. She denies any abdominal pain, loss of fluid, trauma, or recent intercourse. Her past medical history is significant for two prior cesarean sections. On exam, her vital signs are stable, and there is no abdominal tenderness. Speculum exam shows a closed cervix with a small amount of bright red blood at the external os. A digital vaginal exam is deferred.

Evaluation/Tests	Ultrasound shows an anterior placenta that partially covers the internal cervical os. CBC shows an Hgb of 11.2 mg/dL, which is stable from a previous CBC.
Treatment	Pelvic rest. Cesarean delivery at 36–37 weeks gestation or sooner if patient hemodynamically unstable.
Discussion	Placenta previa is the implantation of the placenta over the internal os of the cervix. Bleeding from a placenta previa may occur after 20 weeks gestation, and it is characterized by painless bleeding typically caused by tearing of the placental attachments at or near the cervical os. Risk factors for placenta previa include previous uterine surgery like cesarean section, multiparity, and advanced maternal age. Patients suspected of having a placenta previa should have a vaginal ultrasound to determine position of the placenta. Digital examination of the cervix should be avoided until the diagnosis is excluded. Treatment of a bleeding placenta previa depends on maternal hemodynamic stability, gestational age, and fetal condition. Expectant management may be reasonable if the maternal patient is hemodynamically stable, bleeding has resolved, and the pregnancy is preterm. Delivery will always be by cesarean section due to the placental obstruction of the cervix. Placenta accreta, or abnormal invasion of the placenta into the myometrium due to the absence of the decidua basalis, should be considered in the presence of placenta previa. With a **morbidly adherent placenta**, patients present with postpartum bleeding (predisposing to Sheehan's syndrome). The placenta is abnormally attached, and it does not separate after delivery. **Placenta accreta** is the most common type of morbidly adherent placenta. This stands in contrast to a retained placenta or retained products of conception, in which only a focal area of the placenta remains attached. **Vasa previa** is a rare condition in which the fetal umbilical vessels run over, or in close proximity to, the cervical os. Vessel rupture may result in fetal exsanguination and death. Presentation is often painless vaginal bleeding, fetal bradycardia, and membrane rupture. It is associated with velamentous umbilical cord insertion. Management of a bleeding vasa previa includes prompt delivery by emergency cesarean section.

Hypertension in Pregnancy

Hypertensive disease in pregnancy spans a spectrum of severities and symptoms. The diagnosis can be determined by the timing of onset of elevated blood pressures (>140/90) and other associated symptoms. Symptoms or signs consistent with end organ damage include headache, right upper quadrant pain, vision changes, renal failure, abnormal liver enzymes, hemolysis, DIC, and proteinuria. **Chronic hypertension** is elevated blood pressure before 20 weeks gestation or persistent 12 weeks after delivery.

    Gestational hypertension is elevated blood pressure after 20 weeks gestation in a patient with previously normal blood pressures, and it occurs typically in the absence of proteinuria or end-organ damage. Severe gestational hypertension implies severe range blood pressures (≥160 systolic and/or ≥110 diastolic) after 20 weeks gestation in the absence of proteinuria.

    Preeclampsia is a hypertensive disorder of pregnancy that presents after 20 weeks gestation (<20 weeks may suggest molar pregnancy), and it is usually accompanied by proteinuria (≥300 mg/dL of protein in 24 hours). It is also linked to abnormal invasion of the placental spiral arteries, causing widespread endothelial dysfunction and vasospasm.

    HELLP syndrome is a subset of preeclampsia; the patient presents with the following constellation of symptoms: **H**emolysis, **E**levated **L**iver enzymes, **L**ow **P**latelet count.

    Eclampsia is preeclampsia plus maternal seizures.

	Chronic Hypertension	Gestational Hypertension	Preeclampsia	Eclampsia	HELLP Syndrome
Systolic BP ≥140 and/or diastolic BP ≥90	Before 20 weeks gestation	After 20 weeks gestation, no previous history of HTN, no proteinuria or end-organ damage	After 20 weeks gestation and proteinuria or end organ damage	Preeclampsia and seizures	Severe preeclampsia with hemolysis, elevated liver enzymes, low platelets

(continued)

	Chronic Hypertension	Gestational Hypertension	Preeclampsia	Eclampsia	HELLP Syndrome
Risk factors			HTN, diabetes mellitus, chronic kidney disease, multifetal gestation, advanced maternal age, autoimmune disease, first pregnancy		
Complications			Placental abruption, coagulopathy, pulmonary edema, renal failure, eclampsia, uteroplacental insufficiency, or HELLP	Stroke, intracranial hemorrhage, ARDS, maternal death	Schistocytes, DIC, hepatic rupture from hepatic subcapsular hematomas
Treatment	Antihypertensives (hydralazine, methyldopa, labetalol, nifedipine)	Antihypertensives and deliver at 37–39 weeks	Antihypertensives; if severe range BPs can use IV magnesium; delivery at 37 weeks without severe features, 34 weeks (or time of diagnosis) if severe features are present	Antihypertensives, IV magnesium, immediate delivery	Immediate delivery

CASE 6 | Eclampsia

An 18-year-old G1P0 at 41 weeks gestation presents with headache and new swelling of her lower extremities. She has no known medical problems. Admission blood pressure is 160/90 mmHg. During the exam, she has a tonic-clonic seizure.

Evaluation/Tests	Urine protein is elevated.
Treatment	Magnesium sulfate, antihypertensive medications, and prompt delivery.
Discussion	Eclampsia is one of the most serious complications of preeclampsia, and it is characterized by maternal seizures. **Preeclampsia** is new hypertension after 20 weeks gestation with proteinuria and/or end-organ damage due to abnormal remodeling of the spiral arteries, causing endothelial dysfunction, vasoconstriction, and ischemia. Risk factors include DM, CKD, existing HTN, and autoimmune disorders. Complications include pulmonary edema, renal failure, coagulopathy, HELLP syndrome, uteroplacental insufficiency, and placental abruption. Eclampsia is preeclampsia plus seizures. Magnesium sulfate is the anticonvulsant of choice. Severe hypertension must also be controlled with antihypertensive medication like labetalol or hydralazine because there is a risk for CVA with high BP in preeclampsia. Delivery is the definitive treatment.
Additional Considerations	**HELLP syndrome** is on the spectrum of hypertensive disorders of pregnancy, and it is an extreme manifestation of severe preeclampsia. It is characterized by hypertension, hemolysis, elevated liver enzymes, and low platelets. The clinical presentation includes abdominal pain, headaches, vomiting, hypertension, and proteinuria. If left untreated, it can progress to DIC and subcapsular hematoma of the liver. Delivery is the only known treatment. Initial evaluation should include CBC, reticulocyte count, peripheral smear (to assess for schistocytes indicative of microangiopathic hemolytic anemia), liver function tests, PT, INR, aPTT, urine protein/creatinine ratio (to assess for proteinuria), and abdominal US. The diagnosis of HELLP syndrome requires the presence of the following: 1. Hemolysis, related to microangiopathic hemolytic anemia diagnosed by the presence of schistocytes on peripheral smear 2. Elevated Liver enzymes at least above two times the upper limit of normal 3. Low Platelet count <100,000/mm³ 4. Elevated bilirubin, usually indirect hyperbilirubinemia related to hemolysis

Abnormal Genetic Screening in Pregnancy

Genetic screening and diagnostic tests of pregnancy are offered during prenatal care to screen for aneuploidy; typically, this includes the trisomies (13, 18, 21) and sometimes monosomy X. While any patient at any age can have a pregnancy with aneuploidy, the risk increases with higher maternal age. Ultrasound is the most commonly used method of prenatal assessment, and it is valuable in the screening and diagnosis of many congenital anomalies. Five serum markers (described next) in maternal blood are typically utilized in conjunction with ultrasound to aid in screening for fetal aneuploidies, fetal abdominal wall defects, and neural tube defects. Screening can also be completed via prenatal cell-free fetal DNA, a maternal serum test that can detect the fetal fraction of DNA in the maternal circulating volume. Abnormal genetic screening tests typically prompt discussion of further diagnostic testing with chorionic villus sampling (CVS) or amniocentesis for diagnosis.

Maternal Serum Markers for Autosomal Trisomies in Pregnancy

Serum Marker	Description	Trisomy 21	Trisomy 18	Trisomy 13
First Trimester				
β-hCG	Human chorionic gonadotropin, β subunit—produced by placenta, β subunit is unique from other hormones (compared to α subunit, which is identical to that in TSH, LH, and FSH), signals to corpus luteum to produce progesterone, most sensitive method of detecting pregnancy	↑	↓	↓
PAPP-A	Pregnancy-associated plasma protein A—produced by fetus and placenta, multiple functions including limiting maternal immune system recognition of fetus, angiogenesis, and more	↓	↓	↓
Second Trimester—QUAD screen				
AFP	α-fetoprotein—produced by fetus, levels increase with gestational age, elevated in NTDs, decreased in chromosomal aneuploidies	↓	↓	Normal
β-hCG	Previously described	↑	↓	Normal
Estriol	One type of estrogen, produced by placenta, normally sees a large increase in estriol during pregnancy and is viewed as an indicator of fetal well-being	↓	↓	Normal
Inhibin A	Gonadal hormone produced by placenta, corpus luteum, and fetus; exerts negative feedback on FSH secretion from the anterior pituitary gland	↑	↓ or Normal	Normal

---

CASE 7 | Genetic Screening in Pregnancy (Trisomy 21)

A 41-year-old G1P0 at 16 weeks gestation presents for routine evaluation and anatomy ultrasound. She is not on any medications, and she denies history of tobacco, alcohol, or illicit drug use. Ultrasound shows a male sex fetus with an atrioventricular defect, bilateral renal pelvis dilation, and echogenic bowel.

Evaluation/Tests	Serum QUAD screen shows low AFP and estriol, high β-hCG and inhibin A. HbA1c and serum glucose are within normal limits.
Treatment	Offer genetic counseling, diagnostic testing, and discuss option of induced abortion. If the patient does not want to discontinue pregnancy, perform fetal ultrasound and surveillance throughout pregnancy. Plan for a prenatal neonatal consult.
Discussion	The results of this genetic screening in pregnancy suggest a diagnosis of **Down syndrome (trisomy 21)**, an autosomal trisomy involving the presence of three copies of chromosome 21. This abnormal number of chromosomes (aneuploidy) is the most common viable chromosomal disorder and the most common cause of noninherited genetic intellectual disability, most often due to maternal meiotic nondisjunction (see "Biochemistry" chapter for more information). In addition to trisomy 21, the other two potentially viable autosomal trisomies include trisomy 13 (Edwards syndrome) and 18 (Patau syndrome). Risk of aneuploidy increases with advancing maternal age. All pregnant patients should be offered first and second trimester aneuploidy screening based on their gestational age at presentation. Classically, the QUAD test is performed in the second trimester, and it is a very useful way to screen for genetic abnormalities. Patients older than 35 at delivery should be offered aneuploidy screening with cell-free

CASE 7 | Genetic Screening in Pregnancy (Trisomy 21) *(continued)*

Discussion	fetal DNA vs. diagnostic testing with chorionic villus sampling or amniocentesis. If a diagnosis of trisomy 21 is suspected or confirmed, patients should have a detailed evaluation of the fetal heart. Targeted ultrasound may show major cardiac abnormalities (e.g., tetralogy of Fallot, AV canal defects, septal defects), thickened nuchal fold, echogenic bowel, renal pelvis dilation, shortened long bones, or cardiac echogenic foci. Diagnosis can be confirmed with amniocentesis or CVS. Continued monitoring with serial US for evaluation of fetal growth should occur.
	Trisomy 18 and **13** have more severe clinical manifestations than trisomy 21, and infant survival is usually <1 year. Given no evidence of alcohol use during pregnancy, fetal alcohol syndrome is unlikely. The patient's HbA1c and serum glucose were normal, ruling out gestational diabetes.

Abnormal Fetal Findings

Abnormal fetal findings discovered in the intrapartum period are varied in presentation and origin. Genetic abnormalities, transplacental and other infections, maternal conditions and morbidities, and teratogenic exposures prior to or during pregnancy can all affect the development of the fetus. Teratogens are substances that have the potential to cause anatomic and/or physiologic abnormalities to an exposed fetus. Classically, the risk of congenital anomalies from teratogen exposure is highest during 2–8 weeks gestational age, which is the time of the most intensive fetal organogenesis. In general, the earlier the disturbance in normal embryonic and fetal development occurs, the more severe the abnormalities are. Nonetheless, exposure to medications, illicit substances, and infections can adversely affect the fetus throughout the pregnancy.

Infection (see "Microbiology" chapter)	Prescription Drug Teratogens	Maternal Conditions	Genetic Defects (see "Biochemistry" chapter)

Transplacental infections (ToRCHHeS):
  Toxoplasma gondii
  Rubella
  Cytomegalovirus (CMV)
  Human immunodeficiency virus (HIV)
  Herpes simplex virus (HSV)
  Syphilis
Other infections:
  Streptococcus agalactiae
  Escherichia coli
  Listeria monocytogenes
  Tuberculosis
  Parvovirus
  Varicella zoster virus
  Malaria
  Fungal
	ACE inhibitors
	Alkylating agents
	Aminoglycosides
	Antiepileptic drugs (valproate, carbamazepine, phenytoin, phenobarbital)
	Diethylstilbestrol (DES)
	Folate antagonists (trimethoprim, methotrexate, etc.)
	Isotretinoin
	Lithium
	Methimazole
	Tetracyclines
	Thalidomide
	Warfarin
		Lack of prenatal care
		Vitamin deficiency
		Alcohol abuse
		Cocaine use
		Tobacco use
		Diabetes
		Iodine excess/deficiency
		Methylmercury ingestion (seen with some types of seafood)
		Vitamin A excess
		X-ray radiation
			Trisomy 13 (Edward syndrome)
			Trisomy 18 (Patau syndrome)
			Trisomy 21 (Down syndrome)
			Monosomy X (Turner syndrome)

CASE 8 | Warfarin Exposure

A 39-year-old G7P4024 with a history of a mechanical heart valve, hypertension, and acne presents for evaluation after discovering her home pregnancy test was positive. She has been on depot medroxyprogesterone for contraception, but she missed her most recent dose with her last dose 4 months ago. She is on warfarin for chronic anticoagulation, lisinopril for hypertension, and tetracycline for acne. Her exam is normal.

Evaluation/Tests	Fetal US shows a live 19-week fetus with nasal and limb hypoplasia, stippled epiphyses, and microcephaly. Maternal INR is in therapeutic range.
Treatment	Stop warfarin and start low molecular weight heparin. Stop tetracycline, and switch lisinopril to a safer antihypertensive medication.

CASE 8 | Warfarin Exposure (continued)

Discussion	Warfarin presents two clinical concerns in pregnancy. First, warfarin is teratogenic, most commonly associated with bone and cartilage abnormalities. Second, it crosses the placenta, resulting in full fetal anticoagulation. Fetuses exposed to warfarin are at risk for bleeding complications both in utero and during delivery. Warfarin is teratogenic, even if not at therapeutic range dosing. When possible, pregnant patients on warfarin should be transitioned to heparin or low-molecular-weight heparins (e.g., enoxaparin) by 6 weeks gestation as these agents do not cross the placenta. This patient is also on an **ACE inhibitor** and **tetracycline** antibiotic; both are teratogenic, and therefore should be discontinued. ACE inhibitors can result in renal damage in the developing fetus, while tetracyclines can result in discolored teeth and inhibit bone growth.
Additional Considerations	**Diethylstilbestrol (DES) exposure** in utero leads to increased infertility (mostly as a result of tubal and uterine anomalies), cervicovaginal clear cell adenocarcinoma, cervical intraepithelial neoplasia, and congenital Mullerian abnormalities. Exposed patients should have increased pelvic exams and cervicovaginal cytology screening compared to their unexposed peers. Alcohol exposure in pregnancy can lead to **fetal alcohol syndrome**. There is no definitive cutoff for an acceptable amount of alcohol in pregnancy, so abstinence is recommended. Fetal alcohol syndrome occurs from likely repeated or heavy exposure to alcohol in utero, and it presents with increased risk of cognitive abnormalities, microcephaly, and characteristic facies (smooth philtrum, hypertelorism). At its worst, fetal alcohol syndrome can present with heart-lung fistulas and/or holoprosencephaly. **Aminoglycosides** can cause CN VIII toxicity to the fetus and deafness. **Lithium** is associated with the Ebstein anomaly, which is a ventricular displacement of the tricuspid valve. **Methimazole** can cause aplasia cutis congenita, or absence of skin, with first trimester exposure. For pregnant patients with hyperthyroidism, propylthiouracil is recommended in the first trimester, followed by methimazole in the second and third trimesters. **Thalidomide** is now a banned medication in the United States, in part because of its correlation with phocomelia (shortened limbs) in exposed fetuses.

CASE 9 | Maternal Pregestational Diabetes

A 29-year-old G1P0 with a history of poorly controlled diabetes type 2 presents for her initial prenatal visit. She takes metformin inconsistently. On exam, she is obese with a BMI of 45, and she has acanthosis nigricans. Her HbA1c was 11.4% 3 months ago. By her last menstrual period, she is dated at 19 weeks and therefore undergoes anatomy ultrasound, which reveals cardiac abnormalities.

Evaluation/Tests	Clinical diagnosis.
Treatment	Depending on gestation age at diagnosis, counsel on adherence to medications and switch to insulin therapy; can also discuss induced abortion when desired. Planning for possible postnatal surgical correction of cardiac defect.
Discussion	This patient is presenting with maternal diabetes. Patients with either type 1 or type 2 diabetes are at risk for significant abnormal fetal outcomes in pregnancy, particularly when they have poor glucose control at the time of conception. While poor antenatal glucose control is often associated with fetal macrosomia, patients with diabetes prior to pregnancy are also at an increased risk for fetal intrauterine growth restriction. Uncontrolled diabetes also increases the occurrence of miscarriage, polyhydramnios, the need for respiratory support of the neonate at delivery, and fetal anomalies. Fetal cardiac defects are the most common anomalies (e.g., ventricular septal defect, transposition of great vessels). However, neonates born to patients with pregestational diabetes are also at risk for cleft lip/palate, neonatal hypoglycemia, polycythemia, neural tube defects, and caudal regression syndrome (also known as sacral agenesis, which includes anal atresia to sirenomelia).

CASE 10 | Neural Tube Defects

A 35-year-old G2P0010 returns for routine prenatal care at 20 weeks with plan for anatomy ultrasound during her visit. She has a history of obesity and type 2 diabetes. She has not been taking her prenatal vitamins. She denies alcohol or substance abuse. Fetal ultrasound reveals ventriculomegaly, as well as abnormal skull shape and cerebellum.

Evaluation/Tests	Maternal serum α-fetoprotein (AFP), amniotic fluid AFP, and acetylcholinesterase are elevated. Amniocentesis for chromosomal evaluation reveals no abnormalities.

CASE 10 | Neural Tube Defects *(continued)*

Treatment	Offer pregnancy options, including induced abortion (depending on timing of diagnosis) or *in utero* fetal surgery (depending on the defect). Prepare for neonatal surgical intervention, including insertion of a ventriculoperitoneal shunt for ventriculomegaly and hydrocephalus.
Discussion	The fetus in this scenario is likely suffering from an open neural tube defect (ONTD), which is one of the most common congenital abnormalities of the central nervous system (CNS). ONTDs occur due to a failure of the complex and coordinated closure of the neural tube, which begins at just 3–4 weeks after fertilization. In the developing embryo, the notochord induces overlying ectoderm to differentiate into neuroectoderm and form the neural plate. Over time, the neural plate folds to form the neural tube along the cranial–caudal axis. The walls of the neural tube form the tissue of the central nervous system, while the hollow lumen gives rise to the ventricular system and central canal of the spinal cord. Each end of the neural tube has an open neuropore; the cranial and caudal neuropores close around the fourth week of gestation, and failure to fuse results in ONTDs. This occurs fairly early in gestation, so it is important for patients of reproductive age to have adequate prenatal care, including prenatal vitamins such as folic acid, initiated before conception and continued during pregnancy. Depending on whether the ONTD is caused by failure of fusion of the cranial or caudal neuropore, the deficits observed in the fetus or neonate will occur in the cranium or spinal column, respectively. The most benign and common form of ONTD is **spina bifida occulta**, which involves failure of the caudal neuropore to close but without herniation of neural tissue or meninges. Spina bifida occulta is often associated with a tuft of hair or skin dimple at the level of the bony defect, most often at lower vertebral levels. More severe manifestations of failure of the caudal neuropore to close include **meningocele** (herniation of meninges) and **meningomyelocele** (herniation of meninges and neural tissue). Failure of the cranial (or rostral) neuropore to close results in the severe abnormality known as **anencephaly**. A fetus with anencephaly has no forebrain and an open calvarium. While some ONTDs can be attributed to genetic syndromes, most are multifactorial, likely affected by maternal conditions such as maternal diabetes, low folic acid intake, and family history.

Uterine Size Unequal to Dates

A common problem encountered by the clinician during prenatal care is evaluating a pregnant patient whose uterine size does not correlate to the stated or known gestational age. The first step in this evaluation is to determine whether the patient's gestational age is accurate and to rule out multifetal gestation. An ultrasound evaluation (preferably in the first trimester) will help confirm the gestational age and rule out multifetal gestation. Fundal height is a screening tool utilized in prenatal care to track fetal growth in singleton pregnancies. It is typically used after 24 weeks gestation, and it involves measuring the height of the fundus from the pubic symphysis in centimeters, with the centimeter measurement corresponding roughly to the gestational age.

Uterine Size Greater Than Dates	Uterine Size Less Than Dates
Incorrect dating	Incorrect dating
Polyhydramnios	Oligohydramnios
Fetal macrosomia	Intrauterine fetal growth restriction
Multifetal gestation	
Molar pregnancy	

CASE 11 | Oligohydramnios

A 37-year-old G1P0 at 38 weeks gestation presents for routine antenatal testing for advanced maternal age. She is found on ultrasound to have lower amniotic fluid than expected. She has no obstetric complaints, and the remainder of the ultrasound is unremarkable. On exam, blood pressure is 138/86 mmHg, fundal height is 36 cm, and speculum exam is unremarkable.

Evaluation/Tests	Ultrasound evaluation reveals a low amniotic fluid index (AFI) of 3.5 cm; no evidence of rupture of membranes on exam.

CASE 11 | Oligohydramnios *(continued)*

Treatment	Hydrate patient with IV fluids, and recommend delivery if full-term.
Discussion	Oligohydramnios means low amniotic fluid. It most frequently presents in the late third trimester. Oligohydramnios can be associated with placental insufficiency or it may be due to fetal anomalies such as renal agenesis and posterior urethral valves. Longstanding severe oligohydramnios can lead to the Potter sequence, a specific fetal phenotype including clubbed feet, pulmonary hypoplasia, and compressed facial features. Oligohydramnios in the second trimester should be followed up with close anatomic ultrasound. In the late preterm period, it is sometimes successfully managed with fluid hydration of the maternal patient. At term, it is recommended to proceed with delivery. A separate cause of size unequal to dates is that the fetus itself is smaller or larger than expected. In the case of **fetal growth restriction (FGR)**, fetal weight is less than the 10th percentile for gestational age. Several etiologies of fetal growth restriction are divided into three categories: maternal, fetal, and placental. Maternal etiologies for FGR include chronic disorders that cause vascular disease: hypertension, diabetes mellitus, antiphospholipid syndrome, and substance use such as cocaine and tobacco use. Fetal etiologies include multiple gestation, teratogen exposure (valproic acid, antithrombotic drugs), infectious diseases, genetic conditions, or fetal structural issues like congenital heart disease or gastroschisis. Placental or umbilical cord issues that may lead to fetal growth restriction include placental abruption and 2-vessel umbilical cord.
Additional Considerations	**Polyhydramnios** represents too much amniotic fluid and would be indicated by an elevated AFI on ultrasound. Most cases are idiopathic; however, certain conditions such as maternal diabetes mellitus, multifetal gestations, fetal malformations (e.g., tracheoesophageal fistula, esophageal atresia, anencephaly) are also associated with polyhydramnios. Most cases are followed with routine antenatal surveillance, though severe instances may be managed with amnioreduction for symptomatic patients. At the time of labor/delivery, polyhydramnios is associated with an increased risk of malpresentation, umbilical cord prolapse, placental abruption, and uterine atony.

Postpartum Hemorrhage

Postpartum hemorrhage is the leading cause of maternal mortality worldwide. Primary postpartum hemorrhage is defined as blood loss greater than or equal to 1000 mL, or significant blood loss causing signs and symptoms of hypovolemia within 24 hours of delivery. When evaluating a patient with excessive bleeding following delivery, it is important to consider the 4 Ts: Tone (uterine atony), Trauma (maternal lacerations), Tissue (retained placenta), Thrombin (coagulation defects). Uterine atony is the most common etiology, responsible for up to 80% of all cases of postpartum hemorrhage.

CASE 12 | Uterine Atony

A 29-year-old G5P4 at 39 weeks gestation just delivered a large-for-gestational-age neonate vaginally. She had a prolonged labor, and, after the placenta was delivered, brisk vaginal bleeding with blood loss of 1000 mL occurred. Previous pregnancies were without complications. On exam, she is tachycardic, hypotensive, and the uterus is soft, enlarged, and boggy.

Evaluation/Tests	Clinical diagnosis. Immediate postpartum CBC is significant for an Hgb of 7.2 mg/dL. Coagulation factor panel is normal. Bedside ultrasound and examination of the placenta demonstrate no concern for retained placental tissue.
Treatment	Uterine massage, administer uterotonic medication such as oxytocin.
Discussion	This patient is presenting with uterine atony, the most common cause of postpartum hemorrhage. Postpartum hemorrhage is defined as greater than 1000 mL of blood loss at the time of delivery for both vaginal and cesarean routes. The myometrium has not contracted to cut off the uterine spiral arteries that supplied the placental bed. Uterine massage and uterotonics such as oxytocin, prostaglandin F2 alpha, misoprostol, or methylergonovine maleate are the typical first-line treatment options. Risk factors include overdistension from macrosomia, multiple gestation, or polyhydramnios and exhausted myometrium from prolonged labor, grand multiparity, or uterine infection. **Uterine rupture** or lacerations would be detected on physical exam. **Retained placental tissue** may also be detected by exam or ultrasound. **Coagulopathy** is not likely in this scenario, given normal coagulation factors and no prior hemorrhage with the other deliveries.

GYNECOLOGY

A patient with female reproductive organs may also present with a variety of gynecologic concerns that are unrelated to pregnancy. These issues may include pelvic pain, hormonal changes such as puberty and menopause, abnormal vaginal bleeding (or lack thereof), breast concerns, vulvar concerns, and concerns related to sex and sexuality.

Menopause

Menopause is a clinical diagnosis made once a patient has not had menses for 12 months. This is caused by declining estrogen levels due to age-related reduction of ovarian follicles. Some patients enter menopause without any symptoms, while others will have a myriad of symptoms preceding or during the transition. Vasomotor symptoms, or hot flashes, are the most common menopausal symptoms. Other symptoms and concerns during menopause include vaginal atrophy, dyspareunia, and increased risk for osteoporosis and coronary artery disease.

CASE 13	Menopause
A 50-year-old woman presents with intermittent sweats, sleep disturbance, irritability, and dyspareunia. She denies weight loss, fevers, chills, or vaginal discharge. Her menses have become irregular. Previously she had regular monthly menses, but she had been skipping months for the last 3 years; her LMP was 12 months ago. Pelvic examination reveals pale pink and dry-appearing vaginal mucosa with loss of rugae and prominence of the urethral meatus. Patient notes some discomfort on placement of the speculum.	
Evaluation/Tests	Clinical diagnosis. Pregnancy test is negative.
Treatment	The most effective treatment for menopausal symptoms is hormone replacement therapy. Vasomotor symptoms, or hot flashes, can also be treated with lifestyle modifications (relaxation techniques, fans, air-conditioning), herbal remedies (black cohosh), SSRI, or gabapentin. Genitourinary syndrome of menopause or vulvovaginal atrophy can be treated with vaginal moisturizers/lubricants or vaginal estrogen products.
Discussion	Menopause is defined as 12 months of amenorrhea. Symptoms of menopause include hot flashes, sleep disturbances, vaginal dryness, and change in sexual function. Decline in estrogen levels can cause vulvovaginal atrophy (genitourinary syndrome of menopause). Patients may present with vaginal irritation, dryness, dyspareunia, and recurrent urinary tract infections in the setting of atrophic vaginitis. These symptoms and irregular menses may occur for years before complete cessation of menses (perimenopause). The median age of onset is 51 years, and perimenopause begins approximately 4 years before the last period. It is a clinical diagnosis, so no further testing is needed. At times, an FSH level can be drawn. If the patient is between 40 and 45 years, consider checking hCG, prolactin, TSH, and FSH labs as the workup for oligo/amenorrhea. Treatment of symptoms with estrogen should always be paired with progesterone agents to avoid endometrial cancer, if the patient still has the uterus. Benefit of hormonal therapy should be balanced with the risks of endometrial cancer, breast cancer, venous thromboembolism (VTE), stroke, and cardiovascular disease.

Pelvic Pain

Pelvic pain is both a common and complex presenting symptom for patients with female reproductive organs. It can occur as an acute or chronic condition, and, depending on the etiology, pelvic pain may transition from acute to chronic with time. It is important to remember there are multiple possible etiologies that can explain this symptom; in many cases, there may be more than one contributing factor. Pain may be reported in the lower abdomen or during intercourse (dyspareunia), but patients may have difficulty describing the precise location or timing. This means the differential diagnosis may be wide and varied. One way to frame thinking on this topic is to consider the possible "compartments" of pelvic pain.

Compartments of Pelvic Pain

Gynecologic	Urologic	Gastrointestinal	Musculoskeletal	Neuropsychiatric

Pregnancy (normal and abnormal)
Endometriosis
Fibroids
Ovarian masses (benign or cancerous)
Ovarian torsion
Ovarian cyst
Vulvodynia
Infections:
  STIs
  Pelvic inflammatory disease (PID)
  Vaginitis
  Ovarian abscess
	Painful bladder syndrome (interstitial cystitis)
	Infection
	Nephrolithiasis
		Inflammatory bowel disease
		Irritable bowel syndrome
		Diverticulitis
		Appendicitis
		Gastroenteritis
		Constipation
			Osteoporosis of hip and lower back
			Pelvic floor tension myalgia
			Abdominal wall hernia
				History of trauma/abuse
				Neurogenic pain
				Depression
				Nerve entrapment
				Fibromyalgia

Emergent and Nonemergent Causes of Pelvic Pain in the Nonpregnant Patient

Pelvic Pain	Acute	Chronic	Secondary to Infections
Emergent/serious	Ovarian torsion Ectopic pregnancy	Cancers (ovarian, cervical, endometrial, vulvar)	Pelvic inflammatory disease (PID) Ovarian abscess STIs
Nonemergent	Ruptured ovarian cyst	Endometriosis Fibroids Vulvodynia Adenomyosis Asherman syndrome Nonmalignant ovarian masses	STIs Vaginitis

CASE 14 | Ovarian Torsion

A 27-year-old presents with acute onset of right lower abdominal/pelvic pain associated with nausea and vomiting. On exam, temperature is 37.2°C, and there is tenderness in the right lower quadrant and right adnexal area. There is no cervical motion tenderness or vaginal discharge.

Evaluation/Tests	Urine β-hCG is negative. Transvaginal Doppler ultrasound shows an enlarged left ovary with decreased blood flow.
Treatment	Emergent surgery with untwisting of the ovary if still viable, or salpingo-oophorectomy if ovary is nonviable.
Discussion	Ovarian torsion is a gynecological emergency that occurs due to rotation of the ovary on **infundibulopelvic ligament** causing ischemia. The infundibulopelvic ligament, also known as the suspensory ligament of the ovary, connects the ovaries to the lateral pelvic wall and contains the ovarian vessels. Most cases of ovarian torsion occur in patients of reproductive age, and the primary risk factor is enlargement of the ovaries, which can be due to cysts, hormonal stimulation, pregnancy, or other masses such as tumors. A definitive diagnosis is made surgically by direct visualization of the rotated ovary. In addition to its role in ovarian torsion, the infundibulopelvic ligament is important clinically for two reasons: (1) It must be ligated during oophorectomy to avoid bleeding from ovarian vessels, and (2) it lies in close proximity to the ureters, which course retroperitoneally, so there is risk of ureteral injury during ligation of the vessels.

CASE 15 | Endometriosis

A 31-year-old G0P0 presents for infertility. She has been having regular, unprotected intercourse with her male partner for 2 years. She has severe dysmenorrhea and dyspareunia with deep penetration. On exam, the uterus is not enlarged, but it has restricted range of motion, tender nodules, adnexal masses (endometriomas), and uterosacral ligament nodularity.

CASE 15 | Endometriosis *(continued)*

Evaluation/Tests	Blue-black ("raspberry") or dark brown ("gunpowder") lesions, and/or ovarian "chocolate cysts" (endometriomas) directly visualized by laparoscopy or laparotomy.
Treatment	NSAIDs for pain control and continuous combined hormone contraception to decrease endometrium production. Advanced cases benefit from laparoscopic surgical excision of implants. Refractory cases may benefit from other medications.
Discussion	Endometriosis is a condition in which endometrium is found outside the endometrial cavity; frequent sites include ovaries, peritoneum, and pelvis. Patients can present with chronic pelvic pain, dysmenorrhea, dyspareunia, dyschezia (pain with defecation), and infertility. The uterus is typically normal in size. Definitive diagnosis is made by laparoscopy and biopsy of endometriotic lesions. It is reasonable to attempt medical management for endometriosis pain, while endometriosis-related infertility is often managed surgically.
Additional Considerations	Other causes of pelvic pain, infertility, and abnormal bleeding include the following: **Leiomyoma**—A smooth muscle tumor of the myometrium that is benign. It is sensitive to estrogen, sometimes increasing in size with pregnancy and decreasing with menopause. It may be asymptomatic or cause pelvic pain, abnormal bleeding, and anemia. Leiomyomata are characterized by whorled patterns of smooth muscle bundles with well-demarcated borders. The uterus is typically enlarged. Malignant transformation to leiomyosarcoma is very rare but possible. **Leiomyosarcoma**—A malignant tumor arising from uterine smooth muscle. As opposed to leiomyomas, leiomyosarcoma demonstrates mitotic activity, cellular atypia, areas of necrosis, and local invasion of nearby tissues. **Adenomyosis**—An extension of glandular endometrial tissue into the myometrium due to endometrial hyperplasia. This condition typically presents with a uniformly enlarged, globular uterus. **Asherman syndrome**—Characterized by adhesions/fibrosis of endometrium associated with uterine cavity procedures like dilation and curettage. This may also present with infertility, pelvic pain, abnormal bleeding, and recurrent pregnancy loss. **Endometritis**—An inflammation of the endometrium, typically due to retained products of conception after delivery, miscarriage, or intrauterine procedure. The causative organisms are typically polymicrobial. Treatment is via evacuation of any retained products in the uterus and antibiotics (clindamycin and gentamicin). **Endometrial carcinoma**—Cancer will often present with abnormal or postmenopausal uterine bleeding. Biopsy results would reveal neoplastic proliferation of endometrial tissue, not smooth muscle bundles.

Vaginal Discharge and Pelvic Infections

The normal vaginal ecosystem in the reproductive age patient can vary greatly depending on the timing of the menstrual cycle, pregnancy, use of hormonal contraception or medication, hydration status, and infections. Alterations in the ecosystem can result in variations in the amount, color, and consistency of the usual normal physiologic vaginal discharge. (See "Microbiology" chapter for more information.)

Vulvar Dermatoses

While many presenting vulvar concerns can be attributed to dermatologic manifestations that can occur anywhere on the skin (dermatitis, infection, psoriasis, etc.), the vulva is also prone to a unique group of conditions classified as the vulvar dermatoses. These three "lichens" (sclerosus, planus, and simplex chronicus) typically cause at least one, but often all of the symptoms in the classic vulvar triad: vulvar pruritis, burning, and dyspareunia. Vulvar biopsy is not always required for confirmation because diagnosis is often made by history and exam. However, it can be done to delineate the diagnosis or if the patient is unresponsive to initial treatment.

CASE 16 | Lichen Sclerosus

A 56-year-old postmenopausal patient presents with a 4-month history of worsening vulvar itching and irritation. The symptoms can occur anytime, but they are most bothersome at night. She denies any vaginal discharge or postmenopausal bleeding, but she is having dyspareunia. On exam, the labia minora are fused to the labia majora, and the skin appears fragile, with porcelain-white plaques and a red border.

Evaluation/Tests	Clinical diagnosis. Vulvar biopsy is not required, but it is definitive and recommended if there is poor or no response to treatment.

CASE 16 | Lichen Sclerosus *(continued)*

Treatment	Ultrapotent topical steroids (clobetasol).
Discussion	Lichen sclerosus is typically symptomatic (often with worsening of symptoms at night) with vulvar irritation and/or dyspareunia. There are several pathognomonic physical exam findings, including parchment-paper appearance of the skin, hourglass distribution with sparing of the perineal body, labial agglutination, and phimosis of the clitoral hood. About 5% of cases will undergo malignant transformation, most often to squamous cell carcinoma. **Lichen planus** may occur on the vulva but also occurs on the oral mucosa, scalp, nails, and skin. The condition is poorly understood, but it is proposed to be immune mediated. It occurs in female and male patients. The vulvar variant commonly shows violet/red erosive-appearing plaques with potential for overlying Wickham striae, or reticulated white lines. **Lichen simplex chronicus** is characterized primarily by intense itching, leading to excoriations causing scaling and a lichenified, thick, leathery plaque due to chronic scratching. It is typically caused by environmental factors such as heat, moisture, irritation, or long-standing topical infection. It presents with hyper- or hypopigmentation and thickened, hyperkeratotic skin. As with lichen sclerosus, first-line treatment is with ultrapotent topical steroids. **Vulvar cancer** is rare, and it often presents with leukoplakia. It can be related to HPV infection or from chronic lichen sclerosis, especially in patients over 70 years of age.

Vaginal Masses

When a patient presents with a vaginal mass or bulge, a comprehensive history and focused pelvic exam is typically sufficient to make a diagnosis. Vaginal and vulvar cancers are exceedingly rare, but biopsy of the lesion is indicated if there is ever a question. Most nonmalignant "lesions" of the vagina are listed here, but they may not truly be vaginal in origin due to the proximity of structures from the GI and GU systems.

Cystic Lesions of the Vagina	Solid Lesions of the Vagina
Inclusion cyst	Leiomyoma
Gardner duct cyst	Condyloma
Suburethral diverticulum	Endometriosis
Bartholin's cyst	Uterine prolapse
Cystocele or rectocele	Cervical elongation
Skene's gland cyst	

CASE 17 | Bartholin's Cyst

A 23-year-old presents for evaluation of labial swelling for 3 days. She has one sexual partner, uses protection, and is now noting mild pain during sexual intercourse. She denies any other pain, including when walking or sitting. On physical exam, she is afebrile, her vital signs are normal, and there is a unilateral, fluid-filled mass near the introitus.

Evaluation/Tests	Clinical diagnosis based on physical examination.
Treatment	Sitz bath in warm water may help. Antibiotics are only indicated if there is surrounding cellulitis.
Discussion	This patient is presenting with a Bartholin's cyst, a fluid accumulation due to blockage of the Bartholin's gland duct. The Bartholin glands (also known as greater vestibular glands) are small glands located slightly posterior to the opening of the vagina on each side that develop from the urogenital sinus. Bartholin cysts are fairly common in patients of reproductive age and are often asymptomatic, requiring no intervention. There may be labial swelling or mild dyspareunia (pain during intercourse). They are diagnosed clinically and typically do not need medical treatment unless they become infected. Infection and subsequent inflammation of a Bartholin's cyst can lead to a **Bartholin abscess**. Bartholin abscesses present with increased pain on the side of the cyst, which is exacerbated by particular positions, and dyspareunia. Patients may be febrile and should be treated with incision and drainage as well as consideration of antibiotic therapy.
Additional Considerations	**Vulvar squamous cell carcinoma** is rare but much more concerning and typically presents with leukoplakia, or white patches or spots on the vulva. It may be associated with human papillomavirus (HPV) in patients of reproductive age or long-standing lichen sclerosis in elderly patients.

Abnormal Uterine Bleeding

The normal menstrual cycle is 28 days (+/− 7 days), with menses lasting from 2 to 7 days in length and ranging from light to moderate passage of blood. One way to quantify the amount of blood loss is to determine the number of pads or tampons used or frequency of menstrual cup change in a day at the peak of menses.

Abnormal uterine bleeding (AUB) encompasses a broad range of patterns:

- *Heavy menstrual bleeding (formerly called menorrhagia)*—Menstrual bleeding that lasts over 7 days duration and/or with blood loss of greater than 80 mL over the menstrual event; it may be cyclic or noncyclic; heavy menstrual bleeding can also be defined by what the patient considers to be too heavy.

- *Irregular menses*—Noncyclic/unpredictable occurrence of the menstrual cycle; it may represent anovulatory bleeding that occurs without ovulation or effect from medications or comorbid conditions.

- *Intermenstrual bleeding*—Episodes of vaginal/uterine spotting or bleeding that occur outside of the cyclic menstrual period.

- *Frequent or infrequent menses (formerly called poly- or oligomenorrhea)*—Menses occurring less than 21 days or greater than 35 days apart, respectively.

- *Postcoital bleeding*—Bleeding that occurs after vaginal intercourse.

Often, patients may have more than one of these patterns. While these definitions exist, AUB is ultimately defined as anything the patient feels is abnormal, and it should be assessed accordingly.

Differential for AUB

PALM (Structural)		COEIN (Nonstructural)	
P	Polyp (endometrial)	C	Coagulopathy
A	Adenomyosis	O	Ovulatory dysfunction
L	Leiomyoma (fibroid)	E	Endometrial dysfunction
M	Malignancy/hyperplasia	I	Iatrogenic
		N	Not yet classified

CASE 18	Leiomyoma (Fibroids)
	A 25-year-old G1P0010 presents with heavy menses and occasional intermenstrual spotting. She reports that her menses have always been heavy and that she uses about 8 overnight pads every day. She recently had a miscarriage at 12 weeks. She started noticing increased rectal pressure during her pregnancy, but it never resolved after the miscarriage. She denies hematochezia, easy bruising, bleeding from her gums, or any family history of bleeding disorders. She is not currently on any contraception. On exam, the abdomen is soft and nontender, but the uterus is palpable just above the pubic symphysis, and it feels irregular. On bimanual exam, there is a firm, fixed, 3-cm, nontender mass palpated in the posterior cul-de-sac; no adnexal masses are noted.
Evaluation/Tests	Urine pregnancy test is negative. Pelvic ultrasound shows a 3-cm, posterior, subserosal, hypoechoic mass, and several 1- to 2-cm, intramural, hypoechoic masses along the fundus and anterior uterine wall. Findings are consistent with a fibroid uterus.
Treatment	Treatment options include myomectomy, uterine artery embolization, hysterectomy, hormonal treatment, and/or endometrial ablation.
Discussion	This patient is presenting with fibroids (leiomyomas). Treatment will depend on which symptoms (bulk or bleeding) are more bothersome to the patient and the patient's desire to preserve fertility. "Bulk" symptoms commonly present with urinary frequency, bloating, or lower abdominal heaviness. "Bleeding" symptoms are more typically associated with submucosal fibroids, and they classically present as heavy menstrual bleeding. Pathology would show a whorled pattern of smooth muscle bundles with well-demarcated borders. No treatment is necessary if the patient is not bothered by symptoms and fibroids are noted incidentally on exam or imaging. Transformation to leiomyosarcoma is rare.
Additional Considerations	Other cancers that may present with irregular bleeding are as follows. **Squamous cell carcinoma of vagina** is frequently associated with a history of cervical cancer. It can spread hematogenously, lymphatically, or via direct invasion. Staging is clinical. Chemoradiation is the mainstay of treatment, with radical surgery playing a lesser role.

CASE 18 | Leiomyoma (Fibroids) *(continued)*

Additional Considerations	Most cases of **adenocarcinoma** of the vagina are metastatic. Primary vaginal clear cell adenocarcinomas are classically associated with diethylstilbestrol exposure in utero. **Malignant melanoma** is a rare form of vaginal cancer. The mean age at diagnosis is the mid-50s. Radical surgery is the traditional treatment method, with or without postoperative radiation therapy. **Sarcoma botryoides** is a rare embryonal rhabdomyosarcoma variant seen in infants and children. Mean age of diagnosis is 2–3 years, and on exam, a mass resembling a "cluster of grapes" may be noted protruding from the vaginal apex.

Uterine Cancer

Endometrial carcinomas are the most common subtype, and they arise from the glandular cells of the endometrium. Uterine sarcomas are rare, and they arise from the connective tissue of the endometrium. In postmenopausal patients, any vaginal bleeding should be evaluated with an ultrasound and/or an endometrial biopsy. After menopause, the endometrial thickness on transvaginal ultrasonography should be less than 4 mm. With thickness above this level, biopsy should be considered to rule out endometrial hyperplasia or cancer. Although CA-125 may be elevated in uterine cancers, it is not specific and therefore not recommended for routine screening of the general population. Patients known to have Lynch syndrome should have annual exams to assess for abnormalities starting at age 35.

CASE 19 | Endometrial Cancer

A 57-year-old G0P0 presents with vaginal bleeding and mild lower abdominal cramping for the past month. Her last menstrual period was 6 years ago. She has a history of ductal carcinoma *in situ* diagnosed in her 40s treated with lumpectomy, radiation, and tamoxifen for 10 years. She denies weight loss, lack of appetite, and fatigue. Pelvic exam reveals an enlarged uterus.

Evaluation/Tests	Pelvic ultrasound: thickened endometrial stripe. Endometrial biopsy demonstrates abnormal gland proliferation consistent with carcinoma. Staging CT of chest, abdomen, and pelvis reveals no metastatic disease.
Treatment	Early stage disease is treated with total hysterectomy and bilateral salpingo-oophorectomy. Locally advanced disease should be treated with surgery, followed by local radiation therapy. Systemic disease is typically treated with chemotherapy.
Discussion	Endometrial carcinoma, also known as uterine cancer, typically presents in patients in their mid-fifties to sixties (after menopause) as abnormal uterine bleeding, and it is typically preceded by hyperplasia. Risk factors include unopposed estrogen, obesity, diabetes, nulliparity, tamoxifen use, and Lynch syndrome. Any patient with postmenopausal bleeding should be evaluated with an ultrasound to assess endometrial thickness and/or endometrial biopsy. In **endometrial hyperplasia**, excess estrogen stimulation causes abnormal endometrial gland proliferation, predisposing patients to increased risk of endometrial cancer, especially if nuclear atypia is present. Risk factors include granulosa cell tumors, obesity, hormone replacement therapy, anovulatory cycles, and PCOS.

Cervical Cancer

Squamous cell carcinoma arises from the epithelial cells of the cervix. Disordered growth begins at the basal layer of the squamocolumnar junction and grows apically. These premalignant cells are classified as **cervical intraepithelial neoplasia (CIN)** and graded I–III, with grade III being the most severe. Once invasive features are evident, the lesion is classified as a malignancy. HPV 16 and HPV 18 are the types most strongly associated with cervical cancer. Koilocytes are cervical epithelial cells seen on Pap smear that have undergone structural changes due to HPV infection.

Symptoms such as vaginal bleeding or spotting may only occur with advanced disease, and they can often be ignored. Mainstay of diagnosis is a Pap smear done at regular intervals. Suspicious Pap smear findings should be evaluated further with biopsy of cervical lesion done through colposcopy, a visual examination of the cervix aided by acetic acid to highlight abnormal cells on the surface of the cervix.

The general screening guidelines are as follows: Patients with a cervix aged 21–29 should have Pap smear every 3 years. Those aged 30–65 should be tested with Pap smear and HPV cotesting every 5 years. Alternatively, patients age 25–65 can be screened with a primary HPV test (hrHPV) only every 5 years. When under the age of 21, patients should not be screened regardless of age of onset of coitus. If a patient is low risk, pap smears can be discontinued at age 65.

CASE 20	Squamous Cell Carcinoma of the Cervix
A 42-year-old G2P2002 with a 20-pack-a-year tobacco history presents with postcoital bleeding. She states that almost every time she has intercourse, she has spotting that resolves by the next day. She denies any vaginal or pelvic pain. She denies vaginal itching, discharge, dysuria, or hematuria. She reports her last Pap smear was around 10 years ago, and she never got the results. She was treated for STIs when she was 16 and 24 years old. She is on oral contraceptive pills and uses condoms intermittently. Exam is notable for friable anterior lip of the cervix with inflammatory punctation and abnormal vasculature but no tenderness or masses on bimanual exam.	
Evaluation/Tests	Pap smear shows CIN III and positive HPV 16. Colposcopy with biopsy reveals squamous cell carcinoma with koilocytes. CT of chest, abdomen, and pelvis shows no metastatic disease. Cultures are negative for STIs.
Treatment	Depending on stage, cervical conization or radiation therapy for local disease and chemotherapy for systemic disease.
Discussion	The majority of cervical carcinomas are squamous cell cancers. Pap smears can detect dysplasia before it progresses to invasive cancer. Diagnosis is made by colposcopy and biopsy. Postcoital bleeding is a common symptom of cervical cancer. Patients with invasive cervical cancer may present with foul-smelling brown discharge due to necrosis and possible fistula formation. They may also have postcoital bleeding, sciatica pain, leg swelling, and hydroureter due to compression on surrounding structures. **Cervical dysplasia** begins at the squamocolumnar junction (transformation zone) and extends outward. It is classified as cervical intraepithelial neoplasia (CIN) I, II, or III depending on the extent of dysplasia, and it may progress to invasive cancer if not treated.

Ovarian Masses

Ovarian masses may be found incidentally or during workup of pelvic concerns. They are mostly benign. Many ovarian masses are cystic in nature, and they are considered functional, meaning they arise in response to normal cyclic changes in ovarian physiology; these include follicular and corpus luteum cysts. While these cysts are benign and generally resolve spontaneously, they are a rare cause of acute pelvic pain requiring hospitalization or surgery if they undergo torsion or rupture with intraperitoneal hemorrhage. The ovary is also a site of several nonmalignant cystic lesions, including the mature cystic teratoma (also called dermoid tumor) and the cystadenoma (serous or mucinous). These, along with the functional group, comprise most ovarian masses.

Ovarian cancer is classified by the site of origin: surface epithelium, germ cells, or sex cord-gonadal stromal tissue. Surface epithelial (stromal) tumors are the most common form of ovarian cancers (90%), and they include subtypes such as serous and mucinous cystadenocarcinomas and endometrioid tumors.

Serous cystadenocarcinomas behave aggressively, often present bilaterally, and show psammoma bodies on pathological examination.

Immature teratomas arise from germ cells, also behave aggressively, and are characterized by fetal tissue and neuroectoderm on pathology.

Dysgerminomas occur in adolescents, present with elevation in LDH and β-hCG, and show sheets of fried egg cells on pathological exam.

Granulosa cell tumors usually occur in patients in their fifties, and they are the most common tumors to originate from the stromal tissue of the ovary. They often produce estrogen and/or progesterone, and they can present with postmenopausal or other abnormal uterine bleeding due to the effect of the unopposed estrogen on the endometrium.

Risk factors for ovarian malignancy include increasing age, nulliparity or older age at first pregnancy (>35), endometriosis, PCOS, family history, BRCA1 or BRCA2 mutations, Lynch syndrome (mutation in mismatch repair enzyme), and DES exposure *in utero* (specifically clear cell ovarian cancer). Use of combined oral contraception and increased number of pregnancies and/or time breast-feeding are associated with a decrease in risk. Symptoms are typically nonspecific, and they may present as abdominal or pelvic pain, bloating, fatigue, weight loss with paradoxical increase in waist circumference, and lack of appetite/early satiety. A fixed mass on pelvic exam and nodularity in or loss of the posterior cul-de-sac on rectovaginal exam can all suggest more concerning etiology of an ovarian mass. Many patients are asymptomatic at early stages, and there is not a useful screening tool for early diagnosis at this time. Ultrasound or CT scan findings may include papillary projections, thick septations, and other stigmata of malignancy, including ascites, omental thickening/caking, and paraaortic lymphadenopathy. CA-125 may be useful in creating the differential diagnosis and monitoring for response to treatment and recurrence.

CASE 30 | Hypogonadotropic Hypogonadism: Kallman syndrome *(continued)*

Evaluation/Tests	Semen analysis shows no sperm (azoospermia) and normal volume. FSH, LH, and testosterone levels are decreased. Prolactin level is normal. Brain MRI is normal. Karyotype is normal.
Treatment	The goal is to reestablish the hormonal axis for testicular stimulation with gonadotropin supplementation (human chorionic gonadotropin [hCG]), which acts as an LH analog to stimulate the testes and initiate testosterone production and spermatogenesis.
Discussion	This patient is presenting with Kallmann syndrome, a form of hypogonadotropic hypogonadism that presents with delayed or absent puberty in male or female patients. Secondary gonadal failure occurs due to impaired GnRH-releasing neuron migration from the hypothalamus to the anterior pituitary. This results in failed stimulation of the pituitary by GnRH and subsequent hypogonadism. Kallman syndrome is more common in male patients. Often, male infants will have undescended testicles (cryptorchidism) as testicular descent is driven by the GnRH, LH, and FSH surge that occurs between 0 and 6 months of age. Anosmia is a defining feature of Kallmann syndrome, and this distinguishes it from other causes of hypogonadotropic hypogonadism. In normal embryologic development, GnRH-releasing neurons migrate from the nasal placode (gives rise to olfactory epithelium), through the cribriform plate, and they ultimately synapse in the hypothalamus of the developing forebrain. With Kallmann syndrome, abnormal migration of these neurons results in decreased (hyposmia) or absent (anosmia) sense of smell. In male patients, lack of GnRH results in low levels of LH and FSH, resulting in decreased testosterone and sperm counts. In female patients, lack of GnRH results in decreased LH, FSH, and estradiol. Female patients will have failure of or delayed secondary sexual characteristics, primary amenorrhea, and infertility. Other congenital defects such as midline facial anomalies may be seen. **Prolactinomas** (prolactin-secreting pituitary adenomas) are another cause of hypogonadotropic hypogonadism, and they are associated with erectile dysfunction in men. If the lesion is large enough, visual disturbances (such as bitemporal hemianopsia) due to mass effects on the optic chiasm can occur. Serum prolactin levels will be significantly elevated, and testosterone levels will be low. A normal brain MRI in this case rules out the presence of a prolactinoma. Conversely to Kallmann syndrome, **Klinefelter syndrome** represents hypergonadotropic hypogonadism with elevated FSH and LH due to primary testicular failure. These patients will have an abnormal XXY karyotype. **Hypergonadotrophic hypogonadism**, or primary hypogonadism, is characterized by testosterone level <300 ng/dL and concurrently elevated LH and FSH. Primary causes originate in the testicles, and it can occur in men who have had testicular injury, mumps, orchitis, certain cancer treatments, or radiation to the area or hemochromatosis.

CASE 31 | Orchitis Secondary to Mumps Infection

A 24-year-old male presents with his 25-year-old female partner for failure to conceive after 12 months of unprotected intercourse. His medical history is significant for an episode of low-grade fever, malaise, and nausea with unilateral swelling of the left cheek and protrusion of the ear a few years ago that resolved after a week. His partner had an unremarkable female infertility workup. He denies pregnancy with previous partners. He was not vaccinated as a child. Exam shows normal secondary sexual characteristics, a normal phallus, a normal spermatic cord, and bilateral small and soft testes.

Evaluation/Tests	Semen analysis shows azoospermia with normal volume specimen. Hormone profile shows elevated FSH and LH, low testosterone, normal prolactin, and normal estradiol. Positive IgG serology to the mumps virus.
Treatment	Hormonal testicular stimulation with a selective estrogen receptor modulator or exogenous gonadotropins.
Discussion	This patient is presenting with infertility secondary to **orchitis** caused by previous infection with the **mumps virus**. Mumps is a highly infectious paramyxovirus that classically presents with swelling of the parotid gland (parotitis) in unvaccinated individuals. It is often more severe in adults than in children, and it can result in inflammation of other glandular tissue such as the pancreas (acute pancreatitis) and gonads (testes or ovaries). It can also lead to aseptic meningitis. Inflammation of the gonads, as in this case, can result in subsequent infertility, typically when bilateral. Mumps infection in postpubertal male patients can commonly lead to orchitis. While prepubertal mumps orchitis does not affect fertility, mumps orchitis contracted after puberty may lead to subfertility in 13% of cases or, rarely, infertility, due to injury to the seminiferous tubules and Leydig cells responsible for spermatogenesis and testosterone

CASE 31 | Orchitis Secondary to Mumps Infection *(continued)*

Discussion	production, respectively. While testicular stimulation via manipulation of the hypothalamic-pituitary-testis axis may allow for improvement of semen parameters, couples will often require assisted reproduction due to low sperm counts that are nonresponsive to medical stimulation. It is important not to use exogenous testosterone to treat the infertile male patient attempting to conceive as it will suppress spermatogenesis. **Obstructive azoospermia** classically presents with low volume ejaculate, normal testicular size, and normal gonadotropins (LH and FSH). Spermatogenesis is not impaired; there is simply an abnormality in delivery.

UROLOGY

Urology is the branch of medicine that deals with medical and surgical issues involving the male and female urinary tract systems and the male reproductive organs. Some cases related to the urinary tract system are located in the "Renal" chapter, and the focus of this chapter is on normal and abnormal male reproductive biology.

SCROTAL SWELLING OR MASS

A scrotal swelling or mass can present at any age, and it may or may not be accompanied by pain. Given that testicular cancer is the most common malignancy in men between the ages of 20 and 35 years, cancer should be considered in the differential for any scrotal mass. Patients should have a thorough exam including transillumination by shining a light behind the scrotum. This can help distinguish whether the mass is cystic (light shines through) or solid (light blocked by the mass). An ultrasound can also help determine if a mass is solid or fluid filled. Any solid mass requires immediate evaluation for cancer, including tumor markers LDH, AFP, and β-hCG. A biopsy should never be done if there is concern for testicular cancer because this may cause lymphatic tumor seeding. Instead, an orchiectomy should be performed.

Testicular cancer often presents as a painless mass that is found incidentally. Risk factors include cryptorchidism, a personal or family history of testicular cancer, infertility or subfertility, and HIV. Ultimately, patients with a suspicious testicular mass need ultrasound and orchiectomy. The two broad categories of testicular cancer are seminoma and nonseminoma, which can be differentiated by the tumor markers they secrete. Nonseminomas are more aggressive than seminomas, and they present with multiple different histological subtypes including yolk sac, teratoma, and choriocarcinoma. Treatment consists of a combination of surgery, radiation, and chemotherapy.

Differential Diagnosis of Scrotal Swelling or Mass Based on Patient Age

Neonate/Child	Adolescent/Adult
• Hydrocele • Hernia • Testicular torsion • Testicular tumor	• Hydrocele • Hernia • Testicular torsion • Testicular tumor • Epididymal cyst/spermatocele • Varicocele

Painful swelling of the scrotum warrants emergent evaluation to rule out testicular torsion, which must be corrected within hours in order to keep the testes viable. In contrast, hydroceles and hernias are common causes of painless swelling. One of the first steps for evaluating painless swelling is to differentiate between these two possible diagnoses.

Hydrocele	Hernia
Transilluminate positive	Transilluminate negative
Often able to "get above" when isolating on exam	Unable to "get above" when isolating on exam
Silent auscultation	May have bowel sounds on auscultation
Typically painless	May have pain with Valsalva or if incarcerated (tissue is trapped and cannot return to its original compartment) or strangulated (tissue cuts off blood supply to intestine or testis)
Reducible if communicating	Often reducible (bulge flattens when pushed)

CASE 32 | Hydrocele

A 6-month-old boy is brought to clinic for evaluation of a scrotal bulge that seems to wax and wane. It is largest when he is coughing or crying. It has been noticed since birth, and the mother thinks it may be getting smaller. The infant was delivered at full-term without any complications. On physical exam, both testes are easily palpable in the scrotum. In the upright position, there is a fullness appreciated over the right testis that disappears in the recumbent position. The scrotum transilluminates, and bowel sounds are not heard on scrotal auscultation.

Evaluation/Tests	Clinical diagnosis. Scrotal ultrasound can be obtained if there is concern for tumor, torsion, or trauma.
Treatment	Observation until 2 years of age, then hydrocelectomy if it has not spontaneously resolved.
Discussion	This patient is presenting with a pediatric **hydrocele**. During fetal development, the testicle is initially located intra-abdominally near the kidneys in the posterior abdominal wall and then descends through the inguinal canal into the scrotum, taking along an extension of the peritoneum called the processus vaginalis. The processus vaginalis passes through the anterior abdominal wall through the inguinal canal, carrying with it layers of the abdominal wall that form the spermatic cord. Normally, this processus vaginalis closes, removing the communication between the scrotum and the peritoneum and leaving behind a distal remnant of connective tissue and the tunica vaginalis surrounding the testis. In some instances, the processus vaginalis fails to close, thus allowing the communication of peritoneal fluid with the scrotum, termed a **communicating hydrocele**. Fortunately, most communicating hydroceles are small enough that they only allow communication of fluid, and they close spontaneously. If the defect is large enough to allow the passage of intra-abdominal contents such as bowel or omentum, it is termed a **hernia**.
	In contrast to a communicating hydrocele, **noncommunicating hydroceles** lack communication between the scrotum and peritoneum due to a closed processus vaginalis. However, fluid accumulation can still occur, especially in settings of infection or trauma. Many cases are idiopathic, where the tunica vaginalis produces fluid at a faster rate than it can reabsorb.
	Hernias represent omentum or bowel extending into the inguinal canal or scrotum, would not transilluminate, and may result in bowel sounds on auscultation. Trauma, hematoma, or torsion would have pain on presentation.
	A **testicular tumor** would also not transilluminate.

CASE 33 | Testicular Cancer

A 25-year-old man with a history of bilateral cryptorchidism presents with a "bump" on his left testicle. He is unsure of the duration but noticed it while in the shower approximately 2 weeks ago. There is no associated pain, urinary complaints, or any antecedent trauma. He had bilateral orchiopexies at the age of 8 for his cryptorchidism. On physical exam, there is a nontender, solid, firm, homogeneous mass on the anterior aspect of the left testis that does not transilluminate. The right testis is nontender and palpably normal. There is no inguinal lymphadenopathy.

Evaluation/Tests	Testicular ultrasound shows a well-defined, hypoechoic 2-cm mass without cystic areas. LDH and serum placental alkaline phosphatase (PALP) is elevated, and AFP and β-hCG is normal. CT scan of the chest, abdomen, and pelvis reveals no other abnormalities.
Treatment	Radical inguinal orchiectomy.
Discussion	Primary **testicular cancer** is the most common malignancy in men aged 20 to 35 years and often presents as a firm, unilateral, nonmobile mass that cannot be isolated away from the testicle. They do not transilluminate and are usually painless. Testicular tumors are broadly divided into germ cell tumors (~95%), which develop from sperm-producing germ cells, or sex cord stromal tumors, which develop from derivatives of the embryonic sex cord. In general, most germ cell tumors are malignant, while most sex cord stromal tumors are benign in men. The most common testicular tumor overall and most common germ cell tumor subtype is the **seminoma**, as in this patient. Pathology would show large cells in lobules with a watery cytoplasm and a "fried egg" appearance. Serum tumor markers in testicular tumors can help narrow the differential. Seminomas, by definition, have normal serum AFP and, typically, β-hCG. However, if syncytiotrophoblastic giant cells are present in the tumor, β-hCG may be elevated. PALP is elevated in seminomas. **Cryptorchidism**, or the failure of descent in one or both testes, is a known risk factor for the development of testicular cancer with increasing risk the longer the testes are not descended. Klinefelter syndrome is also a risk factor for testicular tumors. Masses suspected to be testicular cancer should be removed via an inguinal approach as a scrotal approach risks disruption of normal lymphatic drainage, the mechanism by which testicular tumors most commonly spread.

CASE 33 | Testicular Cancer *(continued)*

Discussion	Other types of testicular **germ cell tumors** include teratomas, embryonal carcinomas, yolk sac tumors, and choriocarcinomas. Yolk sac tumors have very high AFP levels, while choriocarcinomas have very high β-hCG levels. Non-germ-cell tumors, or **sex cord stromal tumors**, include Sertoli cell tumors, Leydig cell tumors, and testicular metastatic lymphoma. Following radical inguinal orchiectomy, histology can help identify the specific tumor subtype, and this will help guide subsequent management. A **testicular hematoma** will have a history of trauma. **Varicocele** is typically described as a "bag of worms" feeling in the testicle.

SCROTAL PAIN

It is important to expedite the evaluation of scrotal pain and to rule in or out emergent cases such as testicular torsion from less emergent cases such as epididymo-orchitis or testicular varicocele.

Key Clinical Associations

	Testicular Torsion	Epididymo-orchitis	Varicocele
Onset	Acute	Gradual	Gradual/chronic
Pain	Severe	Severe	Dull ache
Physical Exam	− Cremasteric reflex	+ Cremasteric reflex	Dilated veins of pampiniform plexus (increases with Valsalva), "bag of worms"
	Long axis of testicle is lying horizontally, high riding testicular position in scrotum	Normal testicular lie	Veins decompress in recombinant position
Management	Emergent surgery	Antibiotics/anti-inflammatories	Symptomatic management vs. surgical varicocelectomy

While surgical exploration should not be delayed if testicular torsion is suspected, a testicular Doppler ultrasound can help accurately differentiate various pathologies.

Key Ultrasound Findings	Diagnosis
Lack of blood flow	Testicular torsion
Hypervascular, enlarged epididymis	Epididymitis
Anechoic extratesticular lesion	Spermatocele/epididymal cyst
Retrograde spermatic vein flow with Valsalva	Varicocele
Hypoechoic intratesticular lesion with blood flow	Testicular mass
Inguinal mass, + peristalsis, luminal debris	Inguinal hernia

CASE 34 | Testicular Torsion

A 16-year-old previously healthy boy presents with sudden onset of excruciating left scrotal pain. The pain started suddenly 3 hours ago, and he denies any antecedent trauma and he remembers the exact moment of onset. Pain is rated 10/10, radiates up the left groin, and is associated with nausea and vomiting. His vital signs are within normal limits except for mild tachycardia. On physical exam, the left testicle is exquisitely tender, swollen, and high-riding with a transverse lie. Cremasteric reflex is absent. His right testicle is nontender and lying appropriately in the right hemiscrotum.

Evaluation/Tests	Due to high clinical suspicion, no further tests are necessary. Emergent surgical exploration and treatment are warranted. Doppler ultrasonography would show lack of blood flow through the spermatic cord into the testicle.
Treatment	Emergent surgical correction (orchipexy).

CASE 34 | Testicular Torsion *(continued)*

Discussion	**Testicular torsion** is a urologic emergency presenting with acute scrotal pain, most commonly in teenage years. The sudden onset of pain is caused by the twisting of the spermatic cord and loss of blood supply to the ipsilateral testicle with subsequent ischemia. There are three primary blood supplies to the testicle: (1) the testicular artery from the abdominal aorta, (2) the cremasteric artery from the inferior epigastric artery, and (3) the ductus deferens artery from the inferior vesical artery. All are affected in this condition. Pain is acute and severe. The transverse orientation (lie) and high-riding position are secondary to the twisting of the cord and alteration of the free-hanging orientation. With a transverse lie, the long axis of the testicle is positioned horizontally instead of its normal more vertical positioning within the tunica vaginalis of the hemiscrotum. This change in position often results in the loss of the cremasteric reflex. **Epididymo-orchitis** represents inflammation of both the epididymis and testis. Pain may be severe, but it typically develops gradually and progressively worsens compared to the acute presentation of torsion. There may be associated swelling or hydrocele, and Doppler ultrasonography would show increased blood flow to the epididymis. Common causes include sexually transmitted infections in young men (e.g., *Chlamydia trachomatis*, *Neisseria gonorrhoeae*), *Escherichia Coli*, or *Pseudomonas* infection in elderly men associated with a UTI or benign prostatic hyperplasia, autoimmune disease, adverse effects of medication, or urine reflux associated with straining to void or heavy lifting. While **hernias** may be painless, they may be painful if incarceration (trapped tissue cannot return to original compartment) or strangulation (tissue cuts off blood supply) occur.

CASE 35 | Varicocele

A 29-year-old otherwise healthy man presents with nonradiating left scrotal pain and swelling for the past year. It is described as "dull and heavy," and it is exacerbated with prolonged standing or increased strenuous activity and is relieved with lying down. He also reports that he and his wife have not been able to conceive for the past 2 years. He recently obtained a semen analysis that showed low sperm concentrations, low motility, and abnormal morphology. On physical exam, his left and right testes measure 3.0 cm and 4.0 cm, respectively. His left spermatic cord veins are easily palpable in the standing position, increase with Valsalva, and diminish in the supine position. The spermatic cord is noted to feel like a "bag of worms."

Evaluation/Tests	Clinical diagnosis. Upright scrotal Doppler ultrasonography will show retrograde scrotal vein flow with Valsalva maneuver.
Treatment	Supportive measures (scrotal support, NSAIDs) and observation if no associated infertility or pain. Surgical ligation or embolization when symptomatic.
Discussion	A varicocele is a dilation of the pampiniform venous plexus and the internal spermatic veins due to increased venous pressure. It is the most common cause of scrotal swelling in the adult male and is usually on the left side due to increased resistance to flow from the right-angle insertion of the left gonadal vein into the left renal vein. This is opposed to the right gonadal vein, which flows directly into the inferior vena cava. Dilation of the pampiniform plexus veins is accentuated by standing or performing the Valsalva maneuver. The classic description is a "bag of worms" on palpation. Varicoceles will not transilluminate, and the pain is described as a dull ache. A **hydrocele** would transilluminate. Testicular torsion and epididymo-orchitis often present with more severe, sharp pain. A **spermatocele/epididymal cyst** is due to dilation of the epididymal duct or rete testis, resulting in a paratesticular fluctuant nodule rather than intratesticular location.

URETHRAL DISCHARGE

Urethritis is inflammation of the urethra. Urethritis classically presents with urethral discharge, but some patients may be asymptomatic. Though noninfectious etiologies exist, the term often implies infection-induced urethral inflammation in clinical practice. Urethral infections are typically sexually transmitted. (See "Microbiology" chapter for more information.)

CONGENITAL PENILE ABNORMALITIES

Congenital anomalies of the penis are somewhat common, and they may have characteristic clinical associations. The two main types of congenital penile abnormalities—epispadias and hypospadias—involve abnormal openings of the penile urethra on the dorsal or ventral surface of the penis, respectively. Other congenital penile abnormalities include urethral duplication (rare) and phimosis, the latter of which involves inability to retract tight foreskin that covers the glans penis. Phimosis can be physiologic (normal in young uncircumcised children) or pathologic (due to trauma, scarring, infection, or inflammation).

CASE 36 | Hypospadias

A full-term newborn baby boy is noted to have abnormal genitalia. Prenatal and maternal histories are unremarkable with no intake of exogenous hormones. There is no family history of ambiguous genitalia. Exam is notable for incomplete foreskin on the penis with absence of ventral skin and excess skin on dorsal aspect, causing a hooded appearance. A ventral urethral meatus is located proximally at the midshaft. There is moderate ventral curvature of the penis. The scrotum is bifid. Bilateral testes are palpable in the appropriate hemiscrotum. The child also appears to have an inguinal hernia.

Evaluation/Tests	Clinical diagnosis, however, workup should include karyotype for chromosomal abnormalities, and serum levels of sex hormones (testosterone, LH, FSH), cortisol, and mineralocorticoids to rule out disorders of sexual development.
Treatment	Consider surgical correction, avoid or delay circumcision in case of need for foreskin during reconstruction.
Discussion	**Hypospadias** is among the most common male congenital genitourinary malformations. Embryologically, the penis and clitoris both derive from the genital tubercle. The male urethra forms by progressive fusion of the urethral folds, driven by local dihydrotestosterone (DHT) converted from testosterone by the enzyme 5-α-reductase. Hypospadias results from interruption of this hormonal stimulus and arrested development of the fusion event, leading to the urethral opening on the ventral aspect of the penis. Distal hypospadias does not affect voiding, fertility, or sexual function, but it is often repaired surgically for cosmetic considerations. Conversely, more proximal forms of hypospadias may impair reproduction and the ability to void while standing. Hypospadias is associated with inguinal hernia, cryptorchidism, and chordee (ventral curvature of the penis). While most cases of hypospadias are isolated, one should consider a **disorder of sexual development (DSD)**, especially in cases of more proximal hypospadias with other ambiguous features or a nonpalpable testis. The most common type of DSD is congenital adrenal hyperplasia, which may present in male patients with ambiguous genitalia, undescended testes, and decreased sex hormones and cortisol levels. **Epispadias** is less common. It involves opening of the urethra on the dorsal surface of the penis, and it is associated with bladder exstrophy.

ERECTILE DYSFUNCTION

Erectile dysfunction (ED) is the inability to achieve or maintain an erection sufficient for satisfactory performance. It affects up to 50% of men over the age of 40 with associated perturbations in quality of life. The physiology of normal erections is complex, and, as such, ED tends to be multifactorial in etiology. It can be broadly categorized as either organic or psychogenic, with pure psychogenic causes being rather rare.

The penis is essentially a vascular structure acting as a hydraulic device. Much of understanding erectile dysfunction is understanding the basic physiology of an erection, the underlying pathologies that cause erectile dysfunction, and the treatments. Early-onset erectile dysfunction may be a harbinger for systemic processes. For patients reporting loss of libido, depression, or attenuated secondary sexual characteristic, initial tests include checking testosterone, LH, estradiol, prolactin, TSH, hemoglobin A1c, and basic metabolic panel and lipid profile. Imaging studies are rarely needed unless there is a history of trauma or acute loss of an erection.

The autonomic erection center provides parasympathetic (S2–S4) and sympathetic (T12–L2) input to the pelvic plexus, including the cavernous nerves, which regulate penile blood flow via the cavernous arteries and trabecular smooth muscle. The cavernous nerves deliver high local concentrations of nitric oxide (NO) to the trabecular smooth muscle. NO activates guanylate cyclase to produce cyclic guanosine monophosphate (cGMP), which changes potassium and calcium ion channel permeability, decreasing cytosolic calcium concentrations and resulting in smooth muscle relaxation. With smooth muscle relaxation comes increased blood flow to the penis. One of the key regulators to this biochemical cascade is phosphodiesterase enzymes (PDEs), specifically PDE-5. PDEs inactivate cGMP, resulting in elevated cytosolic calcium concentrations and smooth muscle contraction.

ED Differential Diagnosis

Vascular	Intrinsic	Psychiatric	Miscellaneous
Noncoronary atherosclerosis Cardiovascular disease Penile fracture	Diabetes Neurological conditions (Parkinson's, MS, GBS) Anatomical conditions (Peyronie's, hypospadias)	Performance anxiety Depression	Endocrine disorders Drug interactions (antihypertensives, antidepressants)

Key Findings and ED Differential Diagnosis

ED with Key Associated Findings	Diagnoses
Pain, "pop," acute loss of erection, bruising, swelling; Eggplant deformity	Penile fracture
Pain, "pop," no immediate loss of erection, bruising, swelling	Penile hematoma
History of anxiety/depression	Depression or anxiety disorder
On antidepressants or beta-blockers	Medication side effect
Pain with erections, penile angulation mostly with erections, palpable plaque on penile shaft	Peyronie's disease
Nocturnal erections present, situational erectile dysfunction (e.g., worse with intercourse than with masturbation)	Psychogenic causes

CASE 37 | Erectile Dysfunction (Impotence)

A 58-year-old man with a history of HTN presents with erectile dysfunction. He states that he has had difficulty with attaining and maintaining an erection sufficient for penetration over the last 12 months. He denies any nocturnal erections and states that he is still sexually attracted to his wife. His blood pressure is well controlled with lisinopril. He has not tried any pharmacotherapy for the ED. He has no history of any surgeries or pelvic trauma. On physical exam, both testes are easily palpable in the scrotum, and they are a normal weight and consistency. His penile shaft is without curvature or palpable plaque.

Evaluation/Tests	TSH, HbA1c, lipids, and testosterone levels are normal.
Treatment	Trial of oral phosphodiesterase type 5 (PDE5) inhibitors (i.e., sildenafil).
Discussion	Erectile dysfunction is associated with DM, hypertension, hyperlipidemia, coronary artery disease, depression, and other neurological or endocrine disorders. If no organic causes are apparent, then treatment involves sexual counseling. Otherwise treatment options include oral medications (oral PDE5 inhibitors), injected vasodilators (prostaglandin E1, papaverine, phentolamine), intraurethral suppositories (prostaglandin E1), external vacuum-assisted devices, and surgical implantation of penile prosthesis. The absence of nocturnal erections makes psychogenic etiology less likely. He denies any other neurological complaints that would suggest a neurological etiology such as multiple sclerosis or Parkinson's disease. The absence of penile curvature or plaque rules out **Peyronie's disease**.

URINARY RETENTION

Urinary retention is the inability to completely or partially empty the bladder. It has a wide differential diagnosis spanning multiple organ systems. (Also see "Renal" chapter.) This is opposed to urinary incontinence, or the loss of bladder control, resulting in leakage of urine or constant urge to urinate. However, chronic or unalleviated urinary retention can lead to overflow incontinence as the bladder becomes overfilled, and urine begins to leak out of the urethra. Acute urinary retention is associated with suprapubic pain, occasionally flank pain, and the inability to empty the bladder. Extreme cases will be associated with an inability to urinate at all. In addition to discomfort, there is often resultant acute renal failure with elevated serum creatinine. Chronic urinary retention may present with recurrent urinary tract infections and bladder stones due to urinary stasis, nocturia, or incontinence. Patients with chronic urinary retention can typically urinate but do not empty completely.

Neurogenic causes of urinary retention exist across both sexes. Strokes cause detrusor muscle hyporeflexia, and diabetes causes peripheral neuropathy that may manifest as urinary retention. Bladder dysfunction is present in approximately 80% of those with multiple sclerosis and may be the initial presenting symptom. Issues of outlet obstruction are less common in female patients given the shorter urethra, but strictures may occur, and they should be considered in the setting of a trauma history. More common non-neurologic causes of urinary retention in female patients are related to pelvic organ prolapse. In men, outlet obstruction is more common. The longer urethra provides more locations for potential stricture due to trauma, infection, or urologic manipulation (e.g., transurethral procedures, Foley catheter placement). However, outlet obstruction is far more common secondary to prostate pathology, particularly benign prostatic hyperplasia.

Anticholinergic medications inhibit the actions of the neurotransmitter acetylcholine on the bladder and can result in detrusor muscle hypocontractility with resultant urinary retention. This is sometimes clinically useful because anticholinergic agents may be prescribed to help with urinary incontinence.

Differential Diagnosis for Urinary Retention

Neurogenic	Obstructive	Pharmacologic
• Spinal cord injury • Multiple sclerosis • Stroke • Diabetes mellitus • Cauda equina syndrome • Spinal anesthesia • Parkinson's disease • Spina bifida	• Urethral stricture • Benign prostatic hyperplasia • Prostatitis • Urinary tract infection • Prostate cancer • Pelvic organ prolapse • Pelvic mass • Bladder diverticulum • Constipation • Hematuria (clot retention) • Bladder stone • Bladder cancer	• Anticholinergics • Antihistamines • Antidepressants • Antipsychotics • Anesthetics • Opioids • Benzodiazepines

CASE 38 | Benign Prostatic Hyperplasia (BPH)

A 70-year-old man without significant past medical history presents with severe abdominal pain and inability to urinate. He states that he has only been able to urinate small drops for the entire day. He denies any similar episodes in the past. He does not take any medications. Review of systems is positive for nocturia three times nightly and a several month history of weak stream, frequency, hesitancy, and postvoid dribbling. On physical exam, his vital signs are normal except for mild tachycardia. His bladder is markedly distended, palpable, and tender. His urethral meatus is normal and patent. He does not have any costovertebral angle tenderness. On digital rectal exam (DRE), the prostate is smooth, uniformly enlarged, nontender, and non-nodular.

Evaluation/Tests	Clinical diagnosis based on the presence of lower urinary tract symptoms and absence of other causes. Ultrasound shows a distended bladder with an elevated postvoid residual volume.
Treatment	If bladder obstruction is present, decompress with urinary catheterization. Start α_1-antagonists (e.g., terazosin, tamsulosin) or 5α-reductase inhibitors (e.g., finasteride). Some patients may benefit from bladder outlet obstruction surgery such as transurethral resection of the prostate (TURP).
Discussion	This patient is presenting with **benign prostatic hyperplasia (BPH)**, a non-neoplastic condition caused by hyperplasia of epithelial and smooth muscle cells within the transitional zone of the prostate gland. The transitional zone surrounds the urethra as it passes through the prostate, so hyperplasia in this area can cause difficulties with urination. Other lower urinary tract symptoms include increased urinary frequency, urgency, nocturia, hesitancy, weak stream, and postvoid dribbling. BPH may lead to distension and hypertrophy of the bladder, hydronephrosis, or increased risk of UTIs. BPH is stimulated by circulating androgens, and it is a normal part of aging, with close to half of men having BPH by 50 years of age and more with increasing age. If symptoms are bothersome, they can be managed with pharmacotherapy or surgery for severe cases. It should be noted that prostate-specific antigen (PSA) is frequently elevated in the setting of acute urinary retention, so it should be obtained after resolution of the patient's acute retention. **Urethral stricture** represents a narrowing of the urethra along its course. Etiology can be congenital, infectious, traumatic, or idiopathic. DRE in urethral stricture would be normal. **Prostatitis** may present with similar symptoms as BPH, but it would also have infectious symptoms such as dysuria, fever, and recurrent UTIs. DRE would reveal a tender, swollen prostate, and patients may also have elevated PSA. **Prostate cancer** would likely also have an elevated PSA and on DRE may reveal presence of nodules, areas that are harder than the rest of the gland, or different textures.

CASE 39 | Prostatitis

A 55-year-old man presents with several days of malaise and feelings of incomplete emptying with urination and fevers and chills. He also notes dysuria, urinary frequency, urgency, and, most recently, back pain. His past medical history is significant for diabetes and BPH, which are both controlled on medications. On physical exam, he is febrile and tachycardic. He has mild suprapubic tenderness to palpation. Digital rectal exam reveals an exquisitely tender, enlarged, and boggy prostate. There is no inguinal lymphadenopathy.

Evaluation/Tests	CBC reveals leukocytosis. Urinalysis and urine culture are positive for bacteria, with gram stain revealing gram negative rod bacteria.
Treatment	Antibiotics and supportive measures (NSAIDs, α-blockers, sitz baths).

CASE 39 | Prostatitis *(continued)*

Discussion	Prostatitis refers to either infection or inflammation of the prostate gland. It can be acute or chronic, and it is usually of bacterial origin when it is acute. The symptoms are characterized by lower urinary tract symptoms (dysuria, frequency, urgency, incomplete emptying) and sometimes by back pain. Systemic signs of infection include fever, chills, and malaise. The key to differentiate prostatitis over a urinary tract infection or cystitis is the presence of systemic symptoms (usually not present with a UTI or cystitis) and a tender, edematous prostate on DRE. Acute bacterial prostatitis in older men is usually caused by gram negative organisms such as *E. coli*. In men <35 years, acute prostatitis is usually secondary to an STI such as from *C. trachomatis* or *N. gonorrhea*. Urinalysis and urine culture should guide selected antibiotic treatment. **Chronic prostatitis**, also known as chronic pelvic pain syndrome, can be either bacterial or nonbacterial. It usually has milder symptoms. Nonbacterial chronic prostatitis can be related to prior infections, can be neurological in origin, or can result from chemical irritation from urinary reflux. The key in the differential diagnosis is the chronicity of the symptoms and the lack of an identifiable infection. **BPH** is a clinical diagnosis based on the presence of lower urinary tract symptoms and absence of other causes. It will not have inflammatory or infectious signs such as fever, dysuria, or recurrent urinary tract infections. Though a PSA may be abnormal if checked during acute prostatitis, this would be a transient rise rather than persistent elevation as seen in prostate cancer.

Prostate cancer is the most common cancer in men, especially in men over the age of 65. Screening PSAs are a controversial topic, as most prostate cancers are very indolent and do not require treatment. However, risk factors such as family history may prompt testing. Diagnosis involves PSA level and biopsy of the prostate or suspicious metastatic lesion. Treatment includes surgical resection, radiation, chemotherapy, active surveillance, and testosterone suppression through the use of an LHRH agonist.

CASE 40 | Prostate Cancer

A 78-year-old man with a history of BPH presents with increased difficulty with urination, back pain, and weight loss. He denies dysuria, frequency, or other irritative symptoms. The back pain started 1 month ago, and it has been persistent. The pain wakes him up at night. NSAIDs and rest provide no relief. He denies bowel incontinence, saddle anesthesia, or difficulty walking. He has some mild nausea. His father has a history of prostate cancer. On exam, he is tender to palpation throughout his spine and bilateral pelvis. He has full passive range of motion in both legs and intact flexion and extension of the spine. Genital exam reveals a normal penis without evidence of meatal stenosis. His digital rectal exam reveals an asymmetric prostate with nodules and different textures.

Evaluation/Tests	Urinalysis shows microscopic hematuria with 12 RBCs/HPF. Serum PSA, prostatic acid phosphatase (PAP), and alkaline phosphatase are elevated. Prostate biopsy guided by transrectal ultrasound shows adenocarcinoma arising from the peripheral zone of the prostate. CT imaging of the spine shows multiple blastic lesions in multiple vertebrae. MRI shows no spinal cord compression.
Treatment	Hormone therapy, chemotherapy, palliative radiation.
Discussion	This patient is presenting with prostate cancer. The majority of prostate cancers are adenocarcinomas. They arise from the peripheral zone (posterior lobe) of the prostate, resulting in irregular and asymmetric nodularity on DRE. Prostate cancer typically is seen in older men (>50 years old), and risk is higher in those with a positive family history. In addition to DRE, PSA levels may be used for screening between the ages of 55 and 69 years; however, elevated PSA is not specific because it can also be elevated in BPH and acutely in prostatitis. If there is a concern for prostate cancer, a biopsy should be performed. Positive prostate biopsy results are then followed with histological scoring using the Gleason score, with higher numbers indicating a worse prognosis. Patients with negative prostate biopsy after an elevated PSA will be scheduled for continued PSA monitoring. If identified early, the disease is usually localized to the prostate, and it can be treated with curative intent via radical prostatectomy or radiation. Antiandrogen therapy may be combined with radiation and includes the GnRH analog leuprolide, the GnRH antagonist degarelix, or nonsteroidal androgen receptor inhibitors such as flutamide. Unlike prostatectomy or radiation, antiandrogen therapy is not curative. If identified late, prostatic adenocarcinoma may metastasize, most commonly to pelvic lymph nodes or to the vertebrae of the lumbosacral spine via the prostatic venous plexus, which communicates with the vertebral venous plexus. These metastases may be osteoblastic and result in elevated serum alkaline phosphatase. Compression of the spinal cord may also result in neurologic deficits. MRI of brain and spine could be ordered to help rule this out.

16

Respiratory

Christie Brillante, MD
Ashima Sahni, MD
Anthony Vergis, MD

DYSPNEA

Dyspnea is more commonly known as shortness of breath. It is a subjective experience (symptom) of breathing discomfort from the interactions among multiple physiological, psychological, social, and environmental factors that may induce secondary physiological and behavioral responses. Signs of dyspnea include tachypnea, tripod position, accessory muscle use, and intercostal retractions. Dyspnea can be a normal sensation after heavy exercise, but it becomes abnormal when it is associated with mild exertion or rest. Broadly, dyspnea can be categorized into cardiovascular or respiratory causes. We will review respiratory causes in this section.

Respiratory causes of dyspnea can be broadly divided into the following physiologic causes:

1. Increased respiratory drive involves increased afferent input to the respiratory centers within the brainstem, typically due to stimulation of chemoreceptors in the setting of hypercapnia (elevated CO_2). Hormones, such as elevated progesterone in pregnancy and liver cirrhosis, can also stimulate chemoreceptors. Hypoxia, in the absence of concomitant hypercapnia, *does not usually cause dyspnea*.

2. Impaired ventilatory mechanics due to increased workload on the chest (e.g., obesity, kyphoscoliosis) or neuromuscular weakness (e.g., myasthenia gravis, Guillain-Barré syndrome).

An approach to diagnosing the cause of dyspnea starts with a thorough history and examination. The chronicity, quality of symptoms, triggers, environmental and occupational exposures, and important associated symptoms such as cough, chest pain, wheezing, stridor, fevers or edema will help narrow the differential diagnosis. Determine if symptoms consistent with pulmonary (cough, hemoptysis), cardiac (chest pain), or anemia (blood loss) are present. Determine if physical examination signs consistent with any specific pathology, such as wheezing, crackles, diminished breath sounds, abnormal heart sounds, leg swelling, pallor, nodular liver edge, or kyphoscoliosis, are present.

After thoroughly assessing these, some laboratory tests are crucial in the workup of dyspnea. Initial useful labs and tests include pulse oximetry (SPO_2), CBC to check for anemia, basic metabolic panel (BMP) to evaluate renal function and bicarbonate levels (to clue in on compensated chronic hypercapnia), and TSH. Cardiac enzymes, brain natriuretic peptide (BNP), and D-dimer can also be useful in assessing for cardiac ischemia, heart failure, and pulmonary embolus, respectively. Imaging, such as chest X-rays and CT scans, can show parenchymal pulmonary and cardiac abnormalities. Other useful tests include ECG and echocardiography. Pulmonary function tests can identify obstructive or restrictive lung diseases. Further testing should be tailored based on suspicion; further testing options are listed in the following cases, but differentiating between the major physiologic causes and systems-based causes is always the first step in diagnosis.

Pulmonary function tests (PFT) play a significant role in the diagnosis of pulmonary disease. Spirometry is the initial PFT. A low FEV1/FVC (often defined as <70%) is diagnostic of obstruction. A plateau of the inspiratory and expiratory curves suggests large-airway obstruction in extrathoracic and intrathoracic locations, respectively. A symmetric decrease in both FEV1 and FVC suggests restrictive lung disease. A total lung capacity <80% of the patient's predicted value defines a restrictive defect. The diffusion capacity of the lung for carbon monoxide (DLCO) suggests impaired gas exchange. In the accompanying diagram, note the "scooping" of the *expiratory limb*, which demonstrates slowing of the expiratory flow.

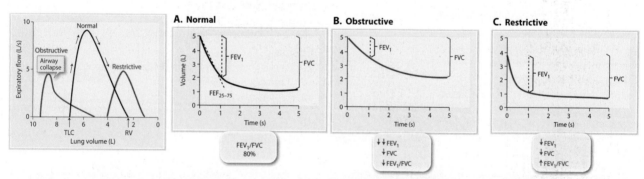

Flow-volume curves in obstructive and restrictive lung diseases. RV, residual volume; TLC, total lung capacity.
Spirograms showing a normal (A), obstructive (B), and restrictive (C) lung diseases. Obstructive and restrictive lung diseases are associated with smaller forced vital capacity (FVC) and forced expired volume in the first second ($FEV_{1.0}$). In obstructive lung disease, the $FEV_{1.0}$:FVC ratio is significantly decreased, whereas in restrictive lung disease, the $FEV_{1.0}$:FVC ratio is normal or increased.
Reproduced with permission from Kibble JD: The Big Picture Physiology: Medical Course & Step 1 Review, 2nd ed. New York, NY: McGraw Hill; 2020.

Dyspnea Differential Diagnoses (See "Cardiovascular" chapter for additional etiologies.)

Pulmonary	Pulmonary-Vascular	Cardiovascular
Airways:	Pulmonary hypertension	Heart failure (HF)
COPD/emphysema	pulmonary embolus	Cor pulmonale
Asthma	(thromboembolic, amniotic, fat)	Cardiomyopathy (CM)
Bronchitis	Hereditary hemorrhagic telangiectasia	Myocarditis (dilated CM)
Bronchiectasis	(pulmonary AVM)	Angina
Aspiration	Alveolar hemorrhage	ACS
Pneumothorax	Vasculitides	Cardiac tamponade
Obstructive sleep apnea (OSA)	Granulomatous polyangiitis (GPA)	Pericarditis
Alveolar:	Eosinophilic granulomatosis	Valvular heart disease
Pneumonia	with polyangiitis (EGPA, formerly	Arrhythmias
Atelectasis	Churg-Strauss)	Congenital heart disease
Acute respiratory distress syndrome (ARDS)	**Rheumatologic**	
Neonatal respiratory distress syndrome (NRDS)	Rheumatoid arthritis	**Neurologic**
Pleural:	Sjögren's	Central sleep apnea
Pleural effusion	Systemic lupus erythematous	Neuromuscular weakness (ALS,
Parenchymal lung disease/interstitial lung disease	Scleroderma	myasthenia gravis)
(ILD):	Polymyositis-dermatomyositis	Phrenic nerve palsy
(Idiopathic pulmonary fibrosis (IPF),	**Miscellaneous**	
pneumoconiosis)	Sarcoidosis	**Hematologic**
Lung cancer (primary or metastatic disease)	Obesity hypoventilation	Anemia
Congenital	Pregnancy	Leukemia
Cystic fibrosis	Panic attack/anxiety	Methemoglobinemia
	Altitude sickness	Acute chest syndrome (sickle cell
	Inhalation injuries	disease)

Key History Findings and Dyspnea Differential Diagnosis

Dyspnea with Key Associated History Findings	Diagnoses
Acute onset	Pneumothorax, pulmonary embolus, flash pulmonary edema due to MI, HF, or mitral regurgitation
Smoking history	COPD, lung cancer, MI
Wheezing	Asthma, COPD, HF
Cough with purulent sputum	Pneumonia, cystic fibrosis, COPD
Occupational exposure (coal miner, metal worker, sand blaster, construction, or shipping)	Pneumoconiosis (coal workers, silicosis), asbestosis
Birdkeeper or farmer	Hypersensitivity pneumonitis
Nocturnal dyspnea and nocturnal cough	Asthma, heart failure, GERD
Chest pain or pressure and dyspnea	Consider acute coronary syndrome, PE
Swelling or fluid retention	Heart failure or ascites (liver disease) or nephropathy
Orthopnea, paroxysmal nocturnal dyspnea, lower extremity edema	Heart failure, pericardial effusion +/− cardiac tamponade, constrictive pericarditis, cirrhosis (ascites), nephropathy
Dyspnea with exertion relieved with rest	Angina
Dyspnea with palpitations	Arrhythmias
History of bleeding, nutritional deficiency, hemolysis	Anemia

Key Exam Findings and Dyspnea Differential Diagnosis (See "Cardiovascular" chapter for additional etiologies.)

Dyspnea with Key Associated Exam Findings	Diagnoses
Pale conjunctiva	Anemia
Clubbing	Chronic hypoxia
Stridor	Foreign body aspiration, epiglottitis, angioedema

(continued)

Key Exam Findings and Dyspnea Differential Diagnosis (See "Cardiovascular" chapter for additional etiologies.) *(continued)*

Dyspnea with Key Associated Exam Findings	Diagnoses
Obesity, large neck	OSA, obesity hypoventilation syndrome
Wheezes	COPD, asthma, heart failure
Expiratory wheezing	Asthma
Bilateral: hyperresonant to percussion and decreased breath sounds, wheezing	COPD
Decrease breath sounds (BS) and dullness to percussion (usually unilateral)	Pleural effusion
Absent BS on affected side, tracheal deviation away from affected side, hyperresonant on percussion	Pneumothorax
Asymmetric chest expansion, diminished breath sounds, inspiratory crackles, bronchophony, egophony, increased tactile fremitus, dullness to percussion, whispered pectoriloquy on affected side	Pneumonia
Inspiratory crackles bilaterally	Pulmonary edema, pulmonary fibrosis
Inspiratory crackles bilaterally, clubbing	Pulmonary fibrosis
Elevated JVP, hepatojugular reflex, displaced apical impulse, crackles, S3, lower extremity edema	Heart failure
Muscular weakness	ALS, myasthenia gravis, GBS, Botulism

CASE 1 | Asthma (Acute Exacerbation)

A 22-year-old woman with no known chronic conditions presents with worsening shortness of breath and wheezing. She has had these symptoms intermittently for several years, but they have become more noticeable after she recently adopted a cat. She has also developed a dry cough at night that has not improved with over-the-counter cough medications. Her family history is remarkable for "breathing problems on her mother's side." She denies smoking cigarettes or use of illicit substances. Her vitals are blood pressure 120/80 mmHg, respirations 22/min, pulse 102/min and regular, SpO_2 98% on room air. Her BMI is 20. She appears to be in respiratory distress because she is unable to finish a full sentence, has alar flaring, and some intercostal rib retractions. On auscultation of her lungs, she has a prolonged expiratory-to-inspiratory ratio and high-pitched expiratory noises on bilateral lung fields (wheezes).

Evaluation/Tests	Clinical diagnosis. CXR shows flattening of the diaphragm, increased spaces between ribs, and no abnormal opacities. Peak expiratory flow rate is 60% of her predicted.
Treatment	Urgent or emergency treatment: short-acting beta 2 agonists (SABA), such as inhaled or nebulized albuterol. Systemic glucocorticoids, either oral or intravenous. IV magnesium can be administered if in severe exacerbation.
Discussion	Asthma is a chronic condition characterized by hyperresponsive bronchi, which causes reversible bronchoconstriction and airway inflammation. Severity of symptoms and exacerbation determine treatment. A severe exacerbation is characterized by inability to complete sentences or phrases, evidence of respiratory distress (alar flaring, supraclavicular and/or intercostal retractions), tripod positioning, and pulsus paradoxus (drop in systolic blood pressure by at least 12 mmHg with inspiration). In an acute setting, such as in this case, measurement of peak expiratory flow rates can help determine the severity of obstruction. A measurement below 200 L/min or ≤50% predicted suggests severe obstruction. The predicted values depend on sex, height, and weight. In a nonacute setting, patients may present with intermittent symptoms of wheezing, cough and dyspnea, typically after exposure to a trigger (dust mites, tobacco smoke, strong smells). Diagnosis is made by history and findings of reversible obstruction on spirometry or methacholine challenge test. On a PFT, the ***pre***bronchodilator flow loops will be either normal (if the patient's asthma is controlled) or show obstruction. The ***post***bronchodilator flow loops will show reversal of obstruction. If the prebronchodilator flow loops are normal, it would be safe to proceed to a **methacholine challenge test**. A patient's FEV1 is measured to establish a baseline, and then the patient is asked to inhale small concentrations of methacholine. In persons with airway hyperresponsiveness, even low doses of methacholine will induce bronchoconstriction. A reduction in FEV1 of at least 20% from baseline suggests asthma.

CASE 1 | Asthma (Acute Exacerbation) *(continued)*

Discussion	The mainstay of nonpharmacologic treatment is avoidance of triggers, which may include allergens (dust mites, pollen, pet dander, cockroaches), extremes of temperatures, or viral URIs. Medications are often started in a stepwise fashion depending on the level of asthma control. All patients should have an as needed inhaled corticosteroid (to reduce exacerbation) and an as needed short acting beta agonist (to relieve symptoms). The next step includes daily inhaled corticosteroids (ICS), which can be up- or down-titrated. For poorly controlled asthma symptoms, additional medications that can be added in a stepwise fashion include long-acting beta 2 agonists (LABA), antimuscarinics or leukotriene modifiers. Cases refractory to usual medications can be treated with biologics (such as omalizumab or dupilumab) or a procedure called bronchothermoplasty. On pathology, airways are characterized by smooth muscle hypertrophy and hyperplasia, Curschmann spirals and Charcot-Leyden crystals.

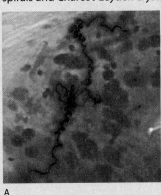 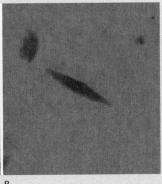

A B

A: Curschmann spirals shed epithelium forms whorled mucous plugs.
B: Charcot Leyden crystals are eosinophilic, hexagonal, double-pointed crystals formed from breakdown of eosinophils in sputum.
Part A used with permission from Dr. Yale Rosen / Wikimedia Commons.
Part B reproduced with permission from Gholamnejad M, Rezaie N. Unusual presentation of chronic eosinophilic pneumonia with "reversed halo sign": a case report, Iran J Radiol 2014 May;11(2):e7891.

COPD typically occurs in smokers, and is characterized by persistent airflow obstruction and accelerated irreversible decline in lung function. **Chronic bronchitis**, is a clinical diagnosis (productive cough >3 months for 2 years). Patients are typically overweight and have early hypercarbia and hypoxia. **Emphysema**, is the destruction and dilatation of terminal airways and affected patients appear thin and cachectic with pursed lips and have late hypercarbia/hypoxia. Smoking typically causes centrilobular destruction, and **low α-1-antitrypsin** activity results in uninhibited elastase in the alveoli, causing panacinar emphysema. In COPD, CXR reveals hyperexpansion as evident by flattened diaphragm, increased retrosternal airspace, and increased anterior-posterior diameter. Pulmonary function tests will show a FEV1/FVC (the ratio of the volume of air forcefully exhaled in 1 second to the total volume forcefully exhaled) <70%. Treatment includes short and long acting beta agonists and muscarinic antagonists, separate or in combination. Acute exacerbations may also treated with steroids, antibiotics and oxygen if needed.

Hypersensitivity pneumonitis (extrinsic allergic alveolitis) presents in patients with exposure to organic dusts from mold, birds (bird fancier's lung), or thermophilic bacteria (hot tube alveolitis).

Additional Considerations	**Exercise-induced asthma** is an asthma variant characterized by coughing and/or dyspnea with onset after about 10 minutes of exercise. Within the first few minutes of exercise, airways will dilate, followed by bronchoconstriction that resolves about 1 hour after exercise. Dyspnea from deconditioning will resolve in <5 minutes postexercise. The treatment includes encouragement of cardiovascular fitness, prophylactic use of SABA 10 minutes prior to exercise or, if refractory, the use of ICS. **Aspirin or NSAID-exacerbated respiratory disease** is characterized by chronic sinusitis with nasal polyps, asthma symptoms, and acute upper and lower respiratory tract symptoms with COX inhibition (leukotriene overproduction results in airway constriction).

CASE 2 | Acute Respiratory Distress Syndrome (ARDS)

A 35-year-old man with a history of alcohol abuse presents with acutely worsening shortness of breath and severe abdominal pain. He notes that the epigastric pain has been increasing in intensity over the past 2 days. He drinks a pint of vodka every day. He has had some nausea and vomiting but no hematemesis. He denies a history of cigarette smoking, vaping, or illicit drug use. On exam, he is anicteric, in respiratory distress, and diaphoretic. His vital signs are blood pressure 100/80 mmHg, respirations 28/min, pulse of 130/min, temp 38°C, and SpO_2 88% on room air. BMI is 28.

He has bilateral diffuse inspiratory crackles and hypoactive bowel sounds and epigastric tenderness. During the evaluation, he decompensates further and becomes cyanotic and progressively hypoxic. He is intubated and started on lung-protective mechanical ventilation.

CASE 2 | Acute Respiratory Distress Syndrome (ARDS) *(continued)*

Evaluation/Tests	The chest X-ray shows diffuse fluffy infiltrates throughout the lung fields. Lipase >3000 U/L. CBC is notable for an elevated WBC count. Blood, sputum, and urine cultures are negative. BNP and PCWP are normal. Arterial blood gas shows hypoxemia. CXR postintubation shows diffuse bilateral opacities. Reproduced with permission from Imanaka H, Takahara B, Yamaguchi H, et al: Chest computed tomography of a patient revealing severe hypoxia due to amniotic fluid embolism: a case report, J Med Case Rep 2010 Feb 18;4:55.
Treatment	Treatment consists of supportive care, maintenance of adequate oxygenation, and treatment of the underlying cause. If oxygenation becomes difficult, intubation and ventilator support should be considered with lung-protective ventilation (low tidal volumes and increased PEEP).
Discussion	This patient is presenting with ARDS in the setting of acute pancreatitis. ARDS is a clinical diagnosis of exclusion and is characterized by progressive dyspnea, increased oxygen requirement, and bilateral lung infiltrates on imaging that occurs within 6–72 hours of insult. A helpful mnemonic is **ARDS**: **A**bnormal imaging (bilateral opacities on CXR or CT) **R**espiratory failure within 1 week of alveolar injury **D**ecreased PaO2/FiO2 (ratio <300) **S**ymptoms of respiratory failure not due to fluid overload from heart failure (noncardiogenic with a normal PCWP). Common causes of ARDS include sepsis, pneumonia, aspiration, trauma, and pancreatitis. The three phases of ARDS are as follows: 1. Exudative (<7–10 days)—Injury results in release of proinflammatory cytokines (e.g., TNF-α, IL-1, IL-6, IL-8). In turn, these cytokines promote neutrophil recruitment into the lungs. Neutrophils can then release proteases and additional inflammatory mediators and produce reactive oxygen species, which then injure epithelial and endothelial cells. Damage to these cells increases vascular permeability, promoting leakage of fluid into the interstitial space and alveoli. 2. Proliferative (1–2 weeks)—Resolution of pulmonary edema, proliferation of type II alveolar cells (stem cell precursors and surfactant-producing cells), early deposition of collagen. 3. Fibrotic (>2 weeks)—This occurs in some patients with resulting diffuse fibrosis and subsequent loss of normal lung architecture. Arrow shows hyaline membrane. Note the pink proteinaceous edema fluid within alveoli. Reproduced with permission from Pires-Neto RC, Del Carlo Bernardi F, et al: The Expression of Water and Ion Channels in Diffuse Alveolar Damage Is Not Dependent on DAD Etiology, PLoS One 2016 Nov 11;11(11):e0166184. The consequences of ARDS can include loss of normal lung compliance and pulmonary hypertension. **Aspiration pneumonia** can precipitate ARDS, but aspiration pneumonia typically presents with lobar distribution of lung opacities, fever, productive cough, chills, and/or rigors. **Pulmonary embolism** can cause hypoxemia; however, the CXR findings are typically normal.
Additional Considerations	**ARDS in children** is most commonly precipitated by respiratory viral or bacterial pathogens. Other risk factors include pulmonary contusion, inhalational injury, near drowning, sepsis, trauma, and burns. Diagnostic criteria are also similar in adult and pediatric groups.

CASE 2 | Acute Respiratory Distress Syndrome (ARDS) *(continued)*

| Additional Considerations | **Neonatal respiratory distress syndrome (NRDS)** is primarily caused by surfactant deficiency. With low or absent surfactant, the surface tension within alveolar walls is high. High surface tension results in low compliance, resulting in collapse of alveoli. This can be seen on CXR as a characteristic "ground-glass appearance."

 Recall the **Law of Laplace: Pressure = 2T/r**, wherein if the surface tension (T) increases or the radius of a sphere decreases, the pressure (P) required to *prevent collapse* of the sphere—the collapsing pressure—increases.

 Surfactant will reduce surface tension in smaller alveoli, preventing their collapse. In conditions such as NRDS with low surfactant, the alveoli collapse more easily. The main risk factor for NRDS is prematurity. Maternal diabetes (due to high fetal insulin) and C-section delivery (due to low fetal glucocorticoid release as compared to vaginal delivery) are other significant risk factors. | 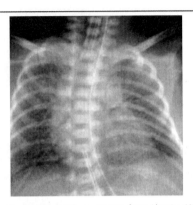 Reproduced with permission from Alorainy IA, Barlas NB, Al-Boukai AA. Pictorial Essay: Infants of diabetic mothers, Indian J Radiol Imaging 2010 Aug;20(3):174-181. |

CASE 3 | Idiopathic Pulmonary Fibrosis

A 65-year-old man with a history of tobacco use presents with increasing dyspnea over a period of 8 months. His symptoms have been slowly worsening, and he presents to the clinic because he can no longer climb one flight of stairs without stopping to catch his breath. He reports a worsening persistent dry cough. He denies extremity swelling. He is a 30 pack year smoker but has no other known medical conditions. He is a retired lawyer. On physical exam, he is not in acute distress, and his vital signs are blood pressure 120/80 mmHg, respirations 22/min, pulse 100/min, temp 37.5°C, and SpO$_2$ 88% on room air. His cardiac examination is normal. Auscultation of the lungs reveals bibasilar fine inspiratory crackles. Extremities exhibit digital clubbing but no edema.

Evaluation/Tests	CXR shows increased bilateral basal reticular markings (Inferior, Peripheral Fibrosis). High-resolution CT shows clustered subpleural bibasilar enlarged air spaces with thick walls ("honeycombing"). 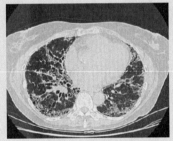 Idiopathic pulmonary fibrosis. CT scan of the lungs showing the typical radiographic pattern of idiopathic pulmonary fibrosis, with a predominantly basilar, peripheral pattern of traction bronchiectasis, reticulation, and early honeycombing. Reproduced with permission from Papadakis MA, McPhee SJ, Rabow MW: Current Medical Diagnosis & Treatment 2021. New York, NY: McGraw Hill; 2021. PFTs reveal decreased FVC and DLCO without a reduction in FEV1/FVC ratio, consistent with restrictive lung disease. Autoimmune panel, including evaluation for rheumatoid arthritis (RA), Sjögren's, SLE, scleroderma, and polymyositis-dermatomyositis were normal.
Treatment	Start oxygen therapy, refer to pulmonary rehabilitation, and vaccinate against influenza and pneumonia. Advise smoking cessation. Medications to decrease fibroblast activation and proliferation, including pirfenidone or nintedanib.
Discussion	Idiopathic pulmonary fibrosis (IPF) is a severe chronic and progressive disease characterized by pulmonary fibrosis and eventual pulmonary hypertension and cor pulmonale. Diagnosis is based on clinical presentation, exclusion of other causes, chest imaging, and sometimes pathologic evaluation. Imaging findings highly suggestive of IPF include subpleural, basilar predominant honeycombing. If the CT scan is consistent, lung biopsy can be avoided. When surgical lung biopsy is performed, it shows a usual interstitial pneumonia pattern. Historically, vaccination, smoking cessation, and oxygen therapy have been used for treatment. Steroids do not have a role in treatment. Treatment is limited to medications that limit fibroblast proliferation among other mechanisms. Lung transplantation is also a possible option for patients with IPF.

CASE 3 | **Idiopathic Pulmonary Fibrosis** *(continued)*

Discussion	Diagnosis is made by excluding other etiologies and characteristic findings on imaging and biopsy. Clinical history and physical examination should focus on occupational history, rheumatologic signs/symptoms (Raynaud phenomenon, joint pain, digital ulcers, fevers, telangiectasia), medications (amiodarone, bleomycin, nitrofurantoin), and family history to rule out other conditions such as pneumoconiosis, hypersensitivity pneumonitis, COPD, or heart failure.

CASE 4 | Sarcoidosis

A 35-year-old woman with no previous medical history presents with a 3-month history of exertional dyspnea and nonproductive cough. She has also had chronic generalized muscle and bilateral ankle joint pain as well as unintentional weight loss. She has occasional chest pain that is not related to exertion. She also reports red and occasionally dry eyes. She takes no medications. She has never smoked and denies alcohol or illicit substance use. She is currently employed as a librarian; prior to that, she had only worked in the college bookstore. She has not traveled outside of her state in 3 years. Her family history is unremarkable.

On physical exam, her vital signs are blood pressure 120/80 mmHg, pulse 80/min, respirations 20/min, and temperature 37.5°C, and BMI is 28. Examination of her head and neck shows a purplish red indurated plaque on the nose and enlarged mobile nontender cervical lymphadenopathy. Her left eye demonstrates ciliary injection (uveitis). Cardiac examination is notable for a loud P2 and bilateral pitting edema on both ankles. Auscultation of the lungs reveals bilateral fine diffuse crackles. General skin examination reveals tender subcutaneous nodules along the extensor surface of both legs (erythema nodosum).

Evaluation/Tests	CBC shows mild anemia and lymphopenia. Urinalysis and serum electrolyte panel were unremarkable apart from a slightly elevated serum calcium. CXR shows diffusely increased reticular markings as well as bilateral enlargement of lymph nodes of the pulmonary hila. A subsequent noncontrast chest CT reveals the extent of lymph node enlargement. 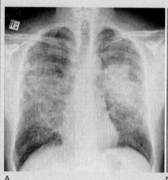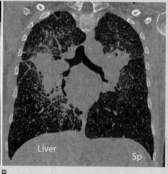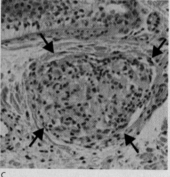 A B C Part A and B reproduced with permission from Lønborg J, Ward M, Gill A, et al: Utility of cardiac magnetic resonance in assessing right-sided heart failure in sarcoidosis, BMC Med Imaging 2013 Jan 11;13:2. Part C reproduced with permission from Kajal B, Harvey J, Alowami S. Melkerrson-Rosenthal Syndrome, a rare case report of chronic eyelid swelling, Diagn Pathol 2013 Nov 13;8:188. A bronchoscopy is performed, and sampling with an ultrasonically guided fine-needle biopsy is performed on an enlarged lymph node. Pathologic studies on the tissue reveal noncaseating granulomas characterized by a collection of modified mononuclear phagocytes with a central area of epithelioid cells sharing cytoplasm with multiple nuclei. There is no debris within the collection of cells. The stains were negative for fungi and mycobacteria. A bronchoalveolar lavage is negative for fungal and mycobacterial elements. The CD4/CD8 ratio is elevated. Additional studies reveal negative PPD, HIV, and negative urine Ab for histoplasma and blastomycosis.
Treatment	Glucocorticoids are first line, followed by methotrexate or TNF alpha inhibitors.
Discussion	Sarcoidosis is an idiopathic disease characterized by multisystem immune-mediated, widespread noncaseating granulomas. The most common symptoms are cough and dyspnea. Nonspecific constitutional symptoms include fatigue, fever, night sweats, and weight loss. Many patients will experience resolution within 5 years. A small percentage of patients can develop restrictive disease characterized by parenchymal fibrosis. Other organs that can be affected include eyes (uveitis), heart

CASE 4 | Sarcoidosis *(continued)*

Discussion	(conduction abnormalities or cardiomyopathy), the CNS (7th nerve palsy, which can be mistaken for Bell's palsy), skin (lupus pernio, erythema nodosum), and joints (rheumatoid arthritis-like arthropathy). There is no single test to diagnose sarcoidosis. Diagnosis is made by a combination of clinical history, physical exam findings, radiologic findings, and biopsy showing noncaseating granulomatous inflammation (figure C). Once a diagnosis is made, evaluation of extrapulmonary involvement should be completed and includes: • Pulmonary function tests to evaluate for restrictive defect and/or reduced DLCO; • Ophthalmologic exam (visual acuity, tonometry, slit lamp, and fundoscopic testing) to evaluate for optic neuritis or uveitis; • ECG to evaluate for heart block and arrhythmias; • Echocardiogram to evaluate for pericardial effusion, valve abnormalities, and right heart complications, including pulmonary hypertension. The loud P2 in this patient suggests elevated right heart pressures. Not all patients require treatment. Those with more severe or persistent symptoms should be treated, typically with systemic steroids. Steroid sparing agents, such as methotrexate, have been used. Serum markers are not helpful to diagnose sarcoidosis but are helpful to exclude other diseases, such as HIV. Although sarcoid is associated with elevated serum angiotensin-converting enzyme, it is not a reliable diagnostic test. Biopsy will help distinguish from other diseases, such as foreign body reaction, leprosy, lymphoma, or mycobacteria. **Berylliosis** also presents with noncaseating granulomas but results from exposure to beryllium and its compounds.

CASE 5 | Silicosis

A 53-year-old man presents with progressive exertional dyspnea, productive cough, fatigue, and some weight loss over the past several years. He smokes an occasional cigarette but otherwise does not drink alcohol or use illicit substances. He is a construction worker and has worked in sandblasting to remove paint from surfaces as well as coal mining. On physical exam, vital signs are temperature 36.5°C, blood pressure 120/80 mmHg, respirations 20/min, pulse 80/min, and SpO_2 90% on room air. His lung exam is notable for diffuse fine crackles. The rest of his exam is unremarkable.

Evaluation/Tests	Chest X-ray shows multiple nodular opacities in the upper lobes and hilar lymphadenopathy (with peripheral calcifications). A CT scan of the chest shows bilateral ground glass opacities predominantly in the upper lobes, hilar and mediastinal lymphadenopathy, and calcification of the lymph nodes at the periphery of the node (eggshell calcification). PFTs reveal FEV1 50%, FVC 48%, normal FEV1/FVC ratio, and TLC 57% with a DLCO 45%.
Treatment	Oxygen therapy as needed, cessation of exposure.
Discussion	This is a classic presentation of silicosis, an occupational pneumoconiosis that is caused by the inhalation of crystalline silicon dioxide (silica). It is the most prevalent chronic occupational lung disease in the world. Occupations associated with this disease are sandblasting, coal mining, stone cutting, and work in foundries. Complications of the disease include cor pulmonale, as well as increased risk of lung cancer, pulmonary tuberculosis, and rheumatoid pneumoconiosis (Caplan's syndrome). Progressive dyspnea is the most common symptom. A productive cough is frequent and is caused by bronchitis from dust inhalation or by compression of the large airways by silicotic nodules. Hemoptysis is not a common presentation and should trigger an evaluation for lung cancer or tuberculosis. The classic imaging findings are "eggshell calcifications" of the hilar lymph nodes, which represent dystrophic calcification. A biopsy is not typically performed as the constellation of occupational exposure and typical chest imaging findings are usually adequate for diagnosis. If biopsy is performed, it would show "silicotic nodules," which are small nodules of fibroblasts and histiocytes with abundant silica. Unfortunately, there is no effective treatment.
Additional Considerations	Other significant occupational pneumoconiosis include: **Asbestosis**—Exposure to asbestos increases the risk for bronchogenic cancer and mesothelioma. It primarily affects the lower lobes, and imaging shows calcified subdiaphragmatic pleural plaques. Sheet metal workers, plumbers, pipefitters, shipbuilders, and building custodians are at risk of exposure.

CASE 5 | Silicosis *(continued)*

Additional Considerations	**Coal workers' pneumoconiosis**, also known as *black lung disease*, is due to prolonged coal dust exposure. Macrophages laden with carbon cause inflammation and fibrosis. This is different from *anthracosis*—an asymptomatic condition caused by repeated exposure to air pollution or carbon, which is common in city dwellers. **Berylliosis**—Nuclear and aerospace industry workers are at risk of developing berylliosis, which also affects the upper lobes and causes noncaseating granulomas, increases the risk of cancer, and complications include cor pulmonale.

CYANOSIS, HYPOXIA, AND HYPOXEMIA

Cyanosis is a symptom and a sign defined as a bluish skin discoloration representing tissue hypoxia that is sometimes associated with shortness of breath. It stems from deoxygenated or reduced hemoglobin in the blood. **Central cyanosis** is evident on the lips, tongue, and sublingual tissues. **Peripheral cyanosis** is a bluish discoloration of the hands and feet and is the result of vasoconstriction and diminished peripheral blood flow. Central cyanosis is due to reduced arterial oxygen saturation or abnormal hemoglobin; it presents later in a disease process, so it is of greater concern.

Hypoxemia is a decrease in the partial pressure of oxygen in the *blood*. It can be diagnosed with an arterial blood gas or pulse oximetry. **Hypoxia** is the reduced level of *tissue* oxygenation. Hypoxia and hypoxemia do not always coexist. In cyanide poisoning, cells are unable to utilize oxygen (hypoxia) despite having normal blood oxygen level (normoxemia).

Determining the etiology of hypoxemia usually includes obtaining an arterial blood gas and calculating the alveolar–arterial (A-a) oxygen gradient. The A-a gradient is the difference between alveolar (PAO_2) and arterial (PaO_2) oxygen levels. In general, the normal A-a gradient is 10 mmHg, but it increases with age. A larger than expected difference between the alveolar and arterial oxygen levels indicates a pathology of the alveolocapillary unit.

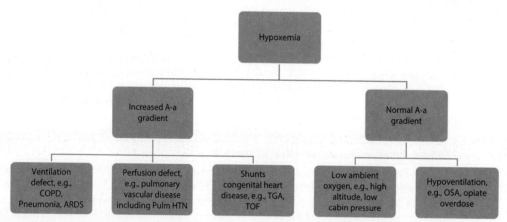

Diseases with increased A-a gradient denote a defect in the alveolocapillary unit, causing a wide difference between oxygen concentration in alveolus vs. artery. Conditions with a normal A-a gradient denote adequate alveolocapillary units.

Another strategy for developing a differential diagnosis of cyanosis, hypoxia, and hypoxemia is to think about different etiologies by age—neonates vs. children vs. adults—or by organ system. Differential diagnosis of cyanosis is often cardiac (see "Cardiovascular" chapter), but noncardiac etiologies include pulmonary and hematologic causes. In order to investigate pulmonary etiologies, it is important to ask about possible exposures like cyanide or carbon monoxide. Lower airway obstruction from smoke particles, for example, in a house fire, and upper airway obstruction from direct thermal injury are also common. Unintentional exposures to asphyxiating gases such as hydrogen sulfide, methane, or hydrocarbons can also occur. Severe upper airway obstruction should also be on the differential when physical exam findings are consistent with stridor, voice changes, or suprasternal retractions. Differential for hematological causes of cyanosis includes methemoglobinemia and acute chest syndrome from sickle cell disease. Neurological diseases that could be contributing to cyanosis include major head trauma or bleeding and seizures. Initial workup of cyanosis should include a complete blood count, basic metabolic panel, arterial blood gas, and chest radiograph; if a congenital heart disease is suspected, then an echocardiogram is warranted.

Differentials for Cyanosis, Hypoxia, Hypoxemia by Organ System

Pulmonary	Cardiac	Hematologic	Toxic	Other
Pneumonia COPD ARDS NRDS Parenchymal lung disease OSA Obesity hypoventilation syndrome (OHS) Pulmonary hypertension Hypoventilation	Heart failure Right to left shunt Eisenmenger syndrome Coarctation of aorta Congenital heart disease (See "Cardiovascular" chapter.)	Acute chest syndrome Hemoglobinopathies	Carbon monoxide poisoning (cherry red skin rather than cyanosis) Methemoglobin Cyanide poisoning	High altitude Hypothermia Arterial or venous obstruction (peripheral cyanosis) Raynaud's

Key Associated Findings and Cyanosis Differential Diagnosis

Cyanosis with Key Associated Findings	Diagnoses
Cyanosis from birth, murmurs or other cardiac abnormalities	Congenital heart disease, cardiac cause (See "Cardiovascular" chapter.)
History of murmurs in childhood presenting with cyanosis older in age and right heart failure symptoms	Eisenmenger syndrome
Bilateral pulmonary infiltrates	Cardiogenic pulmonary edema, pneumonia, ARDS, NRDS
Snoring, nocturnal oxygen desaturation, large tonsils	Obstructive sleep apnea
Old heating system or early winter	Carbon monoxide
Sodium nitroprusside use	Cyanide poisoning
Exposure to nitrates, benzocaine	Methemoglobin
Worsening extremity cyanosis in cold weather	Raynaud's, scleroderma

---

CASE 6 | Inhalational Injury: Carbon Monoxide (CO) Poisoning

A 45-year-old man is brought to the emergency department by EMS after his wife found him unconscious in his garage. The patient was working in the garage, which was being warmed by an old kerosene heater. History is obtained primarily from the wife. Prior to passing out, he had complained of some dizziness and headaches. He is a ½ pack per day (ppd) smoker and occasional alcohol drinker. He does not use illicit drugs. He has no other medical problems. EMS reports his blood glucose level is 150 mmol/L.

On focused exam in the ED, his vitals are blood pressure 98/60 mmHg, temperature 37.5°C, pulse 102/min regular, respirations 22/min, and pulse oximetry on room air 97%.

He regains consciousness and opens his eyes to voice and follows some commands, but he is confused and disoriented. He is able to move all extremities spontaneously and purposefully. His pupils are equally round and reactive to light, and he has very flushed skin (cherry-red skin). His head is atraumatic, and his cardiovascular, pulmonary, and abdominal exams are unremarkable.

Evaluation/Tests	Urine toxicology is negative. CT head noncontrast is negative for hemorrhage or fracture. CBC and comprehensive metabolic panel are unremarkable. Arterial blood gas reveals carboxyhemoglobin of 23%. If done, an MRI may show FLAIR hyperintense foci in bilateral globus pallidus.
Treatment	100% inhaled oxygen.

CASE 6 | Inhalational Injury: Carbon Monoxide (CO) Poisoning (continued)

Discussion	Diagnosis of CO poisoning and carboxyhemoglobinemia requires high index of suspicion based on history. Carbon monoxide is an odorless, tasteless, colorless, nonirritating gas that is one of the leading causes of poisoning in the United States. Although fires remain a significant cause of CO poisoning, gas-powered electric generators, kerosene heaters, charcoal grills, camping stoves, and motor vehicles are also sources of carbon monoxide. Altered mental status and headache are the most common symptoms. Complications include myocardial ischemia and neurocognitive deficits, which may persist. Cyanosis is masked by the cherry red color of carboxyhemoglobin. Pulse oximetry will be normal as it does not differentiate carboxyhemoglobin from oxyhemoglobin. Carboxyhemoglobin measurement by arterial blood gas is the test of choice. Smokers have a baseline CO level of up to 15%, while nonsmokers have up to 3%. The treatment with oxygen administration decreases the half-life of carboxyhemoglobin from 4–5 hours to 60 minutes. Hyperbaric oxygen should be used in situations of severely elevated COHb. Hemoglobin (Hb) has a higher affinity for CO than oxygen; therefore, Hb preferentially binds CO, forming carboxyhemoglobin (COHb). This results in decreased 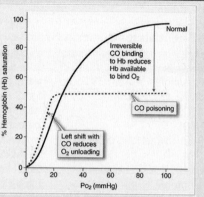 Effect of carbon monoxide (CO) poisoning on oxyhemoglobin dissociation curve. CO binds irreversibly to hemoglobin, decreasing the fraction of total hemoglobin available for oxygen (O_2) saturation. CO binding also causes a left shift in the curve, reducing O_2 unloading from the remaining oxyhemoglobin. Reproduced with permission from Kibble JD, Halsey CR: Medical Physiology: The Big Picture. New York, NY: McGraw Hill; 2009. oxygen saturation and shifts the oxygen–hemoglobin dissociation curve to the left, making it more difficult for hemoglobin to bind oxygen in the lungs and release oxygen to the tissues. This results in tissue hypoperfusion and lactic acidosis. Both carbon monoxide and cyanide (a frequent concomitant poison in housefires) are cellular asphyxiants. They bind to complex IV and prevent oxidative phosphorylation, leading to metabolic acidosis and anaerobic metabolism. Unlike CO poisoning, the oxygen–Hgb curve is normal in cyanide poisoning.
Additional Considerations	**Cyanide poisoning:** Cyanide (CN) is a rapidly acting poison commonly caused by domestic fires (burning insulation, upholstery, plastic, melamine, wool, or silk), but it can come from prolonged sodium nitroprusside infusions. CN can be absorbed through mucus membranes, respiratory tract, GI tract, and skin. Cyanide binds to the ferric ion (Fe^{3+}) of cytochrome oxidase a3, interrupting the electron transport chain and causing histotoxic hypoxia. Typical findings in the right clinical context include lactic acidosis and a high anion gap metabolic acidosis. Treatment is often started empirically based on clinical suspicion because serum cyanide levels (the confirmatory test) is not widely available. Treatments consist of: • Hydroxocobalamin, which binds cyanide and forms cyanocobalamin, which can then be excreted by the kidneys; • Nitrites, which cause oxidation of hemoglobin to methemoglobin (methemoglobin binds cyanide and forms cyanomethemoglobin, which is a less toxic byproduct compared to cyanide); • Sodium thiosulfate, which promotes conversion of cyanide to thiocyanate, which can undergo renal excretion. **Methemoglobinemia** can be a complication of nitrite-based treatment of CN poisoning. Methemoglobinemia is hemoglobin oxidized to its ferric (Fe^{3+}) state, making it incapable of carrying oxygen. Patients may present with dizziness, headache, nausea, and shortness of breath. Clinical diagnosis is suggested by cyanosis despite normal partial pressure of oxygen on ABG. Other clues to diagnosis include known exposure to a precipitating agent (e.g., medications), cyanosis unresponsive to supplemental oxygen, and chocolate-colored blood on arterial blood draw. The diagnosis of acquired methemoglobinemia is with a methemoglobin assay, using either venous or arterial blood. Drugs that may induce acquired methemoglobinemia include sulfonamides (sulfamethoxazole), dapsone, lidocaine, nitrates, nitrogen oxide gases, or phenazopyridine. Treatment is with methylene blue and vitamin C.

CHEST PAIN—PULMONARY CAUSES

Chest pain is often associated with cardiac problems, but it is important to recognize that other organ systems are often involved. The quality of pulmonary chest pain is usually described as pleuritic. Pleuritic pain is usually sharp, sudden onset, and worse with inspiration or expiration and movement. It is caused by irritation of the pleura, which are the linings of the lung. It can also be caused by irritation of surrounding structures like the pericardium, ribs, and intercostal muscles. Pain can also be referred. For example, pain from the diaphragm can be referred to the shoulder or trapezius ridge. Associated symptoms are usually helpful in determining the cause of the chest pain.

Common initial tests and evaluations to confirm or refute diagnoses for patients presenting with chest pain include chest X-ray, CT scan of the chest, pulse oximetry, arterial blood gases (ABG), trial of medications, ECG, cardiac biomarkers, and echocardiogram (ECHO).

Following are some of the key diagnoses. (See "Cardiovascular" chapter for more detailed list.)

Differential Diagnosis for Chest Pain

Pulmonary	Cardiac	Other
Pneumothorax	Acute coronary syndrome	Acute chest syndrome (sickle cell disease)
Pulmonary embolus (PE)	Pericarditis	Gastroesophageal reflux (GERD)
Pleuritis	Heart failure (HF)	Esophageal spasm
Pneumonia/bronchitis	Myocarditis	Peptic ulcer disease (PUD)/gastritis
Chronic obstructive pulmonary disease (COPD)	Vasospasm	Pancreatitis
Asthma	Aortic dissection	Cholecystitis
Sarcoidosis	Valvular heart disease	Mallory-Weiss syndrome
Lung cancer	Arrhythmia	Panic attack
		Trauma
		Referred pain
		Costochondritis
		Muscle strain
		Zoster

Key History Findings and Chest Pain Differential Diagnosis (See "Chest Pain" in "Cardiovascular" chapter for more details.)

Chest Pain with Key Associated Findings	Diagnoses
Sudden onset	Pneumothorax, PE
Radiation to the shoulder or trapezius ridge	Diaphragmatic irritation (e.g., due to pneumonia/effusion)
Fever	Pneumonia, pleuritis
Associated with SOB	Consider pulmonary causes or heart failure
Associated with wheezing	Asthma/COPD
Hemoptysis	PE, pneumonia, cancer
Worse with deep inspiration (pleuritic pain)	PE, pericarditis, pleuritis, pneumonia
Acute pain after prolonged immobilization On oral contraceptive pills	PE
Shoulder pain with radiation to ipsilateral ulnar nerve distribution	Pancoast tumor

Key Exam Findings and Chest Pain Differential Diagnosis (See "Chest Pain" in "Cardiovascular" chapter for more details.)

Chest Pain and Key Associated Exam Findings	Diagnoses
Decrease systolic BP with inspiration (pulsus paradoxus)	Pericardial tamponade, COPD, pneumothorax
Asymmetric absent breath sounds	Pneumothorax or pleural effusion

(continued)

Key Exam Findings and Chest Pain Differential Diagnosis (See "Chest Pain" in "Cardiovascular" chapter for more details.) *(continued)*

Chest Pain and Key Associated Exam Findings	Diagnoses
Tympany upon percussion of chest wall	Pneumothorax
Dullness to percussion of chest wall	Pleural effusion, pneumonia
Focal abnormal lung sounds	Pneumonia
Wheezing	Asthma/COPD

CASE 7 | Primary Spontaneous (Simple) Pneumothorax

A 24-year-old man presents with sudden onset of severe left-sided chest pain and shortness of breath. The pain is sharp and worse with inspiration. He was driving his car when he suddenly felt the pain. He denies any trauma or prior surgeries. He denies cough, fevers, or leg swelling. He smokes 5 cigarettes a day, drinks alcohol occasionally, and smokes marijuana occasionally. On exam, his vitals are temperature 37.4°C, blood pressure 100/70 mmHg, pulse 120/min regular, respirations 24/min, and SpO$_2$ 93% on room air. He is tall, thin, and in acute respiratory distress with alar flaring and breathlessness when speaking. His trachea is midline, his chest wall demonstrates decreased excursion on the left hemithorax compared to the right. There is also hyperresonance on percussion, decreased tactile fremitus, and decreased breath sounds of the left hemithorax. His heart sounds are diminished.

Evaluation/Tests	CXR shows midline trachea, with absent lung markings on the left lung field consistent with pneumothorax. EKG shows sinus tachycardia.
Treatment	Treat with oxygen. In this unstable patient, insert a small-bore chest tube. Stable patients can be treated with oxygen and observation.
Discussion	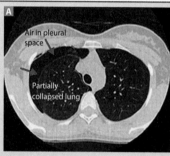 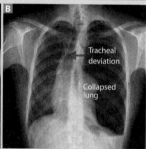 Part A reproduced with permission from Miura K, Kondo R, Kurai M, et al: Birt-Hogg-Dubé syndrome detected incidentally by asymptomatic bilateral pneumothorax in health screening: a case of a young Japanese woman, Surg Case Rep 2015 Dec;1(1):17. Part B reproduced with permission from Rosat A, Díaz C. Reexpansion pulmonary edema after drainage of tension pneumothorax, Pan Afr Med J 2015 Oct 15;22:143. A pneumothorax is caused by rupture of cysts or blebs. The rupture causes air to accumulate in the pleural space, which in turn leads to collapse of the lung on the affected side. Crepitus may be palpated along the chest wall from subcutaneous emphysema. This patient has a **primary pneumothorax**. He has no associated underlying lung disease. It is classically seen in tall thin smokers. **Secondary pneumothorax** occurs in the setting of an underlying lung disease such as emphysema, Marfan disease, or cystic lung disease. In **a tension pneumothorax**, air is able to get into the pleural cavity but has no way to leave, so intrathoracic pressure continually increases with every inspiration. As there is increased pressure on the affected side, the trachea may shift toward the opposite side. The accumulation of positive air pressure within the hemithorax can impinge the great vessels, causing decreased venous return. This results in decreased cardiac output and can lead to shock. Tension pneumothorax is a medical emergency and requires emergent needle decompression. Physical exam and imaging help rule out other conditions such as MI, PE, aortic dissection, muscular pain, or pericarditis.

CASE 8 | Pulmonary Embolism

A 19-year-old woman presents with acute onset, sharp chest pain, shortness of breath, and lightheadedness shortly after a 10-hour flight. The chest pain is worse with inspiration. Her only other symptom is left leg pain and swelling. The symptoms have been persistent since onset 2 hours ago. She reports no significant past medical history, and her only medication is an oral contraceptive medication that she started 6 months ago. On physical exam, her vitals are temperature 37.8°C, blood pressure 110/74 mmHg, pulse 121/min, respirations 28/min, and pulse oximetry on room air shows an oxygen saturation of 90%. She appears anxious and in respiratory distress. On auscultation, her heart and lung sounds are normal. Her left calf is larger than the right, mildly erythematous, tender, and swollen.

CASE 8 | Pulmonary Embolism *(continued)*

Evaluation/Tests	CT scan with IV contrast shows intraluminal filling defects within the pulmonary arteries (consistent with an acute pulmonary embolus). CT angiography is the test of choice to diagnose PE. This figure shows axial cuts with contrast (white) within the pulmonary arteries, and red arrows point out filling defects (dark) that show the emboli. A pregnancy test, which should routinely be performed in women of childbearing age, was negative. ECG usually shows sinus tachycardia, but the classic finding is S1Q3T3, which indicates acute right heart strain. The pattern is characterized by a large S wave in lead I, a Q wave in lead III, and an inverted T wave in lead III. ABG shows low arterial pO_2 (hypoxemia) and low $paCO_2$ (hypocapnia or respiratory alkalosis). V/Q scan, which could be performed in those with contraindications to IV contrast (allergy, renal failure), would be redundant in this case. If performed, it would show a mismatch between areas of ventilation and perfusion. 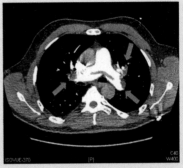 Pulmonary embolism. CT scan revealing bilateral intraluminal filling defects. Reproduced with permission from Oropello JM, Pastores SM, Kvetan V: Critical Care. New York, NY: McGraw Hill; 2017.
Treatment	Treat with oxygen and systemic anticoagulation. Anticoagulation can be done with unfractionated heparin, low molecular weight heparin (e.g., enoxaparin), or direct oral anticoagulants (e.g., rivaroxaban, dabigatran).
Discussion	Pulmonary embolus is important to recognize in all age groups. It is caused by an acute thrombus in the pulmonary arteries. Risk factors for pulmonary embolus include immobility, travel, malignancy, and previous venous thromboembolism. Most pulmonary emboli arise from deep venous thrombosis in the proximal deep veins of the lower extremities. Risk factors can be summed up in Virchow triad (SHE mnemonic): • Stasis (e.g., post-op, long drive/flight) • Hypercoagulability (e.g., defect in coagulation cascade proteins, such as factor V Leiden; oral contraceptive use; pregnancy; malignancy) • Endothelial damage (exposed collagen triggers clotting cascade) Hemodynamically unstable patients (in shock, cardiac arrest) should receive resuscitation with IVF and vasopressors. Thrombolysis (e.g., alteplase, also known as tPA) is indicated in unstable patients, provided there are no contraindications (e.g., intracranial malignancy, history of intracranial hemorrhage). Embolectomy (surgical or catheter directed) can also be performed.
Additional Considerations	Pulmonary emboli are typically thrombi, but types include Fat, Air, Thrombus, Bacteria, Amniotic fluid, Tumor. An embolus moves like a "FAT BAT." **Fat embolism** typically occurs in trauma patients (after fracture of the pelvis or long bones) and the risk increases with the number of bones fractured. It occurs more with open fractures than closed fractures. It can be a complication of orthopedic surgery or liposuction. Symptoms occur 24–72 hours after trauma or surgery. Patients may report dyspnea or vague chest discomfort, and exam findings may include petechiae (especially of the oral mucosa, conjunctiva, and upper half of the body. Tachypnea and fever associated with disproportionate tachycardia are common. Neurological manifestations include drowsiness, confusion, decreased level of consciousness, and seizures. Diagnosis is clinical with supporting history, and CXR shows alveolar infiltrates. If done, a bronchoalveolar lavage (BAL) shows fat droplets, but this lacks specificity. Treatment is focused on prevention with early stabilization of long bone fractures. Treatment is supportive and includes oxygen and possible mechanical ventilation. **Amniotic fluid embolism** is a rare but serious complication of pregnancy. It can occur if amniotic fluid and fetal cells enter the maternal circulation through small tears in the uterine veins. These emboli to the lungs and heart can cause respiratory distress and cardiac dysfunction and activate the coagulation system. The resultant thrombin activates platelets and triggers fibrin formation. This then induces disseminated intravascular coagulation (DIC). Clinically, the disease presents with

CASE 8 | Pulmonary Embolism (continued)

Additional Considerations	abrupt onset of dyspnea, cyanosis, and hypotension that can lead to shock and death. Diagnosis is suspected in women late in pregnancy, often during labor. Treatment is essentially supportive and may include oxygen, mechanical ventilation, and hemodynamic support. To reverse consumed clotting factors and platelets, platelet transfusion, fresh-frozen plasma and cryoprecipitate may be given. Heparin in low doses may be useful in some cases. If amniotic fluid embolism occurs before delivery, the fetus has a poor outcome. Therefore, the fetus should be delivered as soon as the mother is stabilized.

CASE 9 | Malignant Pleural Effusion

A 55-year-old woman with a 30-pack/year smoking history presents with left-sided chest pain and dyspnea for the past month. The pain is worse with deep inspiration, and she is having trouble taking deep breaths. Breathing worsens with exertion and when lying down. She has lost 20 pounds in the last 6 months. She reports decreased appetite and easy fatigability. She denies any recent travel or illness. She denies a history of homelessness or incarceration. She denies prior occupational exposures. On physical exam, her vitals are temperature is 37.8°C, blood pressure is 100/70 mmHg, pulse is 73/min, respirations are 20/min, and pulse oximetry on room air shows an oxygen saturation of 95%. She is cachectic with bitemporal wasting. Her pulse is regular. Chest exam reveals dullness to percussion with decreased tactile fremitus and decreased breath sounds on the left base. There is no wheezing on either lung field. She does not have any cyanosis, edema, or clubbing.

Evaluation/Tests	A CXR shows blunting of the left costophrenic angle and a large pleural effusion on the left side of the lung. A CT scan of the chest shows a spiculated left upper lobe mass measuring 3 × 4-cm mass and enlarged mediastinal lymph nodes. An ultrasound-guided thoracentesis of the left lung drains 800 cc of hemorrhagic fluid. Pleural fluid studies revealed LDH 652 U/L and protein 6 g/dL. Serum LDH is 250 U/L, and serum protein of 2.7 g/dL. Gram stain culture of the pleural fluid is negative for bacteria. Cytology was negative for any malignant cells, but biopsy of the mass shows keratin pearls and intercellular bridges consistent with squamous cell carcinoma.
Treatment	The first step in management of a confirmed pleural effusion is usually a thoracentesis, which can be both diagnostic (via cytology, Light's criteria, and microbiologic studies) and therapeutic (relief from respiratory distress). A pleural effusion is a manifestation of a disease. Thus treatment will always depend on the underlying disease.
Discussion	This patient has a pleural effusion due to squamous cell carcinoma. Pleural effusions are caused by excessive accumulation of fluid between the visceral and parietal pleura. This can lead to restricted lung expansion during inspiration. Light's criteria is a method for differentiating transudates from exudates. Serum and pleural fluid values for LDH and protein are compared. If at least one criterion is fulfilled, the fluid is an exudate and merits aggressive further workup to determine the underlying cause.

	Transudate	Exudate
Pleural protein/serum protein	≤0.5	≥0.5
Pleural LDH/serum LDH	≤0.6	≥0.6
Pleural LDH	≤2/3 upper limit of normal serum LDH	≥2/3 upper limit of normal serum LDH
Common cause	Due to high hydrostatic pressure (e.g., HF, Na+ retention) or low oncotic pressure (e.g., nephrotic syndrome, cirrhosis)	Due to malignancy, inflammation/infection (e.g., pneumonia, collagen vascular disease), trauma (occurs in states of high vascular permeability)

CASE 10 | Malignant Mesothelioma

A 68-year-old man presents with chest pain and progressive shortness of breath. The pain is described as a dull, boring chest pain in his right chest. He denies cough, hemoptysis, fevers, chills, or weight loss. He denies smoking cigarettes, alcohol use, or illicit drug use. He retired a few years ago from his career as a pipefitter on Navy destroyer vessels. On physical exam, his vitals are temperature 37.6°C, blood pressure 110/75 mmHg, pulse 63/min, respirations 20/min, and pulse oximetry on room air shows an oxygen saturation of 94%. There is asymmetric chest wall expansion, dullness to percussion on the right hemithorax up to the midlung field, and diminished breath sounds on right up to right midlung.

CASE 10 | Malignant Mesothelioma *(continued)*

Evaluation/Tests	A CXR shows fluid in the right pleural space (pleural effusion) and widespread dense opacities projecting over both lungs in a nonanatomic distribution (calcified pleural plaques). CT scan of the chest shows right-sided diffuse pleural thickening with areas of calcification and a right pleural effusion. The patient underwent video-assisted thoracoscopic surgery (VATS) and sampling of the pleural tissue, which shows epithelioid cells (polygonal cells with moderate to abundant eosinophilic cytoplasm, vesicular round nuclei, and a prominent nucleolus).
Treatment	Multidisciplinary care and referral to surgery and oncology for treatment.
Discussion	Mesothelioma is the most common primary tumor of the pleura. Approximately 70% of cases are associated with asbestos exposure. There is a long latency between asbestos exposure and disease development. There is not a clear dose–response relationship. Cigarette smoking is not a risk factor for developing malignant mesothelioma. The most common symptom is nonpleuritic chest pain (despite being a disease of the pleura), followed by dyspnea and cough. Pleural plaques themselves do not become mesothelioma but are a marker for asbestos exposure. Diagnosis requires pathologic evaluation. Stains are positive for calretinin and cytokeratin 5/6. Treatment is dictated by stage and requires specialty care. Prognosis is poor, and patients usually die of respiratory failure due to tumor invasion of the ribs and intercostal structures. Disease can spread through the diaphragm, encasing the intraperitoneal organs and causing bowel obstruction.
Additional Considerations	**Asbestosis** is a form of pneumoconiosis associated with shipbuilding, roofing, and plumbing. Asbestos bodies (see figure) can be collected in bronchoalveolar lavage of sputum. Asbestosis is a significant risk factor for bronchogenic carcinoma, which is more common than malignant mesothelioma. **Caplan syndrome** is rheumatoid arthritis plus pneumoconiosis (asbestosis, silicosis, coal workers' pneumoconiosis). Fusiform rods or "dumbbell" fibers, stained with Prussian blue. Reproduced with permission from Kemp WL, Burns DK, Brow TG: Pathology: The Big Picture. New York, NY: McGraw Hill; 2008.

COUGH AND HEMOPTYSIS

Cough is a reflex response to perceived stimuli to the pharynx, larynx, bronchi, lung parenchyma, external auditory meatus (via Arnold's nerve or auricular branch of vagus nerve), and the esophagus. Signals are transmitted via the vagus and superior laryngeal nerves to the brainstem nucleus tractus solitarius (cough center). Impulses are then sent to the glottis, diaphragm, and abdominal wall muscles, which allows generation of force to expel noxious substances from the airway. Dysfunction of the cough reflex arc results in increased likelihood of aspiration of food and saliva and increases the risk of serious infection.

Hemoptysis is the coughing up of blood and is a potentially life-threatening symptom. The first important step in working up hemoptysis is determining clinical stability through history, vital signs, and examination. The next step is determining the source of the bleeding, whether it arises from the respiratory tract or if it is **pseudohemoptysis** (epistaxis, hematemesis). Massive hemoptysis is any volume of blood that is life-threatening and that could lead to airway obstruction and/or asphyxiation. Recall that the lungs have a dual blood supply, with both pulmonary and bronchial circulations. The *pulmonary circulation* is a low-pressure system that participates in gas exchange and is responsible for the majority of blood supply to the lungs. The *bronchial circulation* is a high-pressure system and accounts for very little of the blood supply to the lungs. Life threatening, massive hemoptysis is usually due to problems in the bronchial circulation.

Differential Diagnosis of Cough Based on Duration of Symptoms

Cough	Acute	Subacute	Chronic Cough
Duration	<3 weeks	3–8 weeks	>8 weeks
Common etiologies	Viral, COPD/asthma, pneumonia, irritants or foreign bodies	Postinfectious, COPD/asthma	COPD/asthma, GERD, ACE-I, ILD, cancer, infections (TB, MAI), bronchiectasis

Differential Diagnosis of Cough

Pulmonary	ENT
Chronic obstructive pulmonary disease (COPD)/chronic bronchitis/asthma	Upper airway cough syndrome (postnasal drip)
Allergies	Allergies
Bronchiectasis	Rhinosinusitis
Bronchitis/pneumonia/pertussis	Foreign body
Mycobacteria (TB/MAI)	Croup (acute laryngotracheobronchitis)
Lung abscess	Oropharyngeal cancer
Post infectious cough	**Other**
Cystic fibrosis (CF)	Gastroesophageal reflux disease (GERD)
Sarcoidosis	Medications (ACE-inhibitors)
Primary ciliary dyskinesia	Tobacco and other irritants
Silicosis	Foreign body
Pulmonary fibrosis	Psychogenic cough
Lung cancer	Heart failure
Pulmonary embolus (PE)	

Differential Diagnosis of Hemoptysis

Pulmonary	ENT
Acute bronchitis	Epistaxis (pseudohemoptysis)
Pneumonia	Oropharyngeal mass/lesion
Lung abscess	Foreign body
Fungal infection	**Gastrointestinal**
Tuberculosis	Hematemesis (pseudohemoptysis)
Bronchiectasis	
Lung cancer	**Other**
Pulmonary embolus	Heart failure
Tracheo-innominate fistula	Mitral stenosis
Diffuse alveolar hemorrhage (DAH) (often related to autoimmune lung diseases)	Intrathoracic endometriosis
Arteriovenous malformation (hereditary hemorrhagic telangiectasia, also known as Osler-Weber-Rendu syndrome)	Coagulopathy
	Foreign body

Key Associated Findings and Cough with (+) or without (−) Hemoptysis (H) Differential Diagnosis

Cough with Key Associated Findings	Diagnoses
Sick contacts, congestion, sore throat +/− (H)	Bronchitis, URI
Fevers, purulent sputum production +/− (H)	Pneumonia
Chronic cough, night sweats, weight loss +/− (H), homeless, incarcerated, migrant from endemic country	TB
History of immunosuppression +/− (H)	TB, fungal or atypical infection
History of cystic fibrosis or recurrent lung infections +/− (H)	Bronchiectasis
Significant tobacco use +/− (H)	Malignancy, COPD
Malnutrition, weight loss, purulent sputum, childhood onset, greasy stools	CF
Severe episodes of cough with "whoop" sound	Pertussis
Harsh loud, hoarse cough ("seal barking")	Croup
Exercise association or triggers	Asthma
Worse after certain foods or lying flat	Allergies, upper airway cough syndrome, GERD
Chest pain, elevated D-dimer, unilateral leg swelling	Pulmonary embolus
Recent tracheostomy placement or congenital anomaly	Tracheo-innominate fistula
Shipbuilder, roofer plumber	Asbestosis
Aerospace manufacturer	Berylliosis

(continued)

Key Associated Findings and Cough with (+) or without (−) Hemoptysis (H) Differential Diagnosis

Cough with Key Associated Findings	Diagnoses
Coal worker	Coal workers' pneumoconiosis
Sandblaster, foundry worker, mine worker	Silicosis
After a URI	Postinfectious cough
Infertility in males and females, ectopic pregnancy, bronchiectasis, recurrent sinusitis, chronic ear infections, conductive hearing loss, and situs inversus +/− (H)	Primary ciliary dyskinesia
Difficulty to control asthma, eosinophilia, bronchiectasis +/− (H)	Allergic bronchopulmonary asthma (ABPA)

Key Associated Exam Findings and Cough with (+) or without (−) Hemoptysis (H) Differential Diagnosis

Cough and/or Hemoptysis with Key Associated Exam Findings	Diagnoses
Stridor	Foreign body aspiration, epiglottitis, angioedema, croup
Wheezes	COPD, asthma
Bilaterally: hyperresonant to percussion and decreased breath sounds, wheezing	COPD
Inspiratory crackles, bronchophony, egophony, increased tactile fremitus, dullness to percussion, whispered pectoriloquy on affected side	Pneumonia
Inspiratory crackles bilaterally, digital clubbing	Pulmonary fibrosis
Inspiratory crackles bilaterally, +JVD, edema; S3	Pulmonary edema

Depending on the history and physical examination of a patient, the diagnostic evaluation should be tailored to rule out diagnoses that require urgent intervention (pneumonia, malignancy, PE, and foreign body aspiration).

Initial testing may include CBC (in hemoptysis), creatinine (if suspicion of vasculitis), sputum cultures, TB testing (interferon-γ release assay aka QuantiFERON-TB Gold, sputum AFB, PPD), chest X-ray, pulse oximetry, or pulmonary function testing.

If initial tests are nondiagnostic or the patient has features concerning for other conditions, further tests include:

- CT scans with contrast, useful for diagnosing PE, cancer, or infection.
- High-resolution CT scan, useful for diagnosing ILD or autoimmune and parenchymal lung diseases.

For direct visualization and to obtain biopsy or cultures, refer the patient to obtain bronchoscopy and/or laryngoscopy. For hemoptysis, consider coagulation studies (e.g., PT, PTT) and workup for autoimmune diseases.

CASE 11 | Chronic Obstructive Pulmonary Disease (COPD): Chronic Bronchitis Subtype

A 65-year-old man with a history of 40-pack/year tobacco use presents with persistent cough for several years. Cough is productive of clear sputum, particularly in the mornings. The patient also reports that he has been "slowing down" over the past year, citing having to stop after walking approximately 100 feet. On physical examination, his vital signs are temperature is 37.5°C, respirations are 16/min, pulse is 90/min, pulse oximetry on room air shows an oxygen saturation of 93%. Patient has labored breathing, but he is able to speak in full sentences. Chest percussion reveals hyperresonance. He has diminished breath sounds with bilaterally prolonged expiration and faint crackles and wheezes. His JVP is normal, heart sounds are distant, and he has no lower extremity edema.

Evaluation/Tests	Postbronchodilator spirometry shows a forced expiratory volume in 1 second (FEV1) to forced vital capacity (FVC) of 56. CXR shows hyperinflation of the lungs. CBC, BMP, and BNP are normal. ABG: pH 7.38/$PaCO_2$ 45 mmHg/PaO_2 72 mmHg performed on room air.
Treatment	In acute exacerbations, treatment usually consists of short-acting bronchodilators (e.g., albuterol), systemic steroids, and sometimes a course of macrolides (e.g., azithromycin). Treatment of stable COPD consists of long- and short-acting bronchodilator (beta-agonists and/or muscarinic antagonists). Smoking cessation counseling is always indicated.

CASE 11 | Chronic Obstructive Pulmonary Disease (Copd): Chronic Bronchitis Subtype *(continued)*

Discussion	COPD is characterized by persistent respiratory symptoms and airflow limitation that is due to airway and/or alveolar abnormalities. It is caused by significant exposure to noxious gases and it is a common preventable and treatable disease. The strongest risk factor is cigarette smoking, but indoor biomass exposure (from burning animal dung, wood, or crop residue) is another significant risk factor. **Chronic bronchitis** is a clinical diagnosis and can be a subtype/manifestation of COPD. It is defined as a productive cough for at least 3 months in a year for at least 2 consecutive years, in which other causes have been excluded such as GERD. The majority of patients with chronic bronchitis are smokers. Histologically, there is hypertrophy and hyperplasia of mucus-secreting glands in the bronchi. The diagnosis of COPD is confirmed by the presence of airflow obstruction on postbronchodilator spirometry (FEV1/FVC < 0.7). Characteristic CXR findings of COPD include hyperinflation, increased AP diameter, flattened diaphragms, and increased lung field lucency. COPD can progress to development of pulmonary hypertension and lead to **cor pulmonale**, also known as pulmonary heart disease, which is characterized by right ventricular failure.
Additional Considerations	**Acute bronchitis** is typically caused by viral pathogens, such as rhinovirus, adenovirus, influenza, parainfluenza, RSV, and other viruses. Patients initially may present with upper respiratory tract symptoms such as cough, nasal congestion, sore throat, headache, and/or wheezing. Hemoptysis is mild, self-limited, and caused by irritation of the bronchi from inflammation due to the viral illness. Chest X-ray is usually not needed in the case of bronchitis, but it is a reasonable test to order if a patient presents with hemoptysis to rule out other causes of hemoptysis (e.g., pulmonary cavity, diffuse alveolar hemorrhage). PCR-based testing can determine the specific type of virus causing acute bronchitis. However, this is often not done in an outpatient setting except in vulnerable populations (e.g., transplant recipients) or during an influenza outbreak or pandemic. Conservative treatment with cough suppressants and expectorants is aimed at improving symptoms. In cases of bacterial bronchitis, antibiotics can be prescribed. If the **influenza test** is positive, treat the patient with antiviral therapy (e.g., oseltamivir, which inhibits influenza neuraminidase activity and is most beneficial when started within 48 hours of symptom onset). Bronchodilators may help with wheezing. **Alpha-1 antitrypsin deficiency** is a genetic risk factor for COPD and should be ruled out in those with obstructive lung disease, particularly if the onset is at a younger age, if involvement of the lung bases is seen, and if liver disease is present. In lungs, low α1-antitrypsin results in uninhibited elastase in alveoli. Alveoli become less elastic, resulting in panacinar emphysema.

CASE 12 | Bronchiectasis from Cystic Fibrosis

A 20-year-old woman with a history of cystic fibrosis presents with worsening chronic productive cough for the past week. The cough is productive of green foul-smelling sputum; today, sputum has developed streaks of dark red blood. It has been accompanied by a 5-pound weight loss, fevers, and generalized fatigue. Her only medications are nebulized hypertonic saline. She is hospitalized at least once a year for pneumonia, which usually requires intravenous antibiotics. On physical exam, her vital signs are temperature 38.5°C, respirations 20/min, pulse 110/min; pulse oximetry on room air shows an oxygen saturation of 93%, and BMI is 17 kg/m². Patient has labored breathing, but she is able to speak in full sentences. She has alar flaring and intercostal muscle retractions. Chest percussion reveals dullness over the right lower lobe as well as increased local fremitus. She has crackles over the right lower lobe. Other than tachycardia, her heart and abdomen exam are normal. She has no cyanosis or edema.

Evaluations/Tests	A CBC shows leukocytosis and macrocytic anemia. Her basic metabolic panel is normal. A urine pregnancy test is negative. Chest X-ray shows thickened nontapering airways in bilateral lung fields with lobar consolidation of the right lower lobe. There are no lucencies suggestive of cavities. A noncontrast chest CT reveals dilated airways with dense consolidation of the right lower lobe with air bronchograms. No cavities or endobronchial lesions are noted. Sputum microbial studies show gram negative bacilli and gram positive cocci in chains but no acid-fast bacteria or fungal elements. Two more AFB smears are performed, and these are also negative.
Treatment	Initial antibiotic choice should have coverage for *Pseudomonas aeruginosa* and *Staphylococcus aureus*. The treatment of cystic fibrosis is complex and usually warrants referral to a specialty center for consideration of treatment with a CFTR modulator (ivacaftor, lumacaftor).
Discussion	This patient has cystic fibrosis (CF) and its associated complications of bronchiectasis and frequent pulmonary infections. Hemoptysis in cystic fibrosis usually occurs in the setting of a flare or infection and will typically resolve with treatment of underlying infection.

CASE 12 | Bronchiectasis from Cystic Fibrosis (continued)

Discussion	Bronchiectasis is an irreversible airway dilation that can occur focally or diffusely. The most common etiologies include cystic fibrosis, postradiation fibrosis, recurrent aspiration (as seen in esophageal dysmotility in scleroderma), recurrent infections from immune-deficient states (i.e., common variable immunodeficiency), autoimmune diseases (such as rheumatoid arthritis), foreign object causing obstruction, tuberculosis, or nontuberculous mycobacterial (NTM) infections.
	Bronchiectasis is usually the result of an inflammatory or infectious process. Treatment consists of airway clearance to mobilize secretions through oscillatory positive pressure devices, manual chest percussion, and/or inhalation of hypertonic saline or N-acetylcysteine, pulmonary rehabilitation, and antibiotics to eradicate *Pseudomonas* and MRSA or to suppress bacterial burden.
	Complications of CF include recurrent pulmonary infections, pancreatic insufficiency, malabsorption with steatorrhea, fat-soluble vitamin deficiencies (A, D, E, K), biliary cirrhosis, liver disease, infertility in men (absence of vas deferens, spermatogenesis may be unaffected), and subfertility in women (amenorrhea, abnormally thick cervical mucus). Some may develop nasal polyps and nail clubbing.

CASE 13 | Diffuse Alveolar Hemorrhage (DAH): Anti-GBM (Goodpasture) Syndrome

A 28-year-old man presents with hemoptysis and worsening shortness of breath for 3 days. He initially had small streaks of blood in clear sputum, but the amount is increasing. His only other associated symptom is decreased urine output. He denies smoking cigarettes, use of illicit substances, or alcohol use. He has no medical problems and takes only acetaminophen for the occasional headache. On physical exam, his vitals are temperature 38.1°C, blood pressure 120/80 mmHg, pulse 115/min, respirations 28/min, and SpO$_2$ 90% on RA. He is in respiratory distress with alar flaring and intercostal retractions. His breath sounds reveal crackles on bilateral lung bases.

Evaluations/Tests	Chest X-ray shows diffuse patchy infiltrates. Arterial blood gas shows hypoxemia. Urine toxicology is negative. Serum ANCA, ANA, and anti-dsDNA are negative. Other labs are notable for hemoglobin to 11.2 g/dL and creatinine of 4.5 mg/dL. Anti-GBM antibodies are positive.
	CT scan of the chest shows diffuse bilateral ground glass opacities. Samples of aspirate obtained from bronchoscopy shows >20% hemosiderin-laden macrophages. Gram stain and cultures of the aspirate are negative. Urine analysis shows microscopic hematuria with dysmorphic RBCs. Urine toxicology is negative.
Treatment	This patient is showing signs of impending respiratory failure (severe respiratory distress and a low oxygen saturation) and should be intubated and supported with mechanical ventilation.
	The treatment of anti-GBM disease consists of plasmapheresis, IV steroids, and cyclophosphamide.
Discussion	Diffuse alveolar hemorrhage (DAH) is a syndrome caused by injury or inflammation of the arterioles, venules, or alveolar septal (alveolar wall or interstitial) capillaries. Hemoptysis is usually present but is not a universal symptom, making it a challenging diagnosis.
	Histopathologic patterns of DAH include the following:
	• Pulmonary capillaritis (due to neutrophilic infiltration of alveolar septa) leads to necrosis of septa, resulting in loss of capillary structure and subsequent leakage of blood into alveoli. This is usually associated with autoimmune disorders.
	• Bland hemorrhage is absence of necrosis of alveolar septae. It is usually due to high left ventricular end diastolic pressure, coagulopathies, or anticoagulation.
	• Diffuse alveolar damage is notable for edema of alveolar septa with formation of hyaline membranes. This is seen in ARDS.
	The diagnosis of DAH can be made with bronchoscopy with bronchoalveolar lavage (BAL) fluid showing >20% hemosiderin-laden macrophages. A lavage can be performed on the same lung segment. BAL fluid that becomes progressively hemorrhagic is also diagnostic of DAH.
	Anti-GBM (Goodpasture syndrome) is a pulmonary-renal syndrome and should be suspected in those presenting with concurrent hemoptysis and hematuria or rapidly deteriorating renal function. It is caused by circulating antibodies to the glomerular basement membrane and can result in rapidly progressive (crescentic) glomerulonephritis. Diagnosis is made with a kidney biopsy, which would show crescentic glomerulonephritis on light microscopy. Immunoflourescence microscopy would demonstrate linear deposition of IgG along the glomerular capillaries. Diagnosis can be made quickly (if a kidney biopsy is delayed or contraindicated) using a serum assay for anti-GBM antibodies.

CASE 13 | **Diffuse Alveolar Hemorrhage (DAH): Anti-GBM (Goodpasture) Syndrome** (continued)

Discussion	Other causes of diffuse alveolar hemorrhage include lupus, ANCA-associated vasculitis (e.g., granulomatosis with polyangiitis, microscopic polyangiitis, eosinophilic granulomatosis with polyangiitis), antiphospholipid syndrome, Behçet syndrome, cryoglobulinemia, IgA vasculitis (also known as Henoch-Schönlein purpura), and other causes of systemic vasculitis. Cocaine is an important cause of hemoptysis and DAH, so urine toxicology should be routinely performed.

UPPER RESPIRATORY TRACT

Nasal congestion is a common chief concern that is best assessed by a detailed history and physical examination. When interviewing the patient, consider multiple etiologies including allergic/inflammatory (allergic rhinitis, chronic sinusitis), infection (viral, bacterial), anatomical (deviated septum, turbinate hypertrophy), traumatic, and drug-induced (cocaine, intranasal medications). Duration and timing of symptoms are important factors to consider because causes may vary based on how long the patient has experienced symptoms, precipitating factors, and time of year.

CASE 14 | **Epistaxis**

A 22-year-old man presents to urgent care with nose-bleeding and hemoptysis. He states the bleeding started within the past hour and has not responded to nose pinching. He only started coughing up blood after his nose started bleeding. His medications include intranasal corticosteroid for allergic rhinitis and ibuprofen for a recent knee injury. He does not smoke or use illicit drugs. On focused physical exam, his vital signs are blood pressure 120/80 mmHg, respirations 16/min, pulse 92/min, and temperature 37°C. BMI is 28, and SpO_2 is 100% on room air. Anterior rhinoscopy reveals bleeding coming from the left anterior nasal septum. His breath and heart sounds are normal, and he does not have any abdominal tenderness or organomegaly. Examination of his skin does not reveal any petechiae or hematoma.

Evaluation/Test	Complete cell count shows normal platelet count and hemoglobin of 12. Coagulation panel including PT, INR, and PTT is also within normal ranges. Anterior rhinoscopy can help confirm the location of bleeding.
Treatment	Initial treatment consists of manual compression with nose/alar pinching and intranasal oxymetazoline. If bleeding persists, options include cautery (for discrete bleeding), anterior nasal packing, or posterior nasal packing.
Discussion	Epistaxis is a common condition and is usually due to mucosal trauma or irritation (foreign body, dry weather). Other causes and predisposing factors include medications (aspirin, NSAIDs, warfarin, clopidogrel, intranasal steroids), medical/surgical conditions (bleeding disorders, cirrhosis, recent surgery, head and neck cancer), substance abuse (cocaine), or other hereditary conditions such as hereditary hemorrhagic telangiectasia. Epistaxis is also a differential for hemoptysis and hematemesis. Anterior nosebleeds are the most common, involve the Kiesselbach's plexus in the nasal septum, and are usually self-limited. Kiesselbach's plexus arises from anastomosis of the superior labial artery, anterior and posterior ethmoidal arteries, greater palatine artery, and sphenopalatine artery. Posterior nosebleeds arise from posterolateral branches of the sphenopalatine artery or carotid artery and can be life-threatening. Treatment should first consist of ensuring a secure airway and cardiopulmonary stability. Most anterior epistaxis will respond to conservative measures, such as nose pinching or topical decongestants (oxymetazoline). If the patient is unresponsive, treatment can be escalated to chemical or electrical cautery or nasal packing. Posterior epistaxis is treated with balloon or Foley catheters or cotton packing.

CASE 15 | **Rhinosinusitis: Viral**

A 20-year-old man presents with 7 days of cough, nasal congestion, purulent nasal discharge, and facial fullness. He denies fever, shortness of breath, or chest pain. He has been self-medicating with over-the-counter cold and allergy medications and has some symptom relief. On physical examination, his vital signs are normal. There is no facial tenderness, and his oropharynx is normal, but anterior rhinoscopy shows mucosal edema and rhinorrhea.

CASE 15 | **Rhinosinusitis: Viral** *(continued)*

Evaluation/Tests	Clinical diagnosis.
Treatment	Symptomatic therapy such as analgesics/antipyretics and nasal saline irrigation.
Discussion	Acute rhinosinusitis is most commonly caused by viruses with symptom resolution in 7–10 days but by definition should last <4 weeks. The most common viral etiologies include rhinovirus, influenza, and parainfluenza. Symptoms include nasal congestion/obstruction/discharge, cough, facial pressure, hyposmia, and/or ear fullness.
	When bacteria secondarily infect the inflamed mucosa, it is termed **acute bacterial rhinosinusitis** and is usually caused by *Streptococcus pneumonia*, *Haemophilus influenzae*, and *Moraxella catarrhalis*. Bacterial superinfection has a "double worsening" of symptoms or biphasic symptom profile. Lack of improvement after 10 days or double worsening may indicate bacterial superinfection. However, this is very uncommon and may not always require antibiotic treatment. Very rarely, complications can develop and include periorbital or orbital cellulitis, subperiosteal or intracranial abscess, meningitis, or septic cavernous sinus thrombosis.
	Rhinitis medicamentosa results from prolonged use of topical nasal decongestants such as oxymetazoline. After 3 days of use, patients experience rebound rhinorrhea and thus need more frequent doses of decongestant nasal sprays to experience relief. Patients present with red, swollen nasal mucosa.
	Allergic rhinitis symptoms happen at the same time yearly and are associated with itchy eyes, allergic shiners (dark-gray discoloration under the eye), and a transverse nasal crease (the allergic salute is common in children). Patients may also have other signs of atopy (asthma). Treatment includes allergen avoidance, intranasal glucocorticoids, and intranasal or oral antihistamines.
	Vasomotor rhinitis also occurs at similar times of the year (i.e., during cold weather), but it typically resolves with removal of the offending cause. Symptoms are intermittent and are usually isolated to nasal congestion and rhinorrhea.
Additional Considerations	**COVID-19** is caused by a novel coronavirus called SARS-CoV-2. Patients may be asymptomatic or present with a range of mild to severe symptoms after 2–14 days after exposure. Symptoms include sore throat, loss of taste or smell, nasal congestion, fever, chills, body aches, cough, fatigue, shortness of breath, nausea, vomiting, or diarrhea. Treatment is largely supportive. Patients with severe symptoms such as chest pain, trouble breathing, confusion, should seek immediate medical care.

HEAD AND NECK MASS

The differential diagnosis for a facial or neck mass can be quite broad. Congenital etiologies, neoplastic transformation (e.g., squamous cell carcinoma of the head and neck, lymphoma), trauma (e.g., hematoma), infection (e.g., lymphadenopathy, retropharyngeal abscess), or thyroid masses (e.g., goiter) should be considered. The most immediate consideration is whether the location of the mass or its growth may restrict the airway, in which case the condition may be life-threatening.

Malignancy of the head and neck should always be in the differential diagnoses, and these are more common in smokers over the age of 40. Cancers of the head and neck can present in a variety of ways. In some cases, they present as an enlarging mass with obstructive symptoms and other times as an incidentally found lesion. Symptoms vary based on tumor location. Those with laryngeal cancer may complain of voice hoarseness while those with oropharyngeal cancer often notice a slowly enlarging neck mass. Presenting symptoms may often be attributed to upper respiratory tract infections but persist after completion of antibiotics. Erythroplakia, a red velvety plaque, is a precancerous lesion that may be noticed in those who go on to develop cancer of the oral cavity. Risk factors for head and neck cancers include tobacco, alcohol, HPV-16 (oropharyngeal), and EBV (nasopharyngeal).

The diagnosis of head and neck cancer requires direct visualization and biopsy of the suspicious lesion or mass. Histology of squamous cell carcinoma would be characterized by nests of squamous epithelium arising from the epidermis and extending into the dermis, with large malignant cells and eosinophilic cytoplasm; keratin pearls are often present as well. Staging includes imaging of the head and neck, as well as additional imaging for more extensive disease (for example lung involvement) based on symptoms. Treatment often involves resection if possible, along with chemotherapy and radiation. Patients often require the placement of a feeding tube to obtain nutrition during their therapy.

Key Findings and Head and Neck Mass Differential Diagnosis

Head and Neck Mass and Key Associated Findings	Diagnoses
Older, debilitated persons with dehydration or recent dental procedures, rapid or gradual onset of pain and swelling; local edema, erythema, tenderness, or fluctuance	Acute sialadenitis, abscess
Mild to severe pain of salivary glands, often after meals	Chronic sialadenitis
Kitten or flea exposure, >2-cm near site of inoculation	*Bartonella henselae* infection
URI symptoms; mass is rubbery, mobile; cervical, >2 cm	CMV, EBV
Travel to or immigration from an endemic area, homelessness, immunocompromised	*Mycobacterium tuberculosis* (extrapulmonary)
Cat feces exposure	*Toxoplasmosis*
35- to 55-year-old men with a history of smoking, heavy alcohol use, and multiple sex partners (especially involving orogenital contact)	Human papillomavirus–related squamous cell carcinoma
15–34 years of age or >55 years, constitutional symptoms, later splenomegaly	Hodgkin's lymphoma
History of melanoma or lung, breast, colon, genitourinary cancer	Metastatic cancer
New onset voice hoarseness, smoker	Laryngeal cancer
Children, slow or rapidly growing after URI; acute or subacute. Mass at mandibular angle, anterior to sternocleidomastoid	Branchial cleft cyst
Children, slow or rapidly growing after URI; acute or subacute. Mass at midline, adjacent to the hyoid bone, rises with deglutition	Thyroglossal duct cyst
Very young patients with squamous cell head and neck cancers	DNA repair disorder (e.g., Fanconi anemia)

CASE 16 | Congenital Neck Mass: Infected Branchial Cleft Cyst

A 12-year-old girl with no significant past medical history presents with a tender left neck swelling for 1 week. Her mother notes that she has had a small swelling in the area since birth, but it was not painful. The patient has not traveled recently. They have no pets at home, and she has not been exposed to any animals recently.

On exam, her vital signs are temperature 38°C, pulse 80/min, respiratory rate 18/min, and pulse oximetry of 99% on room air. She has a mass lateral to midline and anterior to the sternocleidomastoid muscle, with overlying erythema of the skin. The mass does not move when the child is asked to swallow. It is moderately tender to palpation. No neck lymphadenopathy is noted.

Evaluation/Tests	Ultrasound of the neck demonstrates a 2-cm cystic structure.
Treatment	The patient should be treated with antibiotics and supportive care during infection and definitive surgical excision after the infection is treated.
Discussion	This presentation is consistent with a branchial cleft cyst with a secondary superinfection. The initial differential for a neck mass can be quite broad. It is important to consider congenital neck masses such as branchial cleft cysts (lateral) or thyroglossal duct cysts (midline), both of which can become superinfected. When a congenital neck mass is identified, it is important to "cool off" the infection prior to any surgical intervention. This is because any incision and drainage will make definitive surgical excision more complex and difficult. Branchial cleft cysts are remnants of the cervical sinus formed temporarily by the second through fourth branchial clefts during embryologic development. They are typically painless, firm, and immobile. **Thyroglossal duct cysts** present similarly but are found midline, often near the hyoid bone and, when large enough, may result in difficulty swallowing. They are painless, firm, and mobile as they move with swallowing. Thyroglossal duct cysts are caused by remnants of the thyroglossal duct, an embryologic remnant of the development of the thyroid gland as it originates from the foramen cecum in the tongue and descends into the neck. Ectopic thyroid tissue (functional or nonfunctional) may develop along this path. Most common etiologies of a pediatric neck mass include infectious etiologies such as **lymphadenitis** (infected lymph node with abscess formation), cat scratch disease caused by *Bartonella henselae*, and atypical mycobacterial infection. Lymphadenitis would likely present with more diffuse lymphadenopathy, and imaging such as ultrasound would demonstrate abscess formation within lymph nodes. Lymphadenitis would be managed with antibiotics, surgical incision, drainage.

CASE 17 | Salivary Gland Mass: Warthin's Tumor

A 65-year-old man with a 40-pack/year smoking history presents with right cheek swelling that has slowly grown in size over the past several months. On exam, a 2-cm cystic mass is palpated in the right preauricular area over the angle of the mandible without overlying skin changes. No palpable neck lymphadenopathy is noted.

Evaluation/Tests	Soft tissue neck CT with contrast demonstrates a 2-cm cystic mass in the superficial parotid gland. Ultrasound-guided fine needle aspiration shows thick, turbid fluid within the mass. Pathology shows abundant lymphocytes and germinal centers within a lymph node–like stroma and epithelial cells.
Treatment	The patient should be evaluated for a parotidectomy.
Discussion	This patient is presenting with a parotid gland mass. In a middle-aged to elderly male smoker, the most likely diagnosis is a benign Warthin's tumor, also known as papillary cystadenoma lymphomatosum. It is a benign cystic tumor almost exclusively seen in the parotid gland. It is associated with smoking and is more common in male patients. On biopsy, characteristic appearance will show epithelial cells along with abundant lymphocytes and germinal centers (lymph node–like appearance). Most are unilateral, but up to 10% can be bilateral. Other salivary gland tumors that should be on the differential include pleomorphic adenoma and malignancies such as mucoepidermoid carcinoma. **Pleomorphic adenoma** is the most common salivary gland tumor and is a benign tumor composed of chondromyxoid stroma and epithelium. They have a high rate of recurrence due to incomplete resection and rarely may transform into carcinoma. **Mucoepidermoid carcinoma** is the most common malignant salivary gland tumor composed of mucinous and squamous cells. Given its malignant nature, it may damage the facial nerve (CN VII) if arising from the parotid gland.

CASE 18 | Nasopharyngeal Cancer

A 58-year-old man with a 40-pack/year smoking history presents with a left neck mass and epistaxis. On exam, his vital signs are normal, and he is not in any distress. He has a nontender enlarged lymph node on the left upper anterior cervical chain. On nasopharyngoscopy, a mass is visible in the left nasopharynx.

Evaluation/Tests	The left nasopharyngeal mass is biopsied and reveals squamous cell carcinoma.
Treatment	Treatment depends on disease stage and usually includes radiotherapy and/or chemotherapy.
Discussion	Nasopharyngeal carcinoma most commonly arises from the posterolateral pharyngeal recess, or fossa of Rosenmüller. Risk factors include tobacco (including smokeless tobacco), EBV, HPV 16, immunodeficiency (solid organ transplant, HIV), and betel nut chewing. Diagnosis is made by biopsy. Nasopharyngeal cancers tend to metastasize early. The workup should include evaluation for cranial nerve involvement, with CN 3, 4, 5, and 6 being most commonly involved because of their anatomic location. HPV-related disease is primarily located in the oropharynx, base of the tongue, or tonsils. Risk factors include multiple sexual partners and oral sex practices. Most cases are associated with high-risk strain HPV16 infection. HPV positive head and neck cancer tend to be chemotherapy responsive, and they have a better prognosis than those who are HPV negative. EBV-associated head and neck cancer is associated with a nonkeratinizing, undifferentiated endemic form of nasopharyngeal carcinoma. There is an increased risk in Southern China.

LUNG CANCERS

Lung cancer is the leading cause of cancer-related deaths in both men and women. Lung cancer encompasses a diverse group of histologically unique tumors and are generally classified as small cell lung cancers (SCLC) and non–small cell lung cancers (NSCLC). NSCLC accounts for the majority of cases. Various molecular abnormalities have been identified that may guide treatment decisions in patients with lung cancer. These abnormalities primarily occur in patients with adenocarcinomas and include mutations in EGFR, ALK, ROS, MET, and BRAF. Targeted therapy is available for patients with tumors that harbor these mutations with stage IV cancers, often with improved outcomes.

Unfortunately, lung cancers are usually diagnosed at an advanced stage. Patients may present with cough, hemoptysis, wheezing, and weight loss. Patients often have an extensive history of tobacco abuse. It is important to ask about exposure to radon, asbestos, or second-hand smoke. On physical exam, wheezing and rhonchi are sometimes heard, and decreased breath sounds may be noted on the affected side due to a large lung mass or effusions. Pleural and pericardial effusions should be considered malignant unless there is an obvious alternative etiology. Hypertrophic osteoarthropathy (clubbing and periostitis of the small hand joints) may be present.

A chest X-ray may reveal a dominant lung mass. If a new mass is seen on X-ray, a CT scan of the chest should be ordered to further characterize the lesion. Any suspicious lesions need to be followed up with a biopsy. Peripheral lesions are more amenable to CT-guided biopsies, but central lesions may require endobronchial ultrasound guided biopsies (EBUS). To complete the workup for a new diagnosis of lung cancer, CT scans of the chest, abdomen, and pelvis with contrast and a bone scan or a PET-CT are done to look for potential sites of distant metastases. Typical sites of metastasis include liver (jaundice, hepatomegaly), adrenal glands, bone (pathologic fracture), and brain. MRI of the brain is generally completed as well, particularly if there is evidence of advanced disease or the patient has neurologic complaints.

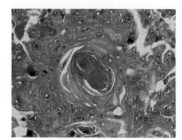

Squamous cell lung cancers are strongly associated with tobacco use, and they are the second most common histology subtype of lung cancer in the non–small cell lung cancer group. Under the microscope, they appear as cells with abundant cytoplasm and pleomorphic nuclei. Keratin pearls and intercellular bridging are seen. These tumors are generally centrally located and tend to cavitate. Squamous cell lung cancers can be associated with neoplastic syndromes, especially hypercalcemia from production of parathyroid hormone–related peptide (PTHrP).

Squamous cell carcinoma. Squamous cell carcinoma is one of the major forms of carcinoma, occurring within many organs including the mouth, upper respiratory tract, and lungs. In the center of the photomicrograph is a keratin pearl, a characteristic feature of a well or moderately differentiated squamous cell carcinoma. Hematoxylin and eosin, 400×.
Reproduced, with permission, from Kemp WL, Burns DK, Travis Brown TG. Pathology: The Big Picture. New York, NY: McGraw Hill; 2008.

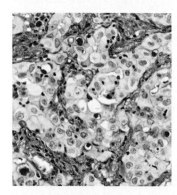

Adenocarcinomas of the lung are the most common histologic subtype of lung cancers found in nonsmokers. They appear in a glandular pattern on histology. Bronchioalveolar carcinomas are also now classified under adenocarcinoma of the lung. Adenocarcinomas tend to occur peripherally and are associated with several molecular mutations including EGFR and ALK. Radon exposure has been associated with adenocarcinomas.

Reproduced with permission from US Department of Health and Human Services and the Armed Forces Institute of Pathology.

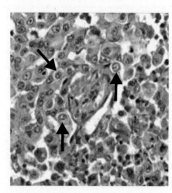

Large cell cancer appears poorly differentiated on pathology. It consists of large cells with abundant cytoplasm and large nucleoli. They may occur centrally or peripherally within the lung parenchyma.

Reproduced with permission from Jala VR, Radde BN, Haribabu B, Klinge CM. Enhanced expression of G-protein coupled estrogen receptor (GPER/GPR30) in lung cancer, BMC Cancer 2012 Dec 28;12:624.

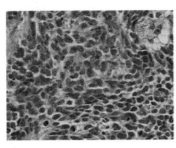

Small cell lung cancer accounts for about 15% of all lung tumors, and they are associated with tobacco use. They may grow and metastasize more quickly than non–small cell lung cancers. Under the microscope, the tumors consist of diffuse sheets of small cells with scant cytoplasm and small hyperchromic nuclei. Neuroendocrine granules can be seen on electron microscopy. These tumors are generally found centrally within the lung parenchyma. Small cell lung cancers are associated with several paraneoplastic syndromes including SIADH, Cushing's syndrome, and Lambert Eaton syndrome.

Light microscopic images of SCLC. Note the small, round, and spindle-shaped cells with hyperchromic nuclei and scant cytoplasm.
Reproduced with permission from Kantarjian HM, Wolff RA: The MD Anderson Manual of Medical Oncology, 3rd ed. New York, NY: McGraw Hill; 2016.

Lung Cancer and Associated Features

Key Feature	Diagnosis
Hoarseness, ipsilateral ptosis/anhidrosis/myosis, upper extremity weakness	Pancoast tumor
EGFR, ALK, MET, ROS, BRAF	Adenocarcinoma
Weakness that improves with use (Lambert Eaton syndrome)	Small cell lung cancer
Hyponatremia in a patient with lung cancer (SIADH)	Small cell lung cancer
Hypercalcemia and/or cavitation in a patient with lung cancer (PTHrP)	Squamous cell carcinoma

CASE 19 | Lung Cancer

A 68-year-old woman with a past medical history of COPD is brought for evaluation of confusion. The patient is a heavy smoker, and her family reports that she has a worsening chronic cough with new onset facial flushing and unintentional weight loss. On exam, her vitals are temperature 98°F, pulse 110/min, respirations 30/min, blood pressure 120/80 mmHg, and pulse oximetry 93% on room air. She appears confused and is oriented to self only. Her face is flushed with blanching after applying gentle pressure (facial plethora) with engorged neck veins and bilateral pitting edema of her arms. On auscultation, breath sounds are diminished bilaterally, but no wheezing is heard.

Evaluation/Tests	Initial blood work shows mildly elevated creatinine and a calcium concentration of 12.8 mg/dL (high). Chest X-ray shows mediastinal opacification. A CT scan of the chest with contrast shows a mass in the right hilar area with compression of the superior vena cava. A biopsy of the mass shows keratin pearls with intercellular bridges suggestive of squamous cell carcinoma of the lung. PTHrP levels are elevated.
Treatment	Immediate treatment consists of correcting her hypercalcemia and relieving obstruction of the superior vena cava (SVC). Hypercalcemia is treated with intravenous hydration and bisphosphonates. The SVC compression can be treated with endovenous stenting, and small cell lung cancer is usually treated with chemotherapy and immunotherapy.
Discussion	This patient is presenting with **superior vena cava (SVC) syndrome** due to **SCC of the lung**. Lung cancer is the most common cause of cancer death, and smoking is the strongest risk factor. However, occupational exposures and chronic lung conditions can increase risk as well. Initial tests to look for metastatic disease include CT scan of the abdomen to evaluate for mediastinal or distant lymph nodes and PET-CT scan. Common sites of spread include liver, adrenals, brain, and bone. Bronchoscopy should also be performed to look for endobronchial lesions, or lesions in the airway. Squamous and small cell carcinomas are typically central and caused by smoking. **Adenocarcinomas** and **large cell carcinomas** are typically peripheral. **Bronchial carcinoid** may be central or peripheral. Treatment may include surgery, radiation, and/or chemotherapy.
Additional Considerations	Complications of lung cancer can result from paraneoplastic syndromes and/or locoregional spread of malignancy. Paraneoplastic syndromes associated with lung cancer are as follows: 1. **Hypercalcemia of malignancy** is a well-known paraneoplastic syndrome in lung cancer, usually non–small squamous cell carcinoma. The best-known mechanism is tumor release of PTH-related protein (PTHrP) aka humoral hypercalcemia of malignancy. Other nonlung tumors release 1,25-dihydroxyvitamin D (calcitriol) or induce bone destruction through osteolytic metastases. 2. **Cushing syndrome**, due to ACTH secretion by tumors, is seen in small cell CA.

CASE 19 | Lung Cancer *(continued)*

Additional Considerations	3. **SIADH**, due to ADH secretion by tumors, is seen in small cell CA. 4. **Lambert-Eaton myasthenic syndrome**. Antibodies against presynaptic (P/Q-type) Ca^{2+} channels at neuromuscular junction, seen in small cell CA. It is characterized by proximal muscle weakness that improves with prolonged exercise (vs. myasthenia gravis, wherein weakness will worsen with prolonged exercise). 5. **Paraneoplastic encephalomyelitis**. Antibodies against Hu antigens in neurons are seen in small cell CA. Locoregional spread of cancer is as follows: 1. **Superior vena cava (SVC) syndrome** is caused by obstruction of venous return to the right atrium and will usually present with face/neck swelling and dyspnea. Severe cases can present with stridor from compromise of the larynx or pharynx. 2. **Pancoast tumor** is also known as superior sulcus tumor. Compression of locoregional structures may cause an array of findings: • Recurrent laryngeal nerve → hoarseness • Stellate ganglion → **Horner syndrome** (ipsilateral ptosis, miosis, anhidrosis), also known as oculo-sympathetic syndrome • Superior vena cava → SVC syndrome • Brachiocephalic vein → brachiocephalic syndrome (unilateral symptoms) • Brachial plexus → sensorimotor deficits • Phrenic nerve → hemidiaphragm paralysis (hemidiaphragm elevation on CXR)

EXCESSIVE DAYTIME SLEEPINESS

The diagnosis of sleep disorders can be difficult, particularly because patients may use "sleepiness" or "fatigue" interchangeably. For clinical purposes, **sleepiness** is the propensity to fall asleep, while **fatigue** is the sensation of low physical or mental energy without the tendency to fall asleep. Excessive daytime sleepiness (EDS) refers to the tendency to fall asleep in inappropriate settings.

The most common cause of EDS is insufficient sleep, which can be caused by poor sleep hygiene (late evening light exposure, TV viewing, video-gaming, smartphone use), family obligations (child care), chronic pain, shift work, or working multiple jobs. Medications commonly associated with EDS include antihistamines, benzodiazepines, opiates, barbiturates, and dopaminergic agents.

Typical Findings and Diagnosis

Key Findings	Diagnosis
Snoring, crowded airway	Obstructive sleep apnea (OSA)
Apnea in heart failure, sleep study showing breathing pattern with apnea and hyperpnea	Central sleep apnea (CSA)
Excessive daytime sleepiness with morbid obesity, chronic respiratory acidosis	Obesity hypoventilation syndrome (OHS)
Sleep paralysis, cataplexy, hypnagogic and hypnopompic hallucinations, sleep study showing reduced sleep latency, hypocretin deficiency in CSF	Narcolepsy

CASE 20 | Adult Obstructive Sleep Apnea (OSA)

	A 55-year-old man with hypertension presents for evaluation of fatigue and snoring. He sleeps 7–8 hours per night, but he wakes up tired and sleepy. He snores very loudly at nighttime, and his wife thinks he sometimes stops breathing in his sleep. He takes his prescribed hypertension medications consistently. His vital signs include blood pressure 160/90 mmHg, pulse 90/min, respiration 16/min, and BMI 40 kg/m². He has a thick neck measuring 18 inches, and his oropharynx is crowded with large tonsils and tongue.
Evaluation/Tests	A polysomnogram shows apnea hypopnea index (AHI) of 35/hour, which is consistent with severe sleep apnea.

CASE 20 | Adult Obstructive Sleep Apnea (OSA) *(continued)*

Treatment	Treatment includes CPAP (continuous positive airway pressure) and lifestyle modification for weight loss.
Discussion	OSA is a sleep disorder characterized by obstructive apneas, hypopneas, and/or arousals caused by repetitive collapse of the upper airway during sleep. Diagnosis is based on either: 1. Symptoms of *nocturnal breathing disturbances* (breathing pauses during sleep, gasping, snoring, or snorting) or *daytime sleepiness* or fatigue that occurs despite adequate opportunities to sleep and is unexplained by other medical conditions; *and* 2. Five or more episodes of hypopnea or obstructive apnea per hour of sleep; *or* 3. Apnea hypopnea index (AHI) is >15 episodes per hour in the absence of symptoms. Each episode of hypopnea or apnea represents a reduction in breathing for at least 10 seconds that commonly results in a ≥3% or 4% drop in oxygen saturation and/or a brain cortical arousal. Witnesses may note snoring, choking or gasping arousals, and apneas. Physical examination usually shows a thick neck and crowded airway. ABG is normal during the daytime. If these patients get hospitalized, the nursing staff might notice nocturnal desaturations on the pulse oximetry. Patients may have adenotonsillar hypertrophy, especially children. Polysomnogram is the gold standard for diagnosis. Treatment usually includes continuous positive airway pressure (CPAP), which keeps the upper airway open during nighttime for effective ventilation.
Additional Considerations	**Central sleep apnea** is impaired respiratory effort due to CNS injuries, heart failure, or opioid usage, which is contrary to OSA in which the respiratory efforts are present. Heart failure causes a typical pattern of central apnea, which is called Cheyne-Stokes respiration (crescendo-decrescendo pattern, oscillation between apnea and hyperpnea). The primary management is to treat the underlying cause: dose reduction or complete cessation of opiates and optimization of heart failure. Other treatment includes positive airway pressure. **Obesity hypoventilation syndrome (OHS)** (also known as Pickwickian syndrome) has a similar presentation to OSA except that these patients have chronic respiratory acidosis on ABG during wakefulness (daytime). They also have high risk of developing pulmonary hypertension. Ideally, other causes of hypercapnia and alveolar hypoventilation should be ruled out before a diagnosis of OHS is made. These include chest wall deformity, neuromuscular disease, metabolic causes, obstructive or restrictive lung disease, and medications. Elevated bicarbonate is due to chronic respiratory acidosis, and erythrocytosis is due to hypoxemia. **Narcolepsy** occurs due to impaired regulation of the sleep-wake cycle characterized by excessive daytime sleepiness, occasional cataplexy (loss of muscle tone due to intense emotion), hallucinations before going to sleep or right before waking, or sleep paralysis. It is caused due to deficiency of hypocretin (orexin) production. Polysomnography (sleep study) and multiple sleep latency tests would show decreased sleep latency and rapid REM onset. Treatment includes good sleep hygiene, daytime stimulants, and occasionally nighttime sodium oxybate. SSRI/SNRIs are used to treat cataplexy.

EDEMA

Edema, or swelling, is noted when excess interstitial body fluid is present. It usually occurs due to an imbalance between the hydrostatic pressure in the capillaries and the colloid oncotic pressure in the interstitial space. Imbalance may be due to inadequate lymphatic drainage, increase in the intracapillary hydrostatic pressure, increased oncotic pressure in the interstitium, reduction in the plasma oncotic pressure, or damage in the endothelial barriers.

When approaching edema, it is important to determine if it is generalized or localized. If localized, identify the local pathology causing the edema. Localized edema could be related to restriction in the lymphatic flow, which occurs in patients with resection of the lymph nodes or filariasis. It may also be due to increased upstream hydrostatic pressure as in varicose veins, thrombophlebitis, and venous thromboembolism. If generalized, evaluate the patient for severe hypoalbuminemia, cirrhosis, protein malnutrition, heart failure, and nephrotic syndrome.

Differential Diagnosis for Generalized Edema

Malnutrition
Heart failure/valvular heart disease/constrictive pericarditis or tamponade/arrhythmias
Liver failure (ascites)
Renal failure/nephrotic syndrome (periorbital edema)
Drug-induced: NSAIDs, calcium channel blockers (CCBs), steroids, cyclosporine
Pulmonary hypertension/OSA
Allergic reaction (may be localized)
Burns (may be localized)

Differential Diagnosis for Lower Extremity Edema

Pitting		Nonpitting
Bilateral Generalized edema causes in preceding table Venous insufficiency	**Unilateral** Deep venous thrombosis (DVT) Ruptured baker cyst Pelvic tumor Pelvic lymphadenopathy Venous insufficiency	Severe hypothyroidism (myxedema): deposition of hyaluronic acid Hyperthyroidism (Graves's disease): pretibial edema Lymphedema Regional lymph node dissection Filariasis Lipedema

CASE 21 | Venous Thromboembolism (VTE): Deep Venous Thrombosis (DVT)

A 58-year-old woman with a past medical history of breast cancer and chronic right knee pain presents with right lower extremity pain and swelling. She does not have chest pain or shortness of breath. She denies any history of leg trauma. On examination, her vital signs show temperature 36.5°C, pulse 100/min, respirations 16/min, and pulse oximetry 99% on room air. Lung exam is clear. There is 1+ pitting edema of the right leg and no edema in the left leg. Pulses are palpable on both extremities.

Evaluation/Tests	D-dimer is elevated. ECG shows sinus tachycardia. CXR unremarkable. Lower extremity venous compression ultrasound with Doppler demonstrates no blood flow detected in the right popliteal vein consistent with deep venous thrombosis (DVT).
Treatment	Anticoagulation.
Discussion	This patient is presenting with a DVT. Though most pulmonary embolisms arise from proximal DVTs of the lower extremities, this patient has no signs or symptoms suggestive of a pulmonary embolus. Virchow's triad effectively characterizes the various clinical states that may predispose a patient to VTE. 1. Stasis (immobility, bed rest, long flight, postoperation) 2. Hypercoagulability (malignancy, estrogen therapy, hypercoagulable states, e.g., Factor V Leiden) 3. Vessel wall injury (from trauma or surgery) ECG findings are generally nonspecific but can include sinus tachycardia. D-dimer is helpful in ruling out DVT (due to its high negative predictive value). There are numerous scoring tools to help determine the pretest probability of a DVT and PE including Wells's and modified Wells's criteria. Anticoagulation is the treatment.

CASE 22 | Pulmonary Hypertension

A 55-year-old woman with hypertension, systemic lupus erythematosus, and a history of pulmonary thromboembolism presents with new onset bilateral lower extremity edema and abdominal bloating over the past 2 weeks. She has had generalized fatigue and progressive dyspnea on exertion over the last 5 months. She reports no fevers, chills, or cough. She denies smoking cigarettes, use of illicit drugs, or alcohol intake. She is on losartan for her hypertension and is not on any medications for SLE or prior PE. On exam, her vital signs are notable for temperature of 36.5°C, respiratory rate 28/min, pulse 100 beats/min, blood pressure 130/80 mmHg, and a pulse oximetry on room air showing blood oxygenation of 87% that increases to 95% after giving oxygen at 2 L/min via nasal cannula. Lungs are clear, and cardiac exam is notable for JVD, a holosystolic murmur at the left sternal border, a loud P2 at the apex, and a parasternal heave. There is hepatomegaly and bilateral lower extremity pitting edema.

CASE 22 | Pulmonary Hypertension *(continued)*

Evaluation/Tests	EKG shows right axis deviation, a prominent P wave >2.5 mm in V1 (indicating right atrial enlargement) and a prominent R wave in V1 (indicating right ventricular hypertrophy). Transthoracic echocardiogram (TTE) shows tricuspid regurgitation and right ventricular systolic pressure estimated to be 50 mmHg. Chest X-ray does not show any pleural effusion or focal pulmonary consolidations. Chest CT scan showed dilated pulmonary artery with enlarged and hypertrophied right ventricle. No interstitial lung disease is noted. Right heart catheterization showed elevated pulmonary systolic pressure with normal pulmonary capillary wedge pressure. Ventilation/perfusion scan was consistent with chronic thromboembolic disease.
Treatment	Treat the patient with diuretics and oxygen. Resume anticoagulation. In the hospital, vasodilators can also be initiated, which can be continued in an outpatient setting. These pulmonary vasodilators include phosphodiesterase inhibitors, endothelin receptor antagonists, and prostacyclin analogs.
Discussion	The World Health Organization (WHO) classifies pulmonary hypertension in five categories: Group 1—Pulmonary arterial hypertension (PAH) is defined as elevated pulmonary arterial pressures (mean pulmonary artery pressure >25 mmHg). It is often idiopathic, can be inherited (heritable PAH due to *BMPR2* gene mutation), and occurs as a primary disease process (pulmonary arterial hypertension). Group 2—Pulmonary hypertension due to left heart disease Group 3—Pulmonary hypertension due to lung disease and/or chronic hypoxia Group 4—Pulmonary hypertension due to blood clots in the lungs Group 5—Pulmonary hypertension due to blood and other disorders The combination of a parasternal heave, loud P2, and narrow splitting of second heart sounds suggest increases in right ventricular afterload likely due to pulmonary hypertension. Chronically elevated pressures lead to right ventricular failure, causing this patient's elevated JVP, bilateral pitting edema, and hepatomegaly. Diagnosis is confirmed with right heart catheterization. Further workup is needed to determine the underlying etiology and may include transthoracic echocardiogram, pulmonary function testing, pulmonary V/Q scan, polysomnography, rheumatological titers, and HIV testing. Treatment varies based on the underlying etiology.
Additional Considerations	WHO groups 1 and 4 of pulmonary hypertension benefit the most from vasodilator therapies including prostacyclin, PDE inhibitors, and endothelin receptor antagonists. WHO group 2 and group 3 benefit the most from the treatment and optimization of the underlying condition. WHO group 4 is potentially curable. Surgery is the definitive therapy, and the procedure of choice is pulmonary thromboendarterectomy.

Index